ADVANCED PRACTICE NURSING:
Essentials for Role Development

SECOND EDITION

ADVANCED PRACTICE NURSING:
Essentials for Role Development

SECOND EDITION

Lucille A. Joel, EdD, APN, FAAN

Professor
Rutgers–The State University of New Jersey
College of Nursing
Newark, New Jersey

 F. A. Davis Company • Philadelphia

F. A. Davis Company
1915 Arch Street
Philadelphia, PA 19103
www.fadavis.com

Printed in the United States of America

Last digit indicates print number: 10 9 8 7 6 5 4 3 2 1

Publisher, Nursing: Joanne Patzek DaCunha, RN, MSN
Director of Content Development: Darlene D. Pederson, MSN, APRN, BC
Developmental Editor: Jennifer Watson
Project Editor: Kim DePaul
Art and Design Manager: Carolyn O'Brien

As new scientific information becomes available through basic and clinical research, recommended treatments and drug therapies undergo changes. The author(s) and publisher have done everything possible to make this book accurate, up to date, and in accord with accepted standards at the time of publication. The author(s), editors, and publisher are not responsible for errors or omissions or for consequences from application of the book, and make no warranty, expressed or implied, in regard to the contents of the book. Any practice described in this book should be applied by the reader in accordance with professional standards of care used in regard to the unique circumstances that may apply in each situation. The reader is advised always to check product information (package inserts) for changes and new information regarding dose and contraindications before administering any drug. Caution is especially urged when using new or infrequently ordered drugs.

Library of Congress Cataloging-in-Publication Data
Advanced practice nursing : essentials for role development / [edited by] Lucille A. Joel. — 2nd ed.
   p. ; cm.
  Includes bibliographical references and index.
  ISBN 978-0-8036-1958-6 (pbk.)
  1. Nurse practitioners. 2. Nursing. I. Joel, Lucille A.
  [DNLM: 1. Nurses. 2. Professional Competence. 3. Nurse's Role. 4. Nursing. WY 16 A244 2009]
  RT82.8.J64 2009
  610.7306'92--dc22

                                       2008055238

Preface

The content of this text was identified only after a careful review of the documents that shape both the advanced practice nursing role and the educational programs that prepare for practice. That review allowed some decisions about topics that were essential to all advanced practice nurses (APNs), whereas others were excluded because they are traditionally introduced during baccalaureate studies. This text is written for the master's-level student in advanced practice and is intended to address the nonclinical aspects of role.

Unit 1 explores *The Evolution of Advanced Practice* from the historical perspective of each of the specialties: the nurse-midwife, nurse anesthetist, clinical nurse specialist, and nurse practitioner. This historical background moves to a contemporary focus with the introduction of the many and varied hybrids of these roles that have appeared over time. These dramatic changes in practice have been a response to societal need. Adjustment to these changes is possible only from the kaleidoscopic view that theory allows. Skill acquisition, socialization, and adjustment to stress and strain are theoretical constructs and processes that will challenge the occupants of these roles many times over the course of a career, but coping can be taught and learned. Our accommodation to change is further challenged as we realize that advanced practice is neither unique to North America nor new on the global stage. Advanced practice roles, although accompanied by varied educational requirements and practice opportunities, are well embedded and highly respected in international culture. In the United States, education for advanced practice had become well stabilized at the master's degree level. Such is no longer true, and the story of our recent transition to doctoral preparation is laid before us, with the subsequent issues this creates.

The Practice Environment, the topic of Unit 2, dramatically affects the care we give. With the addition of medical diagnosis and prescribing to the advanced practice repertoire, we became competitive with other disciplines, deserving the rights of reimbursement, prescriptive authority, clinical privileges, and participation as a member on managed care panels. There is the further responsibility to understand budgeting and material resource management and the nature of different collaborative, responding, and reporting relationships. The APN often provides care within a mediated role, working through other professionals, including nurses, to improve the human condition.

Competency in Advanced Practice, the topic of Unit 3, demands an incisive mind capable of the highest order of critical thinking. This cognitive skill becomes refined as the subroles for practice emerge. The APN is ultimately a direct caregiver, client advocate, teacher, consultant, researcher, and case manager. The APN's forte is to coach individuals and populations so that they may take control of their own health in their own way, ideally even seeing chronic disease as a new trajectory of wellness. The APN's clients are as diverse as the many ethnicities of the U.S. public and the challenge is often to learn from them, taking care to do no harm. The APN's therapeutic modalities go beyond traditional Western medicine, reaching into the realm of complementary therapies and integrative health-care practices that have become expected by many consumers. Any or all of these role competencies are potential areas for conflict, needing to be understood, managed, and resolved in the best interests of the client. The chapters in this section aim to introduce these competencies, not to provide closure on any one topic; the art of direct care in specialty practice is not broached.

When you have completed your course of studies, you will have many choices to make. There are opportunities to pursue your practice as an employee, an employer, or an independent contractor. Each holds different rights and responsibilities. Each demands *Ethical, Legal, and Business Acumen,* which is covered in Unit 4. Each requires you to prove the value you hold for your clients and for the systems in which you work. Cost efficiency and therapeutic effectiveness cannot be dismissed lightly today. The market for APNs among the critical mass that is middle-class America is discussed with concrete examples for spreading the good news of our practice. The nuts and bolts of establishing a practice are detailed, and although these particulars apply most directly to independent practice, they can be easily extrapolated to employee status. Finally, experts in the field discuss the legal and ethical dimensions of practice and how they uniquely apply to the role of the APN to ensure protection for ourselves and our clients.

This text has been carefully crafted based on over 30 years of experience teaching APNs. It substantially includes the nonclinical knowledge necessary to perform successfully in the APN role and raises the issues that still have to be resolved to leave this practice area better than we found it.

LUCILLE A. JOEL

Contributors

Fadwa A. Affara, RN, MA, Msc
International Nurse Consultant, Regulation and
Education Policy
Edinburgh, Scotland, United Kingdom

Judith Barberio, PhD, RN, BC, ANP-C, GNP-C
Clinical Assistant Professor
Rutgers—The State University of New Jersey
College of Nursing
Newark, New Jersey

Deborah Becker, RN, PhD, ACNP-BC
Advanced Senior Lecturer
Director, Adult Acute Care Nurse Practitioner
Program
University of Pennsylvania
School of Nursing
Philadelphia, Pennsylvania

Virginia Trotter Betts, MSN, JD, RN, FAAN
Commissioner
Tennessee Department of Mental Health and
Developmental Disabilities
North Nashville, Tennessee

**Suzanne M. Burns, MSN, RRT, ACNP, CCRN,
FAAN, FCCM, FAANP**
Professor of Nursing
McLeod Hall, School of Nursing
University of Virginia
Charlottesville, Virginia

Ann H. Cary, PhD, MPH, RN, A-CCC
Director, School of Nursing
Loyola University
New Orleans, Louisiana

Pamela F. Cipriano, PhD, RN, FAAN, NEA-BC
Chief Clinical and Chief Nursing Officer
University of Virginia Health System
Charlottesville, Virginia

H. Michael Dreher, DNSc, RN
Associate Professor
Director of Doctoral Nursing Programs
College of Nursing & Health Professions
Drexel University
Philadelphia, Pennsylvania

Lynne M. Dunphy, PhD, APRN, BC
Routhier Chair of Practice
Professor of Nursing, Family Nurse Practitioner
College of Nursing
University of Rhode Island
Kingston, Rhode Island

Mary Lou S. Etheredge, CNS, BC
Director, Nursing Practice Development
Brigham and Women's Hospital
Boston, Massachusetts

Amy Muran Felton, JD
Law Offices
Oak Park, Illinois

Denise Fessler, MSN, RN, CMAC
Manager, Case & Disease Management
Capital Blue Cross
Harrisburg, Pennsylvania

Eileen D. Flaherty, RN, MBA, MPH
Patient Care Services
Director of Financial Management Systems
Massachusetts General Hospital
Boston, Massachusetts

Jane M. Flanagan, PhD, ANP-BC
Assistant Professor
Boston College
Chestnut Hill, Massachusetts

**Donna A. Gaffney, DNSc, RN, APN, C,
PMHCNS-BC, FAAN**
Donna Gaffney Associates
Summit, New Jersey

Rita Munley Gallagher, PhD, RN, C
Senior Policy Fellow
Department of Nursing Practice and Policy
American Nurses Association
Silver Spring, Maryland

Mary Masterson Germain, EdD, ANP-BC, FNAP
Distinguished Practitioner
National Academy of Nursing Practice
Professor, College of Nursing
SUNY-Downstate Medical Center
Brooklyn, New York

Kathleen M. Gialanella, RN, JD, PC
Law Offices
Westfield, New Jersey
Associate Adjunct Professor
Teachers College, Columbia University
New York, New York
Adjunct Professor
Seton Hall University, College of Nursing &
    School of Law
South Orange, New Jersey

Shirley Girouard, PhD, RN, FAAN
Professor and Director
San Francisco State University School of Nursing
San Francisco, California

Christina M. Graf, RN, PhD
Director, Patient Care Services Management
    Systems
Massachusetts General Hospital
Boston, Massachusetts

Patricia M. Haynor, DNSc, RN
Associate Professor
Villanova University
College of Nursing
Villanova, Pennsylvania

Gladys L. Husted, RN, PhD, CNE
School of Nursing, Distinguished Professor
    Emeritus
Duquesne University, School of Nursing
Pittsburgh, Pennsylvania

James H. Husted, Independent Scholar
Pittsburgh, Pennsylvania

Lucille A. Joel, EdD, APN, FAAN
Professor
Rutgers—The State University of New Jersey
College of Nursing
Newark, New Jersey

Dorothy A. Jones, EdD, RNc, FAAN
Professor
Boston College School of Nursing
Chestnut Hill, Massachusetts
Senior Nurse Scientist
Massachusetts General Hospital
Boston, Massachusetts

Anne Keane, EdD, MSN, CRNP, FAAN
Associate Professor Emeritus
University of Pennsylvania
School of Nursing
Philadelphia, Pennsylvania

David Keepnews, PhD, JD, RN, FAAN
Associate Professor
Adelphi University
School of Nursing
Garden City, New York

Phyllis Beck Kritek, RN, PhD, FAAN
Consultation, Training, and Mediation Services
Half Moon Bay, California

Alice F. Kuehn, PhD, RN, BC-FNP/GNP
Associate Professor Emeritus
University of Missouri–Columbia
School of Nursing
Columbia, Missouri
Consultant, North American Mobility Project
University of Minnesota

Irene McEachen, EdD, MEd, MSN, RN
Associate Professor
Department of Nursing
Saint Peter's College
Jersey City, New Jersey

Deborah C. Messecar, PhD, MPH, RN, CNS
Associate Professor
Oregon Health & Science University
School of Nursing
Portland, Oregon

Kammie Monarch, RN, MS, JD
Law Offices
Washington, DC

Sharon E. Muran, RN, MS, CS, Cohn-S
Consultant/Principal
Total Management Solutions, LLC
Bainbridge Island, Washington

Marilyn H. Oermann, PhD, RN, FAAN, ANEF
Professor and Chair, Adult/Geriatric Health
    Division, School of Nursing
The University of North Carolina at Chapel Hill
Chapel Hill, North Carolina

Karen Piren, RN, APN
Psychiatric Nurse Practitioner
Patient Advocate Consultant
State of New Jersey, Division of Mental Health
    Services
Trenton, New Jersey

Susan C. Reinhard, PhD, RN, FAAN
Senior Vice President for Public Policy
AARP International
Washington, DC

Karen R. Robinson, PhD, RN, FAAN
Associate Director for Patient Care
Veterans Affairs Medical Center
Fargo, North Dakota

Mary E. Samost, MSN, RN
Manager, Nursing Quality Improvement
Cambridge Health Alliance
Cambridge, Massachusetts

Madrean Schober, MSN, ANP, FAANP
Senior Visiting Fellow
Alice Lee Centre for Nursing Studies
Yong Loo Lin School of Medicine
National University Singapore
Kent Ridge, Singapore

Nancy K. Smith, APRN-BC, MSN, DNS
Family Nurse Practitioner and Adjunct Faculty
Florida Atlantic University
Christine E. Lynn College of Nursing
Boca Raton, Florida

Thomas D. Smith, MS, RN, CNAA, BC
Senior Vice President, Patient Care Services and
    Chief Nursing Officer
Cambridge Health Alliance
Cambridge, Massachusetts

Mary C. Smolenski, EdD, FNP, FAANP, CAE
Director of Certification
American Nurses Credentialing Center
Silver Spring, Maryland

Christine A. Tanner, RN, PhD, FAAN
Youmans-Spaulding Distinguished Professor
Editor, *Journal of Nursing Education*
Oregon Health & Science University
School of Nursing
Portland, Oregon

Jan Towers, PhD, NP-C, CRNP (FNP), FAANP
Director of Health Policy
American Academy of Nurse Practitioners
Washington, DC

Maria L. Vezina, EdD, RN
Senior Director, Nursing Education, Research
    and Professional Practice
The Mount Sinai Hospital
New York, New York

Marylou Yam, PhD, RN
Vice President of Academic Affairs
Saint Peter's College
Jersey City, New Jersey

Ellis Quinn Youngkin, PhD, ARNP
Professor-Retired
Florida Atlantic University
Christine E. Lynn College of Nursing
Boca Raton, Florida
Emeritus Faculty
School of Nursing
Virginia Commonwealth University–Medical
    College of Virginia
Richmond, Virginia

Rothlyn P. Zahourek, PhD, PMH/CNS-BC, AHN-BC
Clinical Nurse Specialist, Psychiatric Mental
    Health Nursing
Holistic Mental Health Consultation and
    Education Practice
Belchertown, Massachusetts

Reviewers

Michelle A. Beauchesne, DNSc, RN, CPNP, FNAP, FAANP

Associate Professor and Coordinator of PNP
  Programs
Northeastern University
Boston, Massachusetts

Cynthia L. Dakin, RN, PhD

Associate Professor and Assistant Director
Graduate Nursing Studies
Elms College
Chicopee, Massachusetts

Patricia A. Dunn, PhD, RNC

Assistant Professor
Holy Family University
Philadelphia, Pennsylvania

Rose M. Kutlenios, PhD

Board Certified Psychiatric/Mental Health
  Clinical Nurse Specialist and Adult Nurse
  Practitioner
Professor and Chairperson, Department of
  Nursing
Wheeling Jesuit University
Wheeling, West Virginia

Linda Lindeke, PhD, RN, CNP

Associate Professor and Director of Graduate
  Studies
School of Nursing
University of Minnesota
Minneapolis, Minnesota

Denise Lucas, RN, MSN, C-FNP

Assistant Professor of Nursing
Wheeling Jesuit University
Wheeling, West Virginia

Carmen T. Paniagua, EdD, RN, CPC, APN, ACNP-BC

Clinical Assistant Professor
College of Nursing & College of Medicine
Nursing Practice Department Chair
Acute Care Nurse Practitioner Specialty
  Coordinator
Clinical Nurse Geneticist
Winthrop P. Rockefeller Cancer Institute
University of Arkansas for Medical Sciences,
  College of Nursing
Little Rock, Arkansas

Mona P. Ternus, PhD, RN, CNS, CCRN

Associate Professor
University of New Mexico College of Nursing
Albuquerque, New Mexico

Acknowledgments

This book belongs to its authors. I am proud to be one among them. Beyond that, I have been the instrument to make these written contributions accessible to today's students and faculty. I thank each author for the products of his or her intellect, experience, and commitment to advanced practice.

Contents

Preface v

Contributors vii

Reviewers xi

Acknowledgments xiii

UNIT 1
The Evolution of Advanced Practice

1 Advanced Practice Nursing: Doing What Has to Be Done—Radicals, Renegades, and Rebels 2

Lynne M. Dunphy, Nancy K. Smith, and Ellis Quinn Youngkin

The authors chronicle the history of the advanced practice specialties from their earliest days, showing the similarities and differences in their development, the strategic governmental and professional policy choices that enabled survival and growth, and the decisions that gave birth to the title of advanced practice nurse (APN).

2 Emerging Roles of the Advanced Practice Nurse 23

Anne Keane and Deborah Becker

Attention is directed toward the circumstances that have moved the APN role into new and creative models. Examples include the acute care nurse practitioner, the psychiatric/mental health nurse practitioner, nurse practitioners in transitional settings, the psychiatric clinical nurse specialist, population-based clinical nurse specialists, the critical care clinical nurse specialist, the nurse-midwife, and the nurse anesthetist. Several exemplars are provided.

3 Role Development: A Theoretical Perspective 46

Lucille A. Joel

There is only a role for the moment, not any role that will serve for the entire life of a career. Role modifications are dependent on a theoretical body of knowledge, more of it hypothetical than empirical research. These concepts and relationships will allow a comfortable paradigm shift as necessary, with an awareness of the elements of continuity from here to there. This chapter includes a theoretical perspective on the processes of knowledge and skill acquisition and socialization. Also addressed are the consequent stresses and strains that challenge most role occupants, including how to cope with them.

4 Education for Advanced Practice 58

H. Michael Dreher

The author describes the circumstances that have prompted the movement of educational preparation for advanced practice to the doctoral level. The roles played by the traditional research degree (PhD) and the professional practice doctorate (DNP) are explored, and the case for a hybrid academic practice doctorate (DrNP) is presented.

5   **Global Perspectives on Advanced Nursing Practice** 72
  Madrean Schober and Fadwa A. Affara

  Nurses with advanced knowledge and skills, including prescribing, are present in numerous countries. Country context, the complexity of health-care services, and the structure of the health-care system all influence the promotion and support for advanced practice nursing globally. Descriptive information, examples, and models of international development are provided.

UNIT 2

The Practice Environment

6   **Payment for Advanced Practice Nursing Services: Past, Present, and Future** .. 102
  Karen R. Robinson

  Even as we quickly move into a capitated system, reimbursement remains a major issue for all APNs. Today's health-care spending is scrutinized so closely that no APN reimbursement opportunity can be left "untapped." This chapter will assist APNs to understand the reimbursement process, identify existing reimbursement roadblocks, and finally, strategize to improve reimbursement efforts.

7   **Advanced Practice Nurses and Prescriptive Authority** 119
  Jan Towers

  Over 90% of the U.S. public seeking medical attention receives a prescription for medicine at the conclusion of an encounter in the health-care system. Although practice patterns of APNs differ, the authority to prescribe is critical to all. Significant gains have been made over the past several years. The progress has been gradual and methodical, from supervised practice to plenary authority.

8   **Credentialing and Clinical Privileges and the Advanced Practice Nurse** 130
  Ann H. Cary and Mary C. Smolenski

  Is the advanced practice legal credential a second license, deemed status for the profession's certification, or some hybrid of both? To what degree does credentialing guarantee competency? Should title protection be inextricably bound to licensure? And what about clinical privileges? Privileging may allow admitting, treatment, consultation, and visiting rights. We have been slow to realize clinical privileges for nurses, except in rural areas. This is despite the fact that The Joint Commission policies and Medicare regulations permit APNs to hold this status. The authors describe what is, what could be, and how to get there from here.

9   **The Kaleidoscope of Collaborative Practice** 143
  Alice F. Kuehn

  There have been many calls for the design of a new system of health-care delivery for the 21st century focused upon cooperation among professional providers as reflected by active collaboration and open communication. The historic roots of collaboration between physician and nurse, persisting flaws in the relationship, and factors that influence collaborative behaviors are described. A framework for collaboration is presented, listing critical indicators of a highly collaborative practice and comparing and contrasting examples of multi-, inter-, and transdisciplinary practice. Following a brief overview of role development for each of the four APN roles, key strategies for developing a successful collaborative team are given.

10   **Participation of the Advanced Practice Nurse in Managed Care and Quality Initiatives** 172
  Rita Munley Gallagher

  APNs have been notably absent from managed care plan provider panels. In addition, their efforts are not fully recognized in national quality activities. Is this due to their predominately employee status? Are they reticent to take on the full responsibility of a primary care provider, fearful of accepting accountability, hesitant to mobilize consumer support on their own behalf? Or is it a more fundamental issue . . . an issue of respect?

11   Resource Management 191

Christina M. Graf and Eileen D. Flaherty

APNs function within organizations that, whether large or small, must generate a profit to continue to provide services and realize their missions. Effective, quality clinical care that also incorporates efficient resource management is the most desirable outcome for the patient, for the clinician, for the organization, and for society. APNs need a clear understanding of issues and approaches related to resource management to influence organizational deliberations and ensure that clinical considerations are incorporated into fiscal and business decisions.

12   Mediated Roles: Working Through Other People 211

Thomas D. Smith, Maria L. Vezina, and Mary E. Samost

In both direct care and mediated roles, APNs are often dependent on the cooperation of others to achieve their therapeutic goals. These situations may involve formal referral and consultative relationships or working with a variety of health-care personnel, including other nurses. For example, referral involves handing a case over either for management by another specialist or for comanagement among providers. Consultation implies the process of influencing behavior through bringing a higher order of knowledge and experience to a situation. The degree of authority inherent in all of these relationships is an important quality to assess. Exemplars demonstrate these relationships specific to each advanced practice role.

13   Reporting Relationships: Follow the Money 230

Mary Lou S. Etheredge

There is wide variation of opinion regarding the reporting arrangements preferred by APNs. In fact, there may not be any one arrangement that the majority would agree on. Despite the differences, there are common themes that emerge. This chapter explores these themes as they are described by APNs in practice.

UNIT 3
Competency in Advanced Practice

14   Evidence-Based Practice 244

Deborah C. Messecar and Christine A. Tanner

Evidence-based practice is integral to advanced practice nursing. It builds on the process of research use, but includes much more, such as evidence from clinical expertise, the products of reasoning, and patient preferences, to name a few.

15   Advocacy and the Advanced Practice Nurse 261

Karen Piren and Susan C. Reinhard

This chapter defines the concept of advocacy, describing its historical roots, while noting the limited evidence base for its credibility. Three advocacy exemplars are discussed that focus on either the individual or the larger system within which health care and advocacy exist. The process of preparing to be an advocate is described along with the need for further didactic publications and research in this area.

16   Case Management and Advanced Practice Nursing 277

Patricia M. Haynor, Denise Fessler, Irene McEachen, and Marylou Yam

APNs and case management are almost a natural phenomenon. Nursing case management is a hybrid practice that mandates a wide variety of clinical expertise and patient management skills. The APN with additional academic knowledge and clinical practice enhanced by experience-based intuition can make significant contributions toward the coordination of multidisciplinary care. Vignettes are presented.

17   **The Advanced Practice Nurse and Research** 295
Pamela F. Cipriano and Suzanne M. Burns

The APN is a consumer, facilitator, collaborator, and leader in research. The APN develops a research attitude in others and fosters evidence-based practice through the integration of research findings into clinical practice. The APN applies the scientific method to clinical problem solving and provides leadership in the use and conduct of research. Case studies illustrate the APN's role using research methods to influence systems changes and to improve patient outcomes through changes in clinical practice.

18   **The Advanced Practice Nurse and Complementary Therapies** 309
Rothlyn P. Zahourek

Complementary therapies are a $32 billion a year industry for the U.S. public. Additionally, these represent one area in which the APN may assist patients with integrative health-care practices. The relationship between complementary therapies and holistic nursing interventions provides a valuable foundation for advanced practice roles.

19   **Basic Skills for Teaching and the Advanced Practice Nurse** 330
Marilyn H. Oermann

Teaching is an essential component of the APN role. This chapter provides an overview of the basic skills of teaching: assessment of the need for learning, the development of objectives and a teaching plan, instructional strategies for the APN to use in the classroom and clinical setting, and formative and summative evaluation. Additionally, the qualities of effective teachers are discussed. Examples are provided of different teaching methods and a teaching plan.

20   **Culture as a Variable in Practice** 352
Mary Masterson Germain

To fully enter the patient's experience and provide comprehensive care that is respectful of the patient's beliefs and practices, you will need to find ways to bridge the linguistic and cultural challenges that are inherent in caring for an increasingly diverse population. It is uncomfortable to stretch our ethnocentric boundaries—much easier to care for replicas of ourselves. However, if you are open to learning from your patients, the transient discomfort that you experience from having your time-honored interventions and teaching strategies tested and found wanting will be richly rewarded and inform your practice for years to come.

21   **Conflict Resolution: An Essential Competency in Advanced Practice** 381
Phyllis Beck Kritek and Lucille A. Joel

In interpersonal relationships, conflict is a constant, and as an official or symbolic leader, the APN is expected to respond. This chapter explores that reality and its implications for the nurse facing the challenges of advanced practice. It also posits that expanding conflict resolution competency is an opportunity to improve our work environments and a choice worth making.

UNIT 4
Ethical, Legal, and Business Acumen

22   **Evaluation of the Advanced Practice Nurse: Cost Efficiency,
Accomplishments, Trends, and Future Development** 390
Jane M. Flanagan and Dorothy A. Jones

The cost efficiency and therapeutic effectiveness of APNs, including the clinical nurse specialist, nurse-midwife, nurse anesthetist, and nurse practitioner, have been discussed in many forums. This chapter provides a comprehensive synthesis of the contributions made by the APN to improve practice and enhance evidence-based outcomes. Also included is an overview of the work environments employing the APN and a review of salaries and potential directions for expanding practice and using nursing knowledge to affect outcomes across populations and settings.

23   Promoting Advanced Practice Nurses to the Public 403

Donna A. Gaffney

How do we sell the APN to the public? Most of our market has been the poor and disenfranchised. For success and security, APNs need to sell their services to the critical mass that is Middle America.

24   Starting a Practice and Practice Management 421

Judith Barberio

Independent practice allows the APN to maximize patient care, spend time on needed patient education, and encourage patient participation in determining his or her own health-care regimen. But an entrepreneurial spirit, a fine-tuned knowledge base and clinical skill, and the desire to provide quality health care are not enough. Learn how to negotiate the winding road of rules and regulations, strategize for its pitfalls and detours, and ultimately know the rewards of delivering health care your way.

25   The Advanced Practice Nurse as Employee or Independent Contractor: Legal and Contractual Considerations 449

Kathleen M. Gialanella and Kammie Monarch

Employee status confers definite legal rights and responsibilities. The choice of whether to be an employee versus an independent contractor should be informed by knowledge of the differences. The authors explore these differences, as well as the details of executing written practice agreements governing the working relationship between the APN and other parties. This is a relatively new aspect of practice and it is important for the APN to understand the basic, foundational issues that need to be addressed in these written agreements. The authors have identified a number of those issues and also address the relevant case law.

26   The Law, the Courts, and the Advanced Practice Nurse 465

Virginia Trotter Betts, David Keepnews, and Kammie Monarch

The authors present a summary of the legal structures and principles shaping and affecting advanced practice nursing. They illustrate the subtle relationship existing between the legislature, the courts, and the regulatory agencies. Select legal issues are discussed, including scope of practice situations, fraud and abuse, and antitrust law. Case material is used liberally to clarify and explain points.

27   Malpractice Insurance 485

Sharon E. Muran, Amy Muran Felton, and Marie Infante

On the surface, APN malpractice premiums appear low. Is this a reflection of public trust and quality practice? On the contrary, review of societal expectations, practice standards, state and federal governmental regulations, and escalating litigation indicates that financial and professional risks for APNs have increased substantially. APNs can meet these challenges through an ounce of prevention in the form of adoption and integration of professional practices and risk-reduction strategies.

28   Ethics and the Advanced Practice Nurse 510

Gladys L. Husted and James H. Husted

The authors will consider the ethical decision-making competencies of the APN and the barriers that exist to ethical practice. This will be accomplished through a context-based model that concentrates on the professional agreement that exists between nurse and patient. A context-based model actualizes the concept of treating persons as individuals and therefore selecting interactions based on unique patient needs and circumstances. Each patient entering the health-care system hopes to derive some benefit. He hopes to regain his competence to perform his normal functions and to live his life as he chooses. At the very least, he expects to come out better able to live than when he went into that health-care system. Emphasis will be given to the rights of nurse and patient deriving from their implicit commitments and expectations. Case examples will be used in the presentation.

Index 531

Bonus Chapter on DavisPlus

Measuring Advanced Practice Nurse Performance: Outcome Indicators, Models of Evaluation, and the Issue of Value

Shirley Girouard

APNs can no longer assume that it is adequate to be accountable to their patients alone. Consumers, purchasers of care, employers, and policy makers are demanding evidence that APN practice makes a difference in outcomes and is cost effective. This chapter will address reasons for and approaches to measuring performance and establishing the value of advanced practice nursing.

The Evolution of Advanced Practice

1

Advanced Practice Nursing: Doing What Has to Be Done—Radicals, Renegades, and Rebels

Lynne M. Dunphy

Nancy K. Smith

Ellis Quinn Youngkin

Loretta Ford, acknowledged creator of the nurse practitioner (NP) role, noted in 1991 that "the movement thrived because the foundation of the nurse practitioner was deeply rooted in the enduring values and goals of professional nursing" (Ford, 1991, p. 287). This chapter makes the case that, far from being a new creation, advanced practice nurses (APNs) have been around since the founding of modern professional nursing, and in actuality, predate it. A look back into our past reveals legendary figures always responding to the challenges of human need, changing the landscape of health care, and improving the health of the populace. The titles may change, but the essence remains the same. This history contains interwoven strands: the evolution of medicine; changing sociopolitical, economic, and legal horizons; and emerging technologies. The social mandate has been constant: the care of those in need.

Advanced practice is a contemporary term that has evolved to label an old phenomenon: nurses providing care to others in their surrounding communities. As Barbara Ehrenreich and Deidre English (1973) note, "Women have always been healers. They were the unlicensed doctors and anatomists of western history . . . they were pharmacists, cultivating herbs and exchanging the secrets of their uses. They were midwives, travelling from home to home and village to village" (p. 3). Today, with health care dominated by a male-oriented medical profession, APNs are seen as nurses "pushing the envelope"—the envelope of regulated, standardized nursing practice. The reality is that the boundaries of professional nursing practice have always been fluid, with changes in the practice setting speeding ahead of the educational and regulatory environments. It has always been those nurses caring for persons and families who see a need and respond—at times in concert with the medical profession, and at times, at odds—who are the true trailblazers of contemporary advanced practice nursing. The tales that follow are fraught with drama, conflict, and bravery.

PRECURSORS AND ANTECEDENTS

There is a long and rich history of female lay healing with roots in both European and African cultures. Before there was a dominant male medical profession in the United States, and well into the 19th century, the female lay healer was the primary health-care provider for most of the population. As part of this tradition, the sharing of skills and knowledge were seen as one's obligation as a member of a community. Lay healers were not usually formally educated but learned these skills from other female healers. These skills were broad based and might include midwifery, the use of herbal remedies, and even bone setting (Ehrenreich, 2000, p. xxxiii). Laurel Ulrich, in *A Midwives Tale* (1990), notes that when the diary of the midwife Martha Ballard opens in 1785, ". . . she knew how to manufacture salves, syrups, pills, teas, ointments, how to prepare an oil emulsion, how to poultice wounds, dress burns, treat dysentery, sore throat, frost bite, measles, colic, 'whooping Cough,' 'Chin cough,' . . . and 'the itch,' how to cut an infant's tongue, administer a 'clister' (enema), lance an abscessed breast . . . induce vomiting, assuage bleeding, reduce swelling and relieve a toothache, as well as deliver babies" (p. 11).

This was an era of "social childbirth," when female relatives and friends, as well as midwives, attended births. Giving birth to one's own babies was seen as part of the process of becoming a midwife. "There is a tender regard one woman bears to another, and a natural sympathy in those who have gone thro' the Pangs of Childbearing; which doubtless, occasion a compassion for those that labour under these circumstances, which no man can be a judge of," notes one 18th-century midwifery manual (Stone, 1990, p. xiv). Intimate acquaintance with death also enhanced the lay healer's abilities.

Ulrich notes the tiny headstones marking the graves of Ballard's deceased babies and children as further evidence of her ability to provide compassionate, knowledgeable care; she was able to understand the pain and suffering of others. These were autonomous women healers who functioned independently of doctors and hospitals, and these were usually women whose status as healers extended to leadership positions in the general community. The emergence of a male medical establishment in the 19th century marked the beginning of the end of the era of female lay healers, including midwives. There was a profound difference, however, between the lay healers and the emerging medical profession. The lay healers saw their role as intertwined with one's obligations to the community, whereas the emerging medical class saw healing as a commodity to be bought and sold (Ehrenreich & English, 1978).

Hearing of the work of Florence Nightingale in the Crimean War, women of both the South and North were inspired to care for the sick and wounded men of the Civil War. With limited formal structures through which to channel this instinct, in some instances they merely took to the nearby battlefields as the cannon fire ceased, binding wounds, comforting the dying, and providing what scarce succor they could offer. Clara Barton, in her diary, describes how she "broke the shackles and went to the field" (Barton, 1987). Her place, she would write, was "anywhere between the bullet and the hospital" (Pryor, 1987, p. 93).

Nursing histories (O'Brien, 1987) have documented the emergence of professional nursing in the 19th century from women's domestic duties and roles, as an extension of things that women or servants had always done for their families. Modern nursing is usually pinpointed as beginning in 1873, the year of the opening of the first three U.S. training schools for nurses, "as an effort on the part of women reformers to help clean up the mess the male doctors were making" (Ehrenreich, 2000, p. xxxiv). The incoming nurses, for example, are credited with introducing the first bar of soap into Bellevue Hospital in the dark days when the medical profession was still resisting the germ theory of disease and aseptic techniques. Women, rooted in the domestic arts, intuitively understood the need for a clean and safe environment as a mechanism of healing. Having successfully stamped out the lay women healers, doctors, still on uncertain grounds themselves, feared that these new trained nurses might represent a new source of competition, the "female lay healer incarnate" (Ehrenreich, 2000).

The emergence of a strong public health movement in the 19th century, coupled with the founding of the Settlement House Movement, created a new vista for independent and autonomous nursing practice: public health nursing and home visiting. School nursing was another field to emerge from the Henry Street Settlement, a brainchild of Lillian Wald. Wald, a recently graduated trained nurse, created a unique community-based nursing practice on the lower east side of New York City. Along with a dedicated cadre of nurses, Henry Street Settlement remains a beacon of autonomous nursing practice that positively affected the health of an entire generation of New Yorkers and beyond. Wald described these nurses who flocked to work with her at Henry Street Settlement as women of above average "intellectual equipment," of "exceptional character, mentality and scholarship" (Daniels, 1989, p. 24). These nurses, as has been well documented, enjoyed an exceptional degree of independence and autonomy in their nursing practice.

In 1893, Wald described a typical day. First, she visited the Goldberg baby and then Hattie Isaacs, a patient with consumption to whom she brought flowers. Wald spent 2 hours bathing her ("the poor girl had been without this attention for so long that it took me nearly two hours to get her skin clean"). Next, she inspected some houses on Hester Street, where she found water closets that needed "chloride of lime" and notified the appropriate authorities. In the next house she found a child with "running ears," which she "syringed," showing the mother how to do it at the same time. In another room there was a child with a "summer complaint"; Wald gave the child bismuth and tickets for a seaside excursion. After lunch she saw the O'Briens and took the "little one, with whooping cough" to play in the back of the Settlement House yard. On the next floor of that tenement, she found the Costria baby, who had a sore mouth. Wald "gave the mother honey and borax and little cloths to keep it clean" (Coss, 1989, pp. 43–44). This was all before 2 p.m.!

These are just a few of the countless tales that could be told by early healers and nurses. APNs of the 21st century are merely carrying forward a long-standing agenda of response to human need, human suffering, and human want. Sadly, 19th- and 20th-century healers often were at odds with the organized nursing profession; healers were seen as radical, out of the mainstream, not "really" nurses. One and all, they have bravely faced struggles within a male-dominated medical profession, a bastion of scientific and capitalistic power. Far from being some new invention, midwives, nurse anesthetists, clinical nurse specialists (CNSs), and NPs are merely new permutations of long-standing nursing commitments.

NURSE-MIDWIVES

The history of midwifery is long and complex. This chapter focuses on the integration of midwifery into the profession of nursing from 1900 to the present, and what that portended for both professions.

Throughout the 20th century, nurse-midwifery has remained an anomaly in the U.S. health-care system. Nurse-midwives attend only a small percentage of all U.S. births. Since the early decades of this century, physicians laid claim to being the sole legitimate birth attendants in the United States (Dye, 1984). This is in contrast to Great Britain and many other European countries, where trained midwives attend a significant percentage of births. In Europe, homes remain an accepted place to give birth, whereas hospital births reign supreme in the United States. In contrast to Europe, the United States has little in the way of a tradition of professional midwifery.

As late as 1910, 50% of all births in the United States were reportedly delivered by midwives, and the percentage in large cities was often higher. However, the health status of the U.S. population, particularly in regard to perinatal health indicators, was poor (Bigbee & Amidi-Nouri, 2000). Midwives, unregulated, and by most accounts, unprofessional, were easy scapegoats on which to blame the problem of poor maternal and infant outcomes. New York City's Department of Health commissioned a study that claimed that the New York midwife was essentially "medieval." According to this report, fully 90% were "hopelessly dirty, ignorant, and incompetent" (Edgar, 1911, p. 882). There was a concerted movement away from home births. This was all part of a mass assault on midwifery by an increasingly powerful medical elite of obstetricians determined to control the birthing process.

These revelations resulted in the tightening of existing legislation and the creation of new legislation for the licensing and supervision of midwives (Kobrin, 1984). Several states passed laws granting legal recognition of midwives with regulatory control, resulting in the establishment of schools of lay midwifery. One example, the Bellevue School for Midwives in New York City, lasted until 1935, when the diminishing need for midwives made it difficult to justify its existence (Komnenich, 1998). In 1911, the American Society of Superintendents of Training Schools for Nurses passed a resolution to provide for registration, licensure, and training in midwifery. Obstetrical care continued the move into hospitals in urban areas that did not provide midwifery. For the most part, the advance of nurse-midwifery has been a slow and arduous struggle, often at odds with mainstream nursing. For example, Lavinia Dock (1901) wrote that all births must be attended by physicians. Public health nurses, committed to the professionalizing of nursing and adherence to scientific standards, chose to distance themselves from lay midwives. The heritage of the unprofessional image of the lay midwife would linger for many years. A more successful example of midwifery was the founding of the Frontier Nursing Service (FNS) in 1925 by Myra Breckinridge in Kentucky. Breckinridge pursued a vision of autonomous nurse-midwifery practice, having been educated as a public health nurse and traveling to Great Britain to become a certified nurse-midwife (CNM). She aimed to implement the British system in the United States (always a daunting enterprise on any front). In rural settings, where doctors were scarce and hospitals virtually nonexistent, midwifery found more fertile soil. However, even in these settings, professional nurse-midwifery had to struggle to bloom.

Breckinridge founded the FNS at a time when the national maternal death rate stood at 6.7 per 1000 live births, one of the poorest rates in the Western world. More than 250,000 infants, nearly 1 in 10, died before they reached their first birthdays (U.S. Department of Labor, 1920). The Sheppard-Towner Maternity and Infancy Act, enacted to provide public funds for maternal and child health programs, was the first federal legislation passed for specifically this purpose. Part of the intention of this act was to provide money to the states to train public health nurses in midwifery; however, this proved short-lived. By 1929, the bill lapsed; this was attributed by some to major opposition by the American Medical Association (AMA), which advocated the establishment of a "single standard" of obstetrical care, that is, provided by doctors in hospital settings (Kobrin, 1984).

Despite such opposition, the Lobenstine Midwifery Clinic was established in New York in 1931 and joined forces with the Maternity Center Association (MCA) to prepare public health nurses to be midwives, becoming the first recognized nurse-midwifery training program (Bigbee & Amidi-Nouri, 2000). In 1932, the School for Association for the Promotion and Standardization of Midwifery was established. The model of nursing practice that developed from the partnership between the MCA and a school of midwifery was significant. Established in 1918 in response to a study outlining the need for comprehensive prenatal care, the MCA oversaw a network of community-based maternity clinics served by public health nurses and physicians working together. Nurse-midwives began providing services in these centers in approximately 1931, merging nurse-midwifery and public health nursing practice. In 1934, the school merged with Lobenstine Clinic under the MCA and was known thereafter as The Clinic. The emerging role of the nurse in maternity care was quite different than what it is today; it was described in 1937 as a "bedside assistant" and "teacher of health" (Komnenich, 1998, p. 14).

Deep ambivalence persisted in nursing about this new specialty. Breckinridge and her predominantly British staff advocated full recognition of nurse-midwifery as a profession, with certification similar to that required by the English central midwives board. Breckinridge saw nurse-midwives working as independent practitioners and continued to advocate home births. And even more radically, FNS saw nurse-midwives as offering complete care to women with normal pregnancies and deliveries. However, even Breckinridge and her supporters did not advocate the FNS model for cities where doctors were plentiful and middle-class women could afford medical care. She stressed that the FNS was designed for impoverished "remotely rural areas" without physicians (Dye, 1984).

The MCA also took a quite conservative track. Its graduates were not granted any sort of professional certification. The MCA stressed that nurse-midwives were "at best only careful conscientious routine assistants to the physician. None would attempt or pretend to be more" (Hamschmeyer, 1939, p. 1183). Dye (1984) argues that in the end, the possibilities for the establishment of nurse-midwifery as a viable alternative in maternity care were undermined by dominant medical conceptions of childbirth and its management. In a system that emphasized the pathological conditions of birth, nurse-midwives had little role to play. As a result, there were limited opportunities for graduates to practice nurse-midwifery; often they assumed roles in nursing education and administration. As late as 1963, only 11% of CNMs who responded to a national survey were practicing midwifery; a 1977 survey showed 26% of all CNMs actually practicing as midwives. As we know, this is changing. Demands for family-centered, low-tech approaches to birth have led to new opportunities for nurse-midwives. Data published in 1996 showed 70.7% of CNMs practicing as midwives. Settings for practice and reimbursement structures remain contentious. Still, the number of actual CNMs remains small, accounting for only approximately 4% of all masters' enrollees in approximately 30 graduate-level CNM programs (Bigbee & Amidi-Nouri, 2000). The American College of Nurse-Midwives (ACNM) requires a baccalaureate-level education to sit for certification (Kommenich, 1998). The ACNM's requirement is less than the requirement of advanced practice nursing in general to mandate professional commitment by obtaining graduate-level education. This less stringent requirement may be a result of the need that nurse-midwives have to retain their independent midwifery identity. Liability issues plague CNMs as they do physicians in obstetric/gynecological (OB/GYN) practices.

The American Association of Nurse-Midwives (AANM) was founded in 1928, originally as the Kentucky State Association of Midwives, which was an outgrowth of FNS. First organized as a section of the National Organization of Public Health Nurses (NOPHN), the American College of Nurse-Midwifery was incorporated in 1955 as an independent specialty nursing organization when the NOPHN was subsumed within the National League for Nursing (NLN). In 1956, the AANM merged with the college, forming the ACNM. The ACNM sponsors the *Journal of Nurse-Midwifery*, implemented an accreditation process of programs in 1962, and established a certification examination and process in 1971. This body also currently certifies nonnurses as certified midwives and maintains alliances with professional midwives who are not nurses. As noted by Bigbee and Amidi-Nouri, CNMs are distinct from other APNs in that "they conceptualize their role as the combination of two disciplines, nursing and midwifery" (Bigbee & Amidi-Nouri 2000, p. 12).

Breckinridge was an early advocate of evaluative research in tracking the progress of nurse-midwifery. The FNS maintained excellent maternal mortality and morbidity records. Arrangements were made for Louis Dublin, a vice president at the Metropolitan Life Insurance Company and a statistician well known for knowledge of and concern for maternal and infant welfare, to tabulate the FNS medical statistics (Dye, 1984). Breckinridge was ahead of her time in realizing the importance of data.

The International Confederation of Nurse-Midwives (ICNM) was founded in Europe in 1919 with a goal of increasing the health of mothers and infants worldwide. Working closely with the World Health Organization (WHO) and the United Nations International Children's Emergency Fund, ICNM endeavors to bring improved care to mothers and babies in developing countries.

NURSE ANESTHETISTS

Nursing made medicine look good. — *Baer, 1982*

Sister Mary Bernard is recognized as the first nurse anesthetist to practice in the United States (Thatcher, 1953). Church records of 1877 identify her as being called on to function as an anesthetist while enrolled as a student in St. Vincent's Hospital in Erie, Pennsylvania.

Surgical anesthesia was born in the United States in the mid-19th century. Immediately there were rival claimants to its "discovery" (Bankert, 1989). In 1846, at Massachusetts General Hospital, William T. G. Morton first successfully demonstrated surgical anesthesia. Nitrous oxide was the first agent used and adopted by U.S. dentists. Ether and chloroform followed shortly as agents for use in anesthetizing a patient. One barrier to surgery had been removed. However, it would take infection control and consistent, careful techniques in the administration of the various anesthetic agents for surgery to enter its "Golden Age." It was only then that "surgery was transformed from an act of desperation to a scientific method of dealing with illness" (Rothstein, 1958, p. 258). For surgeons to advance their specialty, they needed someone to administer anesthesia with care. However, anesthesiology lacked medical status; the surgeon collected the fee. No incentive existed for anyone with a medical degree to take up the work. Who would administer the anesthesia? And who would administer it reliably, carefully? There was only one answer: nurses.

Marianne Bankert, in her landmark book *Watchful Care: A History of America's Nurse Anesthetists* (1989), explains how the economics of anesthesia changed. Physician-anesthetists "needed to establish their 'claim' to a field of practice they had earlier rejected" (p. 16), and it became necessary to deny, ignore, or denigrate the achievements of their nurse colleagues. The most intriguing part of her study, she says, was "the process by which a rival—and less moneyed—group (in this case, nurses) is rendered historically 'invisible'" (p. 16).

In many settings, one of the younger interns would administer the anesthesia. However, there was not always an intern available. St. Mary's Hospital, later to become known as the Mayo Clinic, played an important role in the development of anesthesia. It was here that Alice Magaw, sometimes referred to as the "Mother of Anesthesia," practiced from 1860 to 1928. In 1899 she published a paper titled "Observations in Anesthesia" in *Northwestern Lancet* in which she reported giving anesthesia in more than 3000 cases (Magaw, 1899). In 1906 she published another review of more than 14,000 successful anesthesia cases (Magaw, 1906). Bigbee and Amidi-Nouri (2000) note, "She stressed individual attention for all patients and identified the experience of anesthetists as critical elements in quickly responding to the patient" (p. 21). She also paid special attention to her patients' psyches: She believed that "suggestion" was a great help "in producing a comfortable narcosis" (Bankert, 1989, p. 32). She noted that the anesthetist "must be able to inspire confidence in the patient" and that much of this depends on the approach (Bankert, 1989, p. 32). She stressed preparing the patient for each phase of the experience and of the need to "'talk him to sleep' with the addition of as little ether as possible" (p. 33). Magaw was also noted for being a meticulous record keeper, recognizing, as had Breckinridge, the value of evaluative research in documenting the clinical effectiveness and productivity of specialty practice, as well as the nurses' performance in that specialty (Komnenich, 1998).

Magaw contended that hospital-based anesthesia services, as a specialized field, should remain separate from nursing service administrative structures (Bigbee & Amidi-Nouri, 2000). This presaged the estrangement that has historically existed between nurse anesthetists and "regular" nursing; again we see a nursing specialty with expanded clinical responsibilities developing outside of mainstream nursing.

It was around the turn of the century that the medical specialty of anesthesiology began to gain a foothold, led largely by women physicians. However, these physicians were unsympathetic to the role of the nurse anesthetists; they wanted to replace them. Different variants of this old power struggle echo today in legislative battles over the need for on-site oversight by an anesthesiologist.

War time in the 20th century was marked by advances in surgical techniques and reliance on the work of nurse anesthetists. Nurses administered anesthesia during the American Civil War, the Franco-Prussian War and World War I (Garde, 1988). Sophie Gran Wilson (1887–1989), having established a record of treating more than 10,000 cases without one fatality, joined the Army Nurse Corp. Wilson, along with a group of other nurses from Minneapolis Hospital Unit No. 26, were assigned to Mobile Hospital No. 1 in the Chateau-Thierry area of France. It was this unit, working with Dr. James T. Gwathmey, that succeeded in using anesthesia in mobile hospitals (Komnenich, 1998, p. 22). World War I saw the advent of the mobile field hospital that provided anesthesia and surgical intervention on, or very near, the battlefield, with great reductions in mortality. One early nurse anesthetist, Sophie Winston, received the *Croix de Guerre* for her service on the battlefield in France. The public's enthusiasm was whetted, but nurse anesthetists' successes raised the hackles of an increasingly male, professionalizing group of anesthesiologists.

World War II further institutionalized the role of nurse anesthetist; it was declared a clinical nursing specialty within the military nursing structure, a move that elevated the stature of nurse anesthetists. By the end of the war in 1945, the American Association of Nurse Anesthetists (AANA) instituted a credentialing examination for nurse anesthetists, far in advance of other nursing specialties. The Army, grasping the value of the nurse anesthetists, established educational programs for nurse anesthetists, including one at Walter Reed Army Hospital.

Nurse anesthetists again played a major role on the battlefield during the Vietnam War; 2 of the 10 nurses killed in Vietnam were male nurse anesthetists. Just as female physician anesthesiologists were replaced by male physicians after the turn of the century, nurse anesthesiology was increasingly a male-dominated specialty. The first class to graduate from the Walter Reed General Hospital in 1961 consisted of only men; another early school, the Letterman General Hospital School of Anesthesia in San Francisco, also graduated an all-male class (Bankert, 1989). At present, there are approximately 28,000 certified registered nurse anesthetists (CRNAs), 42% of whom are males. Interestingly, the inclusion of large numbers of males in their ranks has not eased the advance of this venerable nursing specialty; turf wars between practicing anesthesiologists and nurse anesthetists remain intensely active as of this writing.

Nonetheless, over its lengthy history, there have been medical men in active support of the role, notably Dr. George Crile, who in 1936 praised the role of nurse anesthetists, identifying what he called their "finesse" (Crile, 1947). His ideal of the nurse anesthetist was Agatha Cobourg Hodgins, a native of Canada. Together, Crile and Hodgins founded the Lakeside School of Anesthesia.

The AANA was founded in 1931 by Hodgins and originally named the National Association for Nurse Anesthetists. This group voted to affiliate with the American Nurses Association (ANA), only to be turned away! As early as 1909, Florence Henderson, a successor of Magaw's, was invited to present a paper at the ANA convention, with no subsequent extension of an invitation to become a member of the organization (Komnenich, 1998). Thatcher (1953) speculates that organized nursing was fearful that nurse anesthetists could be charged with practicing medicine. This led the AANA to affiliate with the American Hospital Association. The relationship between nurse anesthetists and anesthesiologists has always been, and continues to be, contentious. Despite a brief period of relative harmony, from 1972 to 1976, when their respective professional organizations issued the "Joint Statement on Anesthesia Practice," their partnership ended when the board of directors of the American Society of Anesthesiologists withdrew their support of this statement, returning to a model that maintained physician control (Bankert, 1989, pp. 140–150). Nonetheless, nurse anesthetists continue to thrive and are increasingly integrated into graduate-level nursing education. Their inclusion in the spectrum of advanced practice nursing is invigorating for us all.

THE CLINICAL NURSE SPECIALISTS

The role of the CNS is the one strand of advanced practice nursing that arose and was nurtured by mainstream nursing education and nursing organizations. Indeed, one could say it arose from the very bosom of traditional nursing practice. As early as 1900, in the *American Journal of Nursing,* Katherine DeWitt wrote that the development of nursing specialties, in her view, responded to a "need for perfection within a limited domain" (Sparacino, 1986, p. 1). According to DeWitt, nursing specialties were a response to "present civilization and modern science [that] demand a perfection along each line of work formerly unknown" (idem). She argued that "the new nurse is more useful, at least to the patient himself, and ultimately to the family and community. Her sphere is more limited, but her patient receives better care" (idem).

Nurses were trained and worked in hospitals that were structured for the convenience of the doctors around specific populations of patients. Early on, nurses initiated guidelines for care for unique populations and often garnered a hands-on kind of intimacy, an expertise in the care of certain patients that was not to be denied. Caring day-in and day-out for patients suffering from similar conditions enabled nurses to develop specialized and advanced skills, not practiced by other nurses, in the care of certain patients. Nurse-midwifery and nurse anesthetists are early exemplars of this specialization. Because of nursing's relative invisibility (Dracup, 1998), areas of early specialty practices are undoubtedly lost. Think of the nurses who cared exclusively for patients with tuberculosis, syphilis, and polio. Because these conditions are no longer common, any nursing expertise that might have been developed has been lost.

In 1943 during a speech, Frances Reiter first used the term *nurse-clinician.* Her philosophy of nursing grounded her concept of the nurse-clinician. She believed that "practice is the absolute primary function of our profession" and "that means the direct care of patients" (Reiter, 1966). Reiter strongly believed that nurses should have complete control over the direct care of the patient. The nurse-clinician, as she conceived the role, consisted of three spheres. Clinical competence, the first sphere, included three additional dimensions of function that she termed *care, cure,* and *counseling.* The nurse-clinician was labeled "the Mother Role" in which the nurse protects, teaches, comforts, and encourages the patient. The second sphere, as envisioned by Reiter, involved clinical expertise in the coordination and continuity of the patient's care. Lastly, she believed in what she called "professional maturity," wherein the physician and nurse "share a mutual responsibility for the welfare of patients" (Reiter, 1966, p. 277). It was only through such working together that the patient could best be served and nursing achieve "its greatest potential" (Reiter, 1966). Although Reiter believed that the nurse-clinician should have advanced expertise and clinical competence, she did not specify that the nurse-clinician should be prepared at the master's level.

In 1943, the National League for Nursing Education advocated a plan to develop CNSs, enlisting universities to educate them (Menard, 1987). Traditionally, advanced education in nursing had focused on "functional" areas: that is, nursing education and nursing administration. Esther Lucile Brown, in her 1948 report *Nursing for the Future,* promoted developing clinical specialties in nursing as a way of strengthening and advancing the profession. The GI Bill was also available. Nurses in the Armed Services were eligible to receive funds for their education.

It took the entrance of another strong nurse leader, Hildegard Peplau, to move these ideas forward to fruition. In 1953, she had both a vision and a plan: She wanted to prepare CNSs at the graduate level who could offer direct care to psychiatric patients, thus helping to close the gap between psychiatric theory and nursing practice (Callaway, 2002). In her first 2 years at Rutgers University in New Jersey, Peplau developed a 19-month master's program that prepared only CNSs in psychiatric nursing. In contrast, existing programs, for example at Teachers College in New York City, attempted to prepare nurses for advanced practice, teaching, and supervision in a 10-month program.

The field of psychiatric nursing was in the process of inventing itself: Before the passage of the National Mental Health Act in 1946, there was no such field as psychiatric nursing. It was the availability of National Institute of Mental Health funds to "seed" such programs as Peplau's that allowed psychiatric nursing to begin and eventually to flourish.

In retrospect, Peplau would note that no encouragement was received from the two major nursing organizations of the day, the NLN and the ANA. She stated "We were highly stigmatized. Any nurse who worked in [the field of mental health] was considered almost certifiable. . . . We were thoroughly unpopular, we were considered queer enough to be avoided" (Callaway, 2002, p. 229). It should be emphasized that at this point in nursing history it was inconceivable that any nurse, under any circumstances, could become a specialist.

The "received wisdom" of the day was the axiom, followed by the vast majority of nurses, that "a nurse is a nurse is a nurse," opposing any differentiation between who was doing what among them. Peplau's rigorous curriculum and clinical and academic program requirements expected that faculty would continue their own clinical practice, do clinical research, and publish the results (Calloway, 2002). This was a radical model for nursing faculty, few of whom were doctorally prepared in the 1950s. In 1956, only 2 years following the initiation of the first clinically focused graduate program, a national working conference on graduate education in psychiatric nursing formally developed the role of the psychiatric clinical specialist.

Most hospital training schools remained embedded in a functional method of nursing well into the 1960s, originally conceptualized by Isabel Stewart in the 1930s. Nurses were "trained." Much of nursing practice was "rule-based and activity-oriented" (Fairman, 1999, p. 312), relying heavily on repetition of skills and procedures. There was little, if any, scientific understanding of the principles underlying care. There was little, if any, intellectual content to be found in nursing care. With the advent of antibiotics in the 1940s and the resulting decline of infectious diseases, nurses were confronted with patients with acute, often rapidly changing exacerbations of chronic conditions. Leaders like Peplau, along with others such as Virginia Henderson, Reiter, and later Dorothy Smith, began developing a theoretical orientation for practice. Students were being taught to assess patient responses to their illnesses and to make analytical decisions. Smith experimented with the idea of a nurse-clinician who had 24-hour responsibility for a patient area and who was on call. Laura Simms at Cornell University-New York Hospital School of Nursing developed a CNS role to provide consultation to more generalist nurses. As opposed to the nurse who might have been expert in procedures, these new clinicians were experts in clinical care for a certain population of patients. This development occurred across specialties and was seen in oncology, nephrology, psychiatry, and intensive care units (Sills, 1983).

Role expansion of the CNS grew rapidly during the 1960s because of several factors. Advances in medical technology and medical specialization increased the need for nurses who were competent to care for patients with complex health needs. Nurses returning from the fields of Vietnam sought to increase their knowledge and skills, continuing to practice in advanced roles and nontraditional areas (such as nurse anesthetists). Role definitions for women loosened and expanded. There was a shortage of physicians. The Nurse Training Act of 1964 allocated necessary federal funds for additional graduate nursing education programs in several different clinical specialties (Mirr & Snyder, 1995).

The terms *nurse-clinician, clinical nurse specialist,* and *nurse specialist,* among others, were used extensively by nurses with experience or advanced knowledge who had developed an expertise within in a given area of patient care. There were no standards in regard to educational requirements or experience. In 1965, the ANA developed a position statement declaring that only those nurses with a master's degree or higher in nursing should claim the role of CNS (ANA, 1965). These trends continued into the 1970s. The number of academic programs providing master's preparation in a variety of practice areas increased. Federal grants including those from the Department of Health, Education and Welfare continued to provide funding for nursing education at the master's and doctoral levels.

In 1976, during the ANA's Congress on Nursing Practice, a position statement on the role of the CNS was issued. The ANA position statement read as follows:

> *The clinical nurse specialist (CNS) is a practitioner holding a masters degree with a concentration in specific areas of clinical nursing. The role of the CNS is defined by the needs of a select client population, the expectation of the larger society and the clinical expertise of the nurse (ANA Congress for Nursing Practice, 1976).*

The statement went on to elaborate that "by exercising leadership ability and judgment," the CNS is able to both affect client care on the individual, direct-care provider level and affect change within the broader health-care system (ANA Congress for Nursing Practice, 1976). The 1970s were a time of growth in academic CNS programs; the 1980s were years in which refinements occurred. In 1980, the ANA revised its earlier policy statement of 1976 to define the CNS as "a registered nurse who, through study and supervised clinical practice at the graduate level (masters or doctorate) has become an expert in a defined area of knowledge and practice in a selected clinical area of nursing" (ANA, 1980, p. 23). This statement was significant because it was the first time that education at the master's level had been dictated as mandatory criteria for entry-level preparation.

The CNS role, more than any other advanced nursing role, was situated in the mainstream of graduate nursing education, with the first master's degree in psychiatric/mental health nursing being offered at Rutgers University in 1955. The inclusion of clinical content in master's degree education was an essential step forward for nursing's advancement. But the implementation and use of the CNS evaded easy categorization and their efficacy was elusive.

In February of 1983, the ANA Council of Clinical Nurse Specialists met for the first time (Sparacino, 1990). The Council grew rapidly throughout the following years, supporting and providing educational conferences for the increasing numbers of CNSs. In 1986, the Council published the Clinical Nurse Specialist's role statement. This statement identified the roles of the CNS as specialist in clinical practice and as educator, consultant, researcher, and administrator. This role statement by the Council depicted the changing role of the CNS, notably delegating and overseeing practice, as its primary focus (Fulton, 2002). The year 1986 was also notable for the publication of the journal *Clinical Nurse Specialist: The Journal for Advanced Nursing.*

In 1986, the ANA's Council of Clinical Nurse Specialists and the Council of Primary Health Care Providers published an editorial comparing the similarities of the CNS and NP roles. Discussion surrounding the commonalities of both specialties occurred throughout the decade. In 1989, during the annual meeting of the National Organization of Nurse Practitioner Faculty (NONPF), the 10-year-old debate regarding the merger of the two roles reached a crescendo without resolution (Lincoln, 2000). It remains an issue of contention to the present day. Despite this, the two ANA councils did merge in 1990, becoming the Council of Nurses in Advanced Practice (Busen & Engleman, 1996; Lincoln, 2000). Following the merger of the councils, several studies were published comparing CNS and NP roles, finding the education for practice generally comparable (Joel, 2003). The 1990s was an era of health-care "reform." Health-care costs were skyrocketing; hospital stays were shorter, with acutely ill patients being discharged quicker and sicker. As a result of fiscal mandates, hospitals were downsizing the number of beds and personnel. The historically hospital-based CNS was considered too expensive and unproven, and the focus of health care shifted from hospital-based to ambulatory care within the community and home. CNSs all over were losing positions.

In 1993, the American Association of Colleges of Nursing (AACN) met to discuss educational needs and requirements for the 21st century. In December 1994, at the AACN's annual conference, members voted to support the merging of the CNS/NP roles in the curricula of graduate education in nursing. Although the structure of the curricula suggested in The Essentials of Graduate Education (AACN, 1995) has been widely adopted, the lived reality of role adaptation and its implementation in the marketplace has been less uniform and more divisive. Sparacino (1990) defined the scope of the CNS as "client-centered practice, utilizing an in-depth assessment, practiced within the domain of secondary and tertiary care settings" (p. 8). The NP role is defined by Sparacino (1986) as being responsible for providing a full range of primary health-care services using the appropriate knowledge base and practicing in multiple settings outside of secondary and tertiary settings. The other side of this story of advanced practice nursing is addressed in the next section of this chapter. The future of these various roles remain on some level intertwined and are further complicated as of this writing by the emergence of a new role and title: the doctor of nursing practice (DNP), and in the case of the CNS, the role of the clinical nurse leader (CNL).

THE EVOLUTION OF THE NURSE PRACTITIONER ROLE: "A DISRUPTIVE INNOVATION"

The history of the NP "movement" has been well documented (Brush & Capezuti, 1996; Fairman, 1999; Jacox, 2002). A lesser known story involves Dr. Eugene A. Stead, Jr., of Duke University, who in 1957 conceived of an advanced role for nurses, somewhere between the role of the nurse and the doctor. A nursing faculty member, Thelma Ingles, on a sabbatical, worked with Stead, rounding with the interns and residents, seeing patients, and managing increasingly ill patients with acumen and sensitivity. Ingles shared Stead's ideas and returned to the Duke Nursing School to create a master of science in nursing program modeled on her experience with Stead. Stead was gratified and anxious to impart this expanded role to other nursing faculty, envisioning a new role for nurses, with, in his view, expanded autonomy. He was shocked at the "lukewarm" response of the dean of nursing at Duke and the nonsupportive stance of a number of prominent nurses at the university. On top of that, the NLN, the school's accrediting body, did not approve of Ingle's new program for clinical nurse specialization and withheld the program's accreditation. They found the program "unstructured," and criticized the use of physicians as instructors to teach courses for nurses in a nursing program. They disavowed the study of the esteemed discipline of medicine that Stead was so anxious to impart (Holt, 1998). Instead, they wanted the students to study "nursing!" Stead could not understand this. What was there in nursing to study? Rejected and disheartened, Stead eventually turned to military corpsmen to actualize this new role, which he named *physician assistant*. He insisted that they be male. In his view, nurse leaders were very antagonistic to innovation and change (Christman, 1998). This was a missed opportunity for organized nursing.

In some ways, Stead's proposal was quite prescient. Gender roles were loosening, as were hierarchical structures in general; nurses were better educated and well able to assume the role responsibilities that Stead envisioned. Yet, it came at a time when nursing was merely a fledgling discipline, new to the university, new to development as an academic discipline, and new to doctoral education. Academic nursing was fixated on defining its own knowledge base and developing its own unique science. Along with expanded opportunities for women came ideas of an autonomous nursing role, separate and distinct from medicine. All these factors were in play when the first NPs emerged in the 1960s.

However, the NP was not really a new role for nurses. Examining our history, it is apparent that nurses functioned independently and autonomously before the rise of organized medicine. If medicine was ambivalent about the emergence of this new role, nursing itself has been no less conflicted.

In 1978 the following statement appeared in the *American Journal of Nursing:*

> *The nurse practitioner movement has become an issue in nursing, a topic on which there is no consensus. One question about the movement is whether the development of the nurse practitioner role adds to, or detracts from, the development of nursing as a distinct scientific discipline (Roy & Obloy, 1978, p. 1698).*

This statement was issued more than 13 years since the initiation of the first NP program at the University of Colorado. In February 2002, *Clinician News* ran a feature titled, "Some Physicians Seeing Red Over the Term *Provider*" (*Clinician's Review*, 2002). The article documents the discomfort of the AMA regarding physicians, NPs, and physician assistants being grouped under the term *provider*. This was seen as yet another infringement on rapidly eroding physician authority. Considering the assaults from competing groups, both from within the profession of nursing and without, it is nothing short of amazing that NPs as a group have grown, been mainstreamed into graduate education, and continue to thrive. It is a testament to their hardiness, their courage, and their commitment. If, as Sparacino (1990) spells out, the domain of the CNS is situated in the secondary and tertiary setting, the domain of the NP originally arose as a role situated in primary care. From this perspective, the role is not nearly as new as it might appear. If anything, it is the 100 years or so of physician domination of this field that is the aberration.

In 1923, physician Francis Peabody called for the return of the generalist physician who would give comprehensive, *personal* care (Peabody, 1930). This call fell on deaf ears, as specialty practice in medicine continued to flourish. It was only in the 1960s that leaders in the field of general practice began advocating a seemingly paradoxical solution to reverse the trend and correct the scarcity of general practitioners: the creation of still another specialty. In 1969, the American Board of Family Practice came into being as the 20th medical specialty board, thus giving birth to the specialty of family practice (Rakel, 1995).

Broadly defined, *primary care* means basic, initial health care for general complaints, frequently given in an ambulatory setting such as an office or clinic, and usually representing a person's first contact with the health-care system. Primary care is continuous, comprehensive, family-centered care that focuses on managing current health-care needs, preventing future problems, and referring to specialists when appropriate. Primary care providers are the gatekeepers to the health-care system (ANA, 1993; Rakel, 1995).

The ANA *Nursing Facts* published a document in 1993 titled "Primary Health Care: The Nurse Solution." This pamphlet defines essential primary care services as the following (ANA, 1993):

- Performing physical examinations and taking health histories
- Assessing and evaluating common symptoms of acute illnesses such as colds, infections, and asthma
- Prescribing and managing medication regimens for common or acute conditions
- Managing chronic health problems such as diabetes, hypertension, and depression
- Providing screening and preventive services such as blood pressure screening, nutrition counseling, immunizations, and smoking cessation
- Providing prenatal care, family care, and delivery of normal pregnancies
- Identifying health needs that require referral for more specialized care

This same pamphlet promotes the role of the registered nurse as the solution to critical problems of access and accountability in the current health-care systems, problems that have only intensified 10 years later. Thinking back to the public health nurses of the turn of the century, it is clear that all of the elements previously noted have long been aspects of professional nursing practice; in retrospect, what is shocking is how nurses ever lost control of these vital functions.

As discussed previously, in the late 1950s and early 1960s, ideas about nursing care were undergoing big changes. Along with the development of the nurse-clinician and CNS roles that were emerging in a variety of places, Ford, along with Dr. Henry Silver, designed a graduate curriculum for pediatric nurses to provide ambulatory care to poor rural Colorado children. The goal of this program was to bridge the gap between the health-care needs of children and the family's ability to access and afford primary health care (Ford & Silver, 1967; Silver, Ford, & Stearly, 1967). This program was situated in graduate education and included courses such as pathophysiology, health promotion, and growth and development, with the intent of the student understanding the underlying principles of healthy child care and patient education. Nurses would then be able to provide preventive nursing services outside of the hospital setting in collaboration with physicians. Students had to have a baccalaureate degree and public health nursing experience to be admitted to the program.

Ford states the following in an interview: "We looked at the nurse practitioner preparation not as a separate program but as integrated into a role that had already been designed at the graduate level" (Jacox, 2002, p. 155). Ford notes that the lack of organizational leadership in the profession coupled with a lack of responsiveness in academic settings caused a "bastardization of the model" (Jacox, 2002, p. 157). She had envisioned that our professional organization, just like in other professions, would identify, credential, and make public advanced nursing practitioners. However, Ford was to discover that the "ANA in those early years was reluctant to stick its neck out and give some leadership to the nurse practitioner groups that were growing rapidly," and that the lack of leadership in nursing education created "a patchwork quilt" of differently prepared NPs (Jacox, 2002, p. 157).

Despite the infusion of federal funds into nursing education on the graduate level in the 1960s, most existing programs taught nurses to be educators and administrators. Although clinically based programs were growing, there remained resistance to the NP model. Ford says,

I understood that faculty members were supposed to be doing just that—Push the borders of knowledge and publish their work. In my naiveté of faculty politics, I expected that since the NP model grew out

of professional nursing and public health nursing—including primary, secondary, and tertiary prevention and community-based services—it was a perfectly legitimate investigation. Instead, it became a battleground, and even recently was labeled in the Harvard Business Review *as a "Disruptive Innovation." What a compliment (Jacox, 2002, p. 155)!*

The reasons for this resistance on the part of the organized nursing leadership, as well as the groves of academe, are complex and multifactorial, but are nonetheless a familiar story we have heard in each diverse area of advanced practice nursing in this chapter. The terrain may change but the journey remains the same.

In 1975, Martha Rogers, nurse theorist, leader, and educator, summed up the opposition view in colorful prose. She deplored the position of nurses who have succumbed to what she called the "blatant perfidy spawned by such terms as pediatric associate, nurse practitioner, family health practitioner, primary care practitioner, geriatric practitioner, physician extender, and other equally weird and wonderful cover-ups designed to provide succor and profit for the nation's shamans" (Rogers, 1975, p. 1834). Certainly she had a point!

Nonetheless, the movement persisted. Market demand, nursing vision, and bravery on the part of individual practitioners fostered forward movement. Members of the medical field were a major support, as was the federal government. Government support is not surprising; the need to provide primary care for the underserved is a tremendous and growing problem. The American Academy of Pediatrics provided sponsorship and supported the development of the National Association of Pediatric Nurse Associates and Practitioners (NAPNAP) as an organization to lead and certify pediatric NPs, thus providing more access to primary care services (Hobbie, 1998).

As early as 1964, the chairman of the department of obstetrics and gynecology at Harvard Medical School, Dr. Duncan Reid, proposed a family NP role to replace the general family physician ("Family Nurse Practitioner," 1964). Organized nursing and nurse educators were the first to oppose this suggestion. The American College of Obstetricians and Gynecologists (ACOG) similarly supported the development of the OB/GYN NP (now certified as the women's health-care practitioner). Through its certification body, the Nurses Association of the American College of Obstetricians and Gynecologists (now the Association of Women's Health, Obstetric, and Neonatal Nurses and permanently separated from the ACOG) developed its first certification examination for these NPs in 1981. The American College of Family Practice similarly backed the NP evolution, promoting this role in ambulatory primary care to diagnose and manage the most common conditions encountered in primary care, particularly in rural areas.

The collaboration between NP and physician has been analyzed and debated since the advent of the NP role, including the relationship between Ford and Silver (Fairman, 2002). The sticking point of collaboration is that it has included a heavy implication for supervision. In truth, in the early 1970s both NPs and physicians had to give up their traditional roles, tasks, and knowledge to establish this new provider role, often in the face of organizational and societal opposition. Jan Towers describes the growth of her own NP practice as follows: "The area that I perhaps most feared turned out to be the least troublesome, after some initial adjustments between the physician with whom I was working and me were made" (Towers, 1995, p. 269). What could often be impossible on an organizational level was often easily resolvable among professionals with a shared interest and commitment: the good of the patient.

The Great Society entitlement programs significantly influenced the need for NP development to care for people who were covered by Medicare and Medicaid. Predominate social movements—women's rights, civil rights, and the antiwar movement—had a profound impact on the need for groups to assert a place in the society of the 1960s and early 1970s. Nurses were not immune to these uncertain times and took advantage of the opportunities to work with physicians "in relationships that were entrepreneurial and groundbreaking, and to engage in a kind of dialogue that supported new models of care" (Fairman, 2002, p. 165). These nurses were pioneers, rebels, and renegades treading on uncertain ground. The change processes of extension and expansion were evolutionary in the role development of NPs (Murphy, 1970). The nurse's own professional "responsibility and judgment" within the nursing field was seen as "something more" for the patient, in contrast to the physician assistant role that was seen as less comprehensive (Murphy, 1970, p. 383).

The National Advisory Commission on Health Manpower supported the NP movement (Moxley, 1968). The Committee to Study Extended Roles for Nurses in the early 1970s recommended that the expanded role for nurses was necessary to provide the consumer with access to health care and proposed the inclusion of highly developed health assessment skills (Kalisch & Kalisch, 1986; Leininger, Little, & Carnevali, 1972; Marchione & Garland, 1997). Although the committee did stop short of providing a definitive scope of practice statement, it recommended support for licensure and certification for advanced practice, recognition in the nursing practice act, further cost-benefit research, and surveys on role impact. Government and private groups rapidly developed funding support for educational programs (Hamric, Spross, & Hanson, 1996). According to Marchione and Garland (1997), "The traditional role of humanistic caring, comforting, nurturing and supporting was to be maintained and improved by the addition" of new primary care functions that the Department of Health, Education and Welfare approved: total patient assessment, monitoring, health promotion, and a focus that encompassed not only disease prevention but health promotion and maintenance, treatment, and continuity of care.

By 1976, when Dorothy Ozimek, director of the NLN's Department of Baccalaureate and Higher Degrees, reviewed the status of NPs, she found them to be an extension of nursing, not the medical profession (Hahn, 1995). She advised that educational programs for NPs should be baccalaureate or master's level. The Division of Nursing of the Department of Health, Education and Welfare tracked the development of the NP role from 1974 to 1977, during which time the number of NP programs rose from 86 to 178 across the country. Although nurse educators by this time wanted NP education standardized, in 1977 most NP programs were certificate programs, but some were still using continuing education models and accepted less than a baccalaureate degree for entry. However, the number of NP graduates of masters' programs did increase from 20% in 1975 to 26% in 1977. More than 200 NP programs were at the master's level by 1994 (Hahn, 1995). The political voice for NPs was enhanced with the formation of the American Academy of Nurse Practitioners (AANP) in 1985 and the American College of Nurse Practitioners in 1993.

The NP educational programs of the times prepared family, adult, pediatric, maternal, school, geriatric, rural, and emergency NPs and were supported by a number of major federal agencies (Kalisch & Kalisch, 1986). Priscilla Andrews, a nurse, and John Connolly, a pediatrician, directed the Bunker Hill/Massachusetts General Nurse Practitioner program in 1968 (Pulcini & Wagner, 2001). This program, along with the Colorado program founded by Ford and Silver, aimed at producing more primary care providers for underserved children. The University of Washington initiated one of the earliest family NP programs (Pulcini & Wagner, 2001): The Primex program in New York City was a 4-month offering of continuing education that started in 1969 (Leininger et al., 1972; Marchione & Garland, 1997). More than 65 programs were operational by 1973, primarily as postgraduate certificate programs with a few master's programs sprinkled in (Pulcini & Wagner, 2001). At the University of Miami, Brower and Baker (1976) were applying a model of advanced nursing theory in their geriatric NP program, integrating it with the more traditional medical model of the era in an effort to encourage an appreciation for nursing care related to older adults.

The Council of Primary Care Nurse Practitioners was developed in 1974 by the ANA, and for the first time there was an effort to examine NP curricula by NP educators at the University of North Carolina-Chapel Hill (Pulcini & Wagner, 2001). The ANA Congress of Nursing Practice defined the nurse and NP roles in 1974, stating, "Nurse Practitioners have advanced skills in the assessment of physical and psychosocial health-illness status of individuals, families or groups in a variety of settings through health and developmental history taking and physical examination. They are prepared for these special skills by formal continuing education which adheres to ANA approved guidelines, or in a baccalaureate nursing program" (Marchione & Garland, 1997, p. 336).

With funding from the Robert Wood Johnson Foundation and under the direction of Darlene Jelinek, the University of New Mexico began to develop curricular guidelines for family NP programs in 1976; these were published in 1980. A significant outcome of this work was the establishment of NONPF that same year. Jelinek was elected the first president, and the organization had 35 members.

The Nurse Training Acts of 1971 and 1975 were critical in providing federal funding to support NP programs. By 1979, more than 133 programs and tracks existed, and approximately 15,000 NPs were in practice. By 1983 and 1984, NP graduates numbered approximately 20,000 to 24,000; they were primarily employed in sites that served those in greatest need: public health departments, community health centers, outpatient and rural clinics, health maintenance organizations, school-based clinics, and occupational health clinics (Pulcini & Wagner, 2001; Hamric et al., 1996; Kalisch & Kalisch, 1986). NPs were typically providing well-person care, minor acute problem and chronic stable illness management, and the full range of teaching and coaching that nurses have always provided for patients and families. A hindrance to practice in rural areas was finding appropriate physician backup. By 1987, the federal government had spent $100 million to promote NP education, primarily through the U.S. Public Health Service Division of Nursing (Pulcini & Wagner, 2001).

Idaho was the first state to legislate the expanded role in 1971, and other states followed with regulatory and legislative action that allowed a broader scope of practice for nurses with appropriate skills. Some states codified these role refinements through administrative regulations, whereas others sought amendments to the nursing practice act or new legislation. A number of states mandated criteria for the expanded role, such as a master's degree or national certification.

Prescriptive authority was delegated either from the medical practice act and carried out under physicians' standing orders or protocols, or it came directly from the nursing practice acts. Oregon and Washington states allowed nurses the freedom to prescribe independently in 1983 (Kalisch & Kalisch, 1986). Some of the fiercest turf battles have heated up over prescriptive privileges. By 1984, nurses were accused of practicing medicine although they were practicing well within the scope of their expanded role. Physicians remained ambivalent. They pushed NPs to function broadly but did not usually support legislation that authorized an increased scope of practice, especially in the area of prescriptive privileges.

By the 1980s, the master's degree was viewed broadly as the educational standard for advanced practice (Geolot, 1987; Sultz, Henry, Kinyon, Buck, & Bullough, 1983), and by 1989, 90% of programs were master's and postmaster's level (Pulcini & Wagner, 2001). NONPF thrived in the 1980s, developing curriculum guidelines and competencies, surveying faculties, and studying role components.

In the mid-1970s, the Department of Health, Education and Welfare recommended national nonfederal certification to regulate quality for all nonphysician providers (Dunn, 1986). Concurrently, the ANA began offering certification examinations in 1977. Certifying examinations helped to legitimize the NP role, moving NP education toward outcomes that were more uniform. By 1978, 1350 nurses were certified. The purpose of the certifying examinations were expanded to include "assurance of quality beyond basic licensure; identification of nurses who may be directly reimbursable for services; and recognizing achievement and quality of practice" (Hawkins & Thibodeau, 1993, p. 77). By the early 1980s, NP-certified specialties included OB/GYN, psychiatric/mental health, community health, family, adult, gerontological, pediatric, and school NPs. The Nurses Association of ACOG (now the Association of Women's Health, Obstetric and Neonatal Nurses) developed and administered the first OB/GYN certification examination in 1980. The certification organization of this group became the National Certification Corporation (NCC) in 1993, adding the neonatal NP to its certification examinations (Hawkins & Thibodeau, 1993). The ANA's credentialing arm, the American Nurses Credentialing Center (ANCC), NAPNAP, and the AANP, along with NCC, offer certification examinations for nine specialties today.

The decline of the CNS role along with increasing third-party direct reimbursement for NPs, prescriptive privilege, and the financial crisis in health care have all led to astronomical NP growth. Nonetheless, it took well into the 1990s for nursing academic leadership to accept that the NP was here to stay and was becoming an increasingly mainstream part of health care.

In the early 1990s, the National Council of State Boards of Nursing (NCSBN) became concerned that states were using the national certifying examinations as entry into practice examinations. It threatened to write its own certifying examination unless certifying bodies proved that their examinations were "psychometrically sound and legally defensible" (J. B. Collins, personal communication, February 11, 2002). In August 1995, the Delegate Forum of the NCSBN gave the national certifying groups 1 year to establish the credibility of their examinations (Hamric et al., 1996). All four certifying bodies—ANCC, NAPNAP, AANP, and NCC—worked to develop the evidence of their similarities and differences and hired respected external groups to examine their examinations to determine whether they were indeed "pychometrically sound and legally defensible." At this point, NCSBN gave its blessing to the examinations.

In part as an outgrowth of the unifying certification efforts was the birth of the NP task force to look at criteria for quality NP programs. The work in 1995 by NONPF and the NLN was the beginning of the development of a model curriculum for NP education that would be used nationally to form the basis for certification eligibility (Hamric et al., 1996). At that time, the NLN was the only accrediting body for nursing graduate programs, and program standards, curriculum guides, and domains and competencies for NP education from NONPF were often used by the NLN in the accreditation process. In 1998, the Commission on Collegiate Nursing Education, an accreditation arm of AACN, was formed to provide an alternative to the NLN as a source of accreditation to schools offering baccalaureate and higher degrees in nursing. The thrust of the 2001 meeting of the NP task force when it reconvened was for both accrediting bodies to move toward the approval of NONPF guidelines and standards as the reigning accepted standards for accreditation of programs preparing NPs (Edwards, 2003).

As of 2008, a total of 137,178 NPs were reported by states (Pearson, 2008). By 2005, the growth of NP numbers is predicted to equal that of family physicians (Cooper, 2001). In 26 states, NPs have title protection. Pearson (2008) says, "The board of nursing has sole authority in scope of practice and no statutory or regulatory requirements for physician collaboration, directions, or supervision" exist (p. 10). Fourteen states offer the NP sole authority in practice scope with a physician collaboration requirement, and six states offer sole authority with physician supervision. Five states provide NP title protection authorized by joint boards of nursing and medicine. All states offer some type of NP prescriptive authority. Thirteen states authorize NP prescriptive authority without physician involvement, including the authority to prescribe controlled substances. Thirty-three states allow prescriptive authority, including the authority to prescribe controlled substances with some degree of physician involvement. Five states allow prescriptive authority that does not include the authority to prescribe controlled substances (Pearson, 2003).

The gains in legal authority, prescriptive privilege, and reimbursement mechanisms across the 50 states and the District of Columbia show that currently NPs have achieved a degree of autonomy in practice and associated prestige (Pearson, 2008). More victories than failures provide evidence of success, but, as in the late 1970s, today's NP is still battling for autonomy and consumer recognition in practice, especially in states with many physicians. Hayes (1985) stated, "No role in nursing, or for that matter, in any field has been so debated in the literature, and possibly no other nursing function has ever been so obsessed about by those performing it as has been the NP role" (p. 145). Yet, as Hayes asserts, there has been an avalanche of support from satisfied consumers of NPs. As any of us who practice in this role can attest, that is still just as true today.

THE CONTINUATION OF "DISRUPTIVE INNOVATION": THE DOCTOR OF NURSING PRACTICE

However, the future contains clouds on the horizon as well as sunshine. Fairman (1999) cautions that although local negotiations between individual physicians and nurses may have been, in some cases, easily traversed in the interest of the good of the patient, on the professional level hierarchical relationships and power are at stake. Within this highly competitive health-care environment, all groups face hurdles, challenges, and assaults.

In June 2008, the AACN sent a memorandum of concern to the AMA regarding Resolutions 303 and 214 drafted by AMA Reference Committees, set to come before the full AMA House. Specifically Resolution 303 is aimed at the protection of the titles "Doctor," "Resident," and "Residency;" and Resolution 214 calls for a policy that nurses prepared in DNP programs must only be able to practice under the supervision of a physician. AACN's memo, authored by AACN President C. Fay Raines, points out that, "Nursing and medicine are distinct practice disciplines that prepare clinicians to assume different roles and meet different practice expectations." The memo goes on to emphasize that advanced nursing practice is regulated by each respective state nurse practice act, not by physician authority. AMA never took action on these resolutions.

In October 2004, the members of the AACN endorsed the *Position Statement on the Practice Doctorate in Nursing,* which called for the movement of educational preparation for advanced practice nursing roles from the master's degree to the doctoral level by the year 2015. This "new" doctorate would be a "practice" doctorate in contrast to the doctor of philosophy (PhD)—the traditional research degree—and is not intended to "replace" the PhD. There are many reasons for this development. Some master's programs for APNs had become very lengthy, without any change in the credential awarded at the completion of studies. The numbers of credits, in many cases, approaches what is required for a doctoral degree. And many educators believe this is necessary to assure clinical competency. Futhermore, other practice disciplines such as pharmacy, physiotherapy, and occupational therapy have moved on to doctoral-level preparation. The debate continues: Since nursing is a practice discipline, is it not appropriate to require a "practice doctorate" for advanced nursing practice?

The case can also be made that APNs across the country have been expanding their skills, both formally and informally. One example is the role of "intensivist" in the hospital, which is being assumed by many NPs and CNSs (Mundinger, 2005). This is consistent with nursing's lengthy history of moving where the need in health care surfaces. The aging of the population, the increased acuity and complexity of care, the continuation of a dwindling number of primary care physicians, and the decreased hours for residents in the hospital due to legislative and accreditation criteria have fostered the need for these nurses to move well beyond the primary care arena. For example, when Columbia University School of Nursing was asked by Presbyterian Hospital to establish two new ambulatory care clinics to meet the growing demand for primary care among the underserved immigrant populations, the faculty accepted. They also proposed conducting a randomized trial comparing independent NPs and primary care physicians. To reduce the variability among roles a nd strengthen the study, the faculty requested that the hospital's medical board grant the faculty NPs admitting privileges. Mundinger (2005) describes this evolution at Columbia, "Several physician(s) . . . provided additional training for our faculty nurse practitioners in dermatology, radiology, and cardiology and helped mentor them through the process of admitting, and co-managing patients and conducting emergency room evaluation" (p. 175).

The results of the randomized trials, with excellent patient care outcomes achieved by NPs, on a par with primary care physicians, was published in the *Journal of the American Medical Association* (Mundinger et al., 2000). This contributed to a change in hospital bylaws, granting faculty NPs hospital admitting privileges. Mundinger sees the level of service delivered by these faculty NPs as beyond that achieved by colleagues with the traditional master's degree preparation for practice. Based on these observations, comes the call for a formal and standardized curriculum leading to a doctoral degree consistent with the practice needs for advanced competencies and increased knowledge. She states, "We know that thousands of nurses aspire to this level of education and schools are responding by developing the new degree. We know that the research degree is asynchronous with these goals, and we know from every other profession that when you reach the competency associated with doctoral achievement, one should receive a doctorate not another MS degree" (p. 175). See Chapter 4 for more discussion on this issue.

We will need our renegades, rebels, and trailblazers more than ever.

CONCLUSION

The boundaries of practice are always malleable. They are always subject to myriad external forces—political, economic, social, and cultural—and are interpreted in different ways by different practitioners. APNs are a mixed breed; each trajectory under the umbrella of advanced nursing practice has evolved differently and under variable circumstances. This leads to vigor, strength, and diversity. The struggles documented within this chapter have aimed to strengthen each variant of the nursing advanced practice role. The struggles are not over; in many ways they are just beginning. It is our hope that nursing will continue to produce rebels, renegades, and trailblazers, motivated by concern for patients, concern for community, concern for humanity. We have no doubt that we will continue to take on new and challenging roles, using creative and diverse strategies.

References

American Association of Colleges of Nursing. (1995). *Essentials of masters education.* Washington, DC: American Association of Colleges of Nursing.

American Nurses Association. (1965). *Educational preparation for nurse practitioners and assistants to nurses: A position paper.* New York: American Nurses Association.

American Nurses Association. (1980). *Nursing: A social policy statement.* Kansas City, MO: American Nurses Association.

American Nurses Association. (1993). Nursing facts from the American Nurses Association. In *Primary health care: The nurses' solution.* New York: American Nurses Association.

American Nurses Association Congress for Nursing Practice. (1976). *Definition: Nurse Practitioner, Nurse Clinician, and Clinical Nurse Specialist.* Kansas City, Mo: Author.

Baer, E. (1982). The conflictive social ideology of American Nursing, 1893: A microcosm. Unpublished dissertation, New York University, School of Education.

Bankert, M. (1989). *Watchful care: A history of America's nurse anesthetists.* New York: Continuum.

Barton, C. (1987). The story of my childhood. In E. Pryor (Ed.),. *Clara Barton: Professional angel* (p. 92). Philadelphia: University of Pennsylvania.

Bigbee, J. L., & Amidi-Nouri, A. (2000). History and evolution of advanced nursing practice. In A.B. Hamric, J. A. Spross, & C. M. Hanson (Eds.), *Advanced nursing practice: An integrative approach* (2nd ed., pp. 4–32). Philadelphia: WB Saunders.

Brower, T. F., & Baker, B. J. (1976). Using the adaptation model in a practitioner curriculum. *Nursing Outlook, 24*(11), 686–689.

Brush, B., & Capezuti, E. A. (1996). Revisiting "A Nurse for All Settings": The nurse practitioner movement, 1965–1995. *Journal of the American Academy of Nurse Practitioners, 8*(1), 5–11.

Busen, N., & Engleman, S. (1996). The CNS practitioner preparation: An emerging role in advanced practice nursing. *Clinical Nurse Specialist: The Journal of Advanced Nursing, 10*(3), 145–150.

Callaway, B. J. (2002). *Hildegard Peplau: Psychiatric nurse of the century.* New York: Springer Publishing Company.

Christman, L. (1998). Advanced practice nursing: Is the physician's assistant an accident of history or a failure to act? *Nursing Outlook, 46*(2), 56–59.

Clinician's Review. (2002, February). Editorial, p. 1.

Cooper, R. A. (2001). Health care workforce for the twenty-first century: The impact of nonphysician clinicians. *Annual Review of Medicine, 52,* 51–61.

Coss, C. (Ed). (1989). *Lillian D. Wald: Progressive activist.* New York: The Feminist Press.

Crile, G. W. (Ed.) (1947). *George Crile, an Autobiography.* Philadelphia: Lippincott.

Daniels, D. G. (1989). *Always a sister: The feminism of Lillian D. Wald.* New York: The Feminist Press.

DeWitt, K. (1900). Specialties in nursing. *American Journal of Nursing, 1*(1), 14–17.

Dock, L. L. (1901). In I. A. Robb, L. L. Dock, & M. Banfield (Eds.), *The Transactions of the Third International Congress of Nurses with the Reports of the International Council of Nurses* (p. 15). Cleveland, Ohio.

Dracup, K. (1998). The invisible profession. *American Journal of Critical Care, 7*(4), 250–252.

Dunn, B. H. (1986). Legal regulation of advanced nursing practice. *NAACOG Update Series, 4*(8), 1–7.

Dye, N. S. (1984). Mary Breckenridge, the frontier nursing service, and the introduction of nurse-midwifery in the United States. In J. Leavitt & R. L. Numbers (Eds.), *Women and Health* (pp. 336–337). Madison: University of Wisconsin.

Edgar. C. J. (1911). The remedy for the midwife problem. *American Journal of Obstetrics and Gynecology, 63,* 882.

Edwards, J., Oppewal, S., & Logan, C. (2003). Nurse-managed primary care: Outcomes of a faculty practice network. *Journal of American Academy of Nurse Practitioners, 15*(12), 563–569.

Ehrenreich, B. (2000). Introduction: Emergence of nursing as a political force. In D. Mason, J. Leavitt, & M. Chafee (Eds.), *Policy and politics in nursing and health care* (4th ed., pp. xxxiii–xxxvii). Philadelphia: Saunders.

Ehrenreich, B., & English, D. (1973). *Witches, midwives, and nurses: A history of women healers.* New York: The Feminist Press.

Ehrenreich, B., & English, D. (1978). *For her own good—150 years of expert advice to women.* New York: Anchor Books.

Fairman, J. (1999). Delegated by default or negotiated by need? Physicians, nurse practitioners, and the process of clinical thinking. *Medical Humanities Review, 13*(1), 38–58.

Fairman, J. (2002). The roots of collaborative practice: Nurse practitioner pioneers' stories. *Nursing History Review, 10,* 159–174.

Family Nurse Practitioner Proposed by APHA Speaker. (1964). *The American Journal of Nursing, 64*(12), 18–21.

Ford, L. C. (1991). Advanced nursing practice: Future of the nurse practitioner. In L. H. Aikein & C. M. Fagin, (Eds.), *Charting nursing's future: Agenda for the 1990s* (pp. 287–299). New York: JB Lippincott.

Ford, L. C., & Silver, H. K. (1967). The expanded role of the nurse in child care. *Nursing Outlook, 15,* 43–45.

Fulton, J. (2002). Defining our practice. *Clinical Nurse Specialist: The Journal for Advanced Nursing, 16*(4), 1–3.

Garde, J. (1988). Preface. In W. Waugaman, S. Foster, & B. Rigor (Eds.), *Principles and Practices of Nurse Anesthesia* (p. xii). Norwalk, CT: Appleton & Lange.

Geolot, D. (1987). Nurse practitioner education: Observations from a national perspective. *Nursing Outlook, 35,* 132–135.

Hahn, M. S. (1995). The nurse practitioner story: 30th anniversary. *Advance for Nurse Practitioners, 3*(7), 22–27.

Hamric, A. B., Spross, J. A., & Hanson, C. M. (1996). *Advanced nursing practice: An integrative approach.* Philadelphia: WB Saunders.

Hamschmeyer, H. (1939). A training school for nurse-midwives established. *American Journal of Nursing, 32,* 374.

Hawkins, J. W., & Thibodeau, J. A. (1993). *The advanced practitioner: Current practice issues* (3rd ed.). New York: Tiresias.

Hayes, E. (1985). The nurse practitioner: History, current conflicts, and future survival. *Journal of Community Health, 34,* 144–147.

Hobbie, C. (1998). NAPNAP: The first 25 years. *Journal of Pediatric Health Care, 12*(6 supp), S3–S8.

Holt, N. (1998). Confusion's masterpiece: The development of the physician assistant profession. *Bulletin of the History of Medicine, 72,* 246–278.

Jacox, A. K. (2002). Dr. Loretta Ford's observations on nursing's past and future. *Nursing and Health Policy Review, 1*(2), 153–164.

Joel, L. A. (2003). *Dimensions of professional nursing* (9th ed.). New York: McGraw-Hill.

Kalisch, P. A., & Kalisch, B. J. (1986). *The advance of American nursing* (2nd ed.). Boston: Little, Brown.

Kobrin, F. E. (1984). The American midwife controversy: A crisis of professionalization. In J. Leavitt & R. L. Numbers (Eds.), *Women and health* (pp. 318–326). Madison: University of Wisconsin.

Komnenich, P. (1998). The evolution of advanced practice in nursing. In C. M. Sheehy & M. McCarthy (Eds.), *Advanced practice nursing: Emphasizing common roles* (pp. 9–41). Philadelphia: FA Davis.

Leininger, M., Little, D. E., & Carnevali, D. (1972). Primex. *American Journal of Nursing, 72*(7), 1274–1277.

Lincoln, P. (2000). Comparing CNS and NP role activities: A replication. *Clinical Nurse Specialist: The Journal of Advanced Nursing, 14*(6), 1–4.

Magaw, A. (1906). A review of over fourteen thousand surgical anesthesias. *Bulletin of the American Association of Nurse Anesthetists 7,* 62.

Magaw, A. (1899). Observations in Anesthesia. *Northwestern Lancet 19,* 207.

Marchione, J., & Garland, T. N. (1997). An emerging profession? The case of the nurse practitioner. *Image: The Journal of Nursing Scholarship, 29*(4), 335–337.

Menard, S. (1987). The CNS: Historical Perspectives. In S. Menard (Ed.). *The clinical nurse specialist/perspectives on practice* (pp. 2–3). New York: John Wiley & Sons.

Mirr, M. P., & Snyder, M. (1995). Evolution of the advanced practice nursing role. In M. P. Mirr & M. Snyder (Eds.), *Advanced Practice Nursing* (pp. 13–21). New York: Springer.

Moxley, J. H., 3rd. (1968). The predicament in health manpower. *American Journal of Nursing, 68*(7), 1486–1490.

Mundinger, M. O. (2005) Who's who in nursing: Bringing clarity to the doctor of nursing practice. *Nursing Outlook,* 53(4), 173–176.

Mundinger, M. O., Kane, R. I., Lenz, E. R., Totten, A. M, Tsai, W., Cleary, P. D. (2000). Primary care outcomes in patients treated by nurse practitioners or physicians: A randomized trial. *JAMA,* 283(1), 59–68.

Murphy, J. F. (1970). Role expansion or role extension. *Nursing Forum, 10*(4), 380–389.

O'Brien, P. (1987). "All a woman's life can bring": The domestic roots of nursing in Philadelphia, 1830–1885. *Nursing Research, 36*(1), 12–17.

Peabody, F. W. (1930). *Doctor and patient.* New York: Macmillan.

Pearson, L. (2008). The Pearson report. *American Journal of Nurse Practitioners, 12*(2), 9–80.

Pryor, E. B. (1987). *Clara Barton: Professional angel.* Philadelphia: University of Pennsylvania.

Pulcini, J., & Wagner, M. (2001). Perspectives on education and practice issues for nurse practitioners and advanced practice nursing. In *Nurse Practitioner/Advanced Practice Nursing Roles in the United States.* Education/Practice Subgroup of the International Nurse Practitioner/Advanced Practice Nursing Network. Geneva: ICN.

Rakel, R. (1995). The family physician. In R. E. Rakel (Ed.), *Textbook of Family Practice* (5th ed., pp. 3–19). Philadelphia: WB Saunders.

Reiter, F. (1966). The nurse clinician. *American Journal of Nursing, 66*(2), 274–279.

Rogers, M. (1975). Nursing is coming of age . . . through the practitioner movement. *American Journal of Nursing, 75*(10), 1834–1843.

Rothstein, W. G. (1958). *American Physicians in the Nineteenth Century: From Sect to Science.* Baltimore: Johns Hopkins Press.

Roy, C., & Obloy, M. (1978). The practitioner movement—toward a science of nursing. *American Journal of Nursing, 78*(10), 1698–1702.

Sills, G. (1983). The role and function of the clinical nurse specialist. In N. L. Chaska (Ed.), *The nursing profession: A time to speak up.* New York: McGraw-Hill.

Silver, H. K., Ford, L. C., & Stearly, S. G. (1967). A program to increase health care for children: The pediatric nurse practitioner program. *Pediatrics, 39*(5), 756–768.

Sparacino, P. S. A. (1986). The clinical nurse specialist. *Nursing Practice 1*(4), 215–228.

Sparacino, P. S. A. (1990). A historical perspective on the development of the clinical nurse specialist role. In P. S. A. Sparacino, D. M. Cooper, & P. A. Manarik (Eds.), *The clinical nurse specialist: Implementation and impact* (pp. 3–9). Norwalk, CT: Appleton & Lange.

Stone, S. (1990). A complete practice of midwifery. In L. T. Ulrich (Ed.), *A midwife's tale: The life of Martha Ballard* (pp. 12–40). New York: Alfred Knopf.

Sultz, H. A., Henry, O., Kinyon, J., Buck, G., & Bullough, B. (1983). Nurse practitioners: A decade of change. *Nursing Outlook, 31,* 137–141.

Thatcher, V. S. (1953). *History of anesthesia with emphasis on the nurse specialist.* Philadelphia, Lippincott.

Towers, J. (1995). Celebrating our 30th anniversary as nurse practitioners and our 10th anniversary as an academy. *Journal of the American Academy of Nurse Practitioners, 7*(6), 267–270.

Ulrich, L. T. (1990). *A midwife's tale: The life of Martha Ballard, based on her diary, 1785–1812.* New York: Alfred A. Knopf.

U.S. Department of Labor. (1920). Children's Bureau Publication No. 61. Washington, DC: U.S. Government Printing Office.

Emerging Roles of the Advanced Practice Nurse

Anne Keane

Deborah Becker

2

EMERGING ROLES OF THE ADVANCED PRACTICE NURSE

Roles of the advanced practice nurse (APN) have emerged and grown substantially over the last century. This growth has been a result of changing patient needs and expectations, pressures related to reimbursement and managed care, a shift in the delivery of care from hospital to community settings, a growth of patient advocacy, and changing attitudes about the role of the nurse. These events have fostered opportunities for the development of new advanced practice nursing roles. At the same time, the preparation of APNs has moved largely into academic settings, with an emphasis on critical thinking, including clinical reasoning, systems evaluation, changing patterns of practice, and an identification of competencies in the core and relevant areas of specialization.

Because advanced practice nursing requires the implementation of health roles within social settings, these roles will inevitably remain dynamic and evolving as they respond to changing patient needs, health-care advances, and regulatory and social pressures. Already at the beginning of the 21st century, several factors have influenced the emergence and acceptability of advanced practice roles. These factors include the growing numbers of elderly patients, the increased complexity and severity of illness in hospitalized patients, renewed pressures to reduce medical residents' clinical hours, and a major nursing shortage. These factors and others will undoubtedly continue to influence the emergence of the APN role in the coming decades.

The range of current advanced practice roles and the numbers of nurses in these roles demonstrate the success of APNs. Studies evaluating clinical outcomes of care delivered by APNs are overwhelmingly positive (e.g., Brooten & Naylor, 1995; Safriet, 1992), as are surveys of patient satisfaction with the delivery of care by APNs. But advanced practice nursing does not represent a unified force in our society. Currently there are four major groups of APNs in the United States: certified registered nurse anesthetists (CRNAs), certified nurse-midwives (CNMs), clinical nurse specialists (CNSs), and nurse practitioners (NPs). These groups reflect different practice traditions and educational histories. These APNs address the problems of different patient care groups in varied health-care settings, have differing histories of success with reimbursement from third-party payers, and have uneven legislative recognition of their status at the state level.

As specialty organizations representing the four areas of advanced practice have matured in outlook and influence, standards of clinical practice and scope of practice statements for these four advanced practice roles have emerged. These standards guide individual APNs as they develop their professional practice. They direct or set the current boundaries of practice, assist in role delineation, and help to identify areas of concern for these practitioners.

By accepting the responsibilities of the advanced practice role, APNs have understood the need to expand legislative recognition of their professional status, including their ability to achieve prescriptive privileges and receive reimbursement for care delivered. Recognition of APNs in the United States varies across the country, with most states providing some level of legal authority for scope of practice or prescriptive authority. However, CNSs are not officially tracked in some states though they may be acknowledged as advanced practice registered nurses (APRNs). **Table 2-1** identifies the numbers of APN by category.

SCOPE OF PRACTICE

Professional nursing organizations and state bodies have understood the need to describe and interpret the responsibilities of advanced practitioners in their area of specialization. Underlying the recognition of this need is the requirement to provide safe patient care, identify the essential characteristics of advanced practice, and interpret for the practitioner the components of care and competent levels of behavior (American Association of Colleges of Nursing [AACN]/American Nurses Association [ANA], 1995). The scope of practice may be described by the functions performed by the APN and the minimal competencies needed to perform those functions. These descriptions and guidelines direct APNs in the implementation and conceptualization of their roles and responsibilities.

In addition, each state has a legislative/regulatory stance on issues affecting advanced practice within its jurisdiction (Pearson, 2002). The legal scope of practice, including prerogatives for diagnosing, prescriptive authority, and reimbursement, is described within these regulations. Scope and standards of practice are defined by the professional organization and enacted into law at the state level. The actual role is further defined through credentialing of practice responsibilities at the institutional or employment level. Hospitals and other health-care organizations typically define role responsibilities and prerogatives through a review by other practitioners, and this is generally expressed through a contract identifying responsibilities, prerogatives, and limitations of the role. This review results in the granting of institutional or practice-based practice privileges for the APN.

Although scope of practice guidelines are important philosophically, and may even have the weight of law, they do not imply that the roles of APNs are unchanging. When knowledge evolves and different care delivery models become viable, roles also evolve. More commonly, roles change as

TABLE 2-1

Numbers of Advanced Practice Nurses

Clinical nurse specialists[a]	69,000 prepared with proper credentials; approximately 14,000 practicing
Certified registered nurse anesthetists[b]	40,000
Certified nurse-midwives[c]	9,000 CNM; 2,320 CM
Nurse practitioners[d]	137,178

CM, certified midwives; CNM, certified nurse-midwives.
[a]National Association of Clinical Nurse Specialists, personal communication, 2008.
[b]American Association of Nurse Anesthetists, personal communication, 2008.
[c]American College of Nurse-Midwives, personal communication, 2008.
[d]Pearson, L. J. (2008). 2008 Pearson Report Summary. *The American Journal for Nurse Practitioners, 12*(2), 16–17.

different practice settings become available and opportunities for improved patient access to care appear. The nature of advanced practice is broader than individual roles or functions. **Table 2-2** lists scope and standard of practice documents for major APN roles.

Regulation of the Advanced Practice Registered Nurse

Regulation of APRNs occurs at the state level, but there are both educational and certification prerequisites. The graduate level educational preparation of APNs is guided by educators and members of professional organizations who identify essential curricular goals, content, and competencies expected of APN graduates. This includes content and competencies core to all APNs and those specific to a particular specialty role. **Table 2-3** lists major APN organizations and the essential content and competency documents. Once completing an accredited master's-level program, graduates must generally pass a national certification examination in the area of intended practice, before applying for license at the state level.

APNs may be recognized and licensed at the state level in one the four APN roles, or in some states as an APRN, which covers several or all of these roles. In an effort to develop more consistent

---

TABLE 2-2

Scope and Standards of Practice Guidelines

American Academy of Nurse Practitioners	*Standards of practice for nurse practitioners.* Austin, TX: Author, 2007.
American Association of Critical Care Nurses	*Scope and standards of practice for the acute care nurse practitioner.* Aliso Viejo, CA: Author, 2006.
American Association of Critical Care Nurses	*Scope and standards of professional performance for the acute and critical-care nurse.* Aliso Viejo, CA: Author, 2002.
American College of Nurse-Midwives	*Core competencies for basic midwifery practice.* Retrieved May 10, 2008, from the American College of Nurse-Midwives Web site: www.midwife.org/display.cfm?id=137.
American Nurses Association	*Scope and standards of practice.* Washington, DC: Author, 2004.
American Association of Nurse Anesthetists	*Scope and standards for nurse anesthesia practice.* Park Ridge, IL: Author, 2007.
Association of Women's Health Obstetric and Neonatal Nurses and National Association of Nurse Practitioners Women's Health	*The women's health nurse practitioner: guidelines for practice and education* (5th ed.). Washington, DC: Author, 2002.
National Association of Clinical Nurse Specialists	*Statement on clinical nurse specialist practice.* Harrisburg, PA: Author, 2004.
National Organization of Nurse Practitioner Faculties	*Domains and competencies of nurse practitioner practice.* Washington, DC: Author, 2002.
National Panel for Acute Care Nurse Practitioner Competencies	*Acute care nurse practitioner competencies.* Washington, DC: National Organization of Nurse Practitioner Faculties, 2004.
National Panel for Psychiatric Mental Health Nurse Practitioner Competencies	*Psychiatric mental health nurse practitioner competencies.* Washington, DC: National Organization of Nurse Practitioner Faculties, 2003.

TABLE 2-3	
Professional Organizations and Essential Educational Content	
American Association of Colleges of Nursing	*The essentials of master's education for advanced prac tice nursing education.* Washington, DC: Author, 1996.
American Association of Colleges of Nursing	*The essentials of doctoral education for advanced nursing practice.* Washington, DC: Author, 2006.
American College of Nurse-Midwives	*Core competencies for basic midwifery practice.* Retrieved May 10, 2008, from the American College of Nurse-Midwives Web site: www.midwife.org/display.cfm?id=137.
American Association of Women's Health, Obstetric and Neonatal Nurses and National Association of Nurse Practitioners Women's Health	*The women's health nurse practitioner: guidelines for practice and education* (5th ed.). Washington, DC: Author, 2002.
Council on Accreditation of Nurse Anesthesia Educational Programs	*Standards for accreditation for nurse anesthesia educa-tional programs.* Chicago: Author, 1994.
National Association of Clinical Nurse Specialists	*Statement on clinical nurse specialist practice and education* (2nd ed.). Harrisburg, PA: Author, 2004.
National Organization of Nurse Practitioner Faculties	*Domains and competencies of nurse practitioner practice.* Washington, DC: Author, 2000.
National Panel for Psychiatric-Mental Health Nurse Practitioner Competencies	*Psychiatric-mental health nurse practitioner compe-tencies.* Washington, DC: National Organization of Public Health Nurses, 2002.
National Task Force on Quality Nurse Practitioner Education	*Criteria for evaluation of nurse practitioner programs.* Washington, DC: National Organization of Public Health Nurses, 2002.

standards for APRN recognition across states, a draft report developed by the APRN Consensus Work Group and the National Council of State Boards of Nursing, has been circulated nationally (Consensus Model for APRN Regulation: Licensure, Accreditation, Certification & Education, Draft, 2008). The proposed regulatory model acknowledges the traditional four APN roles and argues that APRNs must be regulated in one of the four roles and in at least one of six population foci: psych/mental health, gender specific, adult gerontology, pediatrics, neonatal, and individual families across the life span. In addition, content for all APRNs must include graduate-level courses in advanced physiology/pathophysiology, health assessment, pharmacology, and appropriate clinical experience. **Table 2-4** summarizes the draft working definition of an APRN. The recommendations of this working group, as they gain consensus and acceptance, will likely influence the preparation of future APNs and the relicensing of current APNs. The goal of this working group is to provide a vision and some degree of uniformity in the preparation for APNs in the future.

Clinical Nurse Specialist

CNSs are nurses with a master's- or doctorate-level expertise in a defined area of knowledge and prac-tice. They typically work in unit-based or population-based hospital settings, in offices or clinic-based outpatient settings and in community settings. They have been in demand for their specialized clini-cal knowledge, expertise, and ability to care for complex patients since the 1960s. Their favorable impact on patient care outcomes has been well demonstrated on a broad range of measures including

---

TABLE 2-4

Proposed Advanced Practice Registered Nurse Essential Characteristics*

Completion of an accredited graduate-level program in one of the four areas: nurse midwifery, nurse anesthesia, nurse practitioner, or clinical nurse specialist

Successful completion of national certification examination measuring APRN role and population—focused competencies and maintains competence through recertification

Possession of advanced clinical knowledge and skills needed for direct patient care—a significant component of education and practice focuses on direct care of individuals

Practice builds on RN competencies and demonstrates depth and breadth of knowledge, data synthesis, complex skills, intervention, and role autonomy

Educational preparation for health promotion and maintenance, assessment, diagnosis, and management of patient problems including use and prescription of pharmacologic and nonpharmacologic interventions

Possesses depth and breadth of clinical experience reflecting intended license

Possesses license to practice as APRN as CRNA, CNM, CNS or CNP

APRN, advanced practice registered nurse; CNM, certified nurse-midwife; CNP, certified nurse practitioner; CNS, clinical nurse specialist; CRNA, certified registered nurse anesthetist; RN, registered nurse.

*Adapted from Consensus Model for APRN Regulation: Licensure, Accreditation, Certification and Education (2008). Draft APRN joint dialogue group report, completed through the work of the APRN consensus work group and the National Council of State Boards of Nursing APRN Advisory Committee. Retrieved November 11, 2008, from https://www.ncsbn.org/7_23_08_consensue_APRN_final.pdf.

---

improved education and ability to care for self (Lipman, 1986); expert care and improved patient outcomes post–myocardial infarction (Pozen et al., 1977); expert care and decreased symptom distress (McCorkle et al., 1989); and transitional care and early discharge of low birth weight infants (Brooten, Gennaro, Knapp, Brown, & York, 1989).

Recently however, job openings and opportunities for hospital-based CNSs have suffered as a result of hospital downsizing and the onset of managed care programs. Two important challenges have faced CNSs in recent years, those of role confusion and ambiguity and an inability to demonstrate CNS value in economic terms (Scott, 1999). Decisions to downsize or delete hospital-based CNS positions are the result of pressures to decrease health-care costs, especially hospital-based costs.

Even with evidence of their favorable impact, hospital-based CNSs have been particularly vulnerable to administrative attempts to decrease health-care costs. Multiple studies have demonstrated the favorable contributions of CNSs to patient care outcomes and patient satisfaction, but fewer studies have evaluated their economic impact and their ability to generate income and save costs. Cost-saving measures have been demonstrated, such as CNS impact on early discharge, product evaluation, and nursing practice changes (Scott, 1999). These savings are real, but they may not be returned to the CNSs' home (usually nursing) department. Because of this, the immediate supervisors of CNSs may not appreciate the benefits of expert CNS practice. This reality is compounded by the inability of CNSs to bill directly for services, if they are salaried employees. Hospital-based employees cannot bill third-party payers for services delivered such as consultations, teaching programs, pain management, or wound care activities. Skilled advanced practice nursing care is not directly reimbursed and remains bundled in the hospital's room, food, laundry, and supplies bill. It remains to investigate more creative and appropriate financial models that could remedy the situation. This limitation on role functioning is usually not faced by self-employed or practice-based CNSs, who likely are not institutional employees and generally work in outpatient or community settings.

The observation that CNS practice reflects role ambiguity undoubtedly grows out of the ability of the CNS to adapt to changing patient, family, and nursing staff needs, supported by a broad clinical repertoire of skills and knowledge. The CNS shifts functions dependent on the needs of the situation and participates in a mix of direct and indirect patient care activities. Still, the traditional roles of CNS practice remain, including those of expert practitioner, educator, consultant, manager, and researcher. The recent draft document of the Consensus Model for APRN regulation (2008) argues that graduate nursing roles that do not focus on direct patient care will not be considered APRNs in the future. If this position is embraced nationally, some CNSs may not be granted APRN status.

In an evaluation of CNS practice roles, Scott (1999) reported that CNSs nationwide were involved in clinical practice activities 29% to 91% of the time; in educational activities from 24% to 89% of the time; as consultants from 18% to 96% of the time; and in research activities from 15% to 93% of the time. Scott also reported that CNSs were commonly found in community-based practice (32% of the sample). Community practice included such settings as clinics, private practice, school systems, nursing homes, corporations, and prisons.

The advanced practice skills of the CNSs reported in the Scott (1999) study were grouped into three areas: psychosocial activities, psychomotor nursing skills, and advanced medical skills. The top 10 psychosocial role activities in this survey of 724 CNSs included: family therapy, grief therapy, psychotherapy, crisis intervention, marriage counseling, sex/sex abuse counseling, relaxation therapy, substance abuse therapy, depression therapy, and smoking cessation therapy. Psychomotor nursing skills commonly performed by CNSs included: wound, ostomy, and incontinence management; physical assessment; peripheral central line insertions; pain management; and therapeutic touch. Commonly used advanced medical skills used by CNSs in this survey were: pacemaker programming, management, and discontinuation; suturing and stapling; wound debridement; pelvic, rectal, and prostate examination; central line and chest tube insertion and discontinuation; invasive arterial and venous sheath removal; Swan-Ganz catheter management and discontinuation; and cardiac arrest management. Results of this survey demonstrated that CNSs were involved in a broad range of independent counseling activities in the community and in the provision of acute care therapies once provided solely by the physician and similar to, or overlapping with, those currently performed by the acute care nurse practitioner (ACNP; Scott, 1999).

At the time of this survey only community-based psychiatric and mental health CNSs and CNSs in rural areas were able to bill for their services. Since 1998 Medicare regulations have permitted all CNSs to bill for their services, but this opportunity does not exist for CNSs who are employed by an institution that receives third-party payment for services delivered by its employees. Another important concern was that only 6% of the nurses in this survey could identify ways in which they generated income. As Scott (1999) suggests, CNSs must have preparation in health-care economics if they are to have the requisite skills needed to flourish as independent advanced practice health-care providers **(Boxes 2-1** and **2-2).**

Ambiguity and the Clinical Nurse Specialist Role

There have been several responses to the problem of role ambiguity with in-hospital CNS roles. One has been the development of Scope of Practice and Standards of Professional Performance statements for the acute and critical care CNS (American Association of Critical Care Nurses, 2002). The document provides guidelines for competent and professional care for acutely and critically ill patients. It also reflects the three spheres of CNS influence: patient/family; nursing personnel and other health-care providers; and the organizational system for care delivery in different settings (Medina,

> **BOX 2-1**
> ## The Psychiatric Clinical Nurse Specialist Profile
>
> Jane is a psychiatric clinical nurse specialist (CNS) who is prepared at the master's level and for the past 25 years has worked in a private practice supporting clients with multiple psychological problems. Her clients include children over 10 years of age in the context of their families or support systems. She is certified as a marriage and family therapist, as an adolescent therapist, and in eye movement desensitization reprogramming (EMDR), a technique used in the treatment of clients with posttraumatic stress disorder (PTSD).
>
> Jane describes her practice as taking place in an exciting time with new information and research providing her with a broad repertoire of approaches and skills for her clients. She prefers to work as a solo practitioner without supervisory reporting requirements. She is able to set her own working schedule and see clients for as long as she judges appropriate. She bills directly and is not a member of managed care billing panels. She depends on referrals from physicians, other health-care workers, and school principals for her clients and does not advertise. Jane cannot prescribe medications in her state and relies on cooperation with physician colleagues if medications are necessary. Jane loves the work she is doing and plans to stay in the role as long as she can.

2000). Within this framework the CNS is expected to provide continuous and comprehensive care to improve outcomes for acutely and critically ill patients. This is done in a collaborative model that includes patients, families, significant others, nurses, and other providers and administrators (Medina, 2000).

A contribution of this document is that it sets goals and standards for CNS practice and contributes to further role clarification for hospital-based CNSs. The values identified in this document for continuous and comprehensive care for acutely and critically ill patients suggest that the scope of the critical care CNS's responsibilities are not limited to acute or special care units. Seriously ill patients are found in most hospital units, and their continuing specialized care needs are now frequently required in nonhospital or outpatient settings. It is likely that postdischarge role functions will become more common for the acute or critical care CNSs **(Box 2-3).**

Nurse Practitioner

The NP role originated in the 1960s when the inaccessibility of health care in certain regions of the country and for certain groups of people, coupled with the shortage of primary care physicians, was recognized (Sellards & Mills, 1995). As a result, continuing education programs to educate nurses to provide primary care to underserved populations began to open.

Even with the recognized need for this expanded nursing role, it was over 10 years before the American Nurses Association (ANA) formally defined this advanced practice role and established guidelines for continuing education programs that prepared adult and family nurse practitioners (Sellards & Mills, 1995). The educational preparation of NPs has moved from continuing education programs offering certification on completion to university-based graduate programs granting a master's degree in nursing. Today NPs are the largest group of APNs, and they are recognized and can prescribe medications in all 50 states and the District of Columbia (Pearson, 2008). These APNs assess and manage both medical and nursing problems and serve as both primary and specialty care providers.

BOX 2-2
Population-Based Clinical Nurse Specialist Profile

Alicia is a nurse who has master's level training and has been a clinical nurse specialist (CNS) for the past 12 years in a major teaching hospital. For the first 6 years she was a unit-based specialist providing direct care to seriously ill surgical patients and supervising and directing the care provided by unit-based staff nurses. For the past 6 years she has worked as a CNS in ostomy and wound care. In this capacity she serves as an educator and consultant for patients with ostomies (70%) and problems with wound healing (30%). These responsibilities require her to work directly with patients and their families and also with the nursing and medical staff. Alicia also has responsibility for ongoing in-service educational programs and for orientation for new surgical nurses. She reports to the nurse manager of a surgical nursing unit.

Alicia loves her position because she realizes that she is able to direct and coordinate the needs of these complex patients as she works with physicians, staff nurses, discharge planners, and health insurance representatives. Although her role is hospital based, the ongoing postdischarge needs of these patients require that she provide extended supervision and direction to patients struggling to assume responsibility for the complicated care of their ostomies or problem wounds. This follow-up care includes both phone and in-person evaluation, wound and ostomy product adjustments, education, and counseling.

In her role Alicia faces problems related to her inability to prescribe medications, supplies, and devices commonly required by her patients. Written prescriptions for medications, devices, and supplies are necessary, even if they are available over the counter, if patients are to receive insurance reimbursement. Because CNSs cannot prescribe in her state, Alicia directs residents, house staff, or nurse practitioners to write the necessary prescriptions. Similarly, Alicia cannot bill for the care she provides to her patients, even that provided postdischarge. She also admits to being uninformed about ways to identify the cost of her services. These problems result from lack of title recognition at the state level (CNSs are not recognized as advanced practice nurses [APNs] in her state and therefore cannot become eligible for prescriptive privileges), from the lack of credentialing at the institutional level, and from a need to reconceptualize her role responsibilities to include postdischarge care. Alicia's responsibilities cross inpatient and outpatient settings, but her reporting lines are limited to a specific inpatient setting.

Changing Roles for the Primary Care Nurse Practitioner

The original focus of the NP role was to meet the needs of underserved populations in rural areas of the United States. Because of this, practice areas for NPs were traditionally in community and outpatient settings. Responsibilities for this community-oriented NP included the delivery of primary care to the client, including comprehensive health assessment; follow-up care for presenting problems; health promotion activities; and a change from a disease-oriented focus to one including health promotion, health maintenance, treatment, and follow-up (Berger et al., 1996).

Initially, patient populations cared for by NPs were often uninsured immigrants or low-income individuals who were Medicaid recipients. However, since that time NPs have sought to meet the needs of larger groups of patients and have expanded their practice to include clients from suburban and urban outpatient settings and clinics. This move to highly populated, high-income areas where physicians are also readily available has been supported by the decision of health insurance plans to add NPs to their direct provider lists and to reimburse them on par with physicians (Grandinetti,

BOX 2-3
Critical Care Clinical Nurse Specialist Profile

Janet is a clinical nurse specialist (CNS) who is trained at the master's level and has been a critical care CNS for the past 7 years and before that a CNS for an additional 12 years. She is widely regarded as a clinical expert. Her responsibilities are unit-based on a surgical-trauma intensive care unit where she is responsible for the nursing care delivered to seriously ill surgical patients by 65 to 70 staff nurses. She has no direct patient care assignments but is responsible for assigning patient care to the staff nurses, taking into account the patients' level of acuity and the experience level of the staff. She conducts daily patient care rounds that she uses to assess patients' status and to develop staff teaching opportunities. She reports to, and is evaluated by, the unit-based nurse manager who has bachelor's-level training and who is responsible for the systems and organizational resources of the unit.

Janet's passion for excellent patient care and advocacy is well known. She appreciates the opportunities in her role for independence and self-direction and acknowledges that she thrives on these conditions. Her reputation allows her to direct staff and require standards of excellence in their work. Because she works in a staff versus line position, she must persuade, demonstrate, and negotiate in her efforts to improve patient care. Her relations with the nurse manager are excellent, and as Janet notes, they speak "with the same voice."

Janet struggles to be included in the leadership stream of information and communication. Because she is in a staff position, she does not attend meetings in which pertinent information is presented about planned new programs and the related training that she must develop for her staff. Also, Janet has no ability to prescribe or adjust medications, though she frequently suggests such modification to residents and attending physicians. Janet is extremely enthusiastic about the role of the critical care CNS. She has seen their departure over a 10-year period through downsizing, attrition, and elimination. She applauds the newly identified program in her hospital setting of hiring unit-based CNSs and firmly believes the CNS is here to stay.

1999). This move has supported the delivery of holistic primary care to larger groups of patients in community settings, but sometimes has resulted in competition as primary care NPs and physicians attempt to serve similar populations.

The development of the walk-in "retail clinic" has produced broad recognition of the NP role and led to their "discovery" by the public and has been described as "a significant move to reform U.S. health care by business and other groups outside the traditional medical industry" (Pearson, 2008, p. 10). Recognizing this development, the American Academy of Nurse Practitioners (AANP) has recently published Standards for Nurse Practitioner Practice in Retail-based Clinics (AANP, 2007).

Nurse Practitioners in the Community

Primary care NPs have established unique community-centered practice models. In an effort to develop an independent NP service model and to study the way health care is delivered to various populations in the United States, many schools of nursing have opened Academic Community Nursing Centers (Grandinetti, 1999; Zachariah & Lundeen, 1997). These centers are used as settings in which to study how health care is provided to vulnerable populations with limited access to care, who face a lack of coordination and inefficiencies in health-care delivery; to determine the specific needs of the community in which the center is located; and to provide a means of improving the quality of the care delivered (Zachariah & Lundeen, 1997).

In addition to academic community nursing centers, nurse-run clinics providing specialty care are emerging in both rural and urban areas. These centers specifically target groups of patients with certain diagnoses who are especially vulnerable to a multitude of complications if left untreated. Diabetes, heart failure, and wound care are just a few of the diagnoses that NPs have identified as being of great concern to patients in the communities in which they serve. By providing easier access to assessment, treatment, education, and support, NPs are identifying and treating potentially life-threatening conditions. The NPs working in these settings can provide early intervention, or if the condition is more advanced, can consult with their physician colleagues to determine if more intense treatment or hospitalization is required. Because these clinics are community based, they provide a convenient and easily accessible means for patients to have their health concerns addressed.

Nurse Practitioners in Transitional Care Settings

Hospital-based nurses have traditionally focused their interventions on preparing patients for discharge from the hospital. Because of the success and effectiveness that nurses have demonstrated in coordinating care, in anticipating postdischarge concerns or potential complications, and in developing a means to manage these issues, various roles for NPs in home health-care settings have emerged. The need for APNs who can provide transitional care from hospital to community is particularly evident.

Until recently, home health nurses identified problems and concerns regarding the health of their patients and have had to contact the patient's physician to determine the next course of action, a step that often caused a delay in treatment. The development of APN roles that bridge the acute care and community setting for complex, chronically ill patients or those requiring support in making the transition from the acute care setting to home has promoted favorable patient care outcomes and decreased hospital readmission rates. These APNs can recognize subtle changes in their patients' status and provide prompt care potentially averting a more serious result (Craven & Keene, 2000; Naylor, Bowles, & Brooten, 2000). APNs in home care settings engage in such activities as diagnosis and treatment of acute and chronic conditions, including consulting the physician when necessary; education of patients, families, and home care nurses; provision of cost-efficient and cost-effective care; and coordination of complex health-care services (Craven & Keene, 2000).

Although APNs in these roles have clearly demonstrated favorable patient-centered outcomes and have decreased costs, there is still a need to further develop reimbursement systems for the services of APNs. APNs have traditionally been employees of either hospitals or community-based care programs. If their roles in transitional care are to flourish, more sources of reimbursement are essential. Several viable models of APNs in transitional roles have been demonstrated through research efforts (Naylor et al., 2000; Brooten et al., 1989) and reimbursement from insurance companies, but more work is needed.

The NP as consultant in community health settings is another emerging APN role. Long-term care facilities, nursing homes, and rehabilitation centers are settings having few APNs or professional nurses. However, these settings often have residents with chronic health needs that go untreated or unnoticed until they become serious. In response, some administrators have developed roles for APNs to address health issues more quickly (Neal, 1999). These community-based APNs assess problems and develop plans of care in an attempt to prevent further progression of symptoms or needless suffering. Because the NP consultant role in the community is a new and emerging role, many states continue to require that these NPs work in collaboration with, or under the supervision of, a physician. This restriction may limit the ability of these APNs to function independently or may limit the range of services they can provide. Additionally, there are restrictions on the type of services for which NPs can bill directly. However, as changes in health-care reimbursement policies continue to occur, the consultant role in the community will grow more popular.

The Psychiatric Mental Health Nurse Practitioner

Since the 1950s the APN role of the psychiatric mental health nurse has been conceptualized as a CNS role. With recent developments in the science underpinning mental health and psychiatric illnesses, a shifting emphasis is evolving from a traditional psychosocial approach to care, to a biopsychosocial paradigm. In the latter paradigm, psychopharmacology has assumed a prominent place in the treatment inventory (Moller & Haber, 1997). Recently, national certification examinations for the adult psychiatric and mental health NP and the family and psychiatric mental health NP have been developed (American Nurses Credentialing Center [ANCC], 2008a, 2008b).

Acute Care Nurse Practitioner

NPs are found not only in primary care but also in specialized settings such as neonatal, pediatric, geriatric, women's health, and acute and critical care settings. The ACNP role is an emerging role in both pediatric and adult settings. In the late 1980s and early 1990s, many changes in the health-care delivery system in the United States created gaps in the delivery of health care to acutely ill patients. Changes in reimbursement, hospital restructuring, and a reduction in the number of medical residency programs produced clinical care delivery problems in the acute care setting. But these problems also produced an environment more open to the creation of new APN roles that could address gaps in the delivery of care to acutely ill patients (Kleinpell, 1997; Richmond & Keane, 1996). The establishment of NP roles in acute care settings, unlike that of the CNS, occurred initially in response to an identified patient-centered market need (Sechrist & Berlin, 1998). More recently the ACNP role has expanded to fulfill the diverse needs of acutely or critically ill or injured patients across the continuum of acute care services and for all age populations (Becker & Richmond, 2003).

The term *acute* has always been associated with the type of facility in which patient care is provided, but it is also used to describe the patient who is experiencing either a new onset or exacerbation of an existing illness (Miller, 1998). NPs in acute care settings conduct comprehensive health assessments; possess expert skills in the diagnosis and treatment of complex responses of individuals, families, and communities to actual or potential health problems; and demonstrate a high level of autonomy (Marchione & Garland, 1997).

These specialized or acute care NP roles have been evaluated for their effectiveness and acceptability. For example, several studies have examined the quality of outcomes of care delivered by neonatal NPs compared to that delivered by medical house staff. Results demonstrated that care delivered by NPs was as good as, or better than, that delivered by house staff, on measures of cost effectiveness and quality. In addition, care delivered by neonatal NPs had greater continuity and consistency (Bissinger, Allred, Arford, & Bellig, 1997; Mitchell-DiCenso et al., 1996). Other studies have demonstrated similarly favorable outcomes of NP practice in pediatric, rehabilitative, and inpatient trauma care settings (Silver, Murphy, & Gitterman, 1984; Spisso, O'Callaghan, McKinnon, & Holcroft, 1990; Weinberg, Liljestrand, & Moore, 1983).

These acute and specialized NP roles have flourished in acute care settings. Still, they are facing several systems issues that must still be addressed. For example, many of these NPs do not report to a nursing administrator, nor are they funded through the organization's nursing service department. Because many of these positions were created to fill a medical house staff shortage, funding for these positions comes from the medical and not the nursing department's budget. Accountability is tightly aligned with funding and as a result, professional identification can be more aligned with medicine than with nursing. The place of these APNs within the nursing organization can be unclear, unlike that of the hospital-based CNS who reports through the nursing hierarchy.

Another issue faced by acute and specialized NPs is that of reimbursement for services delivered. If employed by a medical practice group, these acute and specialized NPs can bill directly for their services. However, reimbursement is not equal to that received by physicians in the practice. This limitation requires NPs to bill under the name of their collaborating physician (**Box 2-4**).

The Acute Care Nurse Practitioner in Pediatric Settings

NPs have practiced in neonatal intensive care units (ICUs) since the early 1970s. Until recently though, the role of the pediatric NP had not reached into other acute areas of pediatric care. This was related to the strong role of the CNS in pediatric settings. Clinical nurse specialists have long practiced in all pediatric acute care settings in roles such as case management; developing clinical pathways; participating in research; providing consultation; educating care providers, patients, and families; and collaborating with various members of the health-care team in an attempt to provide cost-efficient and quality patient care (Teicher, Crawford, Williams, Nelson & Andrews, 2001).

In pediatric settings the role of the ACNP has evolved into one that assists with managing patients who are acutely ill or who have exacerbations of chronic health problems (Teicher et al., 2001). This new role in pediatric care can be understood as one that blends the roles of the CNS and the NP in an attempt to provide comprehensive services and direct patient care to pediatric patients and their families. As regulating bodies grow in their influence over APN practice, APNs working in blended roles will face the need to seek national certification and state licensing as both CNSs and NPs. The

---

BOX 2-4
Acute Care Nurse Practitioner Profile

Cathy is an advanced practice nurse (APN) who has master's level training and has worked as an interventional cardiology nurse practitioner (NP) for the past 3 years. She is responsible for managing the care of patients on the NP service from admission through discharge. This patient group includes those needing percutaneous transluminal coronary angioplasty (PCTA) and stenting interventions for blocked coronary arteries, aortic and mitral valvuloplasty, and atrial-septal defect closures. Daily responsibilities include patient rounds, admission histories and physicals, ordering of necessary studies such as blood tests, chest x-rays, electrocardiograms, and echocardiograms. She reports to a collaborating physician on a regular basis and for any emergency situation.

Cathy has seen the NP service grow as the hospital has faced a shortage of medical house staff. She has been granted institutional-level practice privileges that permit her to admit and discharge patients, modify and order protocol medications, and tests. Although she is potentially able to bill for services, her practice group would only recover 85% if the services delivered were billed under the NP's name.

Cathy is enthusiastic about her current responsibilities. She is able to try out new functions, make decisions that she is prepared for, and realizes that her care makes a difference to patient outcomes. Patient lengths of stay and time to discharge have been favorably improved on the NP service. While expected to cover an 8-hour shift, she commonly covers a 12-hour period. She communicates well with the nursing staff who value her expertise and the stability that her role provides.

many responsibilities of the APN in pediatrics include such activities as performing health histories and physical examinations; evaluating clinical data; prescribing treatments; performing invasive procedures, such as tracheal intubation and insertion of arterial lines; educating and supporting patients and families; facilitating patient discharge; participating in interdisciplinary rounds; and providing consultative services regarding such issues as wound care and infant feeding problems (Delametter, 1999; Pelosi, 2000; Rossetto & Fair, 1998; Teicher et al., 2001).

The pediatric NP can be found on specific patient care units such as the medical-surgical floor or the ICU, or the NP can be member of a specialty service such as cardiology, pulmonary, oncology, transplantation, gastrointestinal, and general surgery (Delametter, 1999; Pelosi, 2000; Teicher et al., 2001).

Pediatric ACNPs may also work outside the hospital setting in other areas in which acutely ill pediatric patients are found. Such areas include HIV clinics, centers for the management of mechanically ventilated patients, and transport services (Delametter, 1999; Dwyer, 2000; King, Foster, Woodward, & McCans, 2001; Teicher et al., 2001). The role that each NP assumes depends largely on the specific agenda of the agency employing the NP (Delametter, 1999). The focus of the role, no matter the geographical location in which the pediatric ACNP works, is to provide cost-effective and quality patient care.

Adult Acute Care Nurse Practitioners

Like their pediatric counterparts, the roles of adult ACNPs are also evolving and expanding in the acute care setting. Settings in which ACNPs deliver care include emergency rooms; ICUs; step-down or progressive care units; or medical-surgical floors. ACNPs also deliver care to patients outside the tertiary care institutions in settings such as outpatient surgical centers; centers for the management of mechanically ventilated patients; psychiatric evaluation centers; dialysis units; heart failure centers; and correctional facilities.

Kleinpell (1998, 1999) conducted surveys of ACNPs and found that respondents continued to develop new roles to fulfill identified needs for APNs to manage aspects of patient care in a variety of settings. NPs were found to be practicing in specialty care areas such as the cardiac catheterization laboratory; specialized neurology settings; the medical-surgical wards; specialty ear-nose-throat (ENT) services; plastic surgery services; trauma services; general surgery services; and others (Kleinpell-Nowell, 1999). New areas or roles for ACNPs were in sports medicine practices; as hospitalist or intensivists; in holistic medical practices; in occupational health settings; in preanesthesia settings; in nursing home settings; as wound care specialists; in pain management clinics; in electrophysiology diagnostic and treatment settings; in medical flight programs; and in tropical medicine programs. These new practice areas demonstrate the diversity of practice opportunities available to meet the needs of acutely ill patients.

As of 2001, less than 50% of ACNPs continued to work in teaching hospitals, and this change is projected to continue as the role of the ACNP expands into more rural areas (Kleinpell-Nowell, 2001). As this happens, the practice settings for ACNPs will no longer be defined solely by a hospital's walls but will go far beyond them to wherever the needs of acute care patients can be met (Steinke & Hayes, 2000). This evolution in practice setting parallels that of the CNS who was originally totally hospital based, but now one-third of practicing CNSs are found in community settings (Scott, 1999).

Acute Care Nurse Practitioners on Specialty Services

Richmond and Keane (1996) described ACNPs as nurses who have expanded their scope of practice to incorporate the caring paradigm of nursing and parts of the therapeutic paradigm of medicine. The contributions that NPs make in providing continuity of care to patients in the hospital have facilitated the evolution of the role. ACNPs have been recognized as an invaluable source of standardization and stability in various acute care settings (Hicks, 1998). They have provided educational resources and served as liaisons between patients and families, other nurses, physicians, consultants, and other health-care providers. Complex patients on specialty care services such as transplantation, cardiac surgery, and heart failure services need someone who can provide and direct the services necessary to facilitate the patient's return to optimal health in a timely manner (King et al., 2001).

In tertiary health-care centers, cyclic changing of medical residents from one service to another has contributed to fragmented care. The ACNP can provide much needed stability and continuity known to produce positive patient outcomes. Complex settings, in which the continuous follow-up of patients is necessary, are ideal practice areas for the ACNP. ACNPs can make a positive impact on the health-care delivery system through providing a continuous and comprehensive approach to the management of their patients' needs.

Acute Care of the Elderly

In 1996, the Institute of Medicine recognized the demographic projections reflecting the aging of the population in the United States (Martin, 1999). The aging population is projected to increase by over 70% between the years of 2010 and 2030. Coinciding with this is a projected worsening of the shortage of pulmonary and critical care intensivists and nurses. These shortages provide considerable concern for those working in, or relying on, acute health care services (Angus, Kelley, Schmitz, White, & Popovich, 2000). Undoubtedly, the ACNP working in the acute and critical care areas will be confronted with caring for more elderly patients who are subject to significant physiological, social, psychological, and developmental changes that affect their recovery and survival from an acute illness (Miller, 2001). Additionally, elderly patients often come to the acute care setting with multiple and complex medical needs that confound their care.

At present, most educational programs preparing adult ACNPs focus their curricula on the management of the acutely ill patient throughout the continuum of their adult life, without considerable emphasis on gerontological issues. However, there is a growing need to add additional geriatric content to best prepare the ACNP to manage the medically complex and fragile elderly patient.

In response to the need for more adequately prepared health-care professionals who can meet the growing needs of critically ill older patients, the Critical Care Workforce Partnership has been formed. This partnership collectively represents more than 100,000 health-care professionals who specialize in critical care (Angus et. al., 2000). The organizations represented in this partnership include the American College of Chest Physicians, The American Thoracic Society, The American Association of Critical Care Nurses, and the Society of Critical Care Medicine. Their goals are to help inform policy makers and other key audiences of the complex issues associated with shortages of critical care physicians, nurses, pharmacists, and respiratory therapists trained to care for the critically ill, and especially the critically ill aged; to educate health-care professionals in critical care; to promote effective and safe systems of patient care; and to ensure an adequate workforce of trained critical care professionals.

Although still in its early stage, this partnership will influence the preparation of ACNPs for future practice. These future roles will require preparation to manage the needs of the acutely ill elderly, to understand the growing policy changes that will affect their care; to serve as advocates for this vulnerable population; and to integrate evolving knowledge and technological advances into their care.

Nurse-Midwifery

CNMs are registered nurses who have completed an accredited nurse-midwifery program, passed a national certification examination, and met other criteria for certification set by the American College of Nurse-Midwives (ACNM) or the ACNM Certification Council (Rooks, 1997, p. 8). The ACNM accredits all nurse-midwife programs and requires that these program reflect the ACNM core competencies (2006b). In addition, this group will require a graduate degree for entry into practice by 2010. Today, about 68% of CNMs have a graduate degree, whereas 4% have a doctoral degree (ACNM, 2006a).

Currently there are six types of educational programs available to prepare midwives: three for registered nurses and three for nonnurses. Programs to prepare nurse-midwives include a certificate program that provides registered nurses with the essential components of the nurse-midwifery curriculum incorporated into a program of professional studies that either requires a baccalaureate degree on entrance or awards no less than a baccalaureate degree; a graduate-level academic program for registered nurses that grants a master's or doctoral degree on completion of studies in nurse-midwifery; a precertification program that is a postbaccalaureate course of studies for registered nurses who are already professional midwives and that provides selected components of the nurse-midwifery curriculum (ACNM, 2002).

Although multiple entry options exist, graduate programs predominate in nurse-midwifery preparation (91% of nurse-midwifery programs) versus certificate programs (9% of programs). Of the 39 graduate-level programs preparing nurse-midwives 85% are located in schools of nursing, 5% are in schools of public health, and 4% are in other schools such as allied health (ACNM, 2002).

Nurse-midwifery is recognized in all 50 states, although it is regulated by various agencies in the different states and has varying scopes of practice from state to state. Over 50% of CNMs identify physician practices or hospitals as their primary employer. For nurse-midwives practicing in hospital settings, clinical privileges may be granted through membership in the medical staff or through other privileging routes (Cooper, 1998). The purpose of requiring institutional credentialing and practice privileges is to ensure that nurse-midwives provide patient care within the parameters of professional practice (Cooper, 1998). Presently nurse-midwives practice in hospitals, independent practices, clinics, community-based practices, and birthing centers. However, this was not always the case.

Historical Perspective

At the beginning of the 20th century about 50% of the births in the United States were attended by midwives (Stone, 2000). These women were primarily apprentice trained, with no formal education, and were often referred to as lay or granny midwives (Stone, 2000). At that time the infant mortality rate was extremely high. In response to this, nurse-midwives were trained as attendants at normal births while being supervised by a physician. In 1914, Fred Taussig, a physician from Missouri, suggested that schools of midwifery be established for the advanced training of graduate nurses interested in becoming nurse-midwives (Stone, 2000). The curriculum was to include lectures and demonstrations, thorough hospital training in diagnosis, and special work in the treatment of emergencies. Situations in which the nurse-midwife should call for physician assistance were to be emphasized (Stone, 2000).

Over the 20th century, many changes have been made to the way in which nurse-midwifery was taught and practiced. Nurse-midwives originally focused on providing care to women in poor and rural areas who had limited access to health care. Nurse-midwife practice moved into hospital settings in the 1950s, but the focus remained on providing health care to women of childbearing years in community settings. Childbirth during the mid and late 20th century was characterized by an increasing use of technology affecting the care that women received. During this period most women gave birth in hospital settings.

These social and practice changes influenced the manner in which childbirth was perceived in society. The more natural, family-oriented way of delivering babies had been lost and a medical model of childbirth became the dominant model of practice. In response many women turned to lay midwives for assistance with births. The concept of developing out-of-hospital facilities with the goal of providing a safe, homelike, family-centered environment for low-risk maternity care was developed, thus beginning the advent of birthing centers. As of 1999, there were 160 such centers in operation (Stone, 2000). Still, in 2005 only 1% of CNM-attended births occurred in birthing centers and 1% in homes, whereas the remaining 98% occurred in hospitals (ACNM, 2006a).

A decline in the number of CNM-attended births was reported in 2004 with CNM-attended births accounting for 7.5% of births (Declercq, 2007, p. 87). The growth in cesarean births affected this decline, but it is not yet clear if a decreasing pattern is emerging. CNM-attended births were reported as 310,342 in 2004 and as 306,377 in 2005 (Declercq, 2007; ACNM, 2006a).

Primary Care Focus in Nurse-Midwifery

As nurse-midwives continued to provide obstetrical care to women throughout their childbearing years, they realized that many women did not have access to physician services. It became a natural progression for women to seek their primary health care needs from the health-care provider they had trusted during their childbirths. As a result, nurse-midwives began to provide care to peri- and postmenopausal women, a natural expansion of their scope of practice. As the aging of U.S. Americans evolves in the 21st century, the number of women approaching menopause is growing. Large numbers of women are expected to seek menopausal and postmenopausal care from nurse-midwives.

With the growing numbers of women of all age groups seeking health care from CNMs, nurse-midwives working in clinics and various outpatient settings began to provide care to women with health problems not directly related to their reproductive health (Stone, 2000). A survey conducted in 1994 found that CNMs commonly treated conditions such as earaches, mild hypertension, anemia, viral infections, asthma, and dermatitis (Fullerton, 1994; Oshio, Johnson, & Fullerton, 2002).

Results of this survey validated the profession's recognition that nurse-midwives were primary health-care providers for women and newborns and recommended that educational programs preparing nurse-midwives receive should include content in primary care. This recommendation expanded the scope of practice of the nurse-midwife. The most recent version of the ACNM Core Competencies for Basic Midwifery Practice approved in 2002 reflects this expansion (ACNM, 2002) and includes the management of common health problems, as well as perimenopausal and post-menopausal care. Through addressing the primary care needs of women, nurse-midwives expanded their scope of practice. They also continued their focus on midwifery practice, so as to not lose the essence of nurse-midwifery practice, while acknowledging those aspects of primary care that are part of the services offered to patients and their families (Avery, 2000).

Issues Related to Primary Care Practice

CNMs provide primary and preventive care in clinics and other outpatient settings. The ACNM calls for care delivered by CNMs to include all essential factors of primary care and case management. This focus on the ambulatory care of women and newborns emphasizes health promotion, education, and disease prevention and identifies women as central in providing this care (ACNM, 1997). CNMs have also focused on the care of adolescent women, noting that they are largely a medically underserved group.

Nurse-Midwife as First Assistant for Cesarean Section

Another role of the CNM in birthing emergencies has developed out of necessity, that of the surgical first assistant. As obstetrical residency programs across the nation close and cost containment results in fewer physicians available to serve as first assistants, CNMs have expanded their roles to fill the gap (Moes & Thatcher, 2001). Because in many cases the CNM was already present at the time of an emergency, the delivery could progress without interruption, resulting in better outcomes for both the mother and the newborn, if the CNM was prepared as a surgical first assistant.

Not unexpectedly there is opposition to this expansion of the CNM role. The Association for Perioperative Registered Nurses (AORN) and some surgeons are not convinced that CNMs possess adequate knowledge to perform the first assistant role safely. In response to this criticism, the ACNM (1998) has set guidelines for those CNMs who wish to serve as a first assistant and defined the role of the first assistant in cesarean sections as a frequently performed advanced midwifery skill requiring training and supervision in patient assessment, anatomy and physiology, principles of wound repair, and the development of basic surgical skills such as aseptic technique and suturing. At present, each state is addressing the requirements for CNMs who practice as first assistants. Although the number of CNM-first assistant is still small, this may change as appropriate content and supervision are provided in curricula that prepare CNMs.

As the needs of childbearing women have changed over the years, the practice and skills of the nurse-midwife have expanded to meet them. It is obvious that this trend will continue as additional needs are identified **(Box 2-5).**

Nurse Anesthetist

CRNAs are APNs who are anesthesia specialists with authority to practice in all 50 states. They administer all types of anesthesia and provide anesthesia-related care in the following categories: preanesthetic preparations and evaluation; anesthesia induction, maintenance and emergence; postanesthesia care;

BOX 2-5
Nurse-Midwife Clinical Profile

Carol is the practice director of a busy obstetrical, gynecological, and midwifery care program that includes nine midwives and five physicians. She is responsible for the recruitment and evaluation of staff members and serves as liaison to hospital administrators and to the professional and lay community.

As she has progressed in her role, she has assumed more administrative responsibilities, especially those dealing with the need to "break even" financially. The high costs of health care have forced her to learn the business end of the practice. She completed a midwifery business institute course to learn the intricacies of reimbursement because her practice accepts numerous health-care plans, and she acknowledges a "steep" learning curve.

Billing is done through the clinical care association (CCA) that employs her. Nurse-midwives in her practice were offered an incentive-based contract with the CCA, but refused this opportunity, choosing instead a guaranteed base salary with bonuses.

and perianesthetic and clinical support functions (Department of Health and Human Services [DHHS], Public Health Service [PHS] Division of Acquisition Management, 1995).

Nurse anesthetists provide a significant amount of the anesthesia given for surgical procedures in the United States, including that delivered in federal agencies and military installations (Fehder, 2003). These APNs work in urban, suburban, and rural settings and provide more than two-thirds of the anesthesia administered in rural hospitals and 65% of anesthesia given nationally (DHHS PHS Division of Acquisition Management, 1995; Fehder, 2003). In contrast to the high numbers of women in the other APN categories, 42% of CRNAs are men (American Association of Nurse Anesthetists [AANA], 2008; Waugaman & Lohrer, 2000).

Employment patterns for CRNAs have evolved in recent years as a result of their achievement of independent billing rights under Medicare, decreases in anesthesia reimbursement rates, efforts to reduce hospital-based costs, and the growth of surgicenters and other nonhospital-based surgical settings in which anesthesia is administered. As of 1997, 37% of CRNAs were employed directly by hospitals as staff members, an additional 38% were employed by anesthesiology practice groups, 15% were practicing in CRNA-only groups or were independently contracting for their services, and 3.7% were practicing in surgical centers or physicians' offices (Fehder, 2003).

The American Association of Nurse Anesthetists (AANA) serves as the guiding professional organization for CRNAs, setting the educational and certification standards and identifying a Code of Ethics for CRNAs (AANA, 2001), along with Scope and Standards for Nurse Anesthesia Practice (AANA, 2007) and Standards for Office Based Practice (AANA, 2002). Nurse anesthetist students must enroll in schools accredited by the AANA and upon graduation, they must successfully complete a certification examination. They must also participate in mandatory biennial recertification that includes 40 hours of accredited continuing education (Fehder, 2003).

Since the early years of the 20th century to the present, the educational preparation of CRNAs has evolved from a tradition of hospital-based diploma education to university-based graduate degree programs. In 1998, master's degree preparation was required for all entering nurse anesthetist students. Although the required master's degree does not have to be in nursing, about 50% of graduate CRNA programs are located within schools of nursing (McCarthy et al., 2000).

CRNAs are currently recognized as APNs by mainstream nursing groups, including the American Nurses Association (ANA), but this was not always the case. In the 1930s and in much of the 20th century, nurse anesthetists were viewed by many nurses as practicing medicine and not nursing. Today however, expanded roles for nurses including CRNAs are widely accepted by nursing groups and the public.

Still, CRNAs face significant ongoing difficulties in establishing their practice prerogatives. They face considerable pressures from anesthesiologists who have attempted to limit their scope of practice by conceptualizing the administration of anesthesia as the practice of medicine (Shumway & Del Risco, 2000). In 1982, the American Society of Anesthesiologists (ASA) introduced the concept of an anesthesia care team (ACT), a practice model requiring that all anesthetics be given under the direction and supervision of an anesthesiologist (Shumway & Del Risco, 2000).

These restrictive efforts were inadvertently fostered with the introduction of an insurance reimbursement regulation policy by Medicare in 1982. This policy attempted to reduce fraudulent charges for anesthesia care by establishing specific conditions that held anesthesiologists accountable for services they claimed to perform when working with or employing CRNAs (Fehder, 2003; Shumway & Del Risco, 2002). The Tax Equity and Fiscal Responsibility Act (TEFRA) regulations set specific conditions for reimbursable services that seemed to require physician leadership for the delivery of anesthesia as a standard of care. Later attempts to eliminate the perceived necessity for anesthesiologist supervision for Medicare reimbursement of CRNA services have yielded mixed results, and each state can decide whether to opt out of the supervisory regulations (Fehder, 2003). Currently 14 states have done so.

One result of the struggle for CRNA practice prerogatives and leadership has been the establishment of the ACT as the predominant practice model. To clarify if differences exist between CRNAs who work in ACTs and those who do not, Shumway & Del Risco (2000) evaluated personal and professional characteristics, scope of practice, workload, income, and employment arrangements in a sample of over 400 CRNAs. They found that CRNAs who practiced in ACTs were more likely to be women, have less experience, be younger, have a master's degree, and practice in larger cities. ACT-based CRNAs also had a broader scope of practice and used more airway, regional, and monitoring techniques; and performed more varied cases and services. They placed more laryngeal mask airways and arterial catheters and provided more anesthesia for cardiopulmonary bypass, pediatric, intracranial, and trauma cases than non-ACT anesthetists. However, they were less likely to be involved with the placement of epidural and central venous catheters and to participate in pain management and critical care services (Shumway & Del Risco, 2000).

Non-ACT-based anesthetists worked more hours per week and were reimbursed $40,000 more per year. Finally, 91% of ACT-based anesthetists in this sample were employees compared to 4% who were self-employed, whereas 49% of non-ACT-based anesthetists were employees compared to 43% who were self-employed (Shumway & Del Risco, 2002) **(Box 2-6).**

BOX 2-6
Nurse Anesthetist Clinical Profile

Marcy is a certified registered nurse anesthetist (CRNA) who has master's level training and works as a member of an anesthesia care team (ACT) in a university-related urban medical center. She has been a clinical coordinator for the team for the past 2 years and before that was a team member for 2 years. Her clinical responsibilities involve providing anesthesia for patients requiring ear, nose, and throat (ENT), plastic, neurosurgical, thoracic, cardiac, and orthopedic surgery.

Marcy works in a busy practice setting with 24 operating rooms and plans to expand the practice to two other sites. She typically works four 10-hour days. Three are spent in the operating room and one involves administrative duties. She regularly supervises anesthesia students in the operating rooms and teaches and codirects an accredited educational program for nurse anesthetists.

Marcy's responsibilities include the provision of general, regional, and local anesthesia and conscious sedation. She likes the autonomy and independence of her job, and the opportunity it presents to integrate her skill and knowledge in the clinical setting.

Marcy is an employee of the ACT and does not bill directly for her services. Billing is done through the supervising anesthesiologist to maximize full billing potential. Although she cannot prescribe medications in her state, she uses the unit-supplied medications for her patients. Her choices are guided by the patient's history and needs, the surgeon's preference, the surgical procedure, and the patient's preference when possible.

FUTURE DIRECTIONS FOR ADVANCED PRACTICE NURSES

APN roles are thriving as shown in the increased numbers of practitioners; in the expansion of practice roles and settings; in the growth of prescriptive privileges and opportunity for reimbursement for services; and in the numerous studies demonstrating favorable patient outcomes related to APN delivery of care. The growth and expansion of these roles will undoubtedly continue.

APN roles present exciting challenges, enormous diversity, satisfaction, and rewards. But, they also present challenges that reflect those found in the larger health-care arena, including those related to the high cost of health care, reimbursement, and downsizing. They also have problems unique to those found in a predominantly women's profession including the need to recruit an outstanding new generation of APNs in a climate that offers many role opportunities to women and men.

The future for APNs, although promising, will continue to be affected by knowledge development in the biological and social sciences and in evolving political and social expectations and pressures. The development of the clinical nurse leader role (AACN, 2004) and the call for a practice doctorate in nursing, as a proposed terminal degree for APNs (AACN, 2004), will also provide stimuli for role expansion or contraction and for possible changes in educational programs preparing tomorrow's APNs. The clinical nurse leader, conceptualized as an advanced generalist, has been a source of concern to the National Association of Clinical Nurse Specialists about role overlap (NACNS, 2005). APN organizations have varied in their response to the call for a practice doctorate for APNs by 2015: the American Association of Nurse Practitioners (AANP) has endorsed this call; the AANA has endorsed both the PhD and the DNP by 2025, whereas the ACNM has not endorsed this requirement. Serious debate around these issues and others will benefit the APN of the future.

References

American Academy of Nurse Practitioners. (2007). *Standards for nurse practitioner practice in retail-based clinics.* Austin, TX: Author.

American Association of Colleges of Nursing. (2004). Position Statement on the Practice Doctorate in Nursing. Washington, DC: Retrieved May 10, 2008, from the American Association of Colleges of Nursing Web site: www.aacn.nche.edu/DNP/DNPPositionStatement.htm.

American Association of Critical Care Nurses & American Nurses Association. (1995). *Standards of clinical practice and scope of practice for the acute care nurse practitioner.* Washington, DC: American Nurses Publishing.

American Association of Critical Care Nurses. (2002). *A scope of practice and standards of professional performance for the acute and critical care clinical nurse specialist.* Aliso Viejo, CA: Author.

American Association of Nurse Anesthetists. (2001). *Code of ethics for the certified registered nurse anesthetist.* Park Ridge, IL: Author.

American Association of Nurse Anesthetists. (2002). *Standards for office based anesthesia practice.* Park Ridge, IL: Author.

American Association of Nurse Anesthetists. (2007). *Scope and standards for nurse anesthesia practice.* Park Ridge, IL: Author.

American Association of Nurse Anesthetists. (2008). Nurse anesthetists. Retrieved May 10, 2008, from the Wikipedia Web site: http://inwikipedia.org/wiki/Nurse Anesthetist.

American College of Nurse-Midwives. (1997). Position statement. Certified nurse midwives and certified midwives as primary care providers/case managers. Retrieved May 10, 2008, from the American College of Nurse-Midwives Web site: www.midwife.org.

American College of Nurse-Midwives. (1998). ACNM clinical practice statement: the certified nurse-midwife/certified midwife as first assistant in surgery. Washington, DC: Author.

American College of Nurse-Midwives. (2002). Program types. Retrieved May 10, 2008, from the American College of Nurse-Midwives Web site: www.midwife.org/edu/education.cfm.

American College of Nurse-Midwives. (2006a). Fact Sheet. Essential facts about midwives. Retrieved May 10, 2008, from the American College of Nurse-Midwives Web site: www.midwife.org.

American College of Nurse-Midwives. (2006b). Position statement. Mandatory requirements for entry into midwifery practice. Retrieved May 10, 2008, from the American College of Nurse-Midwives Web site: www.midewife.org.

American Nurses Credentialing Center. (2008a). Adult psychiatric and mental health nurse practitioner certification. Description of practice. Retrieved April 23, 2008, from American Nurses Credentialing Center Web site: www.nursecredentialing.org/cert/eligibility/apmhnp.htlm.

American Nurses Credentialing Center. (2008b). Family psychiatric and mental health nurse practitioner certification. Description of practice. Retrieved April 23, 2008 from American Nurses Credentialing Center Web site: www.nursecredentialing.org/cert/eligibility/fpmhnp.htlm.

Angus, D. C., Kelley, M. A., Schmitz, R. J., White, A., & Popovich, J. (2000). Current and projected workforce requirements for care of the critically ill and patients with pulmonary disease: Can we meet the requirements of an aging population? *Journal of the American Medical Association, (284)*21, 2762–2770.

Avery, M. D. (2000). Historic perspectives: core competencies. The evolution of the core competencies for basic midwifery practice. *Journal of Midwifery and Women's Health, 45*(6), 532–536.

Becker, D., & Richmond, T. S. (2003). Advanced practice nurses on acute care services. In D. O. McGivern, E. M. Sullivan-Marx, & S. A. Greenberg (Eds.), *Nurse practitioners: Evolution of advanced practice* (4th ed., pp. 135–149). New York: Springer.

Berger, A., Eilers, J., Pattrin, L., Rolf-Fixley M., Pfeifer B. A., Rogge J. A., et al. (1996). Advanced practice roles for nurses in tomorrow's healthcare system. *Clinical Nurse Specialist, 10*(5), 250–255.

Bissinger, R. L., Allred, C. A., Arford, P. H., & Bellig, L. L. (1997). A cost-effectiveness analysis of neonatal nurse practitioners. *Nursing Economics, 15*(2), 92–99.

Brooten, D., Gennaro, S., Knapp, H., Brown, L., & York, R. (1989). Clinical specialist pre and postdischarge teaching of parents of very low birthweight infants. *Journal of Obstetrical, Gynecological, & Neonatal Nursing, 18*(4), 316–322.

Brooten, D., & Naylor, M. D. (1995). Nurses' effect on changing patient outcomes. *Image The Journal of Nursing Scholarship, 27*(2), 95–99.

Consensus Model for APRN Regulation: Licensure, Accreditation, Certification and Education. (2008). Draft joint dialogue group report completed through the work of the APRN consensus work group and the National Council of State Boards of Nursing APRN Advisory Committee. Retrieved November 11, 2008, from https://www.ncsbn.org/7_23_08_consensue_APRN_final.pdf.

Cooper, E. (1998). Credentialing and privileging nurse-midwives. *Journal of Nursing Care Quality, 12*(4), 30–35.

Craven, R. F., & Keene, T. L. (2000). The advanced practice nurse and home care. *CARING Magazine, 19*(11), 38–40.

Declercq, E. (2007). Trends in CNM-attended births, 1990–2004. *Journal of Midwifery and Women's Health, 52*(1), 1, 87–88.

Delametter, G. L. (1999). Advanced practice nursing and the role of the pediatric critical care nurse practitioner. *Critical Care Nursing Quarterly, 21*(4), 16–21.

Department of Health and Human Services, Public Health Service Division of Acquisition Management. (1995). Expanding the capacity of advanced practice nursing education. Final report [data file]. Retrieved May 10, 2008, from http://bhpr.hrsa.gov/nursing/lewin95.html.

Dwyer, M. L. (2000). Advanced practice nursing for children with HIV infection. *Nursing Clinics of North America, 35*(1), 115–123.

Fehder, W. (2003). Nurse anesthetists: evolution from critical care practitioners to anesthesia providers. In D. O. McGivern, E. M. Sullivan-Marx, & S. A. Greenberg (Eds.), *Nurse Practitioners: Evolution of Advanced Practice* (4th ed., pp. 269–283). New York: Springer.

Fullerton, J. T. (1994). Reflections on nurse-midwifery roles and functions. *Journal of Midwifery, 39*(2), 107–109.

Grandinetti, D. (1999). NP progress report: How is this practice doing? *RN, 62*(7), 36–38.

Hicks, G. L. (1998). Cardiac surgery and the acute care nurse practitioner—"The perfect link." *Heart and Lung, 27*(5), 283–284.

King, B. R., Foster, R. L., Woodward, G. A., & McCans, K. (2001). Procedures performed by pediatric transport nurses: how "advanced" is the practice? *Pediatric Emergency Care, 17*(6), 410–413.

Kleinpell, R. (1998). Reports of role descriptions of acute care nurse practitioners. *AACN Clinical Issues, 9*(2), 290–295.

Kleinpell, R. M. (1997). Acute care nurse practitioners: Roles and practice profiles. *AACN Clinical Issues, 8*(1), 156–162.

Kleinpell, R. M. (1999). Evolving role descriptions of the acute care nurse practitioner. *Critical Care Nurse Quarterly, 21*(4), 9–15.

Kleinpell-Nowell, R. (1999). Longitudinal survey of acute care nurse practitioner practice: Year 1. *AACN Clinical Issues, 10*(4), 510–520.

Kleinpell-Nowell, R. (2001). Longitudinal survey of acute care nurse practitioner practice: Year 2. *AACN Clinical Issues, 12*(3), 447–452.

Lipman, T. (1986). Length of hospitalization of children with diabetes: effect of a clinical nurse specialist. *The Diabetes Educator, 14*(1), 41–43.

Marchione, J., & Garland, T. (1997). An emerging profession? The case of the nurse practitioner. *IMAGE: The Journal of Nursing Scholarship, 29*(4), 232–237.

Martin, R. K. (1999). The role of the transplant advanced practice nurse: A professional and personal evolution. *Critical Care Nursing Quarterly, 21*(4) 69–76.

McCarthy, E. J., Pearson, J., McCall, W. G., Fault-Callahan, M., Lovell, S., L., & Sanders, B. D. (2000). Education of nurse anesthetists in the United States. *AANA Journal, 68(2),* 111–113.

McCorkle, R., Benoliel, J., Donaldson, G., Georgiadon, F., Moinpour, C. & Godell, B. (1989). A randomized clinical trial of home nursing care for lung cancer patients. *Cancer, 64*(6), 1375–1382.

Medina, J. (Ed.) (2000). *Standards for acute and critical care nursing practice.* Aliso Viejo, CA: American Association of Critical-Care Nurses.

Miller, S. K. (1998). Defining the acute in acute care nurse practitioner. *Clinical Excellence for Nurse Practitioners, 2*(1), 52–55.

Miller, S. K. (2001). Gerontology and geriatrics: Considerations for the acute care nurse practitioner. *Nurse Practitioner Forum, 12*(3), 155–160.

Mitchell-DiCenso, A., Guyatt, G., Marrin, M., Goeree, R., Willan, A., Southwell, D., et al. (1996). A controlled trial of nurse practitioners in neonatal intensive care. *Pediatrics, 98*(6), 1143–1148.

Moes, C. B., & Thacher, F. (2001). The midwife as first assistant for cesarean section. *Journal of Midwifery and Women's Health, 46*(5), 305–312.

Moller, M. D., & Haber, J. (1997). Advanced practice psychiatric nursing: the need for a blended role. *Online Journal of Issues in Nursing, 2*(1). Retrieved May 10, 2008, from www.nursingworld.org/ojin.

National Association of Clinical Nurse Specialists. (2005). *NACNS Update on the Clinical Nurse Leader (CNL).* Harrisburg, PA: Author.

Naylor, M. D., Bowles, K. H., & Brooten, D. (2000). Patient problems and advanced practice nurse interventions during transitional care. *Public Health Nursing, 17*(2), 94–102.

Neal, L. J. (1999). Role of the advanced practical nurse. *Home Healthcare Nurse, 17*(5), 323–325.

Oshio, S., Johnson, P., & Fullerton, J. (2002). The 1999–2000 task analysis of American nurse-midwifery/midwifery practice. *Journal of Midwifery and Women's Health, 47*(1), 35–41.

Pearson, L. J. (2002). Fourteenth annual legislative update how each state stands on legislative issues affecting Advanced Nursing Practice. *The Nurse Practitioner, 27*(1), 10–52.

Pearson, L. J. (2008). The Pearson Report. *The American Journal for Nurse Practitioners, 12*(2), 9–10.

Pelosi, L. (2000). The role of the advanced practice nurse in pediatric general surgery. *Pediatric Advanced Practice Nursing, 35*(1), 159–171.

Pozen, M. W., Stechmiller, J. A., Harris, W., Smith, S., Fred, D. D., & Voight, G. C. (1977), A nurse rehabilitator's impact on patients with myocardial infarction. *Medical Care, 15*(10), 830–837.

Richmond, T. S., & Keane, A. (1996). Acute care nurse practitioners. In J. Hickey, R. Ouimette, & S. Venegoni (Eds.), *Advanced Practice Nursing* (pp. 316–326). Philadelphia: Lippincott.

Rooks, J. P. (1997). *Midwifery and childbirth in America.* Philadelphia: Temple University Press.

Rossetto, C. L., & Fair, J. (1998). Assessing competencies for medical procedures as an advanced practice nurse. *Journal of Pediatric Health Care, 12*(2), 102–104.

Safreit, B. J. (1992). Health care dollars and regulatory sense: the role of advanced practice nursing. *Yale Journal of Regulation, 9*(2), 418–488.

Scott, R. A. (1999). A description of the roles, activities, and skills of clinical nurse specialists in the United States. *Clinical Nurse Specialist, 13*(4), 183–190

Sechrist, K. R., & Berlin, L. E. (1998). Special article: role of the clinical nurse specialist: An integrative review of the literature. *AACN Clinical Issues, 9*(2), 306–324.

Sellards, S., & Mills, M. E.(1995). Administrative issues for use of nurse practitioners. *Journal of Nursing Administration, 25*(5), 64–70.

Shumway, S. H., & Del Risco, J. (2000). A comparison of nurse anesthesia practice types. *AANA Journal, 68*(5), 452–462.

Silver, H. R., Murphy, M. A., & Gitterman, B. A. (1984). The hospital nurse practitioner in pediatrics: A new expanded role for staff nurses. *American Journal of Disease of Children, 138*(3), 237–239.

Spisso, J., O'Callaghan, C., McKennan, M., & Holcroft, J. (1990). Improved quality of care and reduction of house staff workload using trauma nurse practitioners. *The Journal of Trauma, 30*(6), 660–664.

Steinke, E. E., & Hayes, K. (2000). The acute care nurse practitioner: an evolving role in Kansas. *Kansas Nurse 75*(6), 1–2.

Stone, S. E. (2000). The evolving scope of nurse-midwifery practice in the United States. *Journal of Midwifery and Women's Health, 45*(6), 522–531.

Teicher, S., Crawford, K., Williams, B., Nelson, B., & Andrews, C. (2001). Emerging role of the pediatric nurse practitioner in acute care. *Pediatric Nursing, 27*(4), 387–390.

Waugaman, W. R., & Lohrer, D. J. (2000). From nurse to nurse anesthetist: the influence of age and gender on professional socialization and career commitment of advanced practice nurses. *Journal of Professional Nursing, 16*(1), 47–56.

Weinberg, R. M., Liljestrand, J. S., & Moore, S. (1983). Inpatient management by a nurse practitioner: Effectiveness in a rehabilitation setting. *Archives of Physical Medicine and Rehabilitation, 64*(12), 588–590.

Zachariah, R., & Lundeen, S. P. (1997). Research and practice in an academic community nursing center. *Image: Journal of Nursing Scholarship, 23*(3), 255–260.

3

Role Development:
A Theoretical Perspective

Lucille A. Joel

There is only a role for the moment, not any role that will serve for the entire life of a career. Role modifications depend on a theoretical body of knowledge, more of it hypothetical than empirical research. These concepts and relationships allow a comfortable paradigm shift as necessary, with an awareness of the elements of continuity from here to there.

A THEORETICAL PERSPECTIVE ON ROLE: AN OVERVIEW

There are two diametrically opposed theoretical perspectives in the behavioral sciences that provide a context for the study of role performance. These are structural-functionalist and symbolic-interactionist theories. The former is based on the assumption that roles are more or less fixed within the society to which they are attached and that opportunities for individuals to alter patterns of social interaction are limited. This is in contrast to the latter, which proposes the more individualistic perspective, that people do not merely learn responses but organize and interpret cues in the environment and choose those to which they wish to react.

Structural-functionalist theory subordinates the individual to the society; it is deductive in its analysis of role. All situations that arise within a society do so because they fill a social need. One such example is the division of labor. The more complex a society, the more differentiated its labor source will become, readjusting and reconstructing over time. Specialization becomes guaranteed, and associates and assistants are created to share in a domain of the work. This concept is dramatically displayed by the division of labor and reordered roles within the health-care delivery system, each role creating its own cadre of technologists, technicians, associates, and assistants. Why should nursing be different?

Altruism also plays a major part here because individuals subordinate their will to the social order. The social forces in a given society validate the roles and the associated behaviors of the individual. Consensual validation is the vehicle for both the maintenance and change of these norms. In many instances, norms are codified by government; in others, they continue to exist in veritable limbo, changing or resisting change according to time and place. A continuing debate exists about the relationship between the fixed norms of a society and the individual's perception of those norms. Often there is no route to interpretation of the social norm except cues offered by others in the situation, and often those cues may be misleading. From another perspective, where may nonconformity be tolerated, to what degree, and in what areas of social participation? Examples abound both professionally and in life. Consider for a moment the immigrant family whose children are schooled in the United States and socialized to the prevailing culture in this country. Are their new ways accepted at home and to what extent? Must they change like a chameleon from place to place or jeopardize belonging or perhaps even sustenance? To what extent can advanced practice nurses (APNs) feel

---

BOX 3-1
Cues That May Predict Limits on Flexibility in Defining Role Behaviors

- Highly precise and detailed job descriptions
- Management by memorandum in situations in which personal communication would have sufficed
- Guarded interdisciplinary boundaries that hamper smooth operation
- A hierarchy that is an obstacle to work rather than a facilitator
- Policies, procedures, and documentation systems that are cumbersome and even inconsistent with current practice
- Absence of staff nurse autonomy in caring for patients
- Organizational relationships designed for supervision, as opposed to reporting
- Absence of inventiveness and creativity
- Verbalized discontent from staff, but no evidence of any attempt to change things
- High turnover rate among employees
- Maintenance of a "screen" for attitudes, values, and behaviors not supported by historic antecedents

---

confident in establishing their personally preferred values, attitudes, and behaviors in a new role or employment situation? See **Box 3-1** for cues that may predict limits on flexibility in defining role behaviors.

In contrast, the symbolic-interactionist view emphasizes the meaning that symbols hold for actors in the process of role development, rather than the constraints presumed to be exerted by the social structure. The interactionist sees the formation of role identity as inductive and complex. The role is a creative adaptation to the social environment and the result of the reciprocal interaction of individuals. Conway (1988) states, "It is the product of self-conception and the perspective of generalized others" (p. 67). To facilitate communication toward these ends, symbols are essential, and they must be social and hold the same meaning for each actor in the process. In other words, self-identity is shaped by the reflected appraisals of others, and it is desirable that an individual's self-perception should be highly congruent with the way they are perceived by others and the way they see themselves as being perceived by others. Should these pieces show a poor fit, an individual could waste a lifetime of effort creating evidence that justifies his or her personal view of self.

Many have rejected the structuralist approach because it seems limited in accounting for the wide variation in roles and behaviors that we see today. Yet, it is impossible to ignore the effect that the culture and the "collective conscience" have on our development of identity and role behaviors. There is recent interest in building conceptual frameworks that are inclusive of both the interactionist and structural perspectives and promise a greatly enlarged understanding of role development. This eclecticism characterizes this chapter's discussion.

ROLE DEVELOPMENT

The concept of reference groups and the process of socialization are central to role development. Reference groups are the frame of reference for the process of socialization. Through socialization, individual behavior is shaped to conform to the standard of the group in which one chooses to seek membership.

Reference Groups

Reference groups convey a standard of normative behavior in terms of values, attitudes, knowledge, and skills. For an individual, this may be a group to which he or she belongs or aspires. In moving toward a standard that is either consciously or unconsciously desired, discussion of several reference groups is in order, including normative groups, comparison groups, and audience groups. The normative group sets explicit standards and expects compliance, and it rewards or punishes relative to that degree of compliance. The church, community, and family are good examples of normative groups. The behaviors that are expected may have wide or narrow latitude, but somewhere there is a "bottom line." The comparison group sets its own standards and only becomes a comparison group when an individual accepts it as such. The nursing staff of a magnet facility may be a comparison group, demonstrating longevity in employment and satisfaction with work, seeking upward mobility through education, and so on. The nursing staff and their leadership in other facilities may aspire to these qualities, making it a comparison group for them. The audience group is a collective group whose attention an individual wishes to attract. The audience group holds certain values but does not demand compliance from the person for whom they serve as a referent (Lum, 1988). In fact, the audience group may not even be aware of this individual. To be recognized, the individual takes note of the group's values and plays to that audience for attention. Staff nurses may observe that physicians value being able to proceed with the treatment of their patients unencumbered by the bureaucratic constraints of health care. Administrators are overwhelmed by the cost factors in health care. Nurses are best positioned if they are aware of these values and attitudes and try to minimize the obstacles they represent to these groups. In other words, they play to the audience through either word or deed.

Socialization

Socialization refers to the learning of the values, attitudes, knowledge, and skills that enable the behavior prescribed for a specific social position or role. The fact that these components are society specific indicates that there are social norms involved. Values are ideas held in common by members of a social structure that prioritize goals and objectives (Scott, 1970). Values are generally the abstract but relatively stable aspects of a person's belief system. Attitude is the tendency to respond to social objects or events in a favorable or unfavorable way. Opinion is defined as expressed attitude (Katz, 1960). Behaviors are observable social acts performed by an individual. Attitudes guide judgement and subsequently behavior, but this assumption of a relationship between attitude and behavior is controversial.

Operationally, the concept of socialization refers to individuals acquiring the necessary knowledge and skills, as well as internalizing and shaping the values and attitudes of a particular social system, in preparation for fulfilling a specific role in that system (Lum, 1988). This process is no less true for the roles of nurse and APN than it is for the role of mother, father, husband, or wife. Further, whereas some roles or statuses have highly specific role prescriptions, others are extremely vague and open to wide variation of interpretation. This latitude may be observed in the setting in which the role is played out, the society in which it is placed, or both. Harmony among these systems enhances role execution. There is often significant discrepancy between the public, professional, legal, and institutional definitions of the role of the nurse. Even if the society and role occupant are bound by the legal role as defined, discrepancies among the other definitions cause problems in recruitment, retention, job satisfaction, and more.

Socialization is a continuous and cumulative process that evolves over time through role-taking and role-making, both of which are techniques of role bargaining. Social behavior is not simply a learned response, but depends on the processes of interaction and communication. Role-taking to be successful requires skill in empathic communication. There is a requirement to project oneself into the circumstances of another and then to step back to imagine how one would feel in the other's situation. If there is accurate determination of the motives and feelings of the other, the actor can modify his or her own behavior to sustain or alter the other's response (Hardy & Hardy, 1988a). The process here is unidirectional. The APN "reads" his or her peers and supervisor as seeing staff development as the major focus of the APN role, although she or he had preferred to carry a significant personal case load of the most complex patients. Staff development is accepted as the priority, but the APN takes on cases as vehicles for teaching at every opportunity.

Put in another way, the less desirable activities are accommodated (first-order change) and even eventually assimilated (second-order change), becoming an integral part of the role. First-order changes are *behavioral shifts* that do not' permanently achieve a desired result. Old preferences keep returning like antagonists because we shift our behaviors but not the core values or attitudes causing the behaviors. Second-order changes are *permanent attitude shifts that cause new behaviors*. The "old ways" stay gone and are not replaced by a new version (like giving up alcohol and starting a nicotine or work addiction).

In contrast, role making is bidirectional and interactive, with both actors presenting behaviors that are interpreted reciprocally for the purpose of creating and modifying their own roles. This process is analogous to a dance, each partner seeking to complement the other while maintaining his or her own uniqueness. The APN notices surprise from the physician when she or he suggests a modification in treatment for a patient. The APN supplies cogent and sophisticated reasoning, and the physician agrees, although skeptical of this behavior. Over time, the physician becomes comfortable with the APN's prescriptions and actually looks for the clinical input. Both role-taking and role-making depend on success in reading role partners correctly. This skill is enhanced by broad social experience, rehearsal of the role anticipated, the recentness of those experiences, attentiveness to role behaviors, and good memory skills. These skills can be developed and honed during the educational experience.

As challenging as internalizing role behaviors is the movement from one role or subrole to another. This process is described in **Box 3-2**. Not only must one learn new behaviors, but one must break from old ones. Inadequate socialization predicts marginalization or the inability to either remain in a previous role or move on to another. A case in point is the nurse who hangs on to the periphery of a system, never quite becoming part of it or bothering to know the personalities involved and refusing to assimilate nursing with the other aspects of life. This is particularly common in people who try to juggle multiple aspects of life, keeping each separate—obligations everywhere, multiple lists of things to do, each with a first-place priority, a comprehensive plan nowhere. The wiser strategy is to integrate the dimensions of life, with professional colleagues becoming personal friends, family participating in workplace and professional events, and so on (one list with one rank ordering of priorities).

Role Acquisition

Knowledge and skill acquisition are important aspects of role implementation in nursing, both for the entry-level registered nurse and the APN. This is not to ignore the essential part played by attitudes and values (the belief system) but to acknowledge that knowledge and skill are expected of professionals by the public (audience group), leadership in the field (comparative group), and peers (normative group). The skill acquisition model, developed by Dreyfus and Dreyfus (1977) and later applied to nursing by Benner (1984), tells us that even experts perform as novices when they enter

> **BOX 3-2**
> **Socialization as Continuous**
>
> **Break from Previous Roles**
> - Minimize previous advantage.
> - Break previous peer relationships.
> - Convert previous peer relationships into friendship relationships.
> - Maintain a portfolio or clinical log reflecting on your evolving practice, values, and attitudes.
>
> **Establish a New Peer Group**
> - Clarify new responsibilities that accompany changed status.
> - Consider the values, attitudes, knowledge, and skills that will contribute to success.
> - Develop new peer group associations.
>
> **Movement to the New Role Prescription (Accommodation)**
> - Provide role rehearsal opportunities.
> - Review benefits of mastery.
> - Consider a mentor.
> - Identify support systems among role partners.*
>
> **Assimilation of Role Behaviors**
> - Be aware of change of self-concept.
> - Recognize the rites of passage as more than symbolic.
> - Create opportunities for success.
> - Treat failure as a learning experience.
> - Move on to process and outcome evaluation once the role is established, although not matured.
>
> ---
> *A role partner may hold the same role or a role that is reciprocal but definitely has role expectations of the primary role occupant.

new roles or subroles, although they proceed to acquisition at a quicker pace. This pattern is verified by several authorities, including Brykczynski (2000) and Roberts, Tabloski, and Bova (1997). In observing APN students, they report periods of regression, anxiety, and conflict before the incorporation of new role behaviors. This is not unexpected, and an analogy can be drawn from work with groups. It is common that in the beginning of a group or when a new member is introduced into an established group, there is a loss of confidence among individual members. The introduction of a person into a milieu with new role expectations is a temporary setback, even where some of the behaviors have been well established in a previous role. As a student, the regression and loss of confidence are often followed by anger directed toward faculty and preceptors who they see as guilty of not giving them enough knowledge or skill. In many ways, they are grieving the role they had previously mastered and responding to the anxiety over moving on.

Anticipatory socialization should be a planned goal during the student period and not left to chance. Ample opportunity should be provided for students to get to know APNs who may just be beginning their careers (peer group) and to participate in discussions with seasoned APNs regarding practice issues (accommodation). Both of these goals may be accomplished through the state nurses association, especially if there is a forum or division on advanced practice. Other experiences should be incorporated in the educational program, such as the opportunity to dialogue with employers and practicing APNs about their expectations of the role. **Box 3-3** contains a format for the participation of APNs on a panel describing their practice and role development for students. These anticipatory experiences should facilitate the period of resocialization as a graduate.

It would be remiss not to mention the clinical competency of faculty. Clinically competent faculty are necessary to give credibility to the program and to narrow the gap "between education and practice" (Brykczynski, 2000, p. 121). The best of all worlds would be for faculty to teach using their own panel of patients. This being impossible much of the time, it is still necessary for faculty to have clinical skill to be able to critique practice and provide the proper oversight for preceptors.

Benner describes five levels of skill acquisition: novice, advanced beginner, competent, proficient, and expert. As one proceeds along this continuum, one becomes more involved in the process of caring, until at the expert stage, situations are recognized in terms of their holistic patterns rather than a cluster of component parts, and the context becomes somewhat irrelevant. In the early stages, new behaviors are accommodated, and they later become assimilated in the practice repertoire, until at the highest level they appear intuitive. Movement from accommodation to assimilation or from novice to expert with its intermediate steps is best accomplished through accruing experience with the opportunity to apply both practical and theoretical knowledge and providing situations in which failure is

---

BOX 3-3
Questions to Guide Advanced Practice Nurse Participation in a Panel on Advanced Practice

1. How did you find your first position after graduation?
2. What job-seeking strategies would you advise new graduates to use in today's market?
3. How do any or all of the following fit into your specific position?
4. What is your prescriptive authority?
5. What kind of practice privileges (i.e., admitting, treating, consulting, and discharging) do you have?
6. What system do you have for reimbursement?
7. Do you participate in a managed-care panel?
8. How have your functions or role changed over the years, and were those changes the result of the evolution of the profession, your choices, your advocacy, or the expectations of an employer?
9. Have you been an active participant in developing your role? How so?
10. What are the major stresses and strains in your practice? How do you handle them?
11. Describe your collaborative arrangement with a physician.
12. How do you show outcomes or document the value of your contribution to the practice? (Or to your employer?)
13. How do you maintain your practice credibility?
14. Do you plan to further develop your own role or skill set? If so, how?
15. What were the most valuable aspects of your graduate educational preparation for advanced practice? The least valuable?
16. What do you know now that you wish you had known earlier in your career?
17. What is your experience with mentoring, either as mentor or protégé?
18. How important to your professional development was this mentor(ed) experience?

BOX 3-4
Role-Enhancing Experiences Planned During Education Experience

■ A synthesis semester at the end of the educational program that incorporates, as far as legally possible, all the ingredients of full-time employment

■ Work-study programs that alternate semesters with work placements in your anticipated field

■ A curriculum that progresses toward more independence and personal accountability, with students and faculty moving to a collegial relationship as opposed to superiors and subordinates

■ Service-education partnerships, with faculty teaching students as they practice with their own patients

■ Opportunity for students to work with faculty on their personal research or in their practice

■ Summer externships and new graduate internships or residencies

■ Patient clinical areas with a primary commitment to the clinical learning needs of students

■ Participation in activities suited to advanced practice nurses (e.g., conferences, meetings, and peer review sessions)

■ Preceptor or "buddy" system involving agency staff

■ An experience with interdisciplinary (or at the least multidisciplinary) education (Joel, 2003)

allowed and treated as a learning experience (Roberts et al., 1997). It should be noted that Benner's model is experiential and does not consider education as a variable in distinguishing these skill levels. However, you cannot apply what you do not know. It would be interesting to use Benner's model to compare an APN and a nonmasters' prepared registered nurse, both with similar experience.

It is helpful for the APN student to consciously approach the socialization process knowing the normative, comparative, and audience groups, and being aware of the changes that are expected to take place in their own behavior, values, and attitudes. Socializing experiences, which could be provided during the course of studies, are presented in **Box 3-4.**

Socialization Deficits

One of the most compelling challenges in professional education is to provide adequate socialization. Socialization deficits are guaranteed to inhibit role performance, introducing additional stress into roles that are already by nature stressful.

APNs are increasingly prepared in programs of part-time study. In addition, the movement into the community college and university settings for entry-level education has, to some degree, diluted the intensity of the socialization experience for nursing. Off-campus living arrangements, a cohort of students who depend on full-time or part-time employment or who have family obligations, courses of study that may be protracted over many years, and so on, all reduce the strength of the primary socialization into the profession. What is the result of an incomplete or weak primary socialization into nursing when moving on to the next role transition to advanced practice (Chen, Chen, Tsai, & Lo, 2007)? This remains a serious question yet to be answered. Further, even if the primary socialization is solid, what does incomplete anticipatory socialization as an APN mean for role acquisition?

This potentially could create a situation of "marginal man," in which a person is a member of one or more cultures, but belongs to none. It also presents a strong case for externships and residency programs through which a concentrated exposure to the role is guaranteed (Santucci, 2004; Starr, 2006). Certification also promises to help role acquisition and role progression with its expectation of additional education and investment in practice.

STRESS AND STRAIN

Stress and strain are natural companions of advanced practice, given the chaotic health-care environment and the fact that these roles are evolving and growing in prominence. Hardy and Hardy (1988b) tell us that role stress is primarily located in the social structure, external to the individual, and owing to incompatible normative expectations. It may or may not generate role strain, the feeling of frustration and anxiety internal to the individual.

Antecedents of Stress and Strain

The situations that create stress and strain for the APN are abundant. They are apparent in the educational preparation in which we may overlook opportunities for anticipatory socialization and in a rapidly restructuring health-care delivery system that demands continuous minor or major modification in roles. Specialization and advances in technology make roles that have become well established over time obsolete and require the role occupants to face a new cycle of ambiguity and transition. Beyond this, there is also the growing emphasis on cost efficiency, consumerism, and the demedicalization of health care. None of these trends are surprising to the reader, but the effect they have on role is often unexpected and unintended. The traditional hierarchy of the system is radically changed, and the primary care provider is as likely an APN or physician's assistant as a physician. Consumer is "king," and health-care organizations are competing to corner their market share of clients. Consumer satisfaction is a major outcome measure against which everyone is measured. In fact, consumers often enter the system with as much information about their condition as the professional who attends them. In the midst of this evolving system, we see the slow but decisive movement toward complementary therapies that have not been part of our nursing repertoire in the past, but that are demanded by the public.

To further complicate the situation, reality finds most nurses as employees in health-care systems. One should never lose sight of the fact that systems (i.e., large, small, simple, or complex) exist to secure their goals and preserve their values. They accomplish this by responding to changing conditions, achieving solidarity among their parts, using a division of labor to accomplish work, controlling the environment, maintaining order, and using resources efficiently. Efficiency has caused a move to accomplish many things through "adhocracy"—systems established for a limited goal and then disbanded. Subcontracting as opposed to the creation of internal departments allows greater flexibility to adjust to change. In like manner, the nursing role has been forced to readjust or jeopardize organizational stability, so resocialization becomes a continuing process, and stress and strain a constant by-product of this process.

Classifying Role Stress

After an exhaustive analysis of research on role stress as it existed in 1988, Hardy and Hardy developed the classification system presented in **Box 3-5** that was subsequently expanded by the work of Schumacher and Meleis (1994).

BOX 3-5
Classification of Role Stress

- Role ambiguity—There is vagueness, lack of clarity of the role expectations.
- Role conflict—Role expectations are incompatible.
- Role incongruity—There is a poor fit between the persons' abilities and their expectations or the expectations of the systems with which they interface.
- Role overload—There is too much expected in time available.
- Role underload—Role expectations are minimal and underuse the abilities of role occupant.
- Role overqualification—Role occupant's motivation, skills, and knowledge far exceed those required.
- Role underqualification (role incompetence)—Role occupant lacks the necessary resources (Hardy & Hardy, 1988b).
- Role transition—Person moves to a new role.
- Role supplementation—There is anticipatory socialization (Schumacher & Meleis, 1994).

Stress and strain are predictable in situations that include ambiguity, ambivalence, incongruity, conflict, and underload and overload and in situations in which the role occupants see themselves as underqualified or overqualified or are moving into a new role or engaged in anticipatory socialization. An example of ambiguity is the new APN who accepts a position without an adequate job description in a setting where there has been little experience with advanced practice, and so there are no seasoned peers to provide direction or support. An example of incongruity is the nurse who has been prepared for primary care practice exclusively and accepts a position that requires extensive coaching and teaching of nursing staff in a specialty area. Role conflict may be operating when the staff nurse feels an obligation to provide quality care but then finds it impossible to achieve satisfactory outcomes within the limits of a predetermined length of stay or in a situation in which the nurse believes that his or her clinical judgment is superior to the client's own choices, but the client refuses to comply. Overload and underload often require a more objective opinion, and the self-assurance to revisit goals and objectives to make them more realistic. Being overqualified or underqualified moves into areas of competence. Some individuals may consider themselves overqualified because they never strain to see or are untrained to see the complexities of a situation. The same circumstances may give rise to feelings of underload. Peer discussion of such clinical situations is helpful to verify your opinion of yourself. Feelings of being underqualified must be talked through and validated, or they result in living the life of an "impostor" (Arena & Page, 1992).

The stress and strain that come with most of the service occupations are labeled "*codependency*" or "*burnout*" in the literature. These two terms are related but different. In codependency, a person controls a situation through the assurance that he or she is needed and works to keep things that way. Whereas in burnout there is difficulty determining who owns a problem. The result is anger; the moral imperative to make a difference, yet the inability to succeed. The natural impulse of nurses to feel for their patients and occasionally bring home their frustrations is played out with exaggeration and eventually rejected. With time, where once they felt too much, they now feel too little in defense of their ego. The result is poor judgment, insensitivity, and intolerance (Joel, 1994). This is the end result of burnout. The codependent personality is at particularly high risk for burnout, which eventually results in negativism and the severe loss of self-esteem as one's clinical competence is questioned.

Responding to Role Strain

Kramer (1974), in an extensive longitudinal study that is still relevant after almost 30 years, identified the problems of new graduates in establishing their roles in the midst of bureaucratic-professional conflict and has termed it *reality shock*. Kramer speaks of "the specific shock-like reactions of new workers when they find themselves in a work situation for which they have spent several years preparing and for which they thought they were going to be prepared, and then suddenly find that they are not" (pp. vi). When the new nurse, who has been *in* the work setting but not *of* it, embarks on a first professional work experience, there is not an easy adaptation of previously learned values, attitudes, and behaviors, but the necessity for an entirely new socialization to practice and simultaneous resolution of conflict with the bureaucracy. This process of resocialization from student to graduate can be easily applied to the APN. Kramer describes the steps as follows:

1. *Skills and routine mastery: The expectations are those of the employment setting. A major value is competent, efficient delivery of procedures and techniques to clients. . . . New graduates immediately concentrate on skill and routine mastery.*
2. *Social integration: [Social integration is] getting along with the group; being taught by them how to work and behave; the "backstage" reality behaviors. If individuals stay at stage one, they may not be perceived as competent peers; if they try to incorporate some of the professional concepts brought over from the educational setting and adhere to those values, the group may be alienated.*
3. *Moral outrage: With the incongruence identified and labeled, new graduates feel angry and betrayed by both their teachers and employers. They weren't told how it would be and they aren't allowed to practice as they were taught.*
4. *Conflict resolution: The graduates may and do change their behavior, but maintain their values, or change both values and behaviors to match the work setting; or change neither values nor behavior; or work out a relationship that allows them to keep their values, but begin to integrate them into the new setting (pp. 155–162).*

The individuals who make the first choice have selected what is called *behavioral capitulation*. They may be the group with potential for making change, but they simply slide into the bureaucratic mold, or more likely, they withdraw from nursing practice altogether. Those who choose bureaucracy (value capitulation), may either become "rutters" (staying in a rut), with an "it's a job" attitude, or they may eventually reject the values of both. Others become organization men and women, who move rapidly into the administrative ranks and totally absorb the bureaucratic values. Those who will change neither values nor behavior, what might be called "going it alone," either seek to practice where professional values are accepted or try the "academic lateral arabesque" (also used by the first group), going on to advanced education with the hope of new horizons or escape. The most desirable choice, says Kramer, is biculturalism, as described in the following:

> *In this approach the nurse has learned that she possesses a value orientation that is perhaps different from the dominant one in the work organization, but that she has the responsibility to listen to and seek out the ideas of others as resource material in effecting a viable integration of both value systems. She has learned that she is not just a target of influence and pressure from others, but that she is in a reciprocal relationship with others and has the right and responsibility to attempt to influence them and to direct their influence attempts. . . . she has learned a basic posture of interdependence with respect to the conflicting value systems (1974, p. 162).*

Even though complicated by the bureaucratic-professional conflict, our original paradigm for socialization is visible in biculturalism.

New graduates do indeed go though variations of this experience, including role-taking, role-making, and bargaining. That there was little change in the adjustment process for decades can be seen by reviewing journals in the interim and by the nomadic workplace patterns of nurses, which must reflect deep-seated job dissatisfaction. Turnover may be a response to boredom, lack of involvement, and apathy and may trace its origin to incomplete or ineffective socialization, or more correctly, ignorance of the socialization process. Hardy and Hardy (1988a) propose that strain may be handled by redefining the role or its expectations, by bargaining among role partners to reestablish priorities, or by decreasing or increasing the degree of interaction.

Managing Role Strain

There is no one prescription for coming to terms with an unmanageable personal or professional life. The problems are relative to the personality of the afflicted, and solutions must be individualized. The ultimate goal is to establish control and identity that is driven by internal strength, rather than being captive to the volatility of the environment. Given that your best investment is in self-care, consider the following:

1. *Learn to use distance therapeutically. Allow people to fail and learn from their own mistakes. Find a comfortable and private place to which you can retreat when you are stressed. If you cannot physically distance yourself, try meditation techniques.*
2. *Decide who owns a problem. If you don't own it, you have no obligation to fix it, especially if it requires self-sacrifice.*
3. *Examine the quality of the peer support you give and get, and correct the situation if needed. Sometimes support systems become habits as opposed to helps.*
4. *Invest in upgrading yourself. Expose yourself to new experiences; learn new skills. Plan your self-care as seriously as you plan your patient care.*
5. *Consciously schedule routine tasks and those requiring physical exertion as a break from complex and stressful activities.*
6. *Learn to trust your instincts. Every problem does not have a rational and logical solution.*
7. *Sometimes think in terms of what could be the worst consequence, then anything short of that is a bonus.*
8. *Identify one person willing to serve as your objective sounding board. This may be one way to find out how you come across to people.*
9. *Make contact with your feelings about situations. Feelings are neither good nor bad; they just are.*
10. *Create options for yourself. Identify those circumstances that you need to personally control, those that are just as well controlled for you, and those that you choose to wait out (Joel, 2003, p. 7).*

CONCLUSION

Socialization into role is a major responsibility of the nursing profession, whether at the point of immersion into the student role and anticipatory socialization to the profession or later with transition to registered nurse and for some on to advanced practice. Socialization requires personalizing a role to your preferences while complying with norms established by the government, the profession, the public, and the institution that employs you. These are your normative, comparative, and audience groups, your major referents; there may be others. The norms held by these groups may be broadly or narrowly interpreted and are revealed through the process of role-taking or empathic communication. There is an opportunity to modify these expectations once you are sensitive to the degree of flexibility allowed by each referent system. This process involves skill in reading our role partners and the environment and reciprocally working to make the role to our liking. This skill can be learned.

Stress and strain are natural companions to nurses, given the environment in which we work, and the work we do. Role stress is located in the social structure, and role strain in the person. Not all stressful circumstances produce strain; this depends on the individual and his or her ability to cope, problem solve, and search for meaning in difficult situations. Success in dealing with stress and strain may be related to complete and effective socialization. This observation reinforces the obligation to both provide socialization experiences and to equip nurses with the resources for self-care.

References

Arena, D. M., & Page, N. E. (1992). The impostor phenomena in the clinical nurse specialist role. *Image: The Journal of Nursing Scholarship, 24*(2), 121–125.

Benner, P. E. (1984). *From novice to expert: Excellence and power in clinical nursing practice*. Menlo Park, CA: Addison-Wesley.

Brykczynski, K. A. (2000). Role development of the advanced practice nurse. In A. B. Hamric, J. A. Spross, & C. M. Hanson (Eds.), *Advanced nursing practice* (2nd ed., pp. 107–134). Philadelphia: WB Saunders.

Chen, Y. M., Chen S. H., Tsai C. Y., & Lo L. Y. (2007). Role stress and job satisfaction for nurse specialists. *The Journal of Advanced Nursing, 59*(5), 497–509.

Conway, M. E. (1988). Theoretical approaches to the study of roles. In M. E. Hardy, & M. E. Conway (Eds.), *Role theory* (2nd ed., pp. 63–72). Norwalk, CT: Appleton & Lange.

Dreyfus, H. I., & Dreyfus, S. E. (1977). *Uses and abuses of multi-attribute and multi-aspect model of decision-making*. Unpublished manuscript. Department of Industrial Engineering and Operations Research. Berkeley: University of Calfornia.

Hardy, M. E., & Hardy, W. L. (1988a). Managing role strain. In M. E. Hardy & M. E. Conway (Eds.), *Role theory* (2nd ed., pp. 241–255). Norwalk, CT: Appleton & Lange.

Hardy, M. E., & Hardy, W. L. (1988b). Role stress and role strain. In M. E. Hardy, & M. E. Conway (Eds.), *Role theory* (2nd ed., pp. 159–239). Norwalk, CT: Appleton & Lange.

Joel, L. A. (1994). Maybe a pot watcher but never an ostrich. *American Journal of Nursing, 94*(46), 7.

Joel, L. A. (2003). *Kelly's dimensions of professional nursing* (9th ed.). New York: McGraw-Hill.

Katz, D. (1960). The functional approach to the study of attitudes. *Public Opinion Quarterly, 24*, 163–204.

Kramer, M. (1974). *Reality shock*. St. Louis: Mosby.

Lum, J. L. J. (1988). Reference groups and professional socialization. In M. E. Hardy & M. E. Conway (Eds.), *Role theory* (2nd ed., pp. 257–272). Norwalk, CT: Appleton & Lange.

Roberts, S. J., Tabloski, P., & Bova, C. (1997). Epigenesis of the nurse practitioner role revisited. *Journal of Nursing Education, 36*(2), 67–73.

Santucci, J. (2004). Facilitating the transition into nursing practice. *Journal for Nurses in Staff Development, 20*(6), 274–286.

Schumacher, K. L., & Meleis, A. I. (1994). Transitions: A central concept in nursing. *Image: The Journal of Nursing Scholarship, 26*(2), 119–127.

Scott, W. R. (1970). *Social processes and social structure: An introduction to sociology*. New York: Holt, Rinehart & Winston.

Starr, K. (2006). Becoming a registered nurse: the nurse extern experience. *The Journal of Continuing Education in Nursing, 37*(2), 86–92.

4

Education for Advanced Practice

H. Michael Dreher

THE QUESTION: IS THE DOCTOR OF PHILOSOPHY OR DOCTOR OF NURSING PRACTICE THE RIGHT DEGREE MODEL FOR FUTURE ADVANCED PRACTICE NURSES?

The advanced practice nursing landscape is changing. Some might even say that it is in upheaval. And when *U.S. News & World Report* featured a cover reading "Who needs doctors? Your future physician might not even be an M.D.—and you might be better off" (Levine & Marek, 2005), or the *Wall Street Journal* features an article called "Making room for 'Dr. Nurse'" (Landro, 2008), you know the health-care environment is actively evolving. In reality, it has not been for too long that the master's degree has been required for the advanced practice nurse (APN). Today the master's is the standard for nurse practitioners (NPs), certified nurse-midwives (CNMs), certified registered nurse anesthetists (CRNAs), and clinical nurse specialists (CNSs). Ann O'Sullivan, past president of the National Organization of Nurse Practitioner Faculty (NONPF), at the recent 2008 national convention in Louisville, Kentucky, reminded the audience that it has taken some 40 years to move from the origins of the NP certificate to the requirement of the master's degree for entry into advanced practice. And now we have the arrival on the scene of a new practice doctorate in nursing.

There is no specific "grandfathering" clause remaining in any state that would allow the NP to enter practice without an actual advanced degree (master's degree in nursing). However, because advanced practice nursing is regulated by individual state statute, older nurses with an advanced practice certificate have often been able to continue practice so long as their status is recognized by the state, and in some situations, specialty certifying bodies. For the CNS, in states where this status is recognized, the master's degree in nursing is required. The American Midwifery Certification Board and the American College of Nurse-Midwives (ACNM) recognize the legitimacy of the postbaccalaureate certificate in midwifery, but the number of certificate programs has declined dramatically as a result of the lack of access to federal funding. Simultaneously, other professional forums such as the American Board of Nursing Specialties (ABNS) and the National Council of State Boards of Nursing (NCSBN) continue to advocate for the master's requirement for practice. As more states adopt the master's requirement, graduates of certificate programs find their ability to practice limited to fewer and fewer states. In 1990, the Council on Accreditation of Nurse Anesthesia Educational Programs (2003, 2004) moved to require the master's degree for entry into nurse anesthesia practice (however, in this case the master's degree is not mandated to be in nursing). But the Council included a "grandfather clause" and never required current CRNAs to obtain a master's degree to continue to practice (Kinslow, 2005). Unfortunately, this makes for 50 different state laws under which the advanced practice roles are each treated somewhat differently. Nonetheless, despite the continuing disparity over the educational standard for entry into practice between the four advanced practice nursing specialties, in October 2004 the American Association of Colleges of Nursing (AACN) membership voted to support the doctor of nursing practice (DNP) degree as the entry level educational credential for advanced practice by 2015. The actual vote was 162 for, 101 opposed, and 13 abstentions.

Impressively, and despite controversy that continues to this day, some 70+ DNP programs (and two DrNP programs) have been developed and are admitting or in the process of admitting students. Many more are also under development. The central question is whether the DNP is a good idea. There are some 240,000 U.S. APNS—140,000 NPs, 70,000 CNSs (although only 1 in 6 CNSs are practicing in direct care positions), 33,000 CRNAs, and 14,000 CNMs, with most overwhelmingly prepared with the minimum of a master's degree (Center for Nursing Advocacy, 2005). The migration of some 240,000 APNs to the doctorate is certainly an ambitious undertaking, and some might question whether this is a realistic goal for the future preparation of all APNs. In reality, the movement to require the entry-level doctorate for advanced nursing practice will be a complex process because the AACN has no legal authority to enforce this on the various state nursing regulatory bodies nor on the respective advanced practice specialty organizations. Further, the two chief accrediting bodies in nursing, the Commission on Collegiate Nursing Education (CCNE) and the National League for Nursing Accrediting Commission (NLNAC) have taken different positions on the approval of DNP programs. The CCNE has elected to only accredit practice doctorate programs with the initials DNP, whereas the NLNAC has stated "As advanced practice nursing moves in new directions, NLNAC will accredit the nursing practice doctorates, whatever their title. We believe that the interests of nursing and health care are best served by focusing on competencies and curriculum content, rather than degree title, and learning outcomes rather than specific curriculum mandates" (2005, p. 1).

Traditionally, APNs who pursued the doctorate pursued the doctor of philosophy (PhD), although historically there have been APNs also pursue the doctor of nursing science (DNSc), doctor of nursing services (DNS), doctor of science in nursing (DSN), doctor of education (EdD), or even sometimes doctorates in another field. However, most of these various nursing doctoral degrees are finally converting to the PhD (Dreher, Fasolka, & Clark, 2008), leaving the PhD in nursing or nursing science as the gold standard research doctoral degree in nursing. And so we enter a new conundrum with the sudden emergence of the DNP degree. Will it become a fully integrated and permanent doctoral degree in the nursing discipline, unlike the nursing doctorate (ND) degree model, which failed as an idea and lasted some 25 years but only had four schools ever adopt it? The central focus of this chapter is whether this new DNP degree can or should become a credible alternative to the PhD for the next generation of APNs. There are lots of implications for our profession with the rise of the DNP. Will the PhD diminish in importance? Will this new nonresearch, practice doctorate negatively affect the expansion of nursing knowledge and erode the major progress nursing has made as a scientific discipline over the past three decades (Dracup, Cronenwett, Meleis, & Benner, 2005)? If our future APNs are required to pursue the DNP, will any of them ever accede to the PhD? And if few APNs obtain the PhD, who will be conducting research and contributing to the evidence base of advanced practice nursing? These are important issues, and many contemporary critics of the DNP believe the future of nursing as a science is literally at stake (Meleis & Dracup, 2005) and that the sudden rise of the DNP has untold implications for our profession as it takes hold and proliferates. This chapter will examine this tension between the PhD and the DNP degree and pose the question whether it is the PhD or the DNP that is the best doctoral degree model for the future of advanced practice nursing. Further, this chapter will question whether these two degrees should be the profession's only two doctoral degree alternatives. Perhaps the more basic question is whether advanced practice nursing should move to the doctorate at all. But in many respects, "this train has left the station." There are just too many internal and external forces driving the DNP degree (some good and some bad) to inhibit its current progression. But just because there is this sudden surge of growth does not guarantee that this degree is ultimately a good idea for advanced practice nursing. Will the DNP take hold in the marketplace and ultimately assuage concerns over health-care cost and quality?

The Doctorate of Philosophy in Nursing: A Degree in Crisis?

Recent data on doctoral nursing enrollment and graduation rates (**Fig. 4-1**) indicate that despite a surge in the number of new PhD programs in the last decade, there has been a decline in overall enrollment and graduation numbers remain flat. With a rapid rise in the number of nursing faculty retirements and a projected shortfall of new PhDs on the supply side, the current nursing faculty shortage is more than critical, it is on "life support" (American Association of Colleges of Nursing [AACN], 2003, 2005a; Smith & Dreher, 2003). According to testimony by Theresa Valiga (2004) of the National League for Nursing at a congressional briefing on the nursing faculty shortage, it takes a registered nurse (RN) an average 8.3 years to complete the doctorate versus 6.8 years for other fields of study! When the endpoints are from the beginning of master's study to the awarding of the doctorate, a RN takes an astounding 15.9 years versus 8.5 years for other disciplines! The AACN (2005b) reported that despite a slight increase in research-focused doctoral program enrollment, there was only a net gain of eight graduates nationally! This is not just disappointing, it is frightening. Even more recent data from the AACN, displayed in Figure 4-1, indicates the depth of this problem.

Although there has been a proliferation of new PhD in nursing programs (over 20 since 2000), there is limited support to properly socialize and mentor students in the nurse scientist role, leaving many unprepared for the rigors of conducting research post-dissertation (AACN, 2005b). This is a criticism offered by the University of Washington's project on *Re-envisioning the PhD* (Nyquist & Wilff, 2000). Similar commentary can be found in "How Business Schools Lost Their Way" from

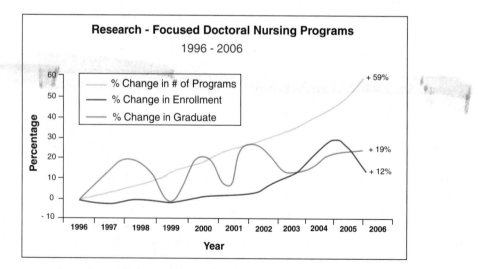

FIGURE 4-1 Research-focused doctoral nursing programs, 1996–2006. *(Data from AACN 1996–2006. Analyzed by H. M. Dreher.)*

the *Harvard Business Review* (Bennis & O'Toole, 2005). The parallels between business education and nursing are striking. Professional business schools have recently come under intense criticism for failing to impart useful skills, instill norms for ethical business behavior, and even lead graduates to good corporate jobs. Part of the problem is that many graduate business schools measure their success by the rigor of the scientific research of their faculty and hire and promote research-oriented professors who have not spent much time working in industry. Many business school faculty seem more comfortable teaching methodology than competently providing experiential discourse on the messy, multidisciplinary issues that are at the very core of contemporary business management. To regain relevancy, Bennis and O'Toole say business schools must rediscover the *practice* of business and find a way to do both: educate the practitioner and create knowledge through research.

Like business, nursing similarly finds itself trying to replicate the academic and scientific traditions of fields such as chemistry and psychology. Consequently, PhD nursing education is often divorced from contemporary nursing practice. This is particularly common when PhD faculty have themselves often left actual clinical nursing practice perhaps decades earlier. The mission to educate the doctorally prepared practitioner/scholar seems to have been lost or at least severely mismanaged in the rush to create the proper nurse scientist. Or perhaps that was never the early vision of doctoral nursing education (i.e., to prepare a practitioner/scholar), but instead to educate the nurse more in the mold of a typical bench scientist. This is quite unfortunate because historically nursing probably shares more in common with another practice discipline, social work, than say developmental biology—and yet our PhD programs seem to operate more like we are preparing a developmental biologist (post-doctorate and all!) rather than a scientist working in a practice and professionally oriented discipline. And so this is where both nursing and business share common challenges in graduate education. Thus, it should not be surprising why so many practicing APNs in particular are not that attracted to their own socially constructed vision of what a PhD prepared nurse is and does. They do not want to forgo employment to attend full-time PhD study and thereby weaken their clinical skills.

Nursing science that contributes critical, high impact translational health research can distinguish the profession of nursing, raise our credibility, and better position our discipline within the community of science. However, nursing research at this point is insufficiently visible and insufficiently supported. As Aaronson (2005) points out, the National Institute of Nursing Research (NINR) remains the lowest funded institute at the National Institutes of Health (NIH) by far, with only $139 million requested for the fiscal year 2006 President's Budget and remained just slightly more funded than the National Center for Complementary and Alternative Medicine (NIH, 2005). With such a comparatively low level of funding, unless more nurse scientists extend the boundaries of their research questions and submit successful proposals to the other NIH institutes (certainly in addition to the NINR), our discipline and science will suffer. Given the move by government to fund more interdisciplinary translational research, the need for well-trained nurse scientists is more apparent than ever (National Academy of Sciences, 2005). Our field needs more properly mentored PhD-prepared researchers who can move into faculty positions in research intensive universities where they can quickly embark on research careers. However, given the nature of the discipline, it is clear that we also need to give nurses who do not necessarily want full-time research careers the training to contribute to knowledge generation in the context of practice.

The Rapid Emergence of the Doctor of Nursing Practice Degree

DNP or DrNP is a *new* degree that was first offered by the College of Nursing at the University of Kentucky in 2001 with their first nine students graduating in 2005. It is confusing that a couple of schools today claim to have had "practice doctorate graduates" in the 1980s or 1990s. This is a historical fallacy. These degree programs were either ND or DNSc programs that converted to the DNP in 2005 or later and then had their university board of trustees approve the conversion of the previously awarded degree to the new DNP. **Table 4-1** indicates the historical progression of the first DNP programs starting in 2001.

So where did this degree suddenly come from? It is probably historically accurate to describe the first DNS and DSN programs as degrees originally designed to be clinical or practice doctorates. The original intent was that they would be different than the two research degrees in the profession, the PhD and the DNSc (also a Doctor of Nursing Science degree, but a research doctorate unlike the DNS and DSN; Apold, 2008). Other authors have previously identified that some of the early DNSc programs were not permitted to be founded as PhD programs often as a result of prejudice by many university faculty in other disciplines who did not fully recognize nursing as a science and thus ineligible to award the PhD. Only recently have all the remaining DNSc degrees in the country (Yale, Columbia, and Widener) completed conversion to the PhD (Dreher et al., 2008). But retrospectively, although the DNS and DSN were originally designed as clinical or practice doctorates and an alternative to the research-focused PhD or DNSc, they ultimately became de facto research degrees and analogous to the PhD. And thus, the first attempt in nursing education to create a practice or clinical doctorate was not successful.

The origin of today's DNP degree model can be traced to Dean Mundinger of the Columbia University School of Nursing. In 2000, Mundinger and colleagues published a clinical trial in the *Journal of the American Medical Association* titled "Primary care outcomes in patients treated by nurse practitioners or physicians: a randomized trial." It was this seminal work on the NP model at Columbia that ultimately led to development of the clinical doctorate or DrNP degree at that institution. Columbia's DrNP was finally approved in 2005. But even the Columbia DrNP model went through an evolution where the faculty first described the degree as a "DrNP in Primary Care," later simply the "first clinical doctorate" (instead of a "practice doctorate" as the DNP is commonly referred to), and then in 2008, the degree was changed to the DNP to satisfy CCNE accreditors. It should be noted that despite the University of Kentucky initiating their DNP in 2001, the degree did not provide any clinical experiences neither within the doctorate nor in the master's degree that preceded it. Instead the Kentucky DNP was designed for the clinical executive with a focus on leadership and management. So some might wonder why the AACN voted in 2004 to endorse the DNP degree awarded through the University of Kentucky while rejecting the DrNP model at Columbia University, which prepared for direct care roles.

Dean Donnelly of the Drexel University College of Nursing and Health Professions (personal communication June 11, 2008) recalls that the AACN sponsored a speaker at their annual meeting some years ago to present pharmacy's movement toward the doctorate (PharmD) for entry into practice. The PharmD is a nonresearch doctorate. According to Donnelly, the membership thought there was a desire by the AACN leadership to move in this direction, but at that time there were no concrete proposals to move advanced practice nursing to the entry-level doctorate. In 2002, a task force was formed by the AACN to explore the practice doctorate (AACN, 2008a). The history of the PharmD model and how it is perhaps not an ideal comparison to the DNP was recently explored by Upvall and Ptachcinski (2007). The AACN Web site presents the DNP as a practice doctorate analogous to doctorates in medicine (MD), dentistry (DDS), pharmacy (PharmD), psychology (PsyD), physical therapy (DPT), and audiology (AudD; AACN, 2008a). The reality is that the DNP is similar in some ways to these degrees and very different in other ways. The MD and DDS are professional practice degrees (nonresearch) like the DNP, but they are required entry-level degrees to practice medicine or dentistry. Although the bachelor of science in nursing (BSN) is preferred by the

TABLE 4-1

Inaugural Doctor of Nursing Practice Programs

School	Year Program Founded	DNP or DrNP	Major	Final Scholarly Work Product
University of Kentucky	2001	DNP	Clinical leadership and executive management tracks	Research utilization project
Case Western Reserve University (OH)	2005	DNP (converted from ND)	Educational leadership and clinical leadership track	Scholarly project—either an independent thesis or applied research project
Columbia University (NY)	2005	DNP (was DrNP 2005–2008)	Clinical doctorate	Portfolio
Drexel University (PA)	2005	DrNP	Clinical research doctorate in nursing science	Clinical dissertation
			Four tracks: practitioner, educator, clinical scientist, and clinical executive	
Rush University (IL)	2005	DNP (converted from ND)	Leadership and the business of health care	Capstone project
Tri-College University ■ Concordia College, Moorhead, MN ■ Minnesota State University ■ North Dakota State	2005	DNP	Family nurse practitioner/generic DNP completion for APNs	None

Continued

TABLE 4-1—cont'd

Inaugural Doctor of Nursing Practice Programs

School	Year Program Founded	DNP or DrNP	Major	Final Scholarly Work Product
University of Colorado at Denver and Health Sciences Center	2005	DNP (converted from ND)	Generic	DNP capstone project
University of South Carolina	2005	DNP (converted from ND)	Multiple primary and nonprimary care options	Research utilization project
University of Tennessee Health Science Center	2005	DNP (converted from DNSc)	Primary care; acute critical care, forensic nursing, gerontology, nursing administration, psychiatric/family nurse practitioner, and public health nursing	Residency project

For a complete list of current programs see www.aacn.nche.edu/DNP/DNPProgramList.htm.

APN, advance practice nurse; DNP, doctor of nursing practice; DrNP, doctor of nursing practice; DNSc, doctor of nursing science; ND, nursing doctorate.

AACN for entry into professional nursing practice, even today there are alternative degree paths to RN licensure. The DPT and AudD are options for entry into physical therapy and speech/audiology practice, respectively, but not required by these disciplines to practice. Further the AudD and in particular the PsyD are not analogous to the DNP (Peterson, 1976, 1982). The DNP was originally conceived as a nonresearch degree by the AACN, stating in their *Essentials for Doctoral Education for Advanced Nursing Practice* that "practice doctorates, requiring a dissertation or other original research are contrary to the intent of the DNP" (AACN, 2008a, p. 20). The AACN's *Essentials* documents have become the standard for designing and assessing master's education programs for advanced practice nursing (AACN, 2008a, 2008b). Some AudD programs require an original research project (Boston University Sargent College of Health and Rehabilitation Science, 2004; University of Washington, 2008) and practically all PsyD programs require a clinical dissertation (Murray, 2000; Wheaton College, 2004; Widener College, 2004). In the literature, these practice doctorates that include some form of original research project or dissertation are termed *hybrid doctorates* as differentiated from the pure research degree (PhD) and nonresearch professional doctorate (PharmD, DPT, or DNP; Dreher, Donnelly, & Naremore, 2005). This is an important distinction. Would the DNP as an alternative to the PhD in nursing result in a decrease in the expansion of nursing knowledge? Will PhD enrollments continue to drop with the concomitant rise in DNP enrollments and graduations?

COMPELLING ARGUMENTS FOR AND AGAINST THE DOCTOR OF NURSING PRACTICE DEGREE

Certainly there are compelling reasons for why the AACN has pushed for an entry-level doctorate for nursing. Three Institute of Medicine reports (1999, 2001, and 2003) have subsequently called for reform in health professions education mainly because of rising health-care errors and patient safety issues, failure of the health disciplines to work collaboratively and deliver optimal health outcomes, and a recognition that the education of students in the health professions, from medicine to nursing to occupational therapy and more, varies too considerably from discipline to discipline. The central arguments for why advanced practice nursing should begin to require the doctorate instead of the master's degree are as follows: (a) master's in nursing degrees, especially those preparing the NP, CRNA, and CNM, often require as many credit hours as some clinical doctorate programs in other disciplines; (b) again, other disciplines like physical therapy and pharmacy are now offering a clinical doctorate and nursing (as the largest health-care profession) should not be any different; and (c) contemporary knowledge is growing exponentially and the master's degree can no longer fully encompass the breadth of coursework necessary for advanced practice (Apold, 2008). As conceptualized by the AACN, the DNP degree prepares the graduate for the highest level of advanced practice in nursing (Lenz, 2005).

As compelling as these arguments are, they are not all based on data. Although the statement about the total number of credits appears to be a salient one, no one would agree that simply the accumulation of credits should merit the attainment of a doctoral degree. Alternatively, perhaps master's degree nursing credits ought to be used more selectively, rather than reflexively moving to a doctoral degree. Second, the issue of whether or not nursing ought to require an entry-level doctorate for advanced practice merely because other health professions have moved to do so is also not necessarily a strong point (Dracup & Brown, 2005). Bloch (2007), in a paper delivered at the first annual conference on the DNP degree in Annapolis, Maryland, argued that the cost and length of new DNP programs will in itself decrease the number of women's health NPs and thus harm access to care for vulnerable populations. Bloch projects a net decrease in the total annual number of Women's Health Nurse Practitioners (WHNP) graduates as the cost to obtain the doctorate instead of the master's will be greater and the time interval from matriculation to graduation will be longer. Indeed, what is missing from the debate on the DNP is a cost-benefit analysis. What is the value of this degree to the health-care system? The strongest argument against the DNP is the decades of strong outcome data supporting the excellence of advanced practice nursing, even in comparison studies to primary medical care. CNMs, CRNAs, CNSs, and NPs are widely recognized by the public and supported in the literature as providing high-quality care. And so the argument that a doctorate instead of a master's is needed to provide high-quality care is fallacious at best. Lending to the confusion, a National Research Council report of the National Academies titled *Advancing the Nation's Health Needs: NIH Research Training Programs*, reads "The need for doctorally prepared practitioners and clinical faculty would be met if nursing could develop a new nonresearch clinical doctorate, similar to the M.D. and Pharm.D in medicine and pharmacy, respectively. The concept of a nonresearch clinical doctorate in nursing is controversial, but some programs of this type exist" (2005, p. 74).

A New Doctoral Nursing Degree Creates Tension: The Doctor of Philosophy Versus the Doctor of Nursing Practice

So it is this new tension over the sudden rise of the DNP at the potential expense of the PhD that serves as a primary concern. New doctoral programs in any discipline are not created without additional resources or the reallocation of resources from other academic programs. Although some universities where both the DNP and PhD are offered report no decline in their PhD enrollment, the trend lines for declining PhD enrollments are clear (see Fig. 4-1). Further, we only have to look at the decline of nursing knowledge development with the near extinction of the master's thesis to imagine that when given a doctoral option requiring a dissertation versus *not requiring a dissertation,* that it is likely many or possibly most graduate students will take the path of least resistance and avoid the research degree. This author anticipates a real risk for decreased expansion of nursing knowledge with the DNP as the primary alternative degree to the PhD and that only the creation of an alternative hybrid degree (a clinical research practice doctorate) will help to avoid this occurrence. The question is whether the public will be confused if the nursing profession promotes a research degree (PhD), a professional/practice nonresearch degree (DNP), and a hybrid degree that combines both research and practice (DrNP). According to Donnelly, the dean where the hybrid doctorate in nursing was first founded in 2005, this is a question she has heard before. She routinely quotes the following "So here is my response to those who say that we may be confusing the public with the proliferation of different types of degrees. 'The public is not confused because they do not care how we structure our degrees. What the public wants is quality, error free evidence-based care; the letters after the name are not the issue; quality of practice is!'" (personal communication, June 11, 2008).

We simply cannot rely solely on nursing PhD graduates to conduct nursing research. That clearly is not in the discipline's best interest. Of course, O'Sullivan, Carter, Marion, Pohl, and Werner (2005) rightly raise the argument that many PhD in nursing graduates never conduct research past their dissertation and perhaps these students may have been better served by a practice doctorate option. The following question is nevertheless posed: if *every* APN in 2015 were to obtain a DNP, who will be *left* to pursue the PhD? Nevertheless, this author also does not believe the DNSc or DSN or DNS should be de facto PhD degrees, which most have become. As mentioned previously, it is unfortunate that university politics and sometimes elitist prejudice against nursing by other scientific disciplines have generally prevented the proper conversion of many of these programs to the PhD.

The University of Alabama at Birmingham is a good example of a DSN program that converted to the PhD in 1999. Most nursing academicians would agree with Fitzpatrick (2003) that the PhD is the proper doctoral degree to prepare the nurse scientist. Therefore, as these other degree models have served their purpose historically, it is time the remaining DNSc, DSN, and DNS programs convert to PhD programs. The critical question posed here, nonetheless, will be whether any future APN will pursue the PhD (instead of a DNP) and who will then be left to expand nursing knowledge if DNP graduates do not have clinical research skills? Right now the diminishing pool of PhD students are *overwhelmingly* recruited from a pool of students who have their master's degree. What will happen when our advanced practice students (CNMs, CRNAs, CNSs, and NPs) pursue the entry-level DNP? This master's pool will thus diminish, and there will likely be few DNP graduates who will make the decision to return to school for yet another doctorate, the PhD.

THE FUTURE OF DOCTORAL NURSING EDUCATION: A NEW VISION

As the advanced practice nursing specialty organizations and other interested parties begin to digest the implications of the AACN 2015 mandate, this chapter offers some suggestions for nursing doctoral education of the future. First, in addition to the DNP, the discipline should adopt a hybrid doctoral degree (DrNP), which requires a clinical dissertation. This would ensure that nursing would always have an academic practice doctorate for clinicians and give graduates more career options, much like the doctor of science of physical therapy degree (DScPT; University of Alabama at Birmingham, Department of Physical Therapy, School of Health Related Professions, 2005). The DScPT degree is physical therapy's hybrid doctorate (all students conduct a clinical research project), the PhD is their research doctorate, and the DPT is their practice doctorate. Second, the DNP degree would be preserved as the professional practice doctorate degree *without* the dissertation. This would establish clinical research preparation as the distinguishing factor between the two practice degree programs: the DNP would be a professional practice doctorate and the DrNP an academic practice doctorate. It is already getting confusing because some DNP programs have already decided to forgo the AACN prohibition against having an original research project. The DNP program at the University of Arizona now requires a "practice dissertation"; the Case Western Reserve University DNP allows a DNP thesis option; Oakland University requires an "original research project"; and Shenandoah University calls for a "clinical research project." At the annual AACN doctoral conference meeting the past few years, the discussion has widened and there has been much questioning as to whether it is wise for the DNP to be an entirely nonresearch degree. The decline in PhD enrollments is becoming more visible and unsettling and challenging the state of knowledge development. This is a very real discussion with implications for our evidence base as both entry-level nurses and APNs.

Although the early developmental work that led to the original Columbia model DrNP in primary care is respected (Mundinger & Kane, 2000), this new degree would have more value if it were an academic practice doctorate (or hybrid) and not an exclusively nonresearch practice doctorate. Whether it is fair or not, if doctorally prepared APNs *truly* want parity or equity with physicians, then their educational preparation needs something that would give them "extra value" *over* the MD. It can be said that this extra value is clinical research skill that physicians learn only through the apprentice model or pursuit of the PhD. Further, O'Sullivan, during her presidency of the NONPF, commented that "many clinicians and faculty have questions about what additional skills and knowledge a NP would have at the practice doctorate level" (2005, p. 12). One obvious answer could be the clinical research competencies gained from the academic practice DrNP rather than the professional practice DNP. A hybrid doctorate model for nursing should be offered with the vision of the NP as a "practitioner/researcher" or "local or field scientist" (a term often used to describe the competencies and role of the PsyD graduate) who would apply research methods to specific problems identified in direct practice. In some ways it is unimaginable that the doctorally prepared APN of the future would not possess the basic clinical research skills to conduct even small-scale studies that would contribute to the evidence-base of nursing practice. From another perspective, will the focus on "outcome evaluation," commonly within the repertoire of the DNP, lead to the expansion of nursing knowledge? I am skeptical that it will. If DNP programs graduate large numbers of students (some are already doing this, which begs the question of quality), will these programs be able to provide sufficient faculty mentoring into the clinical scholar role? Will these students be mentored to publish, present, and disseminate their work? And if not, we must question to what degree these graduates will think, function, and practice differently than the APN with a master's degree?

The discussion of the preparation of the future APN must also include the preparation of the advanced practice nursing educator. To prepare the nurse educator whose primary role is the didactic and clinical teaching of future APNs, colleges and schools of nursing that do not have the resources or the Carnegie classification to seriously compete for NIH funding, should consider establishing a PhD in nursing particularly designed for the student who is inclined to conduct nursing education research. For clarity, however, the degree should be a PhD in nursing (like the Villanova University program) or even nursing education, versus the PhD in nursing science degree reserved for programs geared to preparing the nurse scientist. Despite this intense focus on nursing practice, I still advocate high-quality nursing education research and do not see enough published literature tracking the outcomes of graduates of accelerated bachelor's-entry or master's-entry programs or the efficacy of using personal digital assistants in advanced practice clinical education or whether today's graduate nursing student has an adequate baseline knowledge of genetics to properly counsel patients and their families, and these three issues are listed here only as the beginning of an investigative agenda.

Finally, with few exceptions, I remain very skeptical of BSN-to-PhD programs except for the relatively experienced BSN-prepared RN. Because nursing is a practice discipline, it is futile to graduate doctorally prepared graduates who have had limited exposure to clinical practice. Highly educated, but inexperienced clinicians are not who the nursing profession needs to help alleviate the nursing faculty shortage. In considering admission to any of these doctoral programs, when should we encourage the bachelor's-prepared RNs to matriculate? After 2 years of practice? Three years? More than three? And will we suggest full-time study? If that happens, there really will be few takers. We must be realistic and create programs that accommodate those who need to work full-time to support themselves (although fully funded, full-time PhD study is preferred so nurse scientists can be productive earlier in their careers). These concerns make a strong argument for reserving DNP study as a post-master's option (Dracup et al., 2005).

CONCLUSION

As Broome (2005) has identified, contemporary nursing faces two serious issues: an urgent need for more BSN-prepared nurses and a very severe nursing faculty shortage, which is only going to get worse in the next decade. With these two serious problems facing our profession, only time will tell if the arrival of the DNP was indeed a prudent move by our nursing leadership. In just 3 short years there has been an explosion of largely DNP programs and although the majority are post-master's options (because most current state nurse practice acts still require the master's of science in nursing [MSN] for advanced nursing practice and do not yet consider doctorate-level entry), increasingly we are seeing more BSN-to-DNP program options. With a concomitant decline in PhD enrollments, real questions arise about whether there will be enough doctorally prepared nurses conducting clinical research to provide the evidence for our practice. As Dreher, Donnelly, and Naremore wrote in 2005:

> *What nursing science needs, now more than ever, are more nursing clinicians who will have the skills to conduct meaningful nursing research that will help expedite a greater evidence base for professional and advanced nursing practice. Well-designed, small scale studies can contribute greatly to our science as the number of RNs with an NIH RO1 will always be limited. To better support nursing knowledge development, the PhD needs a better practice-doctorate partner than the DNP. In the end, we believe the Drexel DrNP hybrid (as a clinical research DrNP in Nursing Science, Primary Care, Acute Care or perhaps other iterations like a DrNP in Anesthesia Science or Midwifery—all with a clinical dissertation—is an alternative practice doctorate degree for nursing faculties that do not want to entirely abandon the dissertation or the research enterprise for a new model of non-research based doctoral nursing education. We therefore propose that clinical research preparation serve as the distinguishing factor between the two practice-degree programs: the DNP would be a professional practice doctorate and the DrNP an academic practice doctorate (p. 1).*

Alternatively to the establishment of a hybrid doctorate, the profession is likely to see a real "muddying" of the waters with the DNP in some schools requiring a research project and other schools prohibiting it. And whether the CCNE will be forced to accredit DNP programs that are not truly nonresearch doctorates is another question. There is indeed tension with the new DNP degree and a real level of anxiety about its impact on advanced practice nursing of the future. Will it really have a negative impact on the PhD? Will PhD enrollments plummet further? Will there be no future advanced practice nurses with the PhD? Does that mean future doctorally prepared academic APNs (employed in nursing programs in colleges and universities) will not be hired for tenure-track positions? Will the DNP marginalize the academic APN in the university setting, with other colleagues having the PhD (Gennaro, 2004)? More importantly, will the DNP graduate ultimately practice beyond the scope and skill of the current MSN graduate? Mundinger (2005) of Columbia University has described the ways in which the doctoral role of advanced practice differs from MSN-level practice. She emphasizes that the DNP graduate differs from an APN with a master's degree with the doctoral graduate having "a greater depth and breadth of knowledge and practice. Significant additional science education is provided by courses in genetics, advanced pathophysiology, pharmacology, differential diagnoses, chronic illness, bioinformatics, research methods, and identification and use of medical evidence" (p. 173). The question, however, is how do new DNP programs *really* change their curricula beyond the scope of the MSN? I have served as a consultant to several DNP programs and see uneven attention to skills, knowledge, and competencies beyond the MSN and thus believe this is not the time for rigid adherence to one new practice doctorate degree. The practice doctorate in nursing is so new that there is practically no data on the productivity of its graduates. It is currently impossible to attribute positive outcomes to their practice. What if the DNP fails to improve access to care, cost of care, or quality of care? And what will we do if we see a national decline in the annual number of new APNs as schools begin to drop their MSN and offer only the doctorate? Indeed, the DNP was a bold move, and yet the unfolding of its true impact on the nursing profession and the health of a nation is yet to be seen.

References

Aaronson, L. (2005, January). *The road to interdisciplinary research: NINR and the NIH roadmap.* Paper presented at the 2005 AACN Doctoral Education Conference, Coronado, California.

American Association of Colleges of Nursing. (2003). *White paper: Faculty shortages in baccalaureate and graduate nursing programs: Scope of the problem and strategies for expanding the supply.* Washington, DC: Author.

American Association of Colleges of Nursing. (2005a). *New data confirms shortage of nursing school faculty hinders efforts to address the nation's nursing shortage.* Retrieved March 18, 2005, from the American Association of Colleges of Nursing Web site: www.aacn.nche.edu/Media/NewsReleases/2005/Enrollments05.htm.

American Association of Colleges of Nursing. (2005b). *Institutions offering doctoral programs in nursing and degrees conferred.* Retrieved March 18, 2005, from the American Association of Colleges of Nursing Web site: www.aacn.nche.edu/Education/pdf/DoctoralPrograms05.pdf.

American Association of Colleges of Nursing. (2008a). *Essentials for doctoral education for advanced nursing practice.* Retrieved July 26, 2008, from the American Association of Colleges of Nursing Web site: www.aacn.nche.edu/DNP/pdf/Essentials.pdf.

American Association of Colleges of Nursing. (2008b). *The essentials of master's education for advanced practice.* Retrieved July 26, 2008, from American Association of Colleges of Nursing Web site: www.aacn.nche.edu/education/mastessn.htm.

Apold, S. (2008). The doctor of nursing practice: Looking back, moving forward. *The Journal for Nurse Practitioners, 4,* 101–107.

Bennis, W. G., & O'Toole, J. (2005). How business schools lost their way. *Harvard Business Review, 83*(5), 96–104.

Bloch, J. (2007). *The DNP degree as entry into nurse practitioner practice: Is this nursing's answer to eliminate disparities in health care access to vulnerable populations?* Paper presented at The First National Conference on the Doctor of Nursing Practice: Meanings and Models, Drexel University, Annapolis, Maryland.

Boston University Sargent College of Health and Rehabilitation Science. (2004). *Programs: Audiology, doctor of science.* Retrieved June 8, 2005, from the Boston University Web site: www.bu.edu/sargent/programs/graduate/audiology/research_track.html

Broome, M. E. Constructive debate and dialogue in nursing. *Nursing Outlook, 53*(4), 167–168.

Center for Nursing Advocacy. (2005). *How many nurses are there? And other facts.* Retrieved June 13, 2008, from Center for Nursing Advocacy Web site: http://nursingadvocacy.org/faq/rn_facts.html.

Council on Accreditation of Nurse Anesthesia Educational Programs. (2003). *Trial standards for accreditation of nurse anesthesia programs.* Park Ridge, IL: Author.

Council on Accreditation of Nurse Anesthesia Educational Programs. (2004). *Standards for accreditation of nurse anesthesia programs.* Park Ridge, IL: Author.

Dracup, K., & Brown, C. (2005). Doctor of nursing practice: MRI or total body scan? *American Journal of Critical Care, 14*(4), 278–281,

Dracup, K., Cronenwett, L., Meleis, A. I., & Benner, P. E. (2005). Reflections on the doctor of nursing practice. *Nursing Outlook, 53*(4), 177–182.

Dreher, H. M., Donnelly, G. F., & Naremore, R. C. (2005). *Reflections on the DNP and an alternate practice doctorate model: The Drexel DrNP.* Retrieved December 14, 2008, from Online Journal of Issues in Nursing Web site: www.nursingworld.org/OJIN.aspx.com.

Dreher, H. M., Fasolka, B., & Clark, M. (2008). Navigating the decision to pursue an advanced degree. *Journal of Men in Nursing, 3*(1), 51–55.

Fitzpatrick, J. (2003). The case for the clinical doctorate in nursing. *Reflections on Nursing Leadership, 29*(1), 8–9, 37.

Gennaro, S. (2004). A rose by any other name? *Journal of Professional Nursing, 20*(5), 277–278.

Institute of Medicine. (1999). *To err is human: Building a safer health system.* Washington, DC: National Academy Press.

Institute of Medicine. (2001). *Crossing the quality chasm.* Washington, DC: National Academy Press.

Institute of Medicine. (2003). *Health professions education: A bridge to quality.* Washington, DC: National Academy Press.

Kinslow, K. (2005, September). *Practice doctorate in nursing: American Association of Nurse Anesthetist's perspective.* Paper presented at the Pennsylvania State Nurses Association pre-conference Session on "The Dilemma over the Doctor of Nursing Practice (DNP): Different Perspectives," Harrisburg, Pennsylvania.

Landro, L. (2008). Making room for "Dr. Nurse." *The Wall Street Journal Online,* 4/2/08. Retrieved June 13, 2008, from Physician Assistant Forum Web site: www.physicianassistantforum.com/forums/showthread.php?t=15539.

Lenz, E. R. (2005). The practice doctorate in nursing: An idea whose time has come. The *Online Journal of Issues in Nursing, 10*(3), 1–14.

Levine, S., & Marek, A. (2005). Nurses step to the front. *US News & World Report, 138*(4), 66–71.

Meleis, A. I., & Dracup, K. (2005). The case against the DNP: History, timing, substance, and marginalization. *The Online Journal of Issues in Nursing, 10*(3), 1–8.

Mundinger, M. O. (2005). Who's who in nursing: Bringing clarity to the doctor of nursing practice. *Nursing Outlook, 53*(4), 173–176.

Mundinger, M. O., & Kane, R. L. (2000). Health outcomes among patients treated by nurse practitioners or physicians. *Journal of the American Medical Association, 283*(19), 2521–2524.

Murray, B. (2000, January). The degree that almost wasn't: The PsyD comes of age. *Monitor on Psychology, 31*, 1–5. Retrieved April 4, 2005, from the American Psychological Association Web site: www.apa.org/monitor/jan00/ed1.html.

National Academy of Sciences. (2005). *Advancing the nation's health needs. Committee for monitoring the nation's changing needs for biomedical, behavioral, and clinical personnel.* Washington DC: The National Academies Press.

National Institutes of Health. (2005). *Summary of the FY 2006 president's budget.* Washington DC: Author.

National League for Nursing Accrediting Commission, Inc. (2005). *NLNAC statement on clinical practice doctorates.* Retrieved July 1, 2008, from National League for Nursing Accrediting Commission Inc., Web site: www.nlnac.org/statementClinPrac.htm.

Nyquist, J., & Wilff, D. H. (2000). *Recommendations from national studies on doctoral education: Re-envisioning the Ph.D. Project.* Retrieved March 18, 2005, from the University of Washington Web site: www.grad.washington.edu/envision/project_resources/national_recommend.html.

O'Sullivan, A. L. (2005). The practice doctorate in nursing. *The Mentor, 16*(1), 2–3, 12.

O'Sullivan, A. L, Carter, M., Marion, L., Pohl, J., & Werner, K. (2005). Moving forward together: The practice doctorate in nursing. *The Online Journal of Issues in Nursing, 10*(3), 5.

Peterson, D. R. (1976). Need for the doctor of psychology degree in professional psychology. *American Psychologist, 31*(11), 792–798.

Peterson, D. R. (1982). Origins and development of the doctor of psychology concept. In G. R. Caddy, D. C. Rimm, N. Watson, & J. H. Johnson (Eds.), *Educating professional psychologists* (pp. 19–38). New Brunswick, NJ: Transaction Books.

Smith, M. E., & Dreher, H. M. (2003).Wanted, nursing faculty! If you think the nursing shortage is bad, the nursing faculty shortage is worse. *Advance for Nursing, 5*, 31–32.

University of Alabama at Birmingham Department of Physical Therapy, School of Health Related Professions. (2005). *Doctor of science in physical therapy.* Retrieved June 8, 2005, from University of Alabama at Birmingham Web site: http://main.uab.edu/shrp/default.aspx?pid=80258.

University of Washington. (2008). *Doctor of audiology program.* Retrieved June 13, 2008, from the University of Washington Web site: http://depts.washington.edu/sphsc/aud2/index.html.

Upvall, M., & Ptachcinski, R. (2007). The journey to the DNP program and beyond: What can we learn from pharmacy? *Journal of Professional Nursing, 23*(5), 316–321.

Valiga, T. (2004). *The nursing faculty shortage: A national perspective.* Congressional briefing presented by the A.N.S.R. Alliance, Hart Senate Office Building, Washington, DC.

Wheaton College. (2004). *Clinical dissertation manual for the doctor of psychology degree (Psy.D).* Wheaton College Psychology Department. Wheaton, IL: Author.

Widener University. (2004). *Manual for the clinical dissertation for the doctor of psychology degree (PsyD).* Widener University Institute of Graduate Clinical Psychology. Chester, PA: Author.

5

Global Perspectives on Advanced Nursing Practice

Madrean Schober
Fadwa A. Affara

INTRODUCTION

There is growing international recognition that advanced nursing practice (ANP)[1] should be developed, acknowledged, and legitimized. Factors contributing to a greater willingness to explore ANP options are multifaceted. Physician shortages, increased demand for highly specialized nurses, a greater emphasis on primary health care (PHC) and home-based services, and the increased acuity and complexity of hospitalized patients are motivating decision makers to rethink health service provision. Professional factors are also influencing developments in this field (Bryant, 2005; New Zealand Ministry of Health, 2002; Schober, 2008; World Health Organization [WHO], 2002a, 2002b; WHO-Eastern Mediterranean Region [EMR], 2001). The acquisition of higher professional qualifications as nursing education moves into the higher education sector is matched by a demand for choice in clinical career ladders that acknowledges professional advancement and gives nurses a reason to remain in practice (International Council of Nurses [ICN], 2007a; Zurn, Dolea, & Stilwell, 2005).

The estimated global deficit of 2.4 million doctors, nurses, and midwives has stimulated a renewed examination of skill mix, including options for introducing new types of health-care workers, task shifting and expanding current roles of health professionals (WHO, 2006, 2007). Buchan and Calman (2005) identify several drivers in health systems in countries belonging to the Organization for Economic Co-operation and Development (OECD) contributing to a heightened interest in the advanced practice nursing role. In addition to staff shortages faced by these countries, these authors suggest that health sector reform and new initiatives have stimulated serious consideration of the appropriateness of current role definitions for health-care workers and skill mix. Aspects affecting these deliberations include cost containment measures; actions to improve service quality; the introduction of technological innovations and new therapeutic interventions; and alterations in the legislative/regulatory environment. See **Box 5-1** for a summary of factors contributing to ANP growth.

This chapter will examine some of the issues influencing the development of ANP globally. The emergence of the role in different regions of the world, the International Council of Nurse's (ICN) role in setting international standards, role development, and some of the controversial practice issues affecting the nature of ANP will be explored. Country illustrations will provide examples of growth and progress worldwide.

---

[1]ANP is used as a comprehensive term for the discipline, an umbrella term if you like. Advanced practice nurse (APN) is used in reference to APN roles, APN practice, APN curriculum, or APN positions or individuals who are APNs.

> **BOX 5-1**
> **Factors Contributing to International Growth in Advanced Nursing Practice**
> - Escalating disease burden worldwide
> - Increased inpatient acuity and complexity of treatment
> - Impact of technological innovations and uses of new therapeutic approaches
> - Increased emphasis on primary health-care and community-based services
> - Increasing requests and complexity for home care
> - General global shortage in health-care workers stimulating new consideration of skill mix and task-shifting options
> - Physician shortages
> - Increased demand for specialized nurses
> - Nursing's desire for a clinical career ladder and professional advancement
> - Higher educational qualifications as nursing moves to higher education
> - Better informed health-care consumers
> - Intensified demand for options to address out-of-control health-care costs
> - Search to improve quality of services

THE ROLE OF THE INTERNATIONAL COUNCIL OF NURSES

Since ICN set up the International Nurse Practitioner/Advanced Practice Nursing Network (INP/APNN) in 2000 (see **Box 5-2**), it has consulted intensively to reach consensus on the definition, characteristics, scope of practice, standards, and core competencies for advanced practice nurses (APNs). The ICN position is that the APN is

> . . . a registered nurse who has acquired the expert knowledge base, complex decision-making skills and clinical competencies for expanded practice, the characteristics of which are shaped by the context and/or country in which s/he is credentialed to practice. A master's degree is recommended for entry level (ICN, 2002).

See **Table 5-1** for ICN recommended role characteristics.

Although ICN does not specifically define the scope of practice, it draws on the definition and characteristics previously described and in Table 5-1, in recommending countries to keep the following points in mind when developing scopes of practice for the APN:

- Requires cognitive, integrative, and technical abilities to put into practice ethical and culturally safe acts, procedures, protocols, and practice guidelines
- Has the capacity for delivery of evidence-based care in primary, secondary, and tertiary settings in urban and rural communities
- Practices a high level of autonomy in direct patient care and management of health problems, including case management competencies
- Accepts accountability for providing health promotion, patient and peer education, mentorship, leadership, and management of the practice environment
- Maintains nursing practice current and seeks improvement through the translation, use, and implementation of meaningful research
- Engages in partnerships with patients and health team members for determining resources needed for continuous care and partnering with stakeholders in influencing policies that direct the health-care environment (adapted from ICN, 2008a, p. 13)

BOX 5-2
Goal of the International Council of Nurses International Nurse
Practitioner/Advanced Practice Nursing Network

The key goal of the network is to become an international resource for nurses practicing in nursing practitioner (NP) or advanced nursing practice (ANP) roles and interested others (e.g., policymakers, educators, regulators, and health planners) by:

1. Making relevant and timely information about practice, education, role development, research, policy, and regulatory developments, and appropriate events widely available
2. Providing a forum for sharing and exchange of knowledge, expertise, and experience
3. Supporting nurses and countries that are in the process of introducing or developing NP or ANP roles and practice
4. Accessing international resources that are pertinent to this field

International Council of Nurses. (2002). Definition and characteristics of the role. Retrieved February 27, 2008, from the International Council of Nurses Web site: www.icn-apnetwork.org.

Core competencies have been identified and published in ICN documents *The Scope of Practice, Standards and Competencies of the Advanced Practice Nurse* (ICN, 2008a) and the *Nursing Care Continuum—Framework and Competencies* (ICN, 2008b).

AMBIGUITIES AND ISSUES OF CONTROVERSY

Since 2000, ICN has monitored the progress of ANP globally. In 1999, 33 countries reported nursing roles with advanced practice elements in response to an ICN survey sent to 125 members (Schober & Affara, 2006). In a follow-up, Roodbol (2004) reported 60 countries claiming to be implementing, or in the process of developing, advanced practice roles. This chapter will also draw on data obtained from 18 countries responding to a pilot survey conducted in 2007 to test a new network survey tool. Further information on the state of ANP globally was obtained from a Strength/Weakness/Opportunities/Threats (SWOT) analysis carried out with participants attending the 2006 ICN APN network conference. This analysis highlighted important issues and areas of concern affecting the evolution of ANP in many of the participating countries (Affara, 2006). Issues surfacing were very similar to those uncovered by Schober and Affara (2006) from their survey of key informants and the literature, published and unpublished, on the status of ANP internationally.

An Uncertain Identity Contributing to Poor Role Clarification

The uncertainty of identity appears to center largely on an inability to define, at least at a national level, the scope of practice for the APN. In the absence of a clearly defined scope of practice, it is difficult to delineate accountability and responsibility for the APN. Additionally, as the participants in the SWOT analysis noted, the lack of clear identity affects the ability of APNs to communicate clear messages about the nature of ANP to others, such as clients, policy makers, other health professionals, regulators, and educators.

Proliferation of Titles

ANP is plagued by a proliferation of titles globally. In studying this role internationally, Schober and Affara (2006) found that functions and responsibility vary considerably from one setting to another even when the same title is used in the same country. Extensive confusion has resulted from the

TABLE 5-1		
International Council of Nurses Characteristics for the Advanced Practice Nurse		
Educational Preparation	Nature of Practice	Regulatory Mechanisms (Country-specific regulations that underpin advanced practice nursing practice)
■ Educational preparation at an advanced level ■ Formal recognition of educational programs ■ A formal system of licensure, registration, certification, or credentialing	■ The ability to integrate research, education, and clinical management ■ High degree of autonomy and independent practice ■ Case management ■ Advanced assessment and decision-making skills ■ Recognized advanced clinical competencies ■ The ability to provide consultant services to other health professionals ■ Recognized first point of entry for services	■ Right to diagnose ■ Authority to prescribe medications and treatments ■ Authority to refer to other professionals ■ Authority to admit to hospital ■ Title protection ■ Legislation specific to advanced practice

International Council of Nurses. (2002). Definition and characteristics of the role. Retrieved February 27, 2008, from the International Council of Nurses Web site: www.icn-apnetwork.org.

lack of consensus as to what title should be applied to ANP. Titles currently being used throughout the world include family nurse practitioner (NP), family nurse practitioner (FNP), adult NP, primary care practitioner, nurse-midwife, clinical nurse specialist (CNS), nurse anesthetist (NA), community health NP (CHNP), and women's health NP. Pediatric NP, gerontological NP, emergency room NP, and acute care NP are also titles applied to ANP roles. Some titles indicate the specialty of the APN; other titles have been developed to fit the context of the systems or the situation in which the APN role exists. The pilot survey of 18 countries conducted by the ICN International NP/APN Network discovered 14 different titles being used to designate ANP (Pulcini, Loke, Gul, & Jelic, 2007). The variety of titles being used reveals the explorative nature of advanced practice internationally, with respect to the parameters of the role, and where it sits in relation to other roles in the health-care system.

Lack of Recognition by Others in the Health-Care System

Medical dominance and the control of medicine over health care are cited as some of the main obstacles to implementing advanced nursing roles. Additionally, scope of practice conflicts with other health professionals' scope, especially medicine, contributes to APNs feeling unwelcome within the health-care team. Interestingly, one of the particular problem areas brought up during the analysis was a mistrust that may exist between APNs and other nurses. In many cases it seems that APNs may feel more at ease with medical rather than nursing values. Affara and Schober (2006) uncovered a similar sentiment in information obtained from key informants who reported obstacles to the APN role arising more frequently from nurse, rather than physician, colleagues. In the Netherlands, Roodbol (2005) found that even though physicians believed that the APN presence had a positive effect on the social identity of nurses in general, nurses as a whole did not share this view and were not prepared to accept them into their professional group. This may be a consequence of a perceived fear that this new type of nurse would consider them to be inferior.

Varied Levels of Autonomy

The degree of autonomy afforded to APNs varies from country to country, and even within the country. This appears to be related to the degree of recognition and acceptance of the role and to the type of regulatory mechanisms in place.

Fragmented and Variable Standards and Quality of Education Programs

Historically and up to the present time, educational qualifications for the APN role vary from the awarding of certificates for postbasic courses of various lengths to undertaking a formal university program and obtaining a masters degree. More recent information from the INP/APNN pilot survey indicates that this situation may be improving. In the 18 responding countries, more than 70% reported that APNs were educated at the masters level (Pulcini et al., 2007). Because education beyond the preparation of the generalist nurse is a critical component in the development of the APN role, the ICN Board of Directors approved an organizational position that entry-level education should be set at the master's level (ICN, 2002). See **Box 5-3** for the ICN recommended educational standards.

Issues of Regulation, Credentialing, and Standard Setting

The establishment of standards, regulations, and supportive legislation ultimately provide the underpinnings of successful ANP implementation, but they are also likely to contribute to conflict, discussion, and lengthy debate. The lag between actual APN practice and supportive legislation can be attributed to uneven starts in initiating new roles and the diversity of health issues challenging the communities and countries where these roles seek to grow. Also, restrictive regulations that unnecessarily limit the expertise and scope of practice for APN roles can considerably affect to what extent advanced practice will be embraced by a health system and permit APNs to contribute to their fullest capacity. Thus, a process of evaluation and revision of regulations may be the only option to follow when they are found to hinder optimum professional practice. This in turn poses another set of problems as to who has the authority to initiate and the power to supply leverage in provision of solutions in the credentialing and regulatory arena.

National nursing associations and nursing leadership would seem to be the likely foundation for development and exploration of education requirements and standards, especially because the core of ANP is viewed to be grounded in nursing theory and nursing science. However, there appears to be a lack of consensus among nursing academics and leaders as to what ANP really means, and at times, overt support by nursing bodies is lacking as the roles develop.

BOX 5-3
International Council of Nurses Standards for Education of the
Advanced Practice Nurse

1. Programs prepare the student, a registered/licensed nurse, for practice beyond that of the generalist nurse by including opportunities to access knowledge and skills, as well as demonstrate its integration in clinical practice as a safe, competent, and autonomous practitioner.

2. Programs prepare the authorized nurse to practice within the nation's health-care system to the full extent of the role as set out in the scope of practice.

3. Programs are staffed by faculty who are qualified and prepared at or beyond the level of the student undertaking the program of study.

4. Programs are accredited or approved by the authorized national or international credentialing body.

5. Programs facilitate lifelong learning and maintenance of competencies.

6. Programs provide student access to a sufficient range of clinical experience to apply and consolidate under supervision the theoretical course content.

International Council of Nurses. (2008a). *Nursing care continuum—framework and competencies.* Geneva: Author.

Key decision makers and advisors have begun to provide regulatory and credentialing guidance. International organizations, such as the ICN, are taking official organizational positions regarding ANP and offer publications (ICN, 2008a, 2008b) to facilitate a better understanding of these new nursing roles. **Box 5-4** identifies the minimal regulatory standards recommended by ICN (2008a).

Flexible regulatory language has been encouraged to ensure quality health-care services that are protective of the populations receiving those services. However, at times restrictive regulatory legislation affecting APNs is promulgated or supportive protocols for APN practice are blocked to protect the practice of other health-care professionals. Clarity and consistency in defining the process and structure of credentialing for APNs and accreditation of educational programs worldwide is essential as the APN investigates intercountry choices for employment and educational opportunities. Professional mobility will potentially shape a move toward consensus for credentialing among countries as APNs relocate, immigrate, or accept temporary assignment. The capability of agencies and organizations in addressing legislative issues, standards, and regulations will increasingly come under scrutiny as the international nursing community looks for authorities to provide guidance.

In APN development and implementation, regulation often needs to catch up with innovation, a necessary step if understanding and confidence in the role is to be established for the benefit of key decision makers and the public. However, the setting up of suitable regulatory mechanisms needs to be approached in such a manner that new problems are not created, health-care systems made less efficient, or access is reduced to those who need APN services.

Authority to Prescribe Medicines and Therapeutics

Nurse prescribing of medicines or therapeutics describes various types of nursing practice currently undertaken in different countries or regions of the world. In general, discussion of this issue focuses on the suitability of prescriptive authority for nurses and the appropriateness of nurse

BOX 5-4
International Council of Nurses Minimal Standards for Regulating the
Advanced Practice Nurse

1. Develop and maintain sound credentialing mechanisms that enable the authorized nurse to practice in the advanced role within the established scope of practice.
2. Establish relevant civil legislation or rules to acknowledge the authorized role, monitor the competence, and protect the public through issuance of guidance, assessment processes, and when necessary, fitness to practice procedures and processes.
3. Periodically revise regulatory language to maintain currency with nursing practice and scientific advancement.
4. Establish title protection through rule making or civil legislation.

International Council of Nurses. (2008a). *Nursing care continuum—framework and competencies.* Geneva: Author.

prescribing as it relates to defined characteristics and expected competencies for APN roles. Discourse and comment reveal that nurses have been prescribing medicines, treatments, and other therapies in certain health-care settings, but the reality of carrying out these activities within a legal framework and in a supportive health-care environment such as having enabling workplace policies in place often lag behind the requisites of actual practice. However, as more countries implement APN roles in a variety of settings, the issue of nurse prescribing looks as if it is becoming less of a controversial issue.

It appears that advancement for APN and NP roles necessitates prescriptive authority, but it is worth noting that health-care services in some areas of the world have for some time included nurse prescribing of a range of essential drugs at the first level of practice in primary health-care systems (WHO-EMR, 2001). Thus, nurses may carry prescriptive authority in the absence of the other elements that characterize APN practice.

Buchan and Calman (2004) review nurse prescribing prototypes internationally and provide four models by which nurses may potentially be involved in prescribing. Although nurse prescribing is not always associated with APN or NP roles, countries or regions with authority for nurses to prescribe, such as Sweden, Australia, United States, United Kingdom, Canada, and New Zealand, have well-established community nursing or general nursing roles supportive of this capability. The interest in nurse prescribing continues to grow, and recently Ireland and Spain have reported implementing legislation to promote nurse prescribing (ICN, 2007).

In their appraisal of the key global issues associated with nurses' prescribing. Buchan and Calman (2004), indicate that there is little uniformity as to what role nurses should have with regard to prescriptive authority. Educational programs to prepare nurses for prescribing range from masters degree preparation to a designated program of a few study days. Although these issues are varied, there are common approaches when considering nurses' prescriptive authority. These include the acceptability of nurse prescribing within the health-care setting, designation of which nurses will prescribe, strategies for implementation, and feasibility from an administrative and health policy perspective.

GLOBAL REVIEW—COUNTRY ILLUSTRATIONS

The development of APN and NP roles internationally has progressed to the point where a global review is best accomplished using examples drawn from experiences of specific countries introducing and developing advanced practice nursing roles. Country illustrations are arranged according to regions designated by the World Health Organization (WHO). Descriptions of country progress and expansion in this field are intended to provide representative examples and not meant to portray all activity in a region or a country.

Africa: WHO-AFRO

Botswana

In Botswana, a poorly developed health-care system and a severe shortage of physicians following independence in 1966 triggered the need for nurses with advanced skills and decision making to provide services usually associated with physician practice. Nurses accepted these increased responsibilities but demanded further education to enhance their ability to meet the health-care needs of the country.

The Ministry of Health, through the National Health Institute (NHI), responded by establishing the first FNP program in 1986 with the aim to educate nurses in advanced skills in diagnosis and management of PHC problems common in Botswana. The program evolved to 18 months of postbasic education in 1991, followed by a revision and update in curriculum in 2001 with increased emphasis on comprehensive family health services (NHI, 2002). In 2007, a four-semester format was introduced with implementation in 2007/2008 (Pilane, Neube, & Seitio, 2007).

Because the University of Botswana now offers a master's degree in nursing, a comparative analysis of the masters and FNP curricula is underway to identify how the two programs could articulate common course work, remove redundant or repetitious study while still supporting educational advancement for the FNP. Possibilities for credit transfer and opportunities for challenge examinations or applying for exemption from retaking courses when seeking further study at University of Botswana are being considered (Pilane et al., 2007).

Approximately 250 NPs provide care in outpatient departments, clinics, industry, schools, and private practice throughout the country. The environment in Botswana supports autonomy in provision of PHC services as evidenced in nurse-managed facilities and prescribing privileges. Challenges continue to be lack of specific regulations, the absence of clear qualifications, and no designated career advancement for FNPs (O. Seitio, personal communication, March 13, 2008).

Republic of South Africa

The "key challenges for NPs in South Africa lie in lobbying for enabling legislation, obtaining access to education and training opportunities, and managing risks within the rapidly changing environment" (Geyer, Naude, & Sithole, 2002, p. 11). Even though this statement was made in 2002, the commentary remains true today (N. Geyer, personal communication, March 4, 2008).

The move since 1994 from a mainly hospital-based health-care service to increased emphasis on PHC and community-based services increased the visibility of the NP. The creation of a more unified health-care system while dealing with rapid change in the health-care environment, posed challenges and opportunities for the primary clinical practitioner (PCP). PCP is the title that has been used for NPs in the RSA; however, with the development and introduction of new qualifications in 2008, the title will become FNP (N. Geyer, personal communication, March 4, 2008).

The 2005 Nursing Act and its regulations call for NPs to possess required competencies. Standards for the education and training of nurses and midwives have also been established. Postbasic preparation for FNPs follows either acquisition of 4-year diploma or 4-year degree for general nursing, midwifery, psychiatry, or community health nursing. However, the rapid acceleration in use of nurses in PHC services has resulted in FNPs that have not received specialist education. Therefore, one of the challenges is providing sufficient access to education to ensure nurses in the NP role have the required competence to provide quality care.

The scope-of-practice regulations provided by the South African Nursing Council in 1984 provided practice principles that support nurses and midwives to "perform any acts for which they have been trained" (Geyer et al., 2002, p. 13). The FNP scope of practice is written in such a way that it emphases the provision of comprehensive clinical services such as:

- Comprehensive assessment
- Diagnosis of health and disease, especially diseases common in the Republic of South Africa (RSA)
- Treatment and management (pharmacological and nonpharmacological)
- Referral to other professionals
- Counseling
- Leadership and management
- Health promotion and disease prevention

However, the legal framework for the FNP has not evolved as rapidly as practice. A new scope of practice for nursing has been developed and was promulgated in 2008 (see first numbered item in **Box 5-5**). This scope will make a clear distinction between the roles for professional nurses, staff nurses, and auxiliary nurses while also providing the basis for progression to specialist nurse and NP scope of practice.

The FNP scope of practice overlaps with aspects of scopes of practice for other health practitioners, such as physicians and pharmacists in the case of medicines. Dispensing of drugs falls under the pharmacist's function, and the control of drugs as associated with prescribing is exclusive to the physician, unless the practitioner or professional, such as a nurse, has been authorized to prescribe by their respective councils or regulatory bodies. Nurses are listed as one of these professions (see numbered items 3 and 4 in Box 5-5). A nurse who wishes to dispense medicines must undergo a course accredited with the pharmacy council. Application for a license to dispense medication is made through the national department of health. The license is valid for 3 years, after which reapplication is required.

NPs in RSA are mainly employed in the public health sector at the provincial and local authority level. The majority of health services are provided by nurses and midwives, with nurses identified as the first point of contact for preventive health and minor ailments. With the growing need for home-based care, resulting mainly from the epidemic proportions of HIV and AIDS, nurses and NPs are increasingly holding leadership and supervisory responsibilities for other workers and volunteers in health-care systems.

Establishing collaborative practice in the RSA context is fraught with difficulty because language contained in separate practice acts and regulations governing practice of each category of health-care professionals poses a significant barrier. Health-care practitioners can employ each other, but stipulations within regulations prohibit group practice. Such limitations either discourage formation of multiprofessional groups or require developing involved legal contracts to bypass the rules. Conflict arises when existing scopes of practice are seen to overlap with other professions, thus contributing

> **BOX 5-5**
> **New Developments for the Nurse Practitioners in Republic of South Africa**
>
> 1. The new scope has been structured for three categories of nurses within a framework of professional-ethical practice, clinical practice, and quality of practice. This lends itself to developing a structured scope that progresses to the next levels of specialist nurses and nurse practitioners.
> 2. New educational programs linked to this scope will prepare staff nurses that will be independent/autonomous practitioners able to plan and execute comprehensive care for stable and uncomplicated patients. Professional nurses can specialize in a variety of areas, including family nurse practice. There has been a criterion built in that no nurse can specialize until they have 2-year clinical experience (this includes 1 year of community service after completion of their basic training plus 1 additional year of clinical practice).
> 3. Although there is a new Nursing Act, the profession has not managed to get rid of government control regarding the authorization of nurses to prescribe. Section 56 of the new Nursing Act of 2005 places more controls into the system; nurses will now be licensed to prescribe and reapply for licensing.
> 4. Work is currently in process on regulations for nurse prescribing. The thinking has been that there will be three levels of prescribing where nurses will have access to specified drugs to manage minor injuries and diseases—likely according to protocols. These levels include:
>   - staff nurse = level one
>   - professional nurse = level two
>   - specialist nurse = level three (only access for specialist area)
>
> N. Geyer, personal communication, March 14, 2008.

to lack of agreement supportive of development of advanced nursing roles. This situation has interfered with legislative support for FNP practice and expanded nurse dispensing and prescribing (N. Geyer, personal communication, March 4, 2008).

Western Africa

Madubuko (2001) describes the scope of practice of an NP in West Africa (WA) as very similar to that of registered nurses (RNs) who also possess a postbasic nursing education and clinical training in midwifery (a registered midwife [RM]). Advanced education is not recognized in the nursing register, but hopefully with time, explanation, lobbying, and pressure, the nurses in WA will obtain recognition for advanced education and clinical practice.

All RNs have additional advanced education in at least one specialty area—for instance in the psychiatric, perioperative, nurse education, orthopedic, gynecological, thoracic, or pediatric field. More than 1000 RNs have a master's degree in a nursing specialty. The WA College of Nursing has accredited the University of Benin Teaching Hospitals School of Ophthalmic Nursing for an 18-month master's degree for ophthalmic NPs. Madubuko (2001) considers this to be consistent with the global NP movement.

Madubuko (2001) clarifies that an RN or RM is certified by national certification examination and provides direct PHC. The practice description includes obtaining a history, performing a physical examination, diagnosing and treating common illnesses, performing illness prevention screenings, and health promotion. Education and counseling are provided in collaboration with other health professionals. The reforms globally have supported the concern for more relevant health-care services in WA, providing an opportunity for NPs and other health professionals.

Americas: WHO-AMRO

Canada

The Canadian Nurses Association (CNA) has been instrumental in providing leadership for the development and implementation of ANP in Canada. In 1999, the CNA developed a framework for ANP that was revised in 2002 and 2008. The framework provides the following definition:

> *Advanced nursing practice is an umbrella term describing an advanced level of clinical nursing practice that maximizes the use of graduate educational preparation, in-depth nursing knowledge and expertise in meeting the health needs of individuals, families, groups, and populations. It involves analyzing and synthesizing knowledge; understanding, interpreting and applying nursing theory and research; and developing and advancing nursing knowledge and the profession as a whole (CNA, 2008, p. 5).*

According to this framework, it is the combination of graduate education and clinical experience that allows nurses to develop the competencies required in advanced nursing practice (CNA, 2008, p. 6). Core competencies are described as essential to ANP with a list of competencies in four categories outlined in the framework as clinical, research, leadership, and consultation/collaboration.

During the CNA's 2005 Dialogue on Advanced Nursing Practice that involved 140 nursing leaders, participants identified the framework as a useful tool in the development of curricula, research, policy documents, and interpretation of ANP for multiple stakeholders and the future development of new ANP roles. See **Box 5-6** for a summary of findings from the 2005 Canadian nursing leader's

---

BOX 5-6
Findings from the 2005 Canadian Nursing Leaders Dialogue

- Advanced nursing practice builds on registered nurse practice.
- Canadian advanced practice nurses (APNs) enhance health care in the country.
- Timing is right to ensure APN roles are integrated into the health-care system.
- Expansion of the ANP should be evidence based and reflective of the needs of Canada.
- Continued evolvement of nurses in these roles may require different knowledge and skills.
- Existing and new APN roles need to be understood by the public.
- Pan-Canadian coordination is vital to introducing, developing, and sustaining advanced nursing practice (ANP).
- Strong nursing leadership is needed.
- Nurses must work collaboratively with other professionals.
- The Canadian Nursing Association ANP framework must be updated periodically to reflect changes.

Adapted from a summary of CNPI key messages from International Council of Nurses–APNetwork. (2007). Retrieved March 14, 2008, from APNetwork Web site: www.apnetwork.org.

dialogue. There are currently two recognized ANP roles in Canada: the CNS and the NP. Both the CNS and NP roles are used in all of Canada's 13 provinces and territories.

The implementation of the NP role gained momentum following an 18-month federally funded, CNA-led, Canadian Nurse Practitioner Initiative (CNPI) conducted from 2004 to 2006. This initiative helped in the development of a framework for the integration and sustainability of the NP role in Canada's health-care system. Recommendations for practice, education, legislation, regulation, and health human resources planning were provided as a result of findings from the CNPI.

Nurses in Canada are regulated at the provincial or territorial level. Specific titles used in reference to ANP may vary among provinces and territories. Currently, the only advanced practice nursing role with additional regulation and title protection, beyond RN, is the NP. NPs can autonomously make a diagnosis, order and interpret diagnostic tests, prescribe pharmaceuticals, and perform specific procedures within their legislated scope of practice (CNA, 2008, p. 7).

CNSs in Canada provide expert nursing care for specialized client populations and play a leading role in the development of clinical guidelines and protocols. Additionally, CNSs promote evidence-based practice, provide expert support and consultation, and facilitate system change (Association of Registered Nurses of Newfoundland and Labrador, 2007). Whereas the CNPI brought attention and recognition to the NP role in Canada, a similar national approach has not occurred with the CNS role. The CNA in partnership with its members and the Canadian Association of Advanced Practice Nurses continue to promote understanding and use of the CNS role. Outcomes and the impact of both the CNS and NP role have been highlighted in the new national ANP framework.

Several tools have been developed to assist with the implementation of Canadian ANP roles: the CNPI implementation and evaluation toolkit (CNA, 2006) and the PEPPA framework (Bryant-Lukosius & DiCenso, 2004). These tools serve as a structured and practical guide in assessing the need and readiness for ANP roles based on the population health needs of Canadians.

Although there continues to be a lack of understanding among health professionals in relationship to ANP, the professional and policy environment in Canada is generally receptive and looking to integrate a variety of ANP roles into the health-care system. Policy makers, decision makers, and nursing are working together to face future challenges as they refine and coordinate what this means in terms of services for the country (C. Buckley, personal communication, March 26, 2008).

Jamaica

The NP program in Jamaica started in 1977 as a response to the shortage of physicians and to provide cost-effective health care to the poor in rural and underserved areas. Since 1978, graduate NPs have been providing nursing and medical care to all age groups within the health-care delivery systems and in communities. Most NPs function from health centers in PHC settings, but some provide health services in hospitals within the public sector. Presently there are three specialties: family, pediatric, and mental health/psychiatric nursing. Qualified NPs come from at least 10 Caribbean countries.

In 2002, the education program was upgraded from certificate to the master's degree level and is now taught by the University of the West Indies (UWI) School of Nursing, Faculty of Medical Sciences. Nurse anesthetists (NAs) are technically classified as NPs; however, even though the NA program started many years before the NP program, it has yet to evolve to the master's level.

Despite these achievements, NPs and NAs are not registered or licensed as APNs and have no prescriptive privileges. Apart from being registered as nurses or midwives, at present and for the past 30 years, these nurses have no other official authority. Prescriptions have to be countersigned by doctors. A group of approximately 70 NPs on the island are working diligently to form a professional association to represent the quality services provided by these nurses, while also trying to move forward an agenda to enact policies supportive of advanced nursing roles (D. Less, personal communication, July 14, 2007, March 11, 2008).

Eastern Mediterranean: WHO-EMRO

In June 2001, the Regional Director for Nursing for the WHO—Eastern Mediterranean Region (EMR) convened the Fifth Meeting of the Regional Panel on Nursing to discuss ANP and nurse prescribing (WHO-EMR, 2001). Countries represented at the 3-day workshop in Islamabad, Pakistan, included Bahrain, Cyprus, Islamic Republic of Iran, Iraq, Jordan, Lebanon, Oman, Pakistan, Saudi Arabia, Sudan, Syrian Arab Republic, United Arab Emirates, and the Republic of Yemen. Twenty-two representatives from nursing, medicine, pharmacy, and ministries of health gathered to begin to develop a regional policy framework for ANP and mechanisms for nurse prescribing. The regional panel highlighted factors leading to development of the roles, as well as identifying strategies for the region (WHO-EMR, 2001). Obstacles and factors identified as supportive of development for ANP and nurse prescribing are provided in **Table 5-2**.

Strategies formulated for ANP development include:

■ Assessment of need and cost effectiveness for APN roles in the region
■ Development of APN curriculum and standards of practice
■ Definition of the role and identification of related revision of nurse practice acts to cover ANP

Significantly, there was consensus that authority for nurse prescribing within a range of essential drugs is an activity that could be allocated at some level to the competent general nurse and does not necessarily depend on the development of ANP. On the other hand, authority to prescribe was acknowledged as one of the many areas of expertise associated with APN roles. Additionally, it was agreed that these nursing roles require advanced education, regulatory changes, and expansion of traditional nursing.

TABLE 5-2	
WHO-EMRO Consensus on Factors Influencing Advanced Practice Nursing Development	
Obstacles	Support
Lack of a regional definition and role ambiguity	Increased population and community needs for health-care services
Absence of country-level educational or regulatory systems to support such roles	Improving levels of nursing education
No feasibility studies for advanced nursing practice needs	Desire in the region to improve quality of care and access
No awareness of the role among the public and health professionals	Research studies from outside the region supportive of advance nursing practice
Absence of nursing leadership at the policy level	Commitment of WHO toward development and use of nursing roles

Adapted from World Health Organization—Eastern Mediterranean Region. (2001). *Fifth meeting of the regional advisory panel on nursing and consultation on advanced practice nursing and nurse prescribing: Implications for regulation, nursing education and practice in the Eastern Mediterranean.* WHO-EM/NUR/348/E/L., Cairo: Author.

Recommendations were made for WHO-EMR (2001) to provide guidelines to assist countries in the region who are in the process of developing and strengthening ANP at all levels of health care. Additional assistance was requested from WHO to initiate and coordinate pilot projects to evaluate the impact and cost effectiveness of related change to realistically consider introduction of new nursing roles and nurse prescribing.

Bahrain

As a result of the WHO-EMR meeting in Pakistan in 2001, Bahrain received additional consultative support coordinated by WHO-EMRO to assess the country's readiness for ANP (Schober, 2007b). Consultation services found a stable organizational structure for health-care service provision within PHC. Two pediatric APNs educated in NP programs in the United States have recently started working in pediatric specialties in a hospital. Additional NPs, also educated in the United States, are faculty at the College of Health Sciences (CHS).

The CHS has had an RN-bachelor of science in nursing (BSN) degree for some years and established a 4-year BSN program in 2003. The BSN is now considered entry-level education for nursing practice in Bahrain. With proper planning, this places the CHS in an ideal position to develop an ANP master's degree program. Although the associate degree (AD) nursing programs have been discontinued, the majority of the current Bahraini nursing workforce are graduates from these programs. Postbasic 1-year education, called advanced practice programs, is available in the country. Lacking a current option for a masters program within Bahrain, nurses interested in obtaining ANP education are sponsored by the Ministry of Health to study in the United States or elsewhere (A. Matooq, personal communication, March 14, 2008).

Bahrain faces certain development challenges in developing an APN role suitable for its health services. They include:

- Identifying services that could be provided by APNs
- Developing an educational plan that meets the needs of the current workforce while properly planning for the potential APN roles
- Constructing strategies to ensure faculty are adequately qualified to deliver ANP education
- Establishing standards and regulations supportive of APN roles

Iran

In Iran, the degree of Masters in Nursing Sciences (MSN) was initiated in 1976, in the areas of nursing education and nursing administration. Graduate students focus on any of four subspecialties: (a) psychiatric, (b) pediatric, (c) community health, and (d) medical–surgical nursing. Fourteen schools of nursing offer graduate nursing degrees, and as of 1995 the 10 PhD programs in Iran have graduated nearly 40 individuals. The majority of these graduates are hired for clinical and educational positions in hospital, community, or academic settings.

The Farsi term *Karshenasae-e-Arshad* translates to advanced specialist. In the urban areas physicians and advanced specialist nurses share role responsibilities and functions. In rural regions of Iran, these nurses work in an autonomous manner much like APNs in the United States.

Nurses in Iran obtain a practice permit from the Ministry of Health and can open a private practice clinic (center for nursing services). Medical supervision by physicians is not required because the state Ministry of Health monitors health-care practices. However, the scope of practice is set and supervised by the physicians. Society needs determine curriculum content in the nursing programs. Recent changes include additional emphasis on geriatric, rehabilitation, women's health, neonatal health, military, and oncology nursing at the graduate level. Short-term continuing nursing education courses are available for school nursing, home health, intensive care, burn care, ostomy care, HIV/AIDS, and geriatric courses are also being developed for graduate nurses (M. Fooladi & F. Sharif, personal communication, March 12, 2008).

Oman

Oman is exploring the possibility of community nursing (CN) and community nurse practitioner (CNP) roles. Consultations, discussions, and reports of a successful nurse home-visiting project preceded WHO-EMRO supported consultation services. External consultation and related recommendations advise that progressing to CN and CNP roles would be a logical approach to strengthen community health-care services in the country (Schober, 2007a).

However, difficulties have arisen as (a) physicians are emphatically lobbying the Ministry of Health for highly specialized nurses to assist them in specialty areas such as diabetic clinics, (b) a lack of qualified people to educate for and supervise community service provision, and (c) limited understanding of the reality of what services a CN or CNP could provide. Nurses in more remote area health centers are already providing NP-like services but lacking the necessary advanced skills and qualifications. This is a major cause of concern for the director of nursing services at the Ministry of Health.

These dilemmas pose challenges for the Ministry of Health and nursing leaders as they consider options for ANP, while at the same time needing to address issues such as bridging the educational gaps of the current nursing workforce and meeting community health-care needs and the demands of the multidisciplinary workforce (Schober, 2007a).

Europe: WHO-EURO

With the aid of European Union funding, 13 universities across Europe ranging from the Republic of Ireland to Slovenia, and from Sweden to Italy, are collaborating with St. Martins College in England to establish a European Nurse Practitioner Masters Program. The program will use a combination of distance learning and classroom contact, with students being able to study at any of the involved universities in addition to their home university. The expected outcome will be a European master's degree delivered at standards set by the NP faculty organization in the United Kingdom. It is anticipated that this will encourage progress of the NP movement throughout the European Union (The Association of Advanced Nursing Practice Educators, 2007).

Finland

A physician shortage in Finland stimulated enhanced clinical roles for nurses in many municipalities and organizations. A Ministry of Education study in 2004 supported the need for APNs who could provide care and follow-up of patients with chronic illness. The APN role within secondary prevention will be increasingly important with an increase in the aging population.

Based on the ICN definition of NP/APN, the educational program is a part-time master's level, lasting 2.5 years, and was developed with a first cohort of 19 students. Curriculum for the program focuses on acute care advanced nursing assessment and follow-up for chronic diseases. The APN known as a clinic expert nurse will be expected to be competent in taking responsibility for comprehensive patient care and treatment and will also be the first point of contact for acute health-care problems. Salaries and legislation continue to be addressed as these nurses in new roles take their place within the Finnish health-care systems (ICN-APNetwork, 2007).

France

Interest in ANP is surfacing in France. In 2007, the Minister of Health appointed two leading health organizations, *Haute Autorité De Santé* (HAS) and *Observatoire National De La Demographie Des Professions De Santé* (ONDPS), to form a working group to explore future education for NPs, or *infirmiere cliniciennes* to generate recommendations. They were asked to examine how roles of health-care professionals may be redefined through the transfer of tasks and competencies with a view of improving care and adapting interventions to actual health-care demands (HAS, 2007). Preceding the formation of this working group, five research pilot projects in dissimilar areas of the country had been completed and 10 more are in progress (ICN-APNetwork, 2007).

Historically, although French nurses did acquire increased autonomy in 1978, they are still not considered a point of entry into the health-care system. Private practice nurses *(infirmières liberales)* depend on a medical order to deliver professional nursing care. Recognizing that the current arrangement of the health-care workforce will be inadequate to respond to future health-care needs, the health authorities are considering alternatives that include implementation of APN roles. Capitalizing on this situation the French nurses association (ANFIIDE) has conducted a public information campaign on ANP targeting nurses, authorities, and the public (Schober & Affara, 2006).

Ireland

The National Council for the Professional Development of Nursing and Midwifery (National Council, 2001) in Ireland provides a framework for establishment of APN and advanced midwife practitioner (AMP) roles and posts. In 1998, the Commission on Nursing acknowledged the need to provide a career pathway for nurses and midwives who wanted to remain in clinical practice and progress from registration to clinical specialization, which is linked to advanced practice. The National Council authored a definition and core concepts for the ANP and AMP posts that facilitate the related clinical pathways. Provision of these pathways was a response to the national and international development of advanced practice in nursing and midwifery.

Core concepts for ANP and AMP practice as defined by the National Council (2001) are autonomy in clinical practice, pioneering professional and clinical leadership, expert practitioner, and researcher. Educational preparation is required to be at least at a master's level. Clinical practice includes conducting comprehensive health assessment, and diagnosis and treatment of acute and chronic illness within a collaboratively agreed on scope of practice.

The National Council for the Professional Development of Nursing and Midwifery links the credential to a job description and the location where the APN or AMP will practice. Both the post and job description require approval by the council's accreditation committee. ANP or AMP titles can only be used after the nurse or midwife completes the certification process; however, even if the nurse or midwife meets the certification criteria, he or she is only eligible to practice when employed in an accredited and approved post. Once credentialed, the APN can hold the credential so long as he or she continues to work at the approved post in the same specialty (Schober & Affara, 2006).

Israel

Almost 100 years ago two U.S. nurses arrived in Israel to help improve the health of the Jewish nation in Palestine and established the Hadassah Medical Organization. The aim was to educate nurses to care for a population desperate for adequate health-care services. This tradition of innovation and professionalism continues to this day.

In 2002, the School of Nursing established a master's degree program in advanced practice nursing, the first of its kind in Israel. Its founders and supporters worked hard for many years to develop and set up a program that took the best of theoretical and clinical nursing knowledge from around the world and implemented it within the framework of the Israeli health-care delivery system.

Changes in Israel have created a demand for health-care practitioners who can provide optimal care within the context of the present health-care system. The graduate of the program, known as an APN, is a clinician who can integrate advanced clinical skills with systems knowledge, educational commitment, and leadership ability using clinical judgment and knowledge gained from graduate studies to promote evidence-based practice at the bedside and to persuade other nurses to integrate this practice. The view of the school of nursing is that master's education in general has been shown to develop and refine analytical skills, broad-based perspectives, articulation of viewpoints and positions, and the ability to more clearly connect theory to practice and clinical professional skills.

Economic and professional processes have led to the development of a new model of practice that combines characteristics of the roles of both the NP and the CNS. The new nurse practice role is called the APN. Nursing practice according to this model applies to the entire continuum of health-care delivery (from the hospital to the community) and requires learning and a knowledge base gleaned from both roles. The model attempts to create a balance between the responsibility and authority associated with direct patient care of individuals and groups with an advanced professional role at the level of change agent, teacher, and researcher. A list of clinical competencies for the entry-level graduate of a clinical master's program has been delineated. However, certain aspects of an APN role, such as diagnostic and prescriptive authority, are not possible in Israel at this time. The master's program is based on a combination of the NP and CNS roles, taking into account the realities of the Israeli health-care system.

At present there is no formal standing in Israel for any of the ANP models. Program graduates assume roles in a variety of settings, using their increased knowledge in leadership capacities to clinically improve health-care provision (B. Reznick & M. Rom, personal communication, March 10, 2008).

Netherlands

As of March 2008, there are approximately 1500 NPs working in the Netherlands in all fields of practice, including general practice. Since 2002, nursing education has had bachelor and master programs for nursing education. Currently there are master's educational programs in nine cities.

The shortage of physicians that prompted the introduction of NP roles in the Netherlands has been resolved, but the numbers of NPs continue to increase in contrast to physician assistant (PA) numbers. At one point in time it was thought introduction of PAs would threaten NP development, but that has not been the case.

NPs have been accepted as professionals providing quality care and friendly advice. Each year the government financially supports the education of 250 new NP students, including 20% of their salary and the cost of their preceptors. Legislation has progressed as well, including title protection and prescriptive authority. In 2008, the national description of the NP will be completed, resulting in the opening of an official national register. NPs who are registered will have the option for prescribing and will be allowed to work independently from physicians. In this capacity the NP will be responsible for a well-described patient category. The financial structure in the country is not yet accustomed to the NP services, but the insurance companies are becoming more powerful. It is envisioned they will contract with NPs in the near future (P. Roodbol, personal communication, March 16, 2008).

Sweden

Sweden is exploring the use of NPs as a strategy to improve access to PHC, along with improving care to the elderly in the community. With these targets in mind, educational programs have been established for these two areas. In Skaraborg, the PHC authorities worked with the University of Skovde to develop a model and educational program that met the requirements of the National Board of Health and Welfare. Community PHC needs and the educational preparation of the NP were taken into consideration (Schober & Affara, 2006).

The initial batch of students enrolled in 2003 faced challenges to introduce a new nursing role that fits the Swedish health-care system and is acceptable to all stakeholders. In the process, a definition for the ANP was negotiated:

> *An Advanced Nurse Practitioner in Primary Health Care is a registered nurse with special education as a district nurse with the right to prescribe certain drugs, and with a post graduate education that enables [the advanced nurse practitioner] an increased and deepened competence to be independently responsible for medical decisions, prescribing of drugs and treatment of health problems within a certain area of health care (Schober & Affara, 2006, p. 6).*

It is interesting to note that prescriptive authority for nurses in Sweden was in place approximately 10 years before the consideration and development of ANP.

Switzerland

The Institute of Nursing Science (INS) at the University of Basel, Switzerland, introduced course material including formal clinical assessment, physical examination skills, and clinical reasoning for bachelor nursing education in 2001. As of 2006, six universities of applied science either offer or plan to offer, the BSN degree including similar content (ICN-APNetwork, 2007). Such changes are significant for APN development as moving from diploma-based education to the BSN will provide a stronger foundation for the generalist nurse, and thus, a sounder educational background for the APN studies.

The INS at the University of Basel has also invested in ANP through a master's degree in nursing science, research, and clinical development activities. The momentum to create APN positions originated with insightful nurse leaders who could envision an advanced nursing role and physicians who showed interest in working with nurses with higher level of clinical skills. Exploration of ANP coincides at a time when attention is also being drawn to expanding nursing roles to work that appears to be more like PAs as the country copes with an anticipated physician shortage. Enlightened decision makers hope to strengthen nursing at this challenging time. However, it should be noted that the drive to ANP development is occurring in the absence of a framework that addresses legal, policy, standards, and reimbursement issues (Schober & Affara, 2006).

United Kingdom (England, Northern Ireland, Scotland, and Wales)

Within the United Kingdom, the countries of England, Northern Ireland, Scotland, and Wales are developing the NP roles in different ways. White (2001) describes the emergence of the NP movement in the United Kingdom as a response to the changing demands within health-care systems and acknowledgment that the traditional medical model alone is not sufficient to provide comprehensive health care for community populations.

A reduction in doctors' hours and an overall shortage of general practitioners in some areas accelerated the move toward NPs in acute- and primary-care settings. Additionally, government-initiated pilot programs to address the needs of special groups, such as refugees, the homeless, the mentally ill, traveling families, and the elderly, have increased the use of NPs and provision of services in a range of settings. All of these changes must be seen in the context of the Labour government's modernization program for the health service and their expectations for clinical effectiveness, service quality, and clinical governance.

The year 2002 represented a milestone in NP roles, celebrating the 10th anniversary of the first graduates from the Royal College of Nursing (RCN) NP program. The initial 15 graduates paved the way for NPs now practicing throughout the United Kingdom. The NP degree program, originally developed by the RCN in 1990, has formed the basis for RCN Accreditation of NP programs, using 15 standards and associated criteria as the basis for approval (RCN, 2008). Currently 13 universities have used this method for explicitly demonstrating the quality of their programs, and among them, deliver 26 pathways, ranging from a generic approach to a more specific focus including primary, acute, emergency, pediatrics, neonatal, and cancer care. However, as demand for NP's and advanced nurses increases, the number of universities providing such programs has escalated. For example, the Association of Advanced Nursing Practice Educators (AANPE) now has 43 higher education institutions in its membership from across the UK (AANPE, 2007).

NPs are present in health-care settings that include general practice, walk-in centers, accident and emergency units, and many other specialties. NP practice in the United Kingdom includes diagnosis with advances in prescribing rights, which increasingly include prescription of medication. The move, originating in England, to enable nurses to undergo a specified nonmedical prescribing program has resulted in over 10,000 nurses who are now classed as *independent prescribers,* and as a consequence, can prescribe almost everything from the British National Formulary (Nursing and Midwifery Council [NMC], 2006).

This has resulted in NPs being able to deliver more autonomous care and greatly opens up the opportunities for NP innovation; however, it is worth noting that not all nurses classed as independent prescribers are NPs.

Despite all this activity, regulation of NP practice has not yet been introduced into the United Kingdom. The Nursing and Midwifery Council (NMC), which has regulatory responsibility for the whole of the United Kingdom, has submitted proposals for regulation of ANPs to provide greater public protection to the department of health and is awaiting a response (NMC, 2007). Within their proposals, it is notable that the NMC have used the term ANP to make explicit the level of practice that should be expected from a nurse working in this role (K. Maclaine, personal communication, March 4, 2008).

South-East Asia: WHO-SEARO

Thailand

The Nursing Council of Thailand adopted the ANP concept in 1998, and in 2003, the first group of 49 APNS were certified and awarded the title APN. There are five specialties for certification: medical/surgical, pediatrics, maternal/child, community, and psychiatric/mental health (ICN-APNetwork, 2007).

In response to an urgent need for community health-care services, the country identified short- and long-term goals to offer 4-month education programs for general NPs to work in the community as primary care providers. Even though one of the first postbasic NP programs was established in the 1970s, it was health-care reform and the drive for a universal health-care coverage system, implemented in the country in 2002, that accelerated the development of NP educational programs.

To develop strategic planning for enhancing capacity among NPs, a study was conducted by Hanucharurnkul, Suwisith, Piasue, and Terathongkum (2007) that explored characteristics and work settings of 1928 NPs and provides a picture of those certified by the Thailand Nursing and Midwifery Council. Strategies derived from this study are:

1. Extend within 5 years the entry-level education to a master level by acknowledging the 4-month programs that were originally initiated to respond to PHC needs of the country.
2. Establish NP positions in the health-care system such that when APNs are master's graduates and certified, they would be eligible for the title of APN/MN and have an associated increase in salary.

Findings are consistent with those in other illustrations in this chapter that confirm the perceived usefulness of the NP role. However, at times NPs were functioning at levels beyond their defined scope of practice; their position was not adequately separated from those of other nurses; and administrators did not support them sufficiently.

Western Pacific: WHO-WPRO

Australia

Australia has been considering the development of NP roles since 1990 (Offredy, 1999). This resulted in the implementation of pilot projects first in New South Wales (NSW) and then in most other states and territories of Australia. The results from the initial projects support the findings that NPs are feasible, safe, and effective in their ability to provide quality health-care services in a range of settings (NSW Health Department, 1998).

In Australia, the NP title is protected and only nurses who have been authorized by the state and territories Nurse's Registration Board may use the NP title. A study by Gardener, Dunn, Carryer, and Gardner (2006) supports master's degree of education as preparation for the role from two perspectives. Findings suggest that a master's education is needed to meet the demands of the role and to also provide the necessary credibility with the community and other health-care disciplines, regarding the professional standing of these clinicians. Most states and territories of Australia agree that a master's of NP, or its equivalent, is the minimal level of education required to practice.

The Mutual Recognition Act of 1992 and the Trans Tasman Mutual Recognition Act of 1999 recognize nurses educated in all states of Australia and those educated in New Zealand, regardless of differences within programs. In 2004, the Australian Nursing and Midwifery Council (ANMC) in conjunction with the Nursing Council of New Zealand commissioned a project to develop competency standards for the NP to further ensure delivery of safe and competent care. These competency standards are used in the license renewal process to assess NPs educated overseas and are applied by universities to assess standards when developing curriculum (ANMC, 2006).

In 2008, there were more than 230 authorized NPs in Australia. A recent study by Gardener et al. (2006), found two-thirds of NPs in Australia reported their role is "extremely limited" because of a difference between state and federal governmental laws. At a state level NPs are able to write prescriptions and refer patients to other health-care professionals; however, at a federal level, NPs do not have access to pharmaceutical benefits scheme or Medicare provider numbers. This results in patients having to pay a premium when their prescription is filled at a pharmacy, placing these patients at a disadvantage because they do not have equal access to government subsidies for health care (Queensland University of Technology, 2008).

In Australia, NPs are steadily being introduced throughout the country, while continuing to face country specific challenges. The Australian Nurse Practitioner Association has been established with representation or the facility for representation, from all states and territories of Australia, in the hope of providing a unified voice for NPs in the country (A. Green, personal communication, March 20, 2008).

Hong Kong, China

Hong Kong has been pursuing the concept of the APN/NP for several years, while facing complicated governmental, clinical, and academic challenges. Although there is evidence of strong nurse-led clinics at Queen Elizabeth Hospital, educational initiatives have found it difficult to coordinate appropriate didactic courses and clinical practicum for advanced roles. Hong Kong has still to find a champion for APN roles to catch a foothold within the health-care systems.

The Hospital Authority of Hong Kong, eager to motivate nurses to remain in clinical practice, introduced the nurse specialist position in 1994. The introduction of new nursing roles without regulatory oversight, resulted in uneven clinical, education, and research development (Chang & Wong, 2001). Continued development for APNs continues to be linked to the enhancement of basic nursing education and efforts by the Hong Kong Hospital Authority to introduce a new grading structure and career ladder intended to improve the clinical focus for nursing (Schober & Affara, 2006).

Islands of the Western Pacific (Cayman Islands, Fiji, and Samoa)

NPs and other midlevel practitioners have provided health-care services for the populations of the Pacific island countries for more than 20 years. The rural and remote nature of this region and a shortage of physicians encouraged governments to explore the most appropriate models to provide comprehensive health-care services. Demographics help determine what is the best approach for the Pacific islands in initiating education and practice guidelines for NPs. Reasons for educating nurses for NP roles in the Pacific islands include (WHO-Western Pacific Region [WPR], 2001):

- Nurses are already present in the workforce of most countries and usually compose the largest category of health professionals.
- Nurses are currently living and working in underserved areas.
- Nurses are providing a wide range of preventive and curative services.
- Nurses are considered to be an adaptable, multitalented resource of the workforce.

Strategies recommended by WHO-WPRO for developing and sustaining a midlevel practitioner workforce include:

- Legal protection
- Standard treatment guidelines
- Ongoing clinical supervision
- Continuing education
- Career structure or career ladder (WHO-WPR, 2001)

Cayman Islands

The emergence of ANP services in the Cayman Islands provides an example of how NP-like roles evolve and develop in response to the needs of the people, as well as within geographical circumstances. The initiation of NP-like services started in 1930 with provision of care by a local midwife to meet community health needs. Physician services were scarce and conditions were primitive, with populations residing in remote locations. NPs services progressed with the official employment of a nurse experienced in midwifery and community health to provide PHC. Comprehensive health-care services were provided in homes, schools, and clinic settings (Slocombe, 2000).

Expansion of clinical expertise progressed rapidly during subsequent years, with the nurse as the main health-care provider on the islands. The nurse diagnosed, treated, prescribed, and dispensed what was viewed to be necessary. Conditions receiving care were "whatever walked in through the door" (M. Slocombe, personal communication, 2002). Immunization, antenatal, well-baby, nutritional, diabetic, and hypertensive clinics were held, with backup consultation and collaboration provided by phone call to the nearest hospital or by appointment with periodic visiting physicians. The nurse took on the multifaceted role and duties of counselor, administrator, staff supervisor, health educator, accountant, and secretary. Absence of adequate support by other professionals, lack of resources, and limited educational opportunities created frustration and obstacles to professional development.

The location of the three Cayman Islands, situated in the Caribbean Sea between Jamaica and Cuba, contributes to the diversity, as well as the uniqueness, of presenting conditions. Cuban refugees and rafters trickle in for health screening and health care; periodic care for prison inmates is provided; and hurricane evacuation preparedness is essential for the health centers. The tourist industry with visitors from more than 80 countries requires the nurse to be knowledgeable about trauma and injuries related to deep sea diving (Slocombe, 2000).

Fiji

Fiji is made up of over 300 islands, with over 60% of the population living in rural or remote settings. Through an arrangement of health centers and nursing stations, authorities have attempted to address health-care challenges by providing preventive and PHC services supported by subdivisional and referral hospitals.

Staffing of facilities has been a major problem, especially in rural and remote areas. In 1988, an NP program was developed in response to this difficulty. The Fiji School of Nursing (FSN) is the base for the NP program, admitting RNs and nurse-midwives (NMWs). The first NPs graduated in 1999; and in March 2007, the fourth class completed their academic program and progressed to a 6-month internship. The program has now become regional, including nurses from Tonga and the Marshall Islands. The immediacy of health-care needs prohibited education at the master's level initially, but efforts are being made to increase educational levels. Part of this strategy is enhancing the educational level of the program faculty through a cooperative program with James Cook University in Australia.

NPs in Fiji have an established scope of practice and work under published protocols, allowing them prescriptive privileges. Postings for positions are listed by the Public Service Commission, with most NPs employed by the Ministry of Health. These nurses have been widely accepted by communities and other health-care providers. There is strong support from the directors of health services to continue the educational program. Access to continuing education and career pathways are among the challenges facing NPs in Fiji (ICN-APNetwork, 2007).

Samoa

Education for nurse specialist practice in Samoa is a year of postgraduate study following a generalist nurse preparation. Clinical practice for a nurse specialist reflects in-depth knowledge and relevant skills that are focused on a specific area of nursing and directed toward a defined population or a defined area of activity. Specialist practice may occur at any point along a continuum, from beginning to advanced.

Nurse specialists are considered to be APNs, with practice focusing on health assessment and clinical decision making. Physicians are consulted or accept referrals for confirmation of findings and prescribing of medications. Currently nurses prescribe in life-threatening situations, but the nursing law is being reviewed with respect to wider prescribing rights. Mental health specialist nurses lead community-based family-focused services with minimal of assistance from the volunteer part-time psychiatrist. This service is totally developed and steered by a nurse consultant and her small team of nurses (I. Enoka, personal communication, April 1, 2008).

New Zealand

ANP was initially recognized in 1988 at two levels in New Zealand. The New Zealand Nurses' Organization's (NZNO) credentialing process certified nurses as nurse-clinicians or nurse consultants (clinical). Once the NP model was introduced in 2000, NZNO phased out and ceased its certification process in 2006, when regulation of NPs came under the jurisdiction of the Nursing Council of New Zealand (S. Trim, personal communication, March 11, 2008).

A task force established in 1997 studied barriers to nursing practice and recommended the development of an advanced role. The Nursing Council of New Zealand (NCNZ) then set up a working group to develop a regulatory framework. Following significant consultation, a framework was agreed on and published (NCNZ, 2001). The framework includes standards for the approval of specific master's program and process for such approval, a title (NP), competencies, and a description of the role and a process for endorsement. The role was defined as follows:

> A Nurse Practitioner is a registered nurse practicing at an advanced practice level in a specific scope of practice, who has been recognized at Master's level of education and has been recognized and approved by the Nursing Council as a Nurse Practitioner (NCNZ, 2001, p. 9).

The New Zealand NP model is depicted in **Figure 5-1**.

The requirements for endorsement are:

- Completion of an approved master's program (or approved equivalent)
- A minimum of 4 years clinical experience in a specific specialty area
- Successful assessment against the NP competencies by an approved panel, which includes an NP (or clinical specialist if there are no NPs in the specialty area of practice) and an experienced medical clinician in the same specialty

The applicant formally applies to the council and must present a portfolio that includes a curriculum vitae, transcript of education preparation, research, publications, and evidence of clinical practice that includes descriptions, case studies, case notes from assessments, and endorsements of practice. The panel interview includes a presentation by the applicant describing relevant clinical practice and a response to panel questions that include clinical vitae and scenario testing (M. Clark, personal communication, March 4, 2008).

The first NP in New Zealand was endorsed in late 2001, and initially title protection was achieved through trade-marking. Following the enactment of the Health Practitioners Competence Assurance Act of 2003, the council established a part of the register for NP, and formally stated, as required under the legislation, the following description of the role:

> Nurse Practitioners are expert nurses who work within a specific area of practice incorporating advanced knowledge and skills. They practise both independently and in collaboration with other health care professionals to promote health, prevent disease and to diagnose, assess and manage people's health needs.

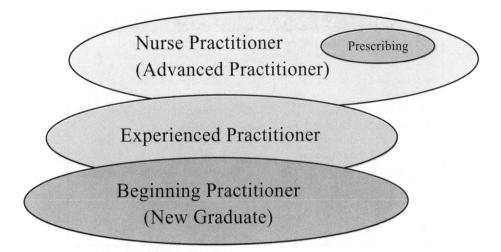

FIGURE 5-1 The New Zealand Framework is depicted in an illustration that portrays a view of the stages of practice that a nurse pursues to become an NP. *(Adapted from Nursing Council of New Zealand, with permission.)*

They provide a wide range of assessment and treatment interventions, including differential diagnoses, ordering, conducting and interpreting diagnostic and laboratory tests and administering therapies for the management of potential or actual health needs. They work in partnership with individuals, families, whanau (indigenous health workers) and communities across a range of settings. Nurse Practitioners may choose to prescribe medicines within their specific area of practice. Nurse Practitioners also demonstrate leadership as consultants, educators, managers and researchers and actively participate in professional activities, and in local and national policy development (New Zealand Government, 2004, p. 2959).

NPs choose their area of practice (scope of practice), which is placed on the register as a condition. This is done to reflect the New Zealand legislation. **Table 5-3** provides details on specialized areas (scopes of practice) in New Zealand.

A report released by the Ministry of Health for district health boards outlined the future use of NPs (New Zealand Ministry of Health, 2002). A variety of activities to assess and provide visibility for advance practice continue to be in progress. A Nurse Practitioner Advisory Committee of New Zealand, composed of four professional groups, NZNO, National Council of Maori Nurses, College of Nurses Aotearoa, and Australia New Zealand College of Mental Health Nurses, is driving the implementation of the role.

In 1999, an amendment to the Medicines Act of 1981 enabled the government to issue regulations allowing prescribing for "designated prescribers," and thus set a pathway for nurses to prescribe. This was followed in 2002 by the requisite regulations to allow NPs to prescribe in child health and aged care. These regulations were very restrictive and only one NP (a U.S. citizen qualified NP in child health) obtained the right to prescribe under them. Extensive lobbying by the profession resulted in much broader regulations in 2005, which allowed all NPs who are authorized by the council to prescribe from an extensive formulary following established and published criteria (New Zealand Gazette, November 10, 2005).

TABLE 5-3

Areas of Nurse Practitioner Specialization in New Zealand

Cardiac care	Ophthalmology
Elective perioperative care	Pain management
Aging care	Palliative care
Mental health	Primary health care
Mental health/intellectual disability	Respiratory care
Child/adolescent health	Solid organ transplantation
Diabetes/related conditions	Urology
Emergency	Women's health
High dependency	Wound care
Neonatal care	

M. Clark, personal communication, March 4, 2008.

The uptake of NPs has been slower than expected but seems to be gaining momentum. As of March 2008, there are 45 NPs (1% of the practicing nursing workforce), 26 of whom are authorized to prescribe (M. Clark & S. Trim, personal communication, March 4, 2008).

South Korea

It could be said that NP-like nursing roles have been in place in Korea since the time of the "medicine lady" in the 15th century. Care provided by the medicine ladies included deliveries, physical examinations, acupuncture, and prescribing of herbal medicines (J. Kang, personal communication, November 15, 2007).

Community health nurse practitioners (CHNPs) have been providing comprehensive primary health-care services in rural communities of South Korea since the health care law for provision of health care for rural residents was legislated in 1980. CHNPs provide PHC to approximately 28% of the rural population in South Korea; however, this number is decreasing because it is more difficult to attract nurses to work in the rural areas (J. Tang, personal communication, November 15, 2007).

Haho Clinic, located 2 hours from Seoul between Yoju and Ichon, has provided clinic services for the community and the surrounding area since 1985. The scope of practice for the CHNPs includes diagnosis, prescriptive authority, and referral to other practitioners. Additionally, home visits, health education, disease management, immunizations, school health services, and care for the elderly are part of the health-care service provision with additional support by nurses and community helpers. The nurse specialist system was formalized in Korea to fulfill changes in the medical environment. Anesthesia, public health, mental health, and home health-care nurses are approved for practice under the Medical Service Law. The Special Law for Agriculture approves the CHNP for practice as a nurse specialist.

Discussions attempting to clarify issues related to APNs began in the 1990s. In 2003, the medical law revision identified qualifications for the APN and designated 13 areas of specialization. Qualifications include master's level education, pass of the certification examination, and experience in a chosen specialty. The first certification examination was given in 2005 (J. Kang, personal communication, 2007). As in many countries, the Korean Nurses Association faces difficulty obtaining consensus from the nursing community on scope of practice, educational requirements, and titling (Schober & Affara, 2006).

Singapore

Singapore established an APN midwife-nurse program in 2003, offering clinical studies in adult care and mental health, while viewing the program as generic in emphasis. In other words, this is considered to be a comprehensive APN degree with no designated specialty as the students exit. The third batch of APNs will graduate in 2008 and complete their internship year before applying for certification with the Singapore Nursing Board. Simultaneously, a new offering for the APN specialty in critical care will be introduced in 2008 in response to a request from directors of nursing who want to add these specialized APNs to the nursing staff in critical care units.

In 2005, the Minister for Health Singapore presented a bill to Parliament to establish a register for APNs. This is expected to help with the systemic development of this category of clinical nurse, educated to a master's level in nursing, in becoming a key player in Singapore's drive to keep health care affordable while maintaining quality services. Consistent with this view, the Singapore nursing board developed a clinical nursing career path for the APN, similar to the career paths that exist for management and education.

Key decision makers in education, policy, and administration are working to adapt models and frameworks from the United States, while at the same time attempting to introduce APN roles, suitable for hospital and community settings in the country. Visibility and support for this advance in nursing is evidenced up to the Ministry of Health level, where a request has been made to have 200 APNs in place in various specialties in Singapore by the year 2017.

Taiwan

ANP development in Taiwan focuses on the acute care nurse practitioner (ACNP) roles. NPs are mainly educated at hospital training programs. Currently there are two universities, Chang Gung University and National Taipei College of Nursing, that offer NP education at the graduate level. NP education will progress to the higher educational system in the future. An NP certification examination was initiated in 2006. For the first examination 1658 attended the test (including both written and mini Objective Structured Clinical Examination [OSCE]) with 582 passing (passing rate = 35.1%). The OSCE is a test of clinical skills such as communication, clinical examination, prescribing, and interpretation of diagnostic evidence.

The Department of Health is trying to estimate the numbers of NPs in Taiwan that will provide an opportunity for the academic community to conduct a national study on role competency, human resources, and clinical practice of NPs in the country. This 2-year study and additional research will help determine scope of practice and guide NP development (J. Tang, personal communication, March 20, 2008).

CONCLUSION

In reviewing country illustrations, it appears that research and description of APN development confirms the usefulness of ANP and supports the view that these nursing roles are feasible, sustainable, and able to provide quality competent health care. Legislation and regulations often lag behind actual practice; disagreement exists among practice acts; and progression presents as more of an intricate maze or puzzle, than a picture of coordinated forward motion. International momentum supportive of ANP services is increasing; however, NP and

APN initiatives are fraught with frustrations, obstacles and challenges as leaders attempt to activate schemes that will ultimately change the profile of the health workforce and care delivery systems worldwide. Role ambiguity and confusion regarding titling, scope of practice, educational preparation, and credentialing continue to present obstacles that must be addressed. A consistent definition and related terminology will enhance possibilities for sound standards for credentialing and legislation, an essential component to legitimatizing the ANP concept globally.

For ANP to thrive in health systems, we believe that a number of areas related to role development need to be confronted and managed successfully. This includes being able to embrace the diversity of health-care systems worldwide without losing ANP core characteristics and reaching international consensus on the scope of practice founded on the core values of nursing. Additionally, we agree that an ideal scope of practice engages APNs in a range of advocacy, illness prevention, treatment of disease, health promotion activities, health planning, and policy development.

Challenges lie in the capacity of ANP advocates and implementers to achieve consistency across clinical and educational models. Continually evaluating and reviewing practice by adding new competencies that reflect dynamic changes in health care will be essential. Finally, APNs will be asked to provide evidence that they are a cost-effective, valued, and a sustainable addition to health-care teams and provision of services. Evidence that demonstrates the ability to provide care in partnership with patients, their families within communities, and in collaboration with other health-care professionals will provide a strong foundation for an innovative addition to comprehensive health-care services.

References

Affara, F. A. (2006). SWOT analysis in relation to advanced nursing practice becoming recognised as a valid part of nursing and health care provision globally. Retrieved February 26, 2008, from the American Academy of Nurse Practitioners Web site: www.aanp.org/NR/rdonlyres/edw7gnx2cgspgvfu6fc23fsp3u456amdanqkeqtde4xg7654qtjkzhzpw7crgr2vsxqsfwkemyjs5vx5lfs ediuowsc/SWOTNPAPNJune2006.ppt#261,2,Strengths.

Association of Advanced Nursing Practice Educators. (2007). Membership Census Autumn 2007: Advanced nursing practice courses results. Retrieved January 10, 2008, from the Association of Advanced Nursing Practice Educators Web site: www.aanpe.org/AANPHome/tabid/448/Default.aspx.

Association of Registered Nurses of Newfoundland and Labrador. (2007). *Advanced practice-clinical nurse specialist.* St. John's: Author.

Australian Nursing and Midwifery Council. (2006). National competency standards for the nurse practitioner. Retrieved November 11, 2008, from the Australian Nursing and Midwifery Council Web site: www.anmc.org.au/docs/ Competency_Standards_for_the_Nurse_Practitioner.pdf.

Bryant, R. (2005). *Regulation, roles and competency development* (ICN global nursing review initiative Issue paper No. 1). Retrieved February 25, 2008, from the International Council of Nurses Web site: www.icn.ch/global/ Issue1Regulation.pdf.

Bryant-Lukosius, D., & DiCenso, A. (2004). A framework for the introduction and evaluation of advanced practice nursing roles. *Journal of Advanced Nursing, 48*(5), 530–540.

Buchan, J., & Calman, L. (2004). *Implementing nurse prescribing: An updated review of current practice internationally* (Monograph No. 16). Geneva: ICN.

Buchan, J., & Calman, L. (2005). *Skill-mix and policy change in the health workforce: Nurses in advanced roles.* (Working paper). Retrieved February 25, 2008, from the Organisation for Economic Co-operation and Development Web site: www.oecd.org/dataoecd/30/28/33857785.pdf.

Canadian Nurses Association. (2006). *Canadian nurse practitioner initiative: Implementation and evaluation toolkit for nurse practitioners in Canada.* Ottawa, Ontario: Author.

Canadian Nurses Association. (2008). *Advanced nursing practice: A national framework.* Ottawa, Ontario: Author.

Chang, K. P. K., & Wong, T. (2001). The nurse specialist role in Hong Kong: Perceptions of nurse specialists. *Journal of Advanced Nursing, 36*(1), 32–40.

Gardner, G., Dunn, S., Carryer, J., & Gardner, A. (2006). Competency and capability: Imperative for nurse practitioner education. *Australian Journal of Advanced Nursing, 24*(1), 8–14.

Geyer, N., Naude, S., & Sithole, G. (2002). Legislative issues impacting on the practice of the South African nurse practitioner. *Journal of the American Academy of Nurse Practitioners, 14*(1), 11–15.

Hanucharurnkul, S., Suwisith, N., Piasue, N., & Terathongkum, S. (2007). Characteristics and working situation of nurse practitioners in Thailand. Retrieved March 14, 2008, from the International Council of Nurses Web site: www.icn-apnetwork.org.

Haute Autorité de Santé. (2007). *Délégation, transfert, nouveaux métiers . . . : Conditions des nouvelles formes de coopération entre professionnels de santé.* Paris: Author.

International Council of Nurses. (2002). Definition and characteristics of the role. Retrieved February 27, 2008, from the International Council of Nurses Web site: www.icn-apnetwork.org.

International Council of Nurses. (2007). *Positive practice environments: Quality workplaces=quality patient care.* Retrieved March 5, 2008, from the International Council of Nurses Web site: www.icn.ch/indkit2007.htm.

International Council of Nurses. (2008a). *Nursing care continuum—framework and competencies.* Geneva: Author.

International Council of Nurses. (2008b). *The scope of practice, standards and competencies of the advanced practice nurse.* Geneva: Author.

International Council of Nurses–APNetwork. (2007). Retrieved March 14, 2008, from APNetwork Web site: www.apnetwork.org.

Madubuko, G. (2001). *NP/ANP development in West Africa.* Retrieved March 11, 2008, from the International Council Nurses Web site: www.icn-apnetwork.org.

National Council for the Professional Development of Nursing and Midwifery. (2001). *Framework for the establishment of advanced nurse practitioner and advanced midwife practitioner posts.* Dublin: National Council for the Professional Development of Nursing and Midwifery.

National Health Institute. (2002). *Curriculum for the training of family nurse practitioners: Post-basic course.* Gaborone, Botswana: National Health Institute.

New South Wales Health Department. (1998). *Nurse practitioner services in NSW.* Sydney: Author.

New Zealand Gazette. November 10, 2005. No. 188, p. 4750. Notice No. 7428.

New Zealand Government. (2004). *New Zealand Gazette.* Issue No. 120. Wellington: Author.

New Zealand Ministry of Health. (2002). *Nurse practitioners in New Zealand.* Wellington: Author.

Nursing Council of New Zealand. (2001). *The nurse practitioner: Responding to health needs in New Zealand.* Wellington: Author.

Nursing and Midwifery Council. (2006). *Standards of proficiency for nurse and midwife prescribers.* Retrieved March 10, 2008, from the Nursing and Midwifery Council Web site: www.nmc-uk.org/aFrameDisplay.aspx?DocumentID=1312&Keyword=.

Nursing and Midwifery Council. (2007). *Advanced nursing practice update—19 June 2007.* Retrieved March 10, 2008 from the Nursing and Midwifery Council Web site: www.nmc-uk.org/aArticle.aspx?ArticleID=2528.

Offredy, M. (1999). The nurse practitioner role in New South Wales: Development and policy. *Nursing Standard, 13*(43): 38–41.

Pilane, C., Neube, P., Seitio, O. (2007). *Ensuring quality in affiliated health training institutions: Advanced diploma programmes in Botswana.* Retrieved March 17, 2008, from the International Council of Nurses Web site: www.icn-apnetwork.org/.

Pulcini, J., Loke, A. Y., Gul, R., & Jelic, M. (2007). *An international pilot survey on advanced practice nursing: Education, practice and regulatory issues.* Retrieved February 26, 2008 from American Academy of Nurse Practitioners Web site: www.aanp.org/NR/rdonlyres/e26g4jrmksqb2oimumtuxcec2e2ssguacxw2s6h6t3gyxhgxkeabqwwo3srtegsrdftqyhckpgh2sxm6plgefkacw4h/APNpilotsurvey.ppt.

Queensland University of Technology. (2008). *Nurse practitioners hamstrung and patients disadvantaged: Study.* [Media release]. Retrieved May 10, 2008, from Queensland University Web site: www.news.qut.edu.au/cgi-bin/WebObjects/News.woa/wa/goNewsPage?newsEventID=15407.

Roodbol, P. (2004). Survey carried out prior to the 3rd ICN-International Nurse Practitioner/Advanced Nursing Practice Network Conference. Network Conference. Gronigen, The Netherlands.

Roodbol, P. (2005) *Willing o'-the-wisps, stumbling runs, toll roads and song lines: Study into the structural rearrangement of tasks between nurses and physicians.* Unpublished summary of doctoral thesis.

Royal College of Nursing. (2008). *Advanced nurse practitioners—an RCN guide to the advanced nurse practitioner, role, competencies and programme accreditation.* London: Author.

Schober, M., & Affara, F. (2006). *Advanced nursing practice.* Oxford: Blackwell Publishing.

Schober, M. (2007a). Development of advanced community nursing/nurse practitioner roles and educational programmes in Oman, EM/NUR/392/E/R/07.07. Cairo: WHO-EMRO. Unpublished.

Schober, M. (2007b). Development of a framework for advanced practice nursing in Bahrain, assignment report EM/NUR/394/E/R07.7. Cairo: WHO-EMRO. Unpublished.

Schober, M. (2008). *Advanced nursing practice: The global experience, reflections on nursing leadership, first quarter.* Indianapolis: Sigma Theta Tau.

Slocombe, M. (2000). *Development of community health services in the Cayman Islands.* International NP/APN Conference, San Diego, CA.

White, M. (2001). *Emergence of the nurse practitioner in the UK.* Geneva: Centre for Nursing Roles.

World Health Organization—Eastern Mediterranean Region. (2001). *Fifth meeting of the regional advisory panel on nursing and consultation on advanced practice nursing and nurse prescribing: Implications for regulation, nursing education and practice in the Eastern Mediterranean.* WHO-EM/NUR/348/E/L. Cairo: Author.

World Health Organization. (2002a). *Human resources, national health systems: Shaping the agenda for action.* (Final Report). Geneva: Author.

World Health Organization. (2002b). *Nursing and midwifery services: Strategic directions 2002–2008.* Geneva: Author.

World Health Organization. (2006). *Working together for health: World health report 2006.* Geneva: Author.

World Health Organization. (2007). *The global recommendations and guidelines on task shifting.* Geneva: Author.

World Health Organization—Western Pacific Region. (2001). *Mid-level and nurse practitioners in the Pacific: Models and issues.* Manila: Author.

Zurn, P., Dolea, C., & Stilwell, B. (2005). Nurse retention and recruitment: Developing a motivated workforce. Retrieved February 25, 2008, from the International Council of Nurses Web site: www.icn.ch/global/Issue4Retention.pdf.

The Practice Environment

6

Payment for Advanced Practice Nursing Services: Past, Present, and Future

Karen R. Robinson

INTRODUCTION

History has shown that nurse practitioners (NPs), clinical nurse specialists (CNSs), certified nurse-midwives (CNMs), and certified nurse anesthetists (CRNAs), collectively referred to as advanced practice nurses (APNs), have made significant contributions to the health-care delivery system in terms of providing quality, cost-effective, and safe care. With the passage of the Balanced Budget Act of 1997 (Public Law 105-33), APNs achieved Medicare professional provider status. With this status came responsibilities for APNs to develop new skills to meet growing demands in the reimbursement arena. To a certain degree, they have been able to achieve additional reimbursement gains, but they still need to have a thorough understanding of the reimbursement process and develop additional strategies to deal with the reimbursement challenges that lay ahead of them.

BACKGROUND

APNs have been practicing for many years. In fact, nurse anesthesia, the oldest advanced nursing specialty, has been in existence since the mid-1800s when nurses became involved in administering anesthesia (Bigbee & Amidi-Nouri, 2000). Nurse-midwifery became the second major advanced nursing specialty to develop, but its history is intertwined with the ancient practice of midwifery. The establishment in 1918 of the Maternity Center Association in response to study findings indicating a need for comprehensive prenatal care became a landmark event in nurse-midwifery history. A few years later, in 1925, Mary Breckenridge established the Frontier Nursing Service in the Appalachian area of Kentucky, which became a futuristic model of nurse-midwifery advanced nursing practice. The psychiatric CNS is the oldest and perhaps the most highly developed of the CNS specialties. By 1970, graduate-prepared psychiatric CNSs assumed roles as individual, group, family, and milieu therapists and obtained some direct third-party reimbursement for their services.

In the early 1960s, physicians began to mentor nurses who had clinical experience. At the same time, increasing specialization in medicine led to a large number of physicians leaving primary care, creating a shortage of primary care physicians. This led to many areas, especially rural areas, being medically underserved. In addition, in 1965, the Medicare and Medicaid programs began to provide health-care coverage to low-income women, children, the elderly, and people with disabilities; thereby, increasing the demand for more primary care services. Because physicians were unable to meet this demand, nurses answered the call to become NPs. Loretta Ford, a nurse, and Henry Silver, a physician, created the first training program for NPs (O'Brien, 2003).

However, even though these four advanced practice roles have been well established for decades, direct reimbursement for their services has been difficult to obtain. Historically, nurses were not paid directly for their services, but rather this cost was included with the overhead that facilities and medical providers charged their patients. In 1948, the American Nurses Association (ANA) began their campaign for direct reimbursement of nursing services; however, they faced many barriers and did not achieve major success until approximately 40 years later when significant changes in federal laws governing health programs granted direct reimbursement to APNs for their services. These changes assisted in breaking down some barriers for full use of APNs as primary care providers, and they enabled them to have a more direct role in the delivery of health care (Mittelstadt, 1993).

In 1965, Congress amended the Social Security Act to establish Medicare and Medicaid (Frakes & Evans, 2006). Medicare reimbursed home care agencies for skilled nursing services. Physician orders were required to initiate the services, but the reimbursement was specifically for nursing care. In the 1970s, NPs established some success in being reimbursed for primary care and CRNAs began their difficult struggle to secure third-party reimbursement (Bigbee & Amidi-Nouri, 2000). In 1973, the first legislation mandating private insurance reimbursements of nurse-midwifery services was passed in the state of Washington. Since 1979, CNMs have received direct reimbursement for both Medicare and Medicaid (Brucker & Reedy, 2000).

In the early 1980s, 25 states had enacted legislation enabling direct reimbursement for specific groups of nurses; however, little data existed regarding the implementation of these laws. A case study of legislation providing direct third-party reimbursement to NPs in Maryland was conducted in 1983 and in Oregon in 1986 (Griffith, 1986). The study investigated the degree to which NPs in these two states were receiving direct third-party reimbursement and how it affected health-care costs. Findings revealed that 4 years after enactment of legislation in Maryland, 1% of NPs in the study had been directly reimbursed by a third-party payer in contrast to 21% of NPs in Oregon, 7 years after enactment of the law. Additional findings indicated that NPs receiving direct third-party reimbursement charged less for their services than salaried NPs; thereby, discounting a charge by others that providing direct third-party reimbursement for nursing services would increase health-care costs.

In 1983, Congress adopted the prospective payment system (PPS) in an effort to control hospital costs to the Medicare program. All services by providers other than those reimbursed through Medicare Part B were assembled into a hospital diagnosis-related group (DRG) payment (Bruton-Maree & Rupp, 2001). This fixed rate was to cover all costs associated with a hospital admission, including services provided by nonphysician providers. Under this system, CRNAs were placed in considerable jeopardy because, in an effort to cut costs, hospitals had no incentive to hire CRNAs because their cost would come directly from the hospital DRG payment (Faut-Callahan & Kremer, 2000). Congress had created reimbursement disincentives for the use of CRNAs while strengthening incentives for the use of anesthesiologists. Lobbying efforts by CRNAs caused the Health Care Financing Administration (HCFA) to revise portions of this legislation that allowed CRNAs to obtain direct Medicare reimbursement or to sign over their billing rights to their employer.

The Office of Technology Assessment (U.S. Congress Office of Technology Assessment, 1986) issued a report to the U.S. Congress in 1986 that revealed that NPs and CNMs, as well as physician assistants, provided high quality of care and patient satisfaction. The emphasis on health promotion and disease prevention by this group made them potentially good providers for the managed care models in the 1980s (Sullivan-Marx, 2008). However, barriers to the use of APNs were evident in terms of physician resistance, legal restrictions, lack of reimbursement, and limited coverage for health promotion/preventive care (U.S. Congress Office of Technology Assessment, 1986).

The Physician Payment Review Commission (PPRC) was created in 1986 to advise Congress on reforms of the methods used to pay physicians under the Medicare Part B program, a program that includes the payment regulations for health-care professionals who are eligible to receive direct reimbursement through the Medicare program. Nursing groups such as the ANA and the American Association of Nurse Anesthetists (AANA) lobbied the PPRC to consider their contributions when they revised the payment system (Robinson, 2004).

In 1989, Congress, incorporating the PPRC recommendations, passed legislation that changed physician payment from a reasonable charge payment method to a Medicare Fee Schedule based on a resource-based relative value scale (RBRVS). In response to the lobbying done by nurses, the legislative package included a recommendation that the PPRC study the effect of the Medicare Fee Schedule on nonphysician providers (PPRC, 1991; Robinson, Griffith, & Sullivan-Marx, 2001).

In its annual report to Congress, the PPRC made a recommendation that *nonphysician providers,* including NPs, CRNAs, and CNMs, should be paid a percentage of physician payment levels reflecting differences in physicians' and nonphysicians' resource costs: work, practice expense, and malpractice expense (Griffith & Robinson, 1993). The ANA counterproposed that APNs should be paid the same as physicians for the same services (Mittelstadt, 1991).

Anticipating that APNs would be included in the emerging RBRVS payment system, Griffith and Robinson (1993) studied nine nurse specialty groups, including CNMs and family NPs, to demonstrate that APNs were providing some of the current procedural terminology (CPT) coded services being considered by the PPRC and universally used for physician payment by government and private insurers. Findings of these exploratory studies provided documentation of the degree to which family NPs and CNMs performed, with little or no supervision, the same services and procedures for which physicians were being reimbursed.

The Balanced Budget Act of 1997 (Public Law 105-33), which became effective January 1, 1998, amended the Social Security Act to grant direct Medicare reimbursement to NPs and CNSs in all geographical areas and health-care settings at 85% of the physician rate. This enactment precipitated a study by Sullivan-Marx and Maislin (2000) to ensure that there were no significant differences in how NPs and physicians assessed work values for commonly used primary codes. The researchers compared relative work values between NPs and family physicians for commonly used office visit codes and found no significant difference between the two groups for establishing relative work values, thus providing an indication that services provided by NPs could be reliably valued in the Medicare Fee Schedule.

To establish relative values for the practice expense component of CPT codes, the Center for Medicare and Medicaid Services (CMS), formerly the Health Care Financing Administration (HCFA), developed and now relies on recommendations from the American Medical Association's (AMA) Relative Value Practice Expense Advisory Committee (PEAC). Specialty societies that serve on PEAC survey their members to obtain accurate "direct input" data for the CPT codes, and then society representatives present the data to the PEAC. The PEAC members critique the data, making modifications as needed. Following PEAC approval, data are fowarded to the CMS to use to calculate the practice expense relative values (AMA, 2008). The ANA has a voting seat on this committee, and the nurse representative served as chair of the PEAC in 2006 (Sullivan-Marx, 2008).

On March 9, 2000, the HCFA announced that removal of the federal requirement that CRNAs must be supervised by physicians when administering anesthesia to Medicare patients was forthcoming. Delays in the final rule continued to occur until July 5, 2001, when CMS published a proposed rule that would maintain the existing supervision requirement, but allow a state's governor, in consultation with the state's boards of medicine and nursing, to request an exemption from the physician supervision requirement. The AANA expressed concerns and submitted extensive comments to CMS; however, in the November 13, 2001, *Federal Register,* the final rule, virtually identical to the July 5, 2001, proposed rule, was published and became effective immediately on publication (Bruton-Maree & Rupp, 2001; Edmunds, 2002).

States may have regulations about private insurance reimbursement and are required to set the Medicaid reimbursement schedule for CNMs (Dorroh & Kelley, 2000). This variation in state law and regulation can have an impact on midwifery practice as evidenced by a study conducted by Declercq, Paine, Simmes, and DeJoseph (1998). Their study findings revealed that the single best predictor of the distribution and practice activities of CNMs was the degree to which state policies facilitated or restricted CNM practice. When compared with states with restrictive regulatory and reimbursement policies for CNM practice, states with high regulatory support and reimbursement environments had a CNM workforce three times larger, three times the number of midwife-attended births, and two times as many midwife-patient contacts.

Over the past decade, there has been gradual acceptance of pay-for-performance principles (Kennerly, 2007). The health-care community is beginning to recognize the importance of developing and implementing a common set of clinical standards for medical care. In other words, an individual provider's performance and reimbursement potential is more likely to be judged against a national standard for care rather than past individual performance. To ensure accountability and public disclosure in health care, the CMS initiated the physician focused quality initiative that has the following focus areas: (a) assess the quality of care for key illnesses and clinical conditions that affect many individuals with Medicare; (b) support clinicans in providing appropriate treatment of the identified conditions; (c) prevent health problems that are avoidable; and (d) investigate the concept of payment for performance (CMS, 2008).

Kennerly (2007) stresses that the day-to-day practice of APNs will be directly affected by the physician focused quality initiative. A recent addition to this initiative, the physican voluntary reporting program uses quality measures to obtain data about the clinical performance of participating physicians. At this time, participation is optional and no relative value units have been assigned; therefore, fee-for-payment is not based on performance data. It is believed, however, that performance measurement is the foundation for future reimbursement. Even though pay-for-performance studies have not included APNs, it is important that APNs be acutely aware that their practice will be affected either directly or indirectly through data about physician incident-to-billing.

Legislation enacted by Congress in 2006 enabled CRNAs to participate in pay-for-performance quality measures development, reporting, and financial incentives (AANA, 2008). With CRNAs providing 27 million anesthetics per year, it has been reported that anesthesia is 50 times safer than in the early 1980s. However, the 1.5% quality reporting incentive payment does not offset the 8% Medicare payment cut in place.

APNs have been part of the health-care system for decades and are now, with other providers, entering a time of change aimed at revolutionizing care delivery and reimbursement (Kennerly, 2007). This section was intended to provide some of the history behind the various APN roles as well as their gains and challenges over time in terms of reimbursement autonomy.

BILLING OPTIONS AND IMPACT ON ADVANCED PRACTICE NURSES

Most third-party payers, whether a managed care organization (MCO), Medicare, or Medicaid, to name a few, will recognize APNs, in varying degrees, as qualified providers of health care. However, the reimbursement and coverage policies may differ considerably. Finerfrock and Havens (1997) stressed that differences exist between how individual health plans "treat" APNs as well as how they are permitted to practice under state law and the criteria the plan may impose as a precondition for payment. These differences in billing for services still exist today; therefore, this section will detail some of the current billing options and discuss the challenges for APNs within each of those options to include:

1. **Medicare,** created as part of the Social Security Act of 1965, is a federally funded health-care program that consists of four parts, A, B, C, and D. Only parts A and B will be dissussed here. Part D is the pharmacy plan, and Part C is managed care, conforming to the managed care model, as discussed on page 107. Part A includes payment to hospitals, home health agencies, nursing facilities, and hospice services (Frakes & Evans, 2006; Robinson, 2004). Part B provides payment to physicians (i.e., medical doctors, optometrists, dentists, and podiatrists) and nonphysician providers, including NPs, CNSs, CRNAs, and CNMs. Part B also covers laboratory services, outpatient hospital care, medical equipment, and supplies. The Medicare programs are administered by the CMS. If a patient is covered by Medicare but is not enrolled with an MCO, Medicare will reimburse the patient's health-care provider on a fee-for-service basis. However, if the patient is enrolled in a managed care health plan, Medicare pays the health plan on a capitated basis for each patient; the health plan then pays the providers on a fee-for-service or capitated basis (Buppert, 1998).

   The Primary Care Health Practitioner Incentive Act, which was included in the Balanced Budget Act of 1997, removed Medicare Part B restrictions on the settings and practices in which APNs could provide professional services. This allowed direct Medicare reimbursement to the APN, but at 85% of the physician fee rate (Frakes & Evans, 2006).

   Under the current reimbursement system, which allows CRNAs or their employers to receive direct reimbursement from Medicare Part B, a process titled *pass-through* occurs (Broadston, 2001; Robinson, 2004). The pass-through process allows a facility to be reimbursed for its CRNA expense from the Medicare program over and above the DRG payment of the prospective payment system. It was created by Congress in an attempt to restore the equal playing field between anesthesiologists and CRNAs. The pass-through process is available only to small health-care facilities that meet specific criteria. A rural hospital can qualify and be paid on a reasonable cost basis for one full-time employed CRNA providing 500 or fewer inpatient and outpatient anesthesia procedures without anesthesiologist services provided at the hospital. The hospital and/or CRNA receiving pass-through funding is prohibited from billing a Medicare Part B carrier for any anesthesia services furnished to patients of that hospital (AANA, 2008).

   Payment to clinical providers under Medicare fee-for-service or managed care is categorized in the CPT coding system, developed by the AMA in 1966. Approximately 8000 procedures are listed in the CPT publication, which mainly describes physician procedures and is intended to provide a uniform language that accurately describes medical, surgical, and diagnostic services (AMA, 2007). The CPT is used extensively by payers for fee-for-service reimbursement and tracking services in managed care. It is revised annually to reflect changes in medical practice and technology. Reimbursement to a service represented by an individual CPT code is based on the RBRVS, which was originally implemented to establish a Medicare fee schedule for Part B physician payment. This system now extends to payment for services provided by APNs, physician assistants, and other Part B providers (Robinson et al., 2001). In this system, a total relative value that incorporates work, practice expense, and malpractice insurance is established for each CPT code. The total relative value for a code is multiplied by a standard dollar amount and adjusted geographically to determine the allowable Medicare charge for that code (AMA, 2007).

The CPT system has been criticized for confining codes to physicians' services; thereby, limiting its usefulness to the current health-care system that uses multiple providers, many of whom are directly reimbursed by Medicare such as APNs (Robinson, 2004; Robinson, et al., 2001).

2. **Medicaid** provides health insurance coverage for certain groups of individuals and families with specified levels of low income and assets. Even within the groups, certain requirements must be met to include age, whether the person is pregnant, disabled, blind, or aged, income and resources, and U.S. citizenship or a lawfully admitted immigrant. The rules for counting income and resources vary from state to state and from group to group. This program is a state-administered program, and each state sets its own guidelines regarding eligibility and services (CMS, 2008). Medicaid does not pay money directly to the patient; instead, the payments are sent directly to the patient's health-care provider.

As is the case with patients covered by Medicare, some patients covered by Medicaid are enrolled in MCOs and others are not. To provide care to a Medicaid patient not enrolled in an MCO, an APN must apply and be accepted as a Medicaid provider by the state Medicaid agency. However, if the Medicaid patient is enrolled in an MCO, the APN must apply and be admitted to the provider panel of the organization to which the patient is enrolled for the APN to be eligible to provide care.

APN reimbursement is mainly provided under a fee-for-service approach in which the state pays the lesser of the provider's charge or a defined maximum amount for a specific service (Frakes & Evans, 2006). Some states will provide APN reimbursement at a percentage of the physician's fee-for-service reimbursement rate, and some will restrict the reimbursement to a specific patient population (statutorily defined as needy compared with individuals demonstrating medical necessity) or APN speciality (i.e., family, adult, geriatric, or pediatric). There are 36 states that directly reimburse CRNAs under Medicaid (AANA, 2008)

3. **MCOs** are insurers that provide both health-care services and payment for services. MCO is an umbrella term that includes health maintenance organizations (HMOs), provider sponsored organizations (PSOs), preferred provider organizations (PPOs), or physician-hospital organizations (PHOs). Refer to **Table 6-1** for specific details of these four categories.

MCOs are third-party payers that control, direct, and approve access to services and costs by using specific systems and mechanisms for reimbursement. APNs need to be credentialed and privileged by the MCOs, and many MCOs require precertification that must be met before a patient receives services for each new treatment plan. MCOs collect educational, license, malpractice, employment, and certification data on APNs and then decide whether or not they are credible to provide services for them (Finerfrock & Havens, 1997).

If APNs become a member of the provider panel of an MCO, they have a contract for providing care, credentialing, directory listing, and reimbursement (Buppert, 1998). The APN has full responsibility for the patient's primary care, which includes (a) complying with the organization's quality, use, and patient satisfaction standards; (b) coordinating care with specialists or hospitals; (c) approving or disapproving specialty care referrals; (d) providing a system for 24-hour access to care; and (e) keeping costs as low as possible while maintaining quality. MCOs reimburse providers on a fee-for-service basis, a capitated basis, or a combination of both. Each organization negotiates a payment arrangement with each group or provider on its panel.

Hansen-Turton, Ritter, Rothman, and Valdez (2006) express a concern that the majority of managed care companies refuse to credential NPs as primary care providers. They reveal results of a survey in which only 33% of 112 maintenance organizations had a policy for NP

TABLE 6-1	
Managed Care Organizations	
Categories	**Chararacteristics**
1. Health maintenance organizations (HMOs)	One of the oldest forms of managed care. Members are provided comprehensive health care. The primary care provider of the HMO member coordinates all of the medical care for that individual. If specialist care is needed, the primary care provider refers the member to a specialist generally within the HMO. A "capitated" financing system is used. Care is provided to each member of the plan for a fixed amount.
2. Provider sponsored organizations (PSOs)	A managed care contracting and delivery organization that accepts full risk for beneficiary lives. The PSO receives a fixed monthly payment to provide care for Medicare. PSOs may be developed for-profit or not-for-profit entities of which at least 51% must be owned and governed by health-care providers. It must supply all medical services required by Medicare law and must do so primarily through its network. A PSO's owner-providers must deliver at least 70% of the cost of services; the remainder may come from contracts with other providers if necessary.
3. Preferred provider organizations (PPOs)	Composed of physicians, hospitals, or other providers that provide health-care services at a reduced fee. A PPO is similar to a HMO, but care is paid for as it is received instead of in advance in the form of a scheduled fee. PPOs can offer more flexibility by allowing for visits out-of-network professionals at a greater expense to the policy holder. Visits within the network require only the payment of a small fee.
4. Physician-hospital organizations (PHOs)	It may consist of a single hospital and a group, multiple hospitals and groups of physicians, or a "super PHO" structure that owns or controls for a group of other PHOs and involves multiple hospitals and physician groups. Most memberships consist of health-care providers that are rivals with one another—they might be competing hospitals, competing community physicians, or hospital-employed physicians or medical school faculty on the one hand and community physicians on the other.

credentialing as primary care providers. Additionally, only 40% of companies with managed Medicaid credential NPs as primary care providers and only 52% of those with NPs as primary care providers reimburse them at the same rate as primary care physicians.

4. **Incident-to-billing** enables APNs to provide services that are "incident to" those of a physician and applies only to the office setting. Services that qualify as an incident to must be part of the patient's normal course of treatment during which a physician personally performed an initial

service and remains actively involved in the course of treatment. The physician does not need to be present in the examination room, but he or she must be present in the office suite and ready to assist if needed. An example of a qualified incident to services would be cardiac rehabilitation (CMS, 2008). The claim can be submitted under the physician's provider number as if the physician performed the service and is paid at 100% of the physician fee schedule (Kleinpell, French, & Diamond, 2007). Documentation must include that the physician supervised the visit.

5. The **shared visits** provision by Medicare allows groups employing APNs to combine services and can occur in an office or inpatient setting. A stipulation for shared visits is that the APN and physician must have employment or other type of contractual business relationship (Kleinpell et al., 2007; Magdic, 2006). When the APN services are combined with the physician, the claim bills under the physician's Unique Physician Identification Number at 100% of the payment schedule. Requirements for the shared visits include (a) must be medically necessary, (b) service must be within the APN's scope of practice, (c) service may occur together or independently on the same calendar day, and (d) documentation by the APN and physician should support the level of service reported and be done separately (Magdic, 2006).

6. **Indemnity insurance companies** pay providers on a per visit, per procedure basis. They have fee schedules based on "usual and customary" charges; however, some insurers may pay more than others for the same procedure. If a provider charges more than what an insurer considers to be usual and customary, the insurer will pay only according to their fee schedule; the patient then becomes responsible for the difference between what the provider charges and what the insurance company pays (Barone & Paniagua-Ramirez, 2006). In this case, it then depends on the provider to collect the difference from the patient. Some providers agree to accept the usual and customary payment, whereas others will not (Buppert, 1998; Robinson, 2004). There are approximately 22 states that mandate direct private insurance payment to CRNAs.

7. **TRICARE** is the government's "managed care" program for active and retired members of the military. It includes three options: (a) Tricare Prime is similar to an HMO that provides the lowest out of pocket cost, in return for the requirement that enrollees use only providers and hospitals that are part of the TRICARE network. Enrollees are assigned a primary care provider, known generally as a *gatekeeper,* who supervises all medical care and authorizes referrals for specialty care. (b) Tricare Standard is the name for the health-care option formerly known as CHAMPUS (civilian health and medical program for the uniformed services). Eligible beneficiaries have the greatest flexibility in selecting a health-care provider and the government will pay a percentage of the cost. Individuals and families who have established relationship with civilian providers generally opt for this health-care plan. (d) Tricare Extra is the PPO. It offers choices of providers from a network of civilian health-care providers (Tricare, 2008). NPs, psychiatric CNSs, CNMs, and CRNAs are authorized to provide TRICARE services and are directly reimbursed (Mittelstadt, 1993; Robinson, 2004).

Strategies That Have Been Successful for Advanced Practice Nurses in Their Pursuit of Reimbursement

Over several decades, APNs have strived to achieve reimbursement for their services and over time have achieved some degree of success by using various strategies to include (**Box 6-1**):

1. APNs working in underserved rural areas took advantage of the reimbursement available under the Rural Health Clinic Act of 1977 (O'Brien, 2003). This Act mandated that 50% of services in funded rural health clinics be provided by NPs and CNMs.

BOX 6-1
Advanced Practice Nurse Reimbursement Achievements: The Road Once Traveled

1. Rural Health Clinic Act of 1977 mandated that 50% of services in rural health clinics be provided by nurse practictioners (NPs) and certified nurse-midwives (CNMs).

2. Office of Technology Assessment issued a report to the U. S. Congress in 1986 that revealed that NPs and CNMs provided high quality of care and patient satisfaction.

3. Omnibus Reconciliation Act of 1989 mandated a study of nonphysician providers and Medicare reimbursement.

4. Balanced Budget Act of 1997 granted direct Medicare reimbursement to NPs and clinical nurse specialists (CNSs) in all geographical areas at 85% of the physician rate.

5. Numerous outcomes-based research studies were conducted by advanced practice nurses (APNs) and their colleagues that demonstrated improved patient outcomes and patient satisfaction.

6. APNs established key political contacts and lobbying campaigns.

7. Increased sophistification in grassroots efforts and activities.

---

2. The Omnibus Reconciliation Act of 1989 provided limited reimbursement for NPs collaborating with physicians in rural areas and established Medicaid payments for pediatric or family NPs. Importantly, it mandated a study of nonphysician providers and Medicare reimbursement. These changes were influenced by a NP appointee to the 14-member Physician Payment Review Committee, as well as by nursing organizations (O'Brien, 2003).

3. The various APN organizations as well as the nursing profession established key political contacts and began strategic lobbying campaigns. Many combined their clinical training with political activism through White House fellowships, presidential management internships, and graduate and postgraduate studies in health-care policy (O'Brien, 2003).

4. APNs and nurse researchers conducted numerous outcomes-based research that demonstrated improved patient outcomes and patient satisfaction, as well as improved access and demonstrated cost-effectiveness benefits of APN care. For example, a study conducted by Spitzer (1997) revealed that university community health services NPs delivered health care at 23% below the average cost of other primary care providers with a 21% reduction in hospital inpatient rates, 42% decrease in prescription drug use, and 24% lower lab use rates compared to physicians. Additionally, 82% of patients reported that they were well satisfied with their quality of care. On a scale of 1 to 4, with 4 being the best, patients averaged their services at 3.56.

   Another study revealed an APN-centered discharge planning and home care intervention for at-risk hospitalized elders reduced readmissions, lengthened the time between discharge and readmission, and decreased the costs of providing health care (Naylor, et al., 1999). Another example of NP effectiveness was demonstrated by Mundinger et al. (2000). They studied 1316 primary care patients who were randomly assigned to either NPs or physicians. Their findings revealed patients' outcomes were comparable in the two groups. In yet another example, following an extensive literature review, three Department of Veterans Affairs researchers concluded that NPs compare equally or better than physicians with patients who have various health-care needs. Many studies in their review documented less costly care, while at the same time maintaining quality and effectiveness (Feldman, Ventura, & Crosby, 1987).

In a CNM study, Blanchette (1995) reported lower cesarean section rates and outcomes comparable with a private obstetrics practice in a CNM practice caring for underserved women (13.1% cesaerian section rate for the CNM group versus 26.4% for the physician group). Fewer interventions, including a lower cesarean section rate, for patients of CNMs compared with similar low-risk women cared for by obstetricians and family physicians were found by Rosenblatt et al. (1997). The cesarean rates were 8.8%, 13.6%, and 15.1%, respectively. In addition, CNMs used 12.2% fewer resources than either group of physicians.

Chenowith Martin, Pankowski, and Raymond (2005) analyzed the health-care costs associated with an on-site NP practice for 4284 employees and their dependents. Annualized cost of the NP program was about $83,000. Savings in health-care costs were $1,313,756 per year, yielding a benefit-to-cost ratio of 15 to 1. Paez and Allen (2006) compared NP and physician management of hypercholesterolemia following revascularization. Patients in the NP-managed group were more likely to achieve their goals and comply with prescribed regimen, with decreased medication costs. A collaborative NP/physician group was associated with decreased length of stay and costs and higher hospital profit, without altering readmissions or mortality (Cowan et al., 2006).

In addition to those studies highlighted in this section, there are many other excellent studies that have been conducted that have demonstrated improved patient outcomes and patient satisfaction as well as the cost-effectiveness benefit. However, APNs can not let their guard down; they must continue to conduct quality outcome studies that demonstrate scientific rigor.

5. Nursing professional organizations are becoming more sophisticated in their grassroots activities. They are able to do this through their association journals, seminars, print materials, and more recently, through their Web sites. An example of these efforts took place in the state of Louisiana, where anesthesiologists reportedly hired 18 lobbyists to defeat a bill expanding CRNA practice. Despite their efforts, CRNAs succeeded because of their intensive personal lobbying campaign (Pearson, 2002).

Another example of APN grassroots efforts involved the passage of Public Law 105-33, which included expansion of Medicare reimbursement for NPs and CNSs to all geographical areas. The ANA and APNs came out in force by (a) providing political presence; (b) assembling and packaging outcome data to show how APNs make a difference in terms of cost and quality to include illustrations of the cost effectiveness of APN reimbursement during a 25-year period by the federal government's TRICARE program; (c) establishing political action partnerships; (d) coordinating state and regional legislative volunteers; and (e) visiting "the Hill" to lobby. Despite obstacles, APN legislative efforts are succeeding more often than they are failing by a ratio of 6 to 1, so APNs are on the right track (Haber, 1997; Robinson 2004).

In the 20th Annual Legislative Update edition, Phillips (2008) and Newland (2008) summarized some 2007 milestones that affected one or more APN roles. They highlighted the fact that Texas APNs defeated legislation to limit ability to perform sports physical examinations and South Carolina defeated a bill sponsored by the Board of Medicine to amend the Medical Practice Act to limit CRNAs with giving anesthesia in outpatient office-based surgery and to limit the title of "Dr." to just physicians. Additionally, Arizona passed legislation giving NPs statutory authoriy to provide a variety of services, and California authorized NPs the ability to perform specified Department of Motor Vehicle physical examinations for the purpose of obtaining a drivers license to operate a farm labor vehicle, paratransit vehicle, or bus.

A more recent example that demonstrates how APNs are using their Web sites and the latest technology is encouraging the cosponsorship and support for H.R. 2066 (S. 59) Medicaid Advanced Practice Nurses and Physician Assistants Access Act of 2007. If passed, it would amend title XIX (Medicaid) of the Social Security Act to eliminate the state option to include NPs, CNMs, and physician assistants as primary care case managers. As currently written, it specifies as primary care case managers any NP or CNM that provides primary care case management services under a primary care case management contract. It revises the coverage of certain NP services under the Medicaid fee-for-service program to remove the specification of certified pediatric NP and certified family NP to extend such coverage to services furnished by a NP or CNS. Additionally, it includes NPs, CNSs, CNMs, and CRNAs in the mix of service providers that Medicaid MCOs are required to maintain (Washington Watch, 2008). Nursing organizations have united to encourage their members to contact their senators and representatives to cosponsor and/or support this bill. They are stressing to their respective memberships the importance of pointing out to legislators the need for access to high-quality, cost-effective providers such as APNs. Latest major action taken on this bill was on April 30, 2007, when it was referred to the House Subcommittee on Health. As of December 2008, both H.R. 2066 and S. 59 remain in committee (Library of Congress, 2008).

Although most states reimburse CNMs at the same rate as obstetricrician/gynecologists under Medicaid, as much as 35% difference in reimbursement exists with the Medicare program. CNMs are currently enlisting the support for the passage of the "Midwifery Care Access and Reimbursement Equity Act of 2007" (S.507). If passed, this act will provide for equitable reimbursement for midwifery services under Medicare, which they believe translates into better reimbursement from all payers (American College of Nurse-Midwives, 2008).

FUTURE REIMBURSEMENT CHALLENGES FOR ADVANCED PRACTICE NURSES

Despite many years of providing safe, cost-effective, quality health care and achieving some remarkable reimbursement accomplishments (as detailed in the previous section), APNs are continuing to fight some of the same battles that they were fighting many years ago (**Box 6-2**).

Some of these long-standing battles and new challenges include:

1. Many insurance companies define and restrict the practice of APNs by limiting reimbursable services, not including them on provider panels, defining the environment in which the services may be provided, and refusing to credential them as individual providers (Ashby, 2006;

BOX 6-2
Future Advanced Practice Nurse Reimbursement Challenges: The Road Ahead

1. Insurance companies continue to limit reimbursable services.

2. Need to standardize state and national certification and credentialing.

3. Lack of reimbursement knowledge and skills limits the abilities of advanced practice nurses (APNs) to be key players in practice and business ventures.

4. Pay-for-performance measurement is gaining momentum.

5. Need to continue to inform legislators and consumers about APN education, licensure requirements, and regulatory procedures.

Buppert, 2005; Partin, 2006). Instead they require those individuals who are employed by a physician to bill for their services under the physician's name. One could argue that they are being paid for the services they provided because the practice is being paid; however, one could counter that they are "hidden or shadow providers" when they are not being directly recognized for their services. Refusal to credential APNs does create a problem when they order diagnostic tests or medications. There are some insurance companies that will not pay for the test or medication that is ordered by a provider who is not credentialed by their company. Additionally, some insurance companies refuse to credential an APN who is not employed by a physician; therefore, this can create severe financial problems for a practice owned by an APN.

2. There continues to be a need to standardize state and national certification and credentialing. Each plays a pivotal role in reimbursement for specialty nursing services. Several states require national specialty certification as a requirement for APN licensure (Porcher, 1996). Additionally, Medicaid reimburses only specific certified APNs. Certification is a "process by which a non-governmental agency or association attests that an individual licensed to practice a profession has met certain predetermined standards specified by that profession" (Porcher, 1996, p. 182).

    The American Nurses Credentialing Center (ANCC), a subsidiary of ANA, has been a leader in the development of national credentialing for nurses. ANCC currently certifies NPs and CNSs in 17 areas of advanced practice. Other professional entities offering APN certifications are the Council on Certification of Nurse Anesthetists, the American Council of Nurse-Midwives Certification Council, the National Certification Board of the Pediatric Nurse Practitioners and Nurses, and the American Academy of Nurse Practitioners Certification Program, which recognizes gerontological, family, and adult NPs. There are also advanced practice certification in addictions, acute critial care, AIDS care, hospice, occupational health, oncology, rehabilitation, and urology. Each of these programs was established under the aegis of their respective specialty society, but they ultimately were made independent and insulated from the parent organization for credibility. The professional society establishes standards for practice, and the certification board applies those standards.

    As a result of the influence of the American Board of Nursing Specialties (ABNS), the structure and process of certifiers has become more consistent and 11 advanced practice certifiers awarding 30 specialty and subspecialty credentials have been accredited by ABNS (ABNS, 2008). The model of ABNS was patterned after medicine, in which the 26 approved medical specialties recognized in the United States are monitored by the American Board of Medical Specialties, the American Osteopathic Association Bureau of Osteopathic Specialists, and the American Board of Physician Specialties (ABMS, 2008). The place where inconsistency pervails is the use of professional certification to satisfy governmental or industry requirements for advanced practice. The majority of participants in a survey of NPs reported being certified by a national board or organization (90.4%); however, only 61.5% reported that certification was a requirement of their state board of nursing. Certification as a practice requirement was highest in the Midwest and south central region of the United States and lowest in the West (Running, Calder, Mustain, Foreschler, 2000; Robinson, 2004).

    There are state Medicaid MCOs that refuse to allow NPs/CNSs to function as a patient's primary care provider (Ashby, 2006). By refusing to credential these providers, the companies have forced patients to either seek a new health-care provider or pay out of their own pocket to continue to receive care from their APN. Pennsylvania has a documented shortage of psychiatrists in the state, but psychiatric APNs who have the necessary education and certification are not allowed to do initial psychiatric evaluations for Medicaid patients. Credentialing is the "validation of required education, licensure, and certification" (Porcher, 1996, p. 186). It is necessary for APNs to be credentialed not only to ensure the consumer of safe care delivered by qualified providers, but also to ensure compliance with federal and state laws relating to nursing practice. Credentialing recognizes the APN's scope of practice. A key point regarding reimbursement is for the state to recognize the APN's credentials, which are granted by the state board of nursing. The current state credentialing system for APNs lacks uniformity. In some states, the scope of advanced practice nursing is so restricted that the financial cost and time to become appropriately credentialed is not worth the effort. Standardizing the process for state and national APN certification and credentialing would facilitate gaining reimbursement. It is important for APNs to demand that this standardization take place by lobbying in each and every state.

3. APNs are well prepared for patient care, but they are not prepared for the finanical aspects of practice. A lack of reimbursement knowledge and skills limits the abilities for APNs to be key players in practice and business ventures (Kennerly, 2006; Zuzelo et al., 2004). Rapid changes are occurring in reimbursement because of enhanced federal monitoring of provider billing and coding error rates, piloting of provider pay-for-performance reimbursement measures, and increased public attention to quality outcomes.

    Zuzelo et al. (2004) developed a 46-item multiple choice examination that tested the knowledge of 137 CNSs in the areas of Medicare program structures and reimbursement processes. One-third of the questions were incorrectly answered by 30% or more of the group. Respondents commented that they did have a Medicare knowledge deficit and that graduate studies had not provided them with the knowledge necessary for understanding reimbursement issues. Ament (2000) reported similar reimbursement knowledge deficitis in CNMs.

    If APNs are going to be recognized as strong participants and a group to be "reckoned with" in the business arena of clinical practice, they must increase their knowledge base in terms of reimbursement. Coding and reimbursement must be a part of every APN's practice role and is essential to their continued viability (Barone & Paniagua-Ramirez, 2006). A challenge was issued by Kennerly (2006) to faculty in APN education programs to strengthen their finanical and reimbursement content.

4. There has been a growing acceptance over the past decade of the principles underlying pay-for-performance (Kennerly, 2007). Performance measurement, although not required at this time, is viewed as the foundation of future reimbursement. CMS began federally funded pay-for-performance Medicare health care quality demonstration projects in 2004. Strategies for testing and refining the pay-for-performance reimbursement model have focused on the physician payment system. APN reimbursement has not been studied directly, although it may be indirectly reflected through data about physician incident-to-billing.

    To date, the financial performance incentives have been sparsely used in the private sector and have had limited application in the CMS demonstration projects. Kennerly (2007) stresses that there are indications that the momentum will escalate for pay-for-performance. APNs need to continue to provide and emphasize quality care and at the same time strengthen their understanding of quality measures and the changing reimbursement methodology. Agencies and practices dependent on direct billing for APN services should demand that APNs be included as participants in the pay-for-performance systems for them to be eligible for maximum reimbursement.

5. Continue to focus on informing legislators and consumers about APN education, requirements for licensure, and regulatory procedures in place (Phillips, 2008). If APNs want to influence changes in health care today and protect reimbursement, they must have personal contact with policy makers at the state and federal levels. This goes beyond knowing the names of legislators and what districts or states they represent. APNs must get to know the legislators as well as their staff who manage the local offices or campaign headquarters (Milstead, 1997; Pearson, 2002; Pruitt, Wetsel, Smith, & Spitler, 2002). The majority of local staff members are acutely aware of the wants and needs of their constituents, in other words, the voters. Most staff members have limited knowledge on the many issues that surface, so they often turn to individuals with whom they have developed relationships to obtain reliable, factual information. APNs can provide this vital information by using fact sheets, statistics, case examples, outcomes-based research findings, and other key resource materials. As stated by Pearson (2002), APNs may not have the purchasing power that other groups have, but they are able to succeed with grassroots efforts.

6. Now is the time for APN organizations and other nursing groups to unite in gathering support for the following endorsed bills that target specific programs that continue to deny access to APN services. The first one is H.R. 2066 (S. 59) Medicaid Advanced Practice Nurses and Physician Assistants Access Act of 2007. If passed, it would amend title XIX (Medicaid) of the Social Security Act to eliminate the state option to include NPs, CNMs, and physician assistants as primary care case managers. As currently written, it revises the coverage of certain NP services under the Medicaid fee-for-service program to remove the specification of certified pediatric NP and certified family NP to extend such coverage to services furnished by all NPs or CNSs. (Washington Watch, 2008). Latest major action taken on this bill was on April 30, 2007, when it was referred to the House Subcommittee on Health. Both H.R. 2066 and S. 59 remain in committee as of December 2008 (Library of Congress, 2008).

   The second bill is the Home Health Care Planning Improvement Act of 2007 (S. 1678) which, if passed, would change Medicare law to grant NPs, CNSs, and CNMs the ability to order and certify home health services and to sign home health plans of care (ANA, 2008; McKeon 2008). Currently it is often reported that APNs must delay admitting patients into home health because they need to find a physician who will agree to his or her name being used on the Medicare documents. These delays certainly inconvenience patients and their families and result in increased cost to the Medicare system when patients are left in expensive "institutional" settings when they could be receiving home health care. The most recent major action on this bill was on June 21, 2007, when it was referred to the Senate Committee on Finance where it remains as of December 2008 (Library of Congress, 2008).

   The third bill would allow APNs to be reimbursed for health-care services to be provided to federal employees injured on the job. The Improving Access to Workers' Compensation for Injured Federal Workers Act (H.R. 4651) addresses one of the last remaining federal health-care programs that continue to deny access to APNs (McKeon, 2008). At this time, the Federal Employees Compensation Act (FECA) just recognizes physicians, podiatrists, dentists, clinical psychologists, optometrists, and chiropractors. FECA claims signed by APNs have been denied by the Department of Labor. H.R. 4651 would specifically add NPs, CNSs, CRNAs, and CNMs to the definition of "medical, surgical and hospital services" in FECA law. The most recent major action on this bill was on December 13, 2007, when it was referred to the Committee on Energy and Commerce. H.R. 4651 also remains deadlocked in committee on December 31, 2008 (Library of Congress, 2008).

CONCLUSION

Even though the number of APNs has been increasing and expanding their impact on the health-care system and producing studies that reveal they are able to provide care at a high quality, reimbursement for their valuable work continues to be a struggle. Restrictive policies of programs such as Medicaid and private insurers, as well as numerous state laws and regulations that limit direct reimbursement and supervision required by another health-care provider, result in significant barriers for APN reimbursement. Because health-care spending is so highly scrutinized in today's health-care environments, every APN reimbursement opportunity must be captured. Therefore, it is essential that all APNs be able to understand the reimbursement process and strategize to succeed in removing current and future reimbursement barriers.

References

Ament, L. (2000). Certified nurse-midwives' knowledge of reimbursement issues. *Journal of Midwifery & Women's Health, 45*(2), 157–160.

American Association of Nurse Anesthetists. (2008). Retrieved February 15, 2008, from the American Association of Nurse Anesthetists Web site: www.aana.com.

American Board of Medical Specialties. (2008). Retrieved April 8, 2008, from the American Board of Medical Specialties Web site: www.abms.org.

American Board of Nursing Specialties. (2008). Retrieved April 8, 2008, from the American Borad of Nursing Specialities Web site: www.nursingcertification.org.

American College of Nurse-Midwives. (2008). Retrieved February 28, 2008, from the American College of Nurse-Midwives Web site: www.midwife.org.

American Medical Association. (2007). *Current procedural terminology 2008: Professional edition.* Chicago: American Medical Association.

American Medical Association. (2008). Retrieved January 24, 2008, from the American Medical Association Web site: www.ama-assn.org.

American Nurses Association. (2008). Retrieved February 15, 2008, from the American Nurses Association Web site: www.anapoliticalpower.org.

Ashby, M. (2006). Barriers to nurse practitioner reimbursement. *The Pennsylvania Nurse, 61*(2), 19.

Barone, C. P., & Paniagua-Ramirez, C. T. (2006). Coding and reimbursement. *AACN Advanced Critical Care, 17*(2), 116–118.

Bigbee, J. L., & Amidi-Nouri, A. (2000). History and evolution of advanced nursing practice. In A. B. Hamric, J. A. Spross, & C. M. Hanson (Eds.), *Advanced nursing practice: An integrative approach* (2nd ed., pp. 3–32). Philadelphia: WB Saunders Company.

Blanchette, H. (1995). Comparison of obstetric outcome of a primary-care access clinic staffed by certified nurse-midwives and a private practice group of obstetricians in the same community. *American Journal of Obstetrics and Gynecology, 172*(6), 1864–1868; discussion 1868–1871.

Broadston, L. S. (2001). Reimbursement for anesthesia services. In S. D. Foster & M. Faut-Callahan (Eds.), *A professional study and resource guide for the CRNA* (pp. 287–312). Park Ridge, IL: American Association of Nurse Anesthetists.

Brucker, M. C., & Reedy, N. J. (2000). Nurse-midwifery: Yesterday, today, and tomorrow. *American Journal of Maternal Child Nursing, 25*(6), 322–326.

Bruton-Maree, N., & Rupp, R. M. (2001). Federal healthcare policy: How AANA advocates for the profession. In S. D. Foster & M. Faut-Callahan (Eds.), *A professional study and resource guide for the CRNA* (pp. 357–379). Park Ridge, IL: American Association of Nurse Anesthetists.

Buppert, C. (1998). Reimbursement for nurse practitioner services. *The Nurse Practitioner, 23*(1), 67–81.

Buppert, C. (2005). Capturing reimbursement for advanced practice nurse services in acute and critical care. *AACN Clinical Issues, 16*(1), 23–35.

Centers for Medicare and Medicaid Services. (2008). Retrieved January 23, 2008, from the Centers for Medicare and Medicaid Services Web site: www.cms.hhs.gov.

Chenowith, D., Martin, N., Pankowski, J., & Raymond, L. W. (2005). A benefit-cost analysis of a worksite nurse practitioner program: First impressions. *Journal of Occupational and Environmental Medicine, 47*(11), 1110–1116.

Cowan, M. J., Shapiro, M., Hays, R. D., Afifi, A., Vazirani, S., Ward, C. R., et al. (2006). The effect of a multidisciplinary hospitalist physician and advanced practice nurse collaboration on hospital costs. *The Journal of Nursing Administration, 36*(2), 79–85.

Declercq, E. R., Paine, L. L., Simmes, D. R., & DeJoseph, J. F. (1998). State regulation, payment policies, and nurse-midwife services. *Health Affairs (Millwood), 17*(5), 190–200.

Dorroh, M. W., & Kelley, M. A. (2000). The certified nurse-midwife. In A. B, Hamric, J. A. Spross, & C. M. Hanson (Eds.), *Advanced nursing practice: An integrative approach* (2nd ed., pp. 491–519). Philadelphia: WB Saunders.

Edmunds, M. (2002). Keeping nurses in their place. *The Nurse Practitioner, 27*(2), 11.

Faut-Callahan, M., & Kremer, M. J. (2000). The certified registered nurse anesthetist. In A. B. Hamric, J. A. Spross, & C. M. Hanson (Eds.), *Advanced nursing practice: An integrative approach* (2nd ed., pp. 521–548). Philadelphia: WB Saunders.

Feldman, M. J., Ventura, M. R., & Crosby, F. (1987). Studies of nurse practitioner effectiveness. *Nursing Research, 36*(5), 303–308.

Finerfrock, W., & Havens, D. H. (1997). Coverage and reimbursement issues for nurse practitioners. *Journal of Pediatric Health Care, 11*(3), 139–143.

Frakes, M. A., & Evans, T. (2006). An overview of medicare reimbursement regulations for advanced practice nurses. *Nursing Economic$, 24*(2), 59–65.

Griffith, H. (1986). Implementation of direct third party reimbursement legislation for nursing services. *Nursing Economic$, 4*(6), 299–304.

Griffith, H., & Robinson, K. R. (1993). Current procedural terminology (CPT) coded services provided by nurse specialists. *IMAGE: Journal of Nursing Scholarship, 25*(3), 178–186.

Haber, J. (1997). Medicare reimbursement: A victory for APRNs. *American Journal of Nursing, 97*(11), 84.

Hansen-Turton, T., Ritter, A., Rothman, N., & Valdez, B. (2006). Insurer policies create barriers to health care access and consumer choice. *Nursing Economic$, 24*(4), 204–211, 175.

Kennerly, S. (2006). Positioning advanced practice nurses for financial success in clinical practice. *Nurse Educator, 31*(5), 218–222.

Kennerly, S. (2007). The impending reimbursement revolution: How to prepare for future APN reimbursement. *Nursing Economic$, 25*(2), 81–84.

Kleinpell, R. M., French, K. D., & Diamond, E. J. (2007). Billing for NP provider services: Updates on coding regulations. *The Nurse Practitioner, 32*(6), 16–17.

Library of Congress. (2008). Retrieved April 17, 2008, from Library of Congress Web site: www.congress.gov.

Magdic, K. S. (2006). Acute care billing: Shared visits. *The Nurse Practitioner, 31*(11), 9–10.

McKeon, E. (2008). Headlines from the Hill: ANA works to remove legal barriers to APRN practice. *American Nurse Today, 3*(3), 18.

Milstead, J. A. (1997). Using advanced practice to shape public policy: Agenda setting. *Nursing Administration Quarterly, 21*(4), 12–18.

Mittelstadt, P. (1991, March 1). PPRC recommends payment levels for non-physician providers. *Capitol Update* (pp. 7–8). Washington, DC: American Nurses Association.

Mittelstadt, P. (1993). Federal reimbursement of advanced practice nurses' services empowers the profession. *The Nurse Practitioner, 18*(1), 43–49.

Mundinger, M. O., Kane, R. L., Lenz, E. R., Totten, A. M., Tsai, W., Cleary, P. D., et al. (2000). Primary care outcomes in patients treated by nurse practitioners or physicians. *Journal of the American Medical Association, 283*(1), 59–68.

Naylor, M. D., Brooten, D., Campbell, R., Jacobsen, B. S., Mezey, M. D., Pauly, M. D., et al. (1999). Comprehensive discharge planning and home follow-up of hospitalized elders. *Journal of the American Medical Association, 281*(7), 613–620.

Newland, J. (2008). Immediate action required! *The Nurse Practitioner, 33*(1), 6.

O'Brien, J. M. (2003). How nurse practitioners obtained provider status: Lessons for pharmacists. *American Journal Health-System Pharmacists, 60*(22), 2301–2307.

Paez, K. A., & Allen, J. K. (2006). Cost-effectiveness of nurse practitioner management of hypercholesterolemia following coronary revascularization. *Journal of American Academy of Nurse Practitioners, 18*(9), 436–444.

Partin, B. (2006). Who, if not you, will determine NP scope of practice? *The Nurse Practitioner, 31*(2), 6.

Pearson, L. J. (2002). Fourteenth annual legislative update: How each state stands on legislative issues affecting advanced nursing practice. *The Nurse Practitioner, 27*(1), 10–22.

Phillips, S. J. (2008). After 20 years, APNs are still standing together. *The Nurse Practitioner, 33*(1), 10–34.

Physician Payment Review Commission. (1991). *Annual report to Congress.* Washington, DC: U.S. Government Printing Office.

Porcher, F. K. (1996). Licensure, certification, and credentialing. In J. V. Hicky, R . M. Ouimette, & S. L. Venegoni (Eds.), *Advanced practice nursing: Changing roles and clinical applications* (pp. 179–187). Philadelphia: Lippincott Williams & Wilkins.

Pruitt, R. H., Wetsel, M. A., Smith, K. J., & Spitler, H. (2002). How do we pass NP autonomy legislation? *The Nurse Practitioner, 27*(3), 56–65.

Public Law 105-33. *Balanced Budget Act of 1997.* Washington DC: U.S. Congress.

Robinson, K. R. (2004). Payment for advanced practice nursing services: Past, present, and future. In L. Joel (Ed.), *Advanced Practice Nursing* (1st ed.) (pp. 99–121). Philadelphia: F. A. Davis.

Robinson, K. R., Griffith, H. M., & Sullivan-Marx, E. M. (2001). Nursing practice reimbursement issues in the 21st century. In N. L. Chaska (Ed.), *The nursing profession: Tomorrow and beyond* (pp. 501–513). Thousand Oaks, CA: Sage.

Rosenblatt, R. A., Dobie, S. A., Hart, L. G., Schneeweiss, R., Gould, D., Raine, T. R., et al. (1997). Interspecialty differences in the obstetric care of low-risk women. *American Journal of Public Health, 87*(3), 344–351.

Running, A., Calder, J., Mustain, B., & Foreschler, C. (2000). A survey of nurse practitioners across the United States. *The Nurse Practitioner, 25*(6 Pt. 1), 15–16; 110–116.

Spitzer, R. (1997). The Vanderbilt University experience. *Nursing Management, 28*(3), 38–40.

Sullivan-Marx, E. M. (2008). Lessons learned from advanced practice nursing payment. Manuscript submitted for publication.

Sullivan-Marx, E. M., & Maislin, G. (2000). Comparison of nurse practitioner and family physician relative work values. *IMAGE: Journal of Nursing Scholarship, 32*(1), 71–76.

Tricare. (2008). Retrieved January 23, 2008, from the Tricare Web site: www.victorious.com/tricare/network.htm.

U.S. Congress Office of Technology Assessment. (1986). *Nurse practitioners, physician assistants, and certified nurse-mid-wives: A policy analysis.* (Health technology Case Study 37, OTA-HCS-37). Washington, DC: U.S. Government Printing Office.

Washington Watch. (2008). Retrieved February 20, 2008, from the Washington Watch Web site: www.washingtonwatch.com.

Zuzelo, P. R., Fallon, R., Lang, A., Lang, C., McGovern, K., Mount, L., et al. (2004). Clinical nurse specialists' knowledge specific to medicare structures and processes. *Clinical Nurse Specialist, 18*(4), 207–217.

7

Advanced Practice Nurses and Prescriptive Authority

Jan Towers

DEVELOPMENT OF AUTHORITY TO PRACTICE

As professional nurses expanded their role to cross into traditional medical domains, the ability to prescribe medications became increasingly important. Although certified registered nurse anesthetists (CRNAs), certified nurse-midwives (CNMs), and clinical nurse specialists (CNSs) had practiced in advanced practice roles for some time before the birth of nurse practitioners (NPs), the advent of NP practice in primary care influenced the authorization of advanced practice nurses (APNs) to prescribe medications. Before that time, CRNAs selected and administered anesthesia but not other medications. Likewise, CNMs traditionally focused on childbirth and did not require extensive prescription authority. CNSs functioned in advanced practice nursing roles with diagnosed patients who were under the care of a physician. Although professionals in each of these roles made judgments regarding medications used by patients under their care, they relied mainly on physicians to provide prescriptions for medications when they were needed.

Nurse Practitioners and Prescriptive Authority

As NPs began to provide primary care services, they used these same traditional processes to provide medications for the patients that they served. Although there is an emphasis on health promotion and disease prevention in primary care practice, most patients coming for primary care services do so with a health problem for which they are seeking assistance. As time went on, it became evident that depending on physicians to prescribe medications created problems in the areas of patient access, continuity of care, and patient flow. When providing primary care, NPs assessed and diagnosed patients and needed to prescribe medications and treatments for their problems.

The inability to sign one's own prescription, even if a physician was on site, was inconvenient for NP, physician, and patient alike. It caused interruptions in the physicians interactions with patients, unnecessary delays each time NPs had to wait to get signed prescriptions from physicians, and often interfered with the credibility of NPs by rendering them dependent on physician signatures for medications that were being ordered based on their own diagnostic decision making. These problems were exacerbated when a physician was not on site. Then patients had to wait for prescriptions to be signed before they could be filled. If a physician was not available for a day or more, the implications for patient safety and health care were serious.

Methods were found to get around this stumbling block, such as calling prescriptions in to pharmacies or using other more questionable methods for obtaining a physician signature on the prescription so that the patient could pursue treatment in a timely manner. The need for the authority of NPs to prescribe under their own names became evident and pressing.

In the early days, NPs did not have title recognition other than that of registered nurse (RN) in their state regulatory systems. They were not alone; with the exception of CNMs and CRNAs in a number of states, no APNs had title recognition in statutory or regulatory language in the state nurse practice acts or administrative rules. Likewise, there was no authority to prescribe medications. In fact, many nurse practice acts clearly prohibited the prescribing of medication by nurses regardless of specialty or status. And so began the long journey of convincing legislators and regulators to change state statutes and regulations to give title recognition and prescriptive authority to APNs.

Because licensure for all professions occurs at the state rather than the federal level, the movement to achieve these goals moved unevenly, as states with the most need moved forward to make changes. The movement was enhanced in the early days by an acute shortage of primary care physicians, and some states with higher primary care needs moved forward more rapidly than others. At that time, rural states were more likely to initiate statutory and regulatory adjustments than were states with large urban populations.

Convincing decision makers in the states was not without its problems. Then, as now, NPs had to demonstrate that they had the knowledge base to safely diagnose illnesses and prescribe medications. This meant that educational programs had to demonstrate that their curriculums prepared NPs for an independent prescribing role. Advanced pathophysiology and pharmacology and the development of differential diagnosis and clinical decision-making skills needed to be visible in the programs. With the advent of federal grants to prepare NPs, the content and quality of the preparatory programs was increasingly standardized.

In addition, to be credible in health-care systems, it was necessary for members of the medical community to advocate for the recognition of these professionals and their ability to prescribe medications independently. Many did, and through this window of opportunity, NPs began to gain prescriptive authority state by state over subsequent years.

Initially, the authority to practice and prescribe was limited. In many of the early states where some form of prescriptive authority was conferred, boards of medicine and boards of nursing were authorized to jointly promulgate rules and regulations governing NP actions including prescriptive authority. States such as North Carolina and Idaho were among those first states with jointly promulgated rules. Even today there are a few states that still fall under the regulation of both boards of nursing and boards of medicine. Some of those states (where the highest degree of controversy over scope of practice has traditionally existed) are limited to joint regulation of prescriptive authority. Recent attempts to change that regulatory pattern have been harder to achieve. Pennsylvania is the most recent state to move away from joint promulgation of rules to regulation solely by the board of nursing.

Initially, NPs were authorized to prescribe a limited number of medications under physician supervision. North Carolina was one of the first states to develop a limited drug formulary. Subsequently, states developed combinations of formularies and physician oversight under jointly promulgated rules or under rules developed by boards of nursing. The form of those rules depended largely on the persuasiveness of NPs and the attitudes of the legislators and governors of those states.

Currently, NPs prescribe legend drugs under their own signature in 50 states and the District of Columbia. In addition, they prescribe controlled drugs in 47 states and the District of Columbia. Variation exists among states in the area of the authorization to prescribe controlled drugs and the relationship, if any, that must be maintained with a physician (American Academy of Nurse Practitioners [AANP], 2008). Currently, there exists plenary prescriptive authority (absolutely no requirement for any physician involvement) in 11 states and additionally in Maine after the first 2 years of practice (Pearson, 2008) **(Fig. 7-1).**

NURSE PRACTITIONER

PRESCRIPTIVE AUTHORITY

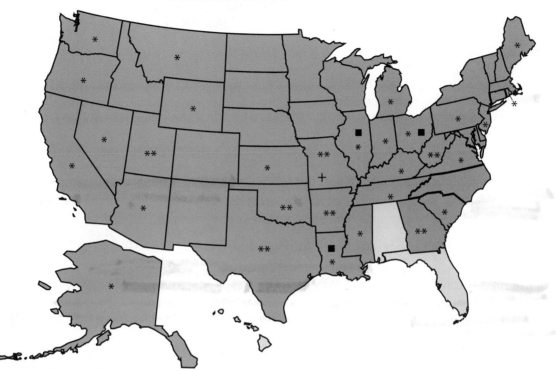

	States That Prescribe Legend Drugs Only
	States Recognized by DEA with Authority to Prescribe Controlled Substances
*	Schedule II–V Only
**	Schedule III–V Only
***	Schedule V Only
■	Schedule II Limitations
+	Pending DEA Approval

FIGURE 7-1 Nurse practitioners authority to prescribe medications. *(Source: Drug Enforcement Administration, Washington, DC, 2007; © American Academy of Nurse Practitioners, 2008.)*

Nurse-Midwives and Prescriptive Authority

CNMs have had to undergo the same process as other APNs to attain prescriptive authority. Because their educational preparation and role developed to include not only obstetrical and newborn care, but also the gynecological management of their patients, the need to prescribe a broader range of medications also increased, making the previously described arrangement for prescribing under the physician's signature unreasonable.

Federal funding of CNM educational programs has helped to implement the standards established by this discipline and facilitate the passage of statutes and rules that allow them to prescribe in 50 states and the District of Columbia with variable limitations in the area of controlled drugs (American College of Nurse-Midwives [ACNM], 2008) **(Fig. 7-2)**. Other factors that have assisted in this endeavor include an enthusiastic consumer population, especially pregnant women, that spread the word about the skills of CNMs. They have often packed hearing rooms and legislative chambers, bringing their babies and children and providing testimony to legislators regarding the worth and skill of the services provided to them by CNMs. CNMs have the same state-to-state variability regarding authorization to prescribe controlled drugs and required relationships, if any, with physicians.

Clinical Nurse Specialists and Prescriptive Authority

CNSs have more recently felt the need to prescribe medications for the patients they serve. Those particularly desirous of the authorization are the psychiatric and mental health CNSs who often have their own practices or function autonomously in mental health clinics and other specialty practices. The prescriptive authority need for practitioners in this field is particularly acute in agencies serving vulnerable populations.

The remainder of the CNS community has mixed responses to the need for authorization to prescribe medications. At the core of this ambivalence is the role played by the CNS in the employment setting, the scope of prescriptive authority needed when working in a particular specialty with patients who have already been diagnosed, the educational preparation required to allow for this authorization, and the risk of being unnecessarily placed under the supervision of physicians in states where such supervision is required. Some states do not provide title recognition for CNSs. There is controversy regarding whether an additional title recognition is actually needed for CNSs. As a result, the issue of prescriptive authority for CNSs has been more cloudy than that of NPs or CNMs.

Nevertheless, CNSs have begun to obtain title recognition (often driven by the need for recognition to receive reimbursement for services), and the authority to prescribe within their scope of practice. Currently a little more than half the states authorize CNSs to prescribe medications in one fashion or another (American Nurses Association [ANA], 2001). Variability in recognizing who may qualify, scope of prescriptive authority, ability to prescribe controlled substances, and required relationships with physicians occur in those states. In some states the statutes and regulations are similar to those of NPs and in others they are not. A few states, such as Florida and Massachusetts, have extended prescriptive authority to psychiatric and mental health CNSs only. Some, such as New Jersey, have grouped all APNs (excepting the CNM) under one set of regulations, whereas others have kept the four clinical groups separated under an APN umbrella that allows for regulatory variability among APNs in their states.

NURSE-MIDWIVES AUTHORITY

TO PRESCRIBE MEDICATIONS

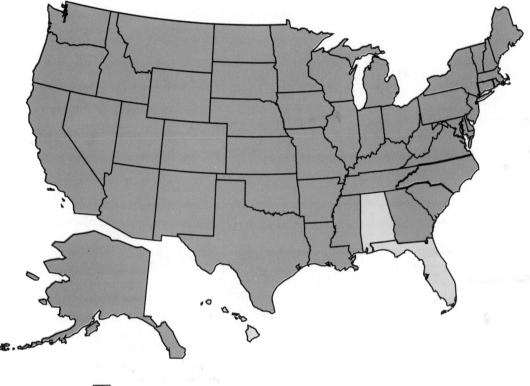

 States in Which Midwives Have Limited Authority to Prescribe Controlled Drugs

States That Authorize Prescription of Controlled Drugs

FIGURE 7-2 Nurse-midwives authority to prescribe medications. *(Source: American College of Nurse Midwives, 2008; © American Academy of Nurse Practitioners, 2008.)*

Nurse Anesthetists and Prescriptive Authority

The authority of CRNAs to select and administer anesthesia has long been recognized. CRNAs have been less involved in the struggle to obtain prescriptive authority than the other three disciplines. Representatives from the CRNA community maintain that ordering and administering anesthesia does not fall under the rubric of prescriptive authority in its traditional sense (American Association of Nurse Anesthetists [AANA], 2003). Increasingly, however, CRNAs are finding themselves involved in pain management of patients in the practices they serve. As with the other APNs, CRNAs have found that they have to work to convince legislators and governors of their knowledge and skills. Their availability in rural areas has enhanced their ability to obtain these privileges in the presence of strong opposition from the medical community. As with NPs, CNMs, and CNSs, they have had to demonstrate the strength of their educational programs and the safety of their practice to obtain privileges in this area.

THE ROAD TO STATUTORY AND REGULATORY CHANGE TO AUTHORIZE PRESCRIPTIVE AUTHORITY

To alter state statutes and regulations, APNs had to educate state legislatures, executive offices, and regulators regarding the role of the APNs they represented. In addition, they had to demonstrate a need for APNs to prescribe and prove that prescribing by APNs was safe and contributed to the well-being of the population.

There are a variety of ways to authorize prescriptive authority within a state. Changes (amendments) may be made to nurse practice acts (statutes); new statutes may be developed separate from nurse practice acts; or changes may be made in states' administrative codes through the development of regulations promulgated by the appropriate regulating board (in most cases the board of nursing).

In the case of new statutes or statutory changes, legislation must be introduced that amends or adds to current law to give title recognition and prescriptive authority to APNs (NPs, CNMs, CNSs, or CRNAs). Once legislation is introduced, it is referred to a committee of jurisdiction (usually a professional licensure committee) for consideration. Once the legislation is in committee, the chair of that committee generally calls for a hearing to allow proponents and opponents of the legislation to give testimony regarding the introduced legislation. After hearings are conducted, at the chair's discretion, the committee votes on the legislation and passes it out of committee. In some states, proposed legislation must also go through the appropriations committee of at least one of the voting chambers to determine cost and evaluate fiscal impact on the state. After passing through all appropriate committees, the legislation, at the discretion of the majority party leadership, is taken to the floor of the voting chamber for a vote. Sometimes this is done simultaneously in both chambers of the state legislature; in others, the legislation passes through one chamber at a time. Once the legislation has been agreed on (passed) by both chambers of the legislature, it is sent to the governor to be signed or, in the case of some states, to be vetoed.

It is during this process that language changes in proposed legislation are often made or negotiated to satisfy other interested parties (i.e, physician collaboration, limits on prescriptive authority, restrictions in the percent of reimbursement allowed to the APN, a role for the board of pharmacy or board of medical examiners in the prescriptive process, or the concerns of certain legislators). For this reason, the language of authorizing statutes vary to a certain extent from state to state. This is particularly true in the sections (a) defining procedures to be followed and requirements that must be met to be recognized as an APN; (b) defining the relationship, if any, that must be held with a physician to prescribe; and (c) determining the scope of prescriptive authority of the APN, particularly the authorization to prescribe controlled drugs schedules I through V. As statutes are passed, much time and energy goes into attempting to negotiate language that is acceptable to the advanced practice community, involved legislators, governors, regulatory bodies, and other interested parties. Once statutes have been passed and signed by the governor of a state, rules and regulations are developed and approved by the authorized regulatory body or bodies.

Many states have not introduced or altered statues to authorize APN prescriptive authority, but rather have developed and instituted regulatory changes in the administrative code by which the advanced practice disciplines must abide. Although regulation cannot override statute, statutes are often worded broadly enough for regulations regarding title recognition and authorization to prescribe drugs to be developed by the regulatory body or bodies without disturbing statutes.

When regulations are developed, they are first written as proposed rules and are placed in a public register for comment. The comment period covers a limited time, after which the promulgating board(s) consider the comments and make appropriate changes in the proposed rule at their discretion before publishing a final rule. In most states, such regulations must then be approved by some arm of the legislature, often committees of jurisdiction, sometimes by one or the other legislative chamber, before approval by the governor. For this reason, APNs and regulatory bodies are often embroiled in negotiations similar to those encountered in the legislative process that result in alterations that make for variance in regulations from state to state. These variations are in the same general areas where there is variability in statute.

Because the purpose of state regulatory bodies, such as boards of nursing, is to protect the public (in this case, the public health), boards of nursing vary in their advocacy of advanced practice roles in the regulatory process. In most states governors appoint the members of the professional licensure boards. Having APNs, who understand the roles of NPs, CNMs, CNSs, and CRNAs, appointed to these positions can help the regulatory process when issues such as prescriptive authority are considered.

Patterns of Statutory and Regulatory Authority

Four basic patterns of regulation regarding prescriptive authority have evolved over time. They include:

- The use of an established formulary or list of drugs that the APN can prescribe
- A negative or exclusionary formulary that allows the APN to prescribe all drugs with a short list of forbidden drugs
- An individualized collaborative formulary established by the APN
- A collaborating physician and an open formulary that sets no prescribing limits on the APN

Regulator Established Formulary

An established formulary was used in the early days of NP prescribing activity to establish an agreed-on list of drugs that NPs could prescribe. As new drugs came onto the market, these formularies had to be updated to allow NPs to prescribe according to current practice standards. Although this quickly became a cumbersome process, it is still in use today for NPs in such states as Oregon and New Hampshire and was even incorporated into regulations recently developed in Pennsylvania. Other APNs have found that acceptance of this kind of formulary has made prescribing more palatable to legislators, regulators, and other interested parties because it can limit the number of drugs or drug types to those who are within a defined scope of practice.

Negative or Exclusionary Formulary

Exclusionary formularies were found to be a more practical approach to regulation of prescriptive authority of NPs. By creating a short list of forbidden drugs (for example, cancer drugs and gold treatments), the NP had more flexibility in choosing appropriate treatments for patients. This has been particularly important in the primary care setting. An example of a state with an exclusionary formulary is Oklahoma.

Collaborative Formulary

More flexible than the established formulary, and to a certain extent more flexible than a negative formulary, a collaborative formulary allows the APN to create a formulary most useful to his or her practice in collaboration with an identified physician who serves as a collaborator. Although this has worked well in some states, in others, where the formulary must be shared with the regulatory board, it has sometimes become a nightmare. Requirements regarding information to be included in formularies and updating formularies can be, to say the least, cumbersome and obstructive. States using this framework in varying degrees include New York, Maryland, California, and New Mexico.

Open Formulary

The most flexible framework for prescriptive authority is the open formulary, in which APNs have no limitations regarding what they can prescribe. In these cases, APNs prescribe according to their own specialty scope of practice, just as physicians prescribe within their own scope of specialty practice. The majority of states have included this framework in their regulations without difficulty or negative repercussion. Examples of states using open formularies include Alaska and Washington.

Advanced Practice Nurse-Physician Relationships in Statute and Regulation

Often, the requirement of some sort of collaborative arrangement with physicians to prescribe is coupled with the prescriptive authority patterns discussed previously. Whereas many states do not require formal collaborative arrangements with physicians, the remainder have some requirement for collaborative or supervisory agreements with physicians to practice or prescribe medication. For NPs, approximately one-third of the state statutes and regulations have no requirements, less than one-fourth require supervision or have delegated authority, and the remainder require some kind of collaborative or consulting arrangement with a physician (AANP, 2008). The arrangements range from identifying a consulting physician to submission of a written agreement to the regulatory board(s) for filing or approval. CNMs have a similar pattern: approximately one-fourth have no requirements; approximately one-fourth require a supervising physician; and the remainder require some kind of collaborative/consulting relationship in statute or administrative rule (ACNM, 2001). CRNAs have supervising or cooperating physicians in most states (AANA, 2003), whereas CNSs tend to have the same requirements as NPs in the states in which they have prescriptive authority (ANA, 2001).

Some of these requirements stem from a desire on the part of legislators or interested and influential parties for physician oversight to prescribe; others have been driven by reimbursement laws and policy that call for physician oversight of APNs. Sadly, sometimes rules are made for APNs that reflect the supervisory relationship required of physician assistants in all states, without considering the fact that APNs are accountable under their own license, carry their own liability insurance, and in the majority of states are not required to be supervised by physicians.

BARRIERS TO PRESCRIPTIVE PRACTICE

The roads traveled by APNs to obtain prescriptive authority have not been without struggle. There is no denying that the majority of barriers to practice have roots in organized lobbying by certain parts of the medical community to limit the autonomy of APNs. This move has often been couched in the language of "protecting the public health." As a result, some legislators and governors have seen fit to set limitations in statute and administrative rules governing APNs. The literature is replete with studies that report on the clinical safety of APNs. In the studies that have been conducted, APNs have been found to be as safe as physicians and often have been found to be safer than physicians (Office of Technology Assessment [OTA], 1986). The ratings on quality of care have been consistently high in the studies that have been conducted over the years. APNs, particularly NPs, have been studied and scrutinized in multiple studies with consistently positive reports (AANP, 2007).

The biggest barriers to practice for all groups have been the limitations set in state statute and regulation. Of those, the requirements for formalized agreements with physicians to prescribe or practice have created the most frustrating barrier for APNs. This has been particularly true for NPs and CNMs who must find physicians who will agree to serve as collaborators to practice and receive reimbursement. CRNAs, particularly in rural areas, suffer from similar problems.

Once a physician has agreed to serve as a consultant, both the APN and physician often find the reporting rules to be frustratingly cumbersome. Although it does not occur in all states, requirements to list types of patients seen, consultation patterns to be maintained, types of drugs to be prescribed, and identification of physicians to serve as backup in the absence of the identified collaborating physician still plague APNs, particularly NPs.

Although, generally speaking, pharmacists have been cooperative and NPs generally report a good working relationship with pharmacists, issues such as continued use of the collaborating physician name as the prescriber on a medicine bottle label and requests for the name of the "supervising physician" before dispensing a prescription have frustrated APNs, physicians, and patients through the years. The requirement of a Drug Enforcement Administration (DEA) number by insurance companies to pay for prescriptions has been problematic in states where APNs are not yet authorized to prescribe controlled drugs. This problem lands on the pharmacists' doorstep when they cannot obtain reimbursement for dispensed drugs from insurance companies without an accompanying DEA number. Although this practice is a misuse of the DEA number, which is to be used for the prescription of controlled drugs only, it has become common practice for insurance companies and pharmacies to use this number as an identifier because of its uniformity for physician identification throughout the country. It is hoped that the institution of the NPI (National Provider Indicator) will resolve some of these issues.

Mail-order pharmacies have sometimes created barriers for APNs. Occasionally patients cannot obtain prescriptions from these entities without the name or signature of a physician. Although this is no longer a problem with most mail-order pharmacies, those with warehouses located in states where laws for this form of dispensing require the order of a physician may still pose difficulties for patients with prescriptions written by APNs.

Confusion about the role and scope of practice of an APN through the grouping of NPs, CNMs, and physician assistants as "midlevel practitioners" has created problems for APNs. It is often assumed that the required supervisory arrangements for physician assistants is the same for NPs and CNMs, so that policies related to practice, including prescriptive authority and ordering of medications for patients, are often based on the statutes and rules governing physician assistants rather than the APNs. Because most regulation of physician assistants stems from a state's medical practice act, insurance companies, institutions, accreditation entities, and pharmaceutical companies sometimes assume that the physician assistant administrative rules apply to all "midlevel practitioners" and do not seek out information regarding APNs from a state's nurse practice act. Because APNs are authorized to practice more autonomously in most instances, this assumption and the actions taken based on it, create barriers for the APN in a variety of venues, including prescriptive authority and ordering medications for patients in both inpatient and outpatient settings.

ADAVANCED PRACTICE PRESCRIBING PATTERNS

The AANP has conducted three national surveys that examined the prescribing patterns of NPs throughout the United States (Goolsby, 2005; Towers, 1989, 1999a, 1999b). In those studies it was found that an NP's prescription patterns reflected the specialty and the practice setting of the NP. In one study (Towers, 1999a), which consisted of 11,000 NP respondents, family NPs wrote an average of 19 prescriptions per day, followed closely by adult and gerontological NPs at 17 and 15 prescriptions per day, respectively. Women's health and pediatric NPs followed with a mean of 12 and 13 prescriptions per day. The mean number of prescriptions written per day increased with years of experience of the NP. In the 2004 study (Goolsby, 2005), the mean number of prescriptions for all NPs was 19. Family, adult, emergency, and psych/mental health nurse practitioners wrote an average of over 20 prescriptions per day, the highest mean being NPs practicing in emergency departments (26), followed by family nurse practitioners (23).

Drugs most frequently prescribed by all specialties in both studies were antimicrobials, anti-inflammatories, and analgesics. Antihypertensives, bronchodilators, and cardiovascular drugs were prescribed most frequently by adult, family, and gerontological NPs. Contraceptives were most often prescribed by women's health NPs, regardless of whether the APN was working in a family planning clinic or a public health department. More than 90% of NPs practicing in emergency department settings prescribed analgesics, anti-inflammatories, and antimicrobials most often. In the Department of Veteran's Affairs (VA) hospital setting, more than 70% of NPs prescribed antihypertensives and cardiovascular drugs most frequently, followed by diabetic medications, gastrointestinal medications, and analgesics. Among NPs authorized to prescribe controlled drugs, the majority of adult, family, gerontological and psychiatric and mental health NPs prescribed them at least once a week, the highest percentages being in the hospital and VA hospital setting (Towers, 1999b).

CNM prescriptive activities center on medications needed for prenatal care, such as vitamins, and intrapartum and postpartum care, such as analgesics. In addition, their prescribing practices are similar to those of women's health NPs. They include contraceptives and other hormone therapies, vaginal preparations, and antimicrobials, followed by anti-inflammatories, analgesics, and vitamin therapies (Towers, 1999a).

The CNSs who most often prescribe medications at this time are the psychiatric and mental health specialists. In a study conducted by Talley and Richens (2001), psychiatric and mental health CNSs authorized to prescribe controlled drugs were reported to most frequently prescribe antidepressants (selective serotonin uptake inhibitors and tricyclic antidepressants). The next most frequently prescribed medications were antiparkinsonian drugs and antihistamines for neuroleptic side effects and sleep, followed by mood stabilizers such as lithium and carbamazepine. In this cohort, CNSs who had practiced longer prescribed fewer drugs, whereas those with less professional experience prescribed more frequently.

Among CNSs of other specialties, prescribing activities appear to function around already diagnosed conditions and altering, adjusting, or refilling physician-prescribed medications in stable patients. The lack of authorization and the desire to maintain autonomy in nursing practice led many CNSs to choose not to obtain authorization in settings in which such authorization is attainable. The position of the National Association of Clinical Nurse Specialists (NACNS) is that CNS prescriptive authority should be optional and that when prescribing is to be undertaken, the CNS should meet the requirements of any other APRN (Lyon & Minarik, 2001; NACNS, 2002).

CONCLUSION

Prescriptive authority is now generally recognized as an integral part of advanced practice nursing. Although totally unfettered authority by all APNs has not yet been achieved, the experience of prescribing medications for patients under the care of these providers has been found to be safe and beneficial. The arguments put forth to limit their prescribing activities grow weaker with each advance that APNs make. The practicality, the enhancement of quality of care, and the cost effectiveness of the practice of these groups has enhanced the logic and desirability to give prescriptive authority to APNs nationwide.

References

American Academy of Nurse Practitioners. (2007). *Cost effectiveness of nurse practitioners.* Washington, DC: Author.

American Academy of Nurse Practitioners. (2008). *Statutory and regulatory authority for nurse practitioners.* Washington, DC: Author.

American Association of Nurse Anesthetists. (2003). *Scope and standards for nurse anesthesia practice.* Chicago: Author.

American College of Nurse-Midwives. (2001). *State laws governing the relationship between CNMs and physicians.* Washington, DC: Author.

American College of Nurse-Midwives. (2008). *Midwives and prescriptive authority.* Washington, DC: Author.

American Nurses Association. (2001). *States which recognize prescriptive authority.* Washington, DC.,: Author.

Goolsby, M. (2005). 2004 AANP National Nurse Pactitiner Sample Survey, Part II: Nurse Practitioner Prescribing. *Journal of the American Academy of Nurse Practitioners, 17*(12), 506–511.

Lyon, B., & Minarik, P. (2001). Statutory and regulatory issues for clinical nurse practitioner practice. *Clinical Nurse Specialist, 15*(3), 30–39.

National Association of Clinical Nurse Specialists. (2002). *Assuring the public's access to CNS services: Model statutory/ regulatory language to regulate CNS practice.* Mission Aliso, CA: Author.

Office of Technology Assessment. (1986). *Nurse practitioners, physician assistants and certified nurse-midwives: A policy analysis.* (Policy No. OTA-HCS-37). Washington, DC: U.S. Government Printing Office.

Pearson, L. (2008). The Pearson report: A national overview of nurse practitioner legislation and healthcare issues. *The American Journal for Nurse Practitioners, 12*(2), 9–80.

Talley, S., & Richens, S. (2001). Prescribing practices of advanced practice psychiatric nurses: Part I—Demographic, educational and practice characteristics. *Archives of Psychiatric Nursing, 15*(5), 205–213.

Towers, J. (1989). American Academy of Nurse Practitioners National Survey. Part II. *Journal of the American Academy of Nurse Practitioners, 1*(4), 137–145.

Towers, J. (1999a). *American Academy of Nurse Practitioners National Survey: Prescribing practices.* Washington, DC: American Academy of Nurse Practitioners.

Towers, J. (1999b). *American Academy of Nurse Practitioners National Survey: Prescribing practices in hospital settings.* Washington, DC: American Academy of Nurse Practitioners.

8

Credentialing and Clinical Privileges and the Advanced Practice Nurse

Ann H. Cary

Mary C. Smolenski

INTRODUCTION

Credentialing and privileging of health-care providers and advanced practice nurses (APNs) in particular, is the initial and ongoing mechanism employed by regulatory and voluntary oversight bodies and delivery systems to ensure protection of the public and quality patient care during the delivery of health-care services. The independence and autonomy of APN services necessitates the same degree of attention to the processes of credentialing and privileging as accorded to physicians. The fact that the process is a critical dimension of any risk management plan is reflected in the level of responsibility for the governing board or top administrator of the institution to assure the public of this accountability.

This chapter discusses credentialing and privileging as separate mechanisms, with the understanding that analysis of the data about the APN's application (credentialing) is a precursor to the decision about the nature of activities for which privileging will be awarded. Issues related to credentialing and privileging for APNs within the health-care arena are also presented.

CREDENTIALING

Credentialing involves the collection, verification, and assessment of information determining the eligibility and qualifications of the APN provider to execute health-care services and includes three categories: current licensure; education and training; and experience, ability, and current competence to perform the privileges (The Joint Commission [TJC], 2008). Whereas privileging decisions are based on evaluation of the applicant's credentials and performance, the credentialing process itself guarantees the integrity of the data on the APN and serves as the basis of decisions regarding authorization for scope of practice and appointment of the APN in a facility or system.

The types of data gathered during the credentialing process are directed by federal and state regulations; professional standards; facility requirements, policies, and procedures; and voluntary oversight bodies. Conditions of participation often drive the federal and state funded and regulated processes; standards of practice guide the professional standards; institutional bylaws, policies, and procedures mandate the specific application of the credentialing and privileging processes for the employed or independent contractor or provider; and voluntary or semiregulatory accreditation standards mandate the institutional processes. Regardless of the particulars of data that must be provided to support the APN application, there are common data elements that the APN can expect to see on the application.

Credentialing Application and Procurement of Data

Regardless of the facility in which the APN seeks credentialing, there are general categories of data required to support the application for APN appointment or reappointment to a clinical position. **Box 8-1** lists the common categories included in the credentialing application process.

Typically, a written application is required to be submitted to the authorized department or person in an institution. The application may be lengthy; and completeness and accuracy of information are critical to ensure timeliness of processing. Review of the application examines both the submission of information by the APN and verifies sources as well as consistency of information among all sources. Any gaps in information or inconsistency are further investigated by the institution before a decision is made for appointment. The APN has the responsibility to add information as needed and to answer queries for incomplete or inconsistent data. In circumstances where changes in status for the APN occur (e.g., licensure renewal, registration, additional education and certifications, recertification, voluntary or involuntary termination of staff membership, reduction or loss of privileges), the provider is obligated to submit the respective information to the credentialing body immediately for review of appointment status. Falsification of information or intentional omission of information on the application may be grounds for termination of the process, disciplinary action, or dismissal.

Verification of Advanced Practice Nurse Application Data

Two types of verification of data sources, primary and secondary, are conducted on an application in accordance with the rules and regulations of the accountable body for credentialing within the institution and as directed by the intsitutional accreditation process. Primary source verification attests to the accuracy of the APN's credentials based on evidence obtained from any source issuing the credential or the attestation of clinical performance. Examples include verification of licensure

---

BOX 8-1
Categories of Data Required to Be Satisfied for Credentialing Application

Personal and practice demographic information
Education and training
Work history
State(s) licensure history (including state-controlled substance licenses)
Certifications
Drug Enforcement Agency certificates
Liability insurance and claims history
History of sanctions and penalties imposed on practice and voluntary relinquishment of licenses/certifications
Disclosures of physical, mental, substance, or criminal problems
Attestation of information completeness and accuracy
Authorizing statement to collect any information necessary to verify application

by state agency and certifications by certifying bodies, letters by authorized personnel at the professional school, letters from individuals personally acquainted with the APN's skills, and database queries. Secondary source verification relies on verification actions of the APN credentials based on data obtained by means other than direct contact with the issuing source of the credential (Utilization Review Accreditation Commission [URAC], 2008a, 2008b). Examples include unofficial copies of documents or reports on patient satisfaction statistics by the applicant.

Some credentialing processes allow for Internet or telephone verification if documented. In addition, some health-care institutions contract with credentialing verification organizations (CVOs) to collect the primary and secondary data on which the decision for appointment will be made. The institution contracting with the CVO has adjunctive accountabilities to monitor the quality of service provided by the CVO and may require the CVO to be accredited by one of the national accrediting bodies such as URAC. The institution is not relieved of liability resulting from decisions based on contracted CVO data and processes for credentialing of APNs. In addition, the institution remains accountable for the accreditation standards issued by its accreditation bodies such as The Joint Commission (TJC).

Analysis of Credentialing Application

On completion of the APN application review and verification processes, the institutional procedures for decision on appointment is the final step. These are guided by institutional policies and procedures related to structure of the decision-making body; roles of the members; risk management and legal reviews; due process mechanisms; documentation requirements for decisions; and reporting mechanisms to the institutional board of directors, clinical directors, and the applicant. In most institutions, the credentialing committee is composed of physicians. The credentialing process is time consuming because of the importance of adhering to principles of good data integrity and decision making. It can often take 90 to 120 days (Monarch, 2002). It behooves the APN to obtain a copy of the policy and procedures for the credentialing process, committee member list, schedule of meetings, anticipated action on the application, and due process mechanisms. Rapid response to queries facilitates the completion of data collection and decision making. Also, alerting primary sources of the impending request by the verification body can facilitate the response for information.

When a credentialing process results in an appointment to the staff, the length of appointment and reappointment procedures are guided by institutional policy. It is wise to obtain copies of the reappointment process and criteria so that the APN can continuously compile the necessary evidence and documents to meet the criteria for reappointment. As new technologies and procedures become common, the APN needs to understand the minimum criteria for credentialing in new procedures as well and document accordingly (Kamajian, Mitchell, & Fruth, 1999; TJC, 2008).

Decisions for emergency credentialing of volunteer licensed independent practitioners (LIPs) have been revisited since 2002 because of national and local emergencies. For example in 2002, TJC created a standard that allows the institutional chief executive officer, medical staff president, or his or her designee to grant emergency privileges when an emergency management plan has been activated. Implications for credentialing focus on data integrity: acceptable sources of identification, including a current license to practice, current hospital identification with the license number, or verification of identity by a current hospital or medical staff member (American Hospital Association [AHA], 2002; TJC, 2008). Time limitations are imposed for credentialing in this status.

Sources of Organizational Standards
for Credentialing of Advance Practice Nurses in Institutions

APN practices can be found in almost all venues of health-care delivery. Appointment and privileging oversight mandates from credentialing organizations have broadened the standards to include LIPs in hospitals, ambulatory care organizations, subacute long-term care, mental health, and managed care organizations (MCOs), regardless of practice structures. Credentialing for other delivery systems is on the horizon. Because the standards of sponsoring organizations can change annually, the reader is advised to consult the list of Web sites related to this chapter on DavisPlus to obtain the most current information possible on their standards for accreditation as they relate to credentialing and privileging of the APN's practice.

Once the application for credentialing is approved, a subsequent decision is made by the institution to authorize the practice activities of the APN. In some instances a separate privileging application is required. Consult institutional policies for their procedures.

PRIVILEGING

Privileging, once only practiced within the realm of the medical staff, is now a process that many APNs are facing as they apply for positions within health-care facilities, MCOs, mental health and substance abuse treatment facilities, and even doctors' offices (if the APN will be following private patients in the acute-care setting). Privileging is used by a facility or employing organization to monitor the clinical activities a provider is authorized to perform in that facility and is the process of authorizing a health-care professional to perform (order) specific diagnostic or therapeutic services within well-defined limits. The granting of privileges is based on the following factors: state practice acts, agency regulations, license, education, training, experience, competence, health status, and judgment (Jones-Schenk, 1998).

Monarch (2002) identifies seven categories of staff privileges within health-care facilities and systems. These are shown in **Box 8-2.**

Rationale and Background

Privileging is a component of the credentialing process of health-care facilities. As mentioned previously, national accrediting bodies such as URAC, the National Committee for Quality Assurance, TJC, and the Accreditation Association for Ambulatory Care establish both the credentialing and privileging standards and processes by which organizations are accredited. In 1984, TJC (then, the Joint Commission on the Accreditation of Healthcare Organizations [JCAHO]) revised its definition of medical staff and broadened scope of practice rules to include permissive language to allow hospitals to include other licensed individuals permitted by law and by the hospital to provide patient care services independently in the hospital. These privileges usually include clinical and admitting practices. TJC also established a mechanism to monitor these privileges and charged the hospital to establish criteria for clinical privileging and a process to ensure that competent individuals are providing patient care (Quigley, Hixson, & Janzen, 1991).

The current TJC (2008) standards speak to the issue of hospital privileging in standards MS 4.0 through MS 4.13 The standards speak to the process itself and to the mechanisms that must be in place and outlined in the hospital bylaws. These processes must include the time frames, the appeals processes, criteria for appointment and determining specific privileges, those responsible for the credentialing and privileging process, the reappointment process, temporary privileging, telemedicine

---

BOX 8-2
Staff Privileges Categories

Active—This level of clinical privileges allows the health-care provider to admit patients and participate in other hospital programs.

Courtesy—This level of clinical privilege is awarded when a limited number of patients will be admitted and when the health-care provider is an active member of another medical staff.

Affiliate—This level of clinical privileges is awarded when the health-care provider is no longer active, but has a long-standing relationship with the hospital.

Outpatient—This level of clinical privileges is awarded when the health-care provider is regularly engaged in the care of patients in outpatient settings or in programs sponsored by or on behalf of the health-care organization.

Honorary—This level of clinical privileges is awarded when the health-care provider is no longer active, but has outstanding accomplishments or reputation. Honorary staff privileges are distinguished from affiliate staff privileges in that honorary staff privileges permit the health-care professional to continue to admit patients to the organization.

House—This level of clinical privilege allows a health-care professional to admit patients within a specialty area with the approval of an active staff member.

Allied Health Professional—This level of clinical privilege permits nonphysician health-care providers to provide specified patient care services.

Reprinted with permission from Monarch, K. (2002). *Nursing and the Law.* Washington, DC: American Nurses Association, p. 246.

---

privileges, disaster privileges, and the quality improvement process. One standard speaks to those individuals providing patient care via telemedicine and introduces the concept of credentialing and privileging by proxy. The proxy approach recognizes the burden of credentialing for the originating site (where the patient is located) when privileges are bestowed to providers at the distant site (where providers of care are located) and for which there is more relevant information to base a decision. Finally the proxy acknowledges that the originating site may have little experience with how to privilege certain specialty providers (TJC, 2008). APNs, as well as other practitioners, providing telemedicine diagnostic and treatment services may be subject to the credentialing process of the organization receiving the telemedicine services. In the case of disaster privileges, an APN may be granted disaster privileges through a modified process. This process is typically granted for two conditions: when a disaster management plan has been activated and when the organization is unable to meet immediate patient care needs. At a minimum, verification of license and oversight of care treatment and services must be provided (TJC, 2008). Continuing education is also mandated in TJC standards, as are four core criteria. These include current licensure, relevant training or experience, current competence, and ability to perform privileges requested.

There are six areas of competence that inform the evaluation of a practitioner in current TJC (2008) standards for the credentialing and privileging process. These include:

1. Patient care
2. Medical and clinical knowledge
3. Practice-based learning and improvement

4. Interpersonal and communication skills
5. Professionalism
6. System-based practice

In addition to incorporating the aforementioned concepts into the overall evaluation of an individual's credentialing and privileging file, there are also two other processes that allow for closer evaluation. The first is a focused professional practice evaluation. This might be used when an individual has the credentials on paper, but there is a need to evalutate the individual more closely to determine competence. The second is ongoing professional practice evaluation that allows for a more evidence-based approach to credentialing rather than just the formal process every 2 years. If any issues are apparent during the ongoing evaluation, a more focused evaluation can be done.

When the process is done correctly, it can provide protection for the facility, the patient, and the practitioner. The process of credentialing and privileging attempts to decrease chances of liability for the facility and the practitioner by ensuring that the practitioners providing care to patients are currently licensed, have been educated for the role in which they are working, and are safe and competent in the scope of care they are authorized to provide. The intent is that patients ultimately benefit from well-educated, safe, competent practitioners. The process in an accredited organization also provides some security for the practitioner in that it requires that credentialing and privileging practices include mechanisms that protect them from any potential bias from economic competitors and ensures a due process mechanism (Jones-Schenk, 1998). The process provides for time frames and feedback to the practitioner and provides mechanisms for temporary or emergency privileging. Finally, privileging provides data for determining economic effect of provider practice on the healthcare system.

As stated in the definition, there are several factors that affect the outcome of privileging: state practice acts, agency regulations, license, education, training, experience, competence, health status, and judgment. The factor that affects APNs most is the scope of practice outlined in the state practice act for the state of licensure and authorization. Each state regulates the practice of APNs differently and the scope of practice outlined in the state regulations or statutes can be broad or narrow. Some practice acts define what APNs can do and what specific drugs they may or may not be able to prescribe, if they have prescriptive authority. The National Council of State Boards of Nursing (NCSBN) Advanced Practice Council worked for several years with stakeholders to draft an advanced practice mutual recognition compact, which was passed by the NCSBN House of Delegates in 2002. This compact outlines uniform criteria that all states might adopt for recognition of advanced practice. As of December 2008, three states have signed on to the compact—Utah, Texas, and Iowa—but no date has been set for implementation. This will provide for more consistency and allow for work mobility across state lines without the task of obtaining a license in each state. In 2008, NCSBN, working with other stakeholder groups, created a vision paper for APN credentialing (NCSBN, 2008).

Agency regulations are usually defined by the medical staff and hospital board and may restrict APNs from performing certain procedures. The license is tied to scope of practice issues outlined in the state practice act. Education provides the theoretical and experiential components to develop specific outcome competencies (as determined by the professional organization and the profession in scope and standards of practice). For example, the outcome competencies for a pediatric nurse practitioner (NP) would not be the same as those for a geriatric NP, although there may be some overlapping competencies.

It is important to document training and experience as practitioners progress in their careers because not everything essential for practice can be learned in the formal education process. However, just because a practitioner learned a particular procedure does not mean he or she is legally allowed to perform it because it may be outside the scope of practice and license. Health requirements (both physical and mental) are evaluated and certain restrictions may apply. Untreated substance abuse problems and physical impairments may interfere with the performance of a particular role. Competence and judgment become a little more subjective when evaluating and reviewing a privileging file. Many of the components of the file are taken into consideration when making an overall determination of competence and judgment, and the credentialing panel may want to establish a period of observation and performance evaluation.

Process

Therapeutic and diagnostic patient care services that fall under the privileging framework are usually defined by the particular medical or surgical specialty area within the health-care facility, and criteria are established that outline safe practice. Delineation of the specific types of privileges may be presented in a variety of ways, and each facility may have its own guide. Among the basic types of approaches are the following: cateogry, "laundry list," severity or complexity of care, and hybrid form. The first, category, usually defines privileges along specialty lines and can vary significantly across types of specialty programs because of curriculum. The listing of privileges and skills, or the laundry list approach, is used mainly for procedures and is less appropriate when specific diseases are referenced because of the variability of presentation. The severity or complexity of care is the third form and the fourth is a variation or hybrid form of those previously mentioned.

The credentialing panel or peer review panel who reviews the credentialing files may also determine the applicant's privileges, or there may be a separate panel composed of members, including peers, from the particular service or area. The ideal panel includes an interdisciplinary group, with APNs represented. This group determines if a candidate applying for particular privileges meets the criteria based on the information submitted in his or her credentialing package and application. They may allow the practitioner independent privileges or supervised privileges depending on the evaluation.

Clinical privileges are reviewed, revised, or updated for a variety of reasons other than at the time of reappointment. Evaluations of performance may warrant privileges being expanded or reduced. Nonuse of privileges may indicate that specific privileges are not needed and competency cannot be maintained. Finally, as technology and innovation emerge across hospital procedures and in the treatment of various diseases, the scope of privileges also change. Privileging is an ongoing process and new privileges may be added and some may be taken away based on performance. Accreditation requires that the privileges and credentials files be reviewed every 2 to 3 years to ensure currency and competence.

As an example, some of the specific tasks or procedures identified by Kleinpell (2002) for which an acute care NP might want to get hospital privileges include ventilator adjustments, managing resuscitation, interpretation of x-ray films, wound debridement, and insertion of arterial or central venous catheters. Another exemplar of clinical privileges is identified in the Guidelines for Clinical Privileges developed by the American Association of Nurse Anesthetists (AANA, 2005). CRNAs, one of the four types of APNs, have been completing credentialing and privileging processes for years, and other APNs can learn from their experience.

Temporary privileging may need to occur from time to time when a particular provider becomes ill or disabled, necessitating that another provider be recognized to take over certain duties of care. Recently recruited providers whose skills are specialized and needed in the facility may be awarded temporary privileges while the formal process of credentialing continues. These privileges are time limited and primary source verification of licensure and competence are allowed through phone calls until the full credentialing process occurs.

The National Practitioner Data Bank (NPDB) serves an important role in the credentialing process. In a survey of NPDB users, Waters, Warnecke, Parsons, Almagor, and Budetti (2006) found that most institutions use this inquiry process to make decisions about credentialing and subsequently privileging in a timely manner. Less than 10% of institutions indicated they had reached a credentialing decision before receiving the NPDB report, whereas up to 30% of respondents receiving a NPDB report did not grant privileging applications as requested. However the issue of incidents not being reported to the NPDB remains a barrier to the NPDB process as a leverage to comprehensive access to provider performance. Clearly multiple methods of data access and analysis are needed to achieve the goals of any credentialing and privileging system.

THE CAREER PORTFOLIO

Portfolios have taken on a new meaning in the world of competence. Portfolios are being used in a variety of ways by facilities, regulators, nursing organizations, certifying bodies, and educational institutions. Hospitals use them for evaluation and career ladder programs. Regulatory agencies use them for ensuring the public of competent practitioners (e.g., in Ontario, Canada). Dietitians use them for their recertification processes. Educational institutions use them for advanced placement of RNs into bachelor of science and graduate programs. Professional portfolios serve as the foundation of the credentialing and privileging application process used in today's health-care system.

Just as evidence-based practice provides a scientific, justifiable rationale for patient care therapeutics, practice-based evidence provides a rationale for authorizing a practitioner to perform specific patient care therapeutics. Documentation of this practice-based evidence provides just the information needed for the credentialing process as currently outlined.

It is difficult to track the events in our own lives as the world gets more and more complex, even though one would think it should be easier with all the technology available. As we add new experiences and roles to enrich our professional careers, work with new practitioners in a variety of settings, learn new skills, and pursue a path of lifelong learning, it becomes more and more difficult to remember where and when we did what, and where and when we learned what from whom. Establishing a professional credentialing portfolio as the APN begins his or her advanced practice education and career can take the agony out of the credentialing and privileging process and save time and money. It may even help the APN to be more adequately compensated by allowing him or her to achieve a higher status within a health-care facility because of practice-based evidence. Many bachelor's- and graduate-level programs in nursing already require the student to develop a portfolio during their educational process. The credentialing and privileging portfolio identified here can build on this process. For students or early professionals building a portfolio consider including some of the following items as suggested by Beauchesne (2007, pp. 34–35):

- Résumé
- Personal statements on practice and scholarship
- Case studies and research activities
- Health-care project descriptions
- Brief papers and assignments
- Publications and presentations
- Evidence-based examples

- Clinical practice logs or reflections
- Video clips
- Certificates of participation
- Letters of support and recommendation
- Continuing education activities
- Evaluations and competency reviews
- Course syllabi and transcripts

An online portfolio is an excellent way to build a professional career history that can serve multiple purposes, including the credentialing and privileging process. Licenses, certificates, transcripts, and documents can be scanned and uploaded to the online portfolio eliminating the need for paper copies. The individual can have access to their file anytime, anywhere they have Internet access. Fear of misplacing documents or having them destroyed by unforseen natural disasters (i.e., floods, hurricanes, or fires) can be eliminated. Stronger security of online materials has resulted from files that can be password protected. In addition, compilation of particular documents can be sent to credentialing committees via e-mail or they may be provided Internet access to them. Updates can be added to the portfolio as new knowledge and skill are acquired, making the portfolio a living document.

The purpose for which a portfolio is used determines the elements it should contain. Although many of the components are similar across portfolio types, some things are unique to the credentialing and privileging portfolio. Keeping the idea of credentialing and privileging in mind, the following format is suggested for developing this type of career portfolio. The career portfolio is composed of four major components: (a) the practitioner contact information page; (b) the practice-based evidence component, used to assist in determining specific privileges; (c) the credentials component section; and (d) the attestation page.

Practitioner Contact Information

An introductory page with name, address, contact information, practitioner's identity, and photo (if desired) is included.

Practice-Based Evidence Component

This area provides evidence to support the six areas of general competencies being evaluated, which include patient care; medical and clinical knowledge; practice-based learning and improvement; interpersonal and communication skills; professionalism; and system-based practice.

The practice-based evidence component should include the following:

1. Copy of the state practice act governing scope of practice in the state of licensure
2. Core competencies for the APN specialty
3. A sampling of references on the cost effectiveness and quality of care provided by APNs
4. Copies of job descriptions held in the past, especially those where clinical privileges were held
5. Specialty procedures or processes learned and verified:
   a. in the educational process
   b. on the job
   c. through continuing education
   (See sample of verification form, **Figure 8-1,** which could be used to validate these procedures.)
6. Letters of support and verification of practice competence in the areas outlined; include both peers and supervisors or employers

Name:

Specialty:

Certification: _____

Procedure(s):

Description/elaboration:

Verification:

I, the undersigned, have observed _____ and can verify
that he/she can safely perform the above outlined procedure(s)
independently/with supervision (circle one).

Provider/verifier: _____

Title: _____

License: _____

Facility: _____

Address: _____

_____

_____

Phone: _____   **Date:** _____

FIGURE 8-1 Sample verification of practice form.

7. Employment history, identifying significant responsibilities
8. Any performance outcome data that may have been collected at places of employment (e.g., number of patients seen per day, revenue generated)

Credentials Component

The credentials component should include the following:

1. Education (transcripts and diplomas)
2. Military history (if any)
3. Licenses (numbers and expiration dates or copies)
4. Certification(s) (national specialty)
5. Certification(s) (e.g., advanced cardiac life support, basic cardiac life support, pediatric advanced life support, trauma nurse coordinator)
6. Drug Enforcement Agency (DEA) and Medicaid numbers
7. Insurance coverage and any liability history
8. Immunizations and dates
9. Languages spoken, written, and understood (identify beginning, average, or advanced levels)
10. Research in progress or completed
11. Publications
12. Continuing education (no more than 5 years worth or length of certification)
13. Professional organization membership and offices held in those organizations
14. References (professional and personal)

Attestation Page

The final page, or the fourth component, should include a statement that is signed and dated by the provider attesting to the information contained in the portfolio. This should be updated every 2 years, as should the entire portfolio.

Sample

I, _____, attest to the authenticity of the information contained in this portfolio and verify that I am in good health and able to perform the clinical privileges I am requesting. I permit the employer or gaining party of this portfolio to verify any of the information provided if necessary.

Signed _____   Date _____

ISSUES

Although APNs are joining the staff of various facilities in greater numbers, there remain several areas that continue to challenge the APN full scope of practice and the process to achieve it in clinical settings. The issues presented here are not exclusive, but provide a springboard for fuller discussion and solution generation in a manner in which APN scope of practice can benefit consumers.

Maintaining Data About Performance

APNs are held to standards of performance that includes clinical practice and administrative standards. Both have economic implications for decisions to appoint or reappoint APNs to an institutional staff. The institution may find that clinical performance falls outside established benchmarks if patients under the APN's care have excessive lengths of stay, repeated and lengthy delays in appointments, and additional exposure to liability resulting from variation in performance. Patient satisfaction may be easily tied to performance. Credentialing is a given in professional and institutional life, with decisions to credential based on financial and performance factors (Kamajian et al., 1999).

APNs are wise to monitor their performance against the targets of the organization and colleagues and use the feedback to initiate personal or systems-wide performance improvement strategies. Maintaining documentation of outputs and accomplishments, patient acknowledgments, and cost savings are important assets for the APN's portfolio. It is also important that APNs are aware of the information and reference data about activities that are required to be verified as part of the credentialing process. Losing track of certification and licensure renewals have immediate repercussions for the credentialing process. Determining the accuracy of any inputs into the NPDB or other databases are important to verify before an institutional query occurs. Opportunities to correct information are less stressful when the APN is not abutting an institutional deadline.

Managed Care Panels

Health-care providers work in a competitive environment where more that one type of provider may be able to provide the same scope of practice or provide partial activities within another scope of practice. The ability to be credentialed and apply for legal scope of practice privileges rests in the hands of the credentialing structure. Professional medical societies are flush with complaints from physicians who perceive they have been excluded from MCO provider panels, and these exclusions present a glass ceiling for APNs as well.

Sometimes the exclusion of APNs is due to lack of knowledge about APN practice parameters, and at other times there is a perception of anticompetitive action (Kendig, 2002). APNs are well advised to provide documentation about APN performance outcomes compared with other providers through the use of evidence-based reports and articles, especially published in the provider's representative journals. Seeking advocates and allies at the institution to which the APN is applying can assist in the politics of selection for worthy candidates. Where warranted, legal consultation may prove helpful to understand the issues and the APN's rights. Six legal cases related to the multiple dimensions of this concern are discussed by Monarch (2002), and more have emerged since the author's publication. Patient advocacy groups can be particularly helpful to informing and creating demand for APN services.

Burden of Credentialing with Multiple Organizational Venues

When working in a health-care system or between two or more entities, the APN may be confronted with replication of the credentialing application process for each entity. This can be extremely time consuming and expensive in opportunity costs. It is important to gather perceptions from other providers and administrators about expectations and ramifications for productivity given duplication in processing of multiple credentialing applications. Create a solution team to construct alternative approaches to reduce redundancy and be prepared to gather support from colleagues on alternative proposals to present to the governing board.

Models for Second Licensure of Advanced Practice Nurses

Credentialing requirements for APNs vary among states as to the mechanism for title protection and scope of practice differences. The NCSBN proposed that it is appropriate for APNs to be legally regulated through a second license because their activities are complex, involve specialized competencies, independence, and autonomy (NCSBN, 2002, 2008). Most models require an application, RN licensure, completion of a graduate degree with a major in nursing or a graduate degree with a concentration in the advanced nursing practice category, and professional certification from a board-approved national certifying body.

All 50 states currently address advanced practice in public policy in some manner. For the most part, state boards of nursing hold authority over advanced practice. Additional education in pharmacology may be required where the prescription of medications is a sanctioned activity. By this arrangement, many state boards of nursing have deferred to the profession's right to recognize its specialists through certification and to develop and promulgate the standards of practice on which certification is based.

As you think about eventual changes in credentialing and privileging, be aware that no change is insignificant. Each readjustment holds both personal ramifications and implications for the profession as a whole. It is always wise to follow the dialogue and planning around national regulatory initiatives that will direct your scope of practice.

References

American Association of Nurse Anesthetists. (2005). *Guidelines for core clinical privileges: CRNA practice.* Park Ridge, Il: Author. Retrieved May 1, 2008, from the American Association of Nurse Anesthetists Web site: www.aana.com/practice/clinical_priv.asp.

American Hospital Association. (2002). Retrieved from the American Hosptial Association Web site: www.ahanews.com.

Beauchesne, M. A. (Ed.). (2007). *NP competency based education evaluation: Using a portfolio approach.* Washington, DC: National Organization of Nurse Practitioner Faculties.

Jones-Schenk, J. (1998). The brave new world of advanced practice: Credentialing and privileging. *Applied Nursing Research, 11*(3), 99–100.

Kamajian, M. F., Mitchell, S. A., & Fruth, R. A. (1999). Credentialing and privileging of advanced practice nurses. *AACN Clinical Issues, 10*(1), 316–336.

Kendig, S. (2002). Managing managed care. *Women's Health Care, 1*(1), 15–20.

Kleinpell, R. M. (2002). *The acute care nurse practitioner: An expanding opportunity for critical care nurses.* Retrieved June 10, 2002, from the Critical Care Nurse Web site: www.critical-care-nurse.org/CCN/ccn.

Monarch, K. (2002). *Nursing and the law: Trends and issues.* Washington, DC: American Nurses Association.

National Council of State Boards of Nursing. (2002). *Credentialing for advanced practice.* Retrieved June 29, 2003, from the National Council State Boards of Nursing Web site: www.ncsbn.org/public/regulation/res/APN_Position_Paper2002.pdf.

National Council of State Boards of Nursing. (2008). *APN vison paper—update and outcomes.* Retrieved May 1, 2008, from the National Council State Boards of Nursing Web site: www.ncsbn.org.

Quigley, P., Hixson, A. K., & Janzen, S. K. (1991). Promoting autonomy and professional practice: A program of clinical privileging. *Journal of Nursing Quality Assurance, 5*(3), 27–32.

The Joint Commission. (2008). *Comprehensive accreditation manuals.* Chicago: Author.

Utilization Review Accreditation Commission. (2008a). *Credentials verification organization standards, Version 3.0.* Washington, DC: Author. Retrieved May 1, 2008 from the Utilization Review Accreditation Commission Web site: www.urac.org/docs/programs.

Utilization Review Accreditation Commission. (2008b). *Provider credentialing organization standards, Version 4.0.* Washington, DC: Author. Retrieved May 1, 2008 from the Utilization Review Accreditation Commission Web site: www.urac.org/docs/programs.

Waters, T. M., Warnecke, R. B., Parsons, J., Almagor, O., & Budetti, P. P. (2006). The role of the national practitioner data bank in the credentialing process. *American Journal of Medical Quality, 21*(1), 30–39.

The Kaleidoscope of Collaborative Practice

Alice F. Kuehn

9

Pearson's (2008) 20th annual legislative update of the status of advanced practice nurse (APN) practice notes that despite opposition from organized medicine, APNs continue to progress toward full practice autonomy, including removal of requirements for physician oversight or supervision. However, this does not preclude the current emphasis on teamwork in health care. Solo practice seems unlikely today in any health-care discipline, and current trends in health care reflect an increasing call for collaborative practice. In the American Nurses Association's (ANA) *Nursing Policy Statement,* collaboration is recognized as the "recognition of the expertise of others within and outside one's profession, . . . some shared functions, and a common focus on the same overall mission" (1995, p. 12). The role of the APN has evolved along a continuum of collaborative inter-active models of increasing complexity (Kuehn, 1998). Just as a kaleidoscope creates a constantly changing set of colors and patterns, collaboration is a constantly changing aspect of health-care practice, moving from little interest to a great demand, from frustration to success, and sometimes back again. The interactions among members of a health-care team present a new picture each time the group, the situation, the time, or the environment changes. This chapter reviews the history and examines the myriad aspects of collaborative practice. It compares and contrasts multi-, inter-, intra-, and transdisciplinary practices, using examples to clarify the distinctions and similar-ities. The value, barriers, and strategies by which collaborative practice is being successfully devel-oped are presented as the continuing evolution of collaborative practice models is examined.

A HISTORY OF CHANGING RELATIONSHIPS

Our world continues to rapidly change to such an extent that change itself has become the con-stant. This sense of change in every aspect of life was described by Alvin Toffler in his classic 1970 publication, *Future Shock,* a term he created to describe the "shattering stress and disorientation" resulting from too much change too quickly. Our response to change has historically been slower than the change itself. However, in today's world of a rapidly increasing pace of change, the lag between the change and our response is growing, and this is what Senge (1994) calls *future shock.* Much of our human behavior flows from our ability to embrace or to fight the pace of life. Ours is a world of transience: a series of short-term relationships with people, things, places, workplaces, and information itself. In a situation in which the duration of relationships has been shortened, our sense of reality and of commitment and our ability to cope are seriously challenged. The flow of change is not linear, and we are being forced to adjust to novel situations for which we have not been prepared. Because we are living in a health-care world demanding collaboration, cost effec-tiveness, and quality care, the relationships among professionals are rapidly changing and we must be flexible and adapt. A key recommendation of the Institute of Medicine report *Keeping Patients Safe: Transforming the Work Environment of Nurses* (2004) was for health-care institutions to move away from a hierarchal approach to decision making and increase their support of interdisciplinary collaboration. "Ultimately, the success of each discipline will be judged by how effectively it participates in a continuum of care that meets the needs of patients and of the health care system overall" (Cooper, 2001, p. 58).

Physician-Nurse Relationships Over Time

In 1859, Florence Nightingale described the role of nursing as a specific set of relationships to medicine and hospital administration set within the social structure of the times. Placing the nurse as a care provider subservient to the physician established and formalized a role structure that, after nearly 150 years, continues to define society's general sense of the nurse role as within the role of the physician (Workman, 1986). The challenges physicians face in understanding, supporting, and embracing the reality of the advanced practice role is a result of "cognitive dissonance," a rejection or denial of information that challenges their preconceptions of the nurse role. In examining the historic roots of collaborative experiences between physician and nurse, the years between 1873 and the 20th century saw the relationship of nurse to physician become more and more a scenario within a hospital setting. The triad of physician-nurse-hospital superintendent never truly evolved in equilibrium as the Nightingale model envisioned because the scenario of a nursing superintendent reporting separately to the hospital trustees challenged the deference given physicians and administrators in practice and would have undermined both their authority and the use of student nurses as workers. Some nurses dissented to this deference, notably Isabel McIsaac, who asked at the turn of the 20th century, "Are we preparing nurses, or assistants to surgeons?" (Roberts, 1959, p. 248). However, according to Reverby (1979), "Hospital superintendents . . . sought the departmental dependence of nursing and their office, in alliance with the physicians, to assure that the nursing school and its female superintendent remained dependent on both the physician and hospital superintendent authority . . . [helping] minimize warfare in the hospital family" (p. 71). Also around the turn of the century, doctors, responding to challenges of low social and economic status and the growing importance of the hospitals, forged medical reforms with the result of power becoming concentrated in the hands of the physicians within a centralized, bureaucratic practice set.

Nurses had argued at the turn of the century that the absolute control by the physician was a shortsighted policy from a business point of view. However, the ongoing development of hierarchical relationships within the hospital between physicians, nurses, and administrators resulted also from changes occurring in nursing itself. Nursing sought to gain more professional status through a rigid hierarchical management style of its own within a continuing hospital management attitude of paternalism (Markovitz & Rosner, 1979; Reverby, 1979, 1987). Change began in the 1920s and 1930s as collaborative relationships with physicians, hospitals, and foundations serving the health-care system began to develop (Roberts, 1959). Evidence of collaboration was seen in cooperative planning during and immediately following the Great Depression, and medical society support of nursing school excellence in New York was affirmed by its participation in the Committee on Nursing of the Association of American Medical Colleges as they endorsed the Committee on the Grading of Nursing Schools. Unfortunately, the medical society withdrew from the committee shortly afterward. In 1935, a manual on hospital nursing service administration was published, sponsored by the American Hospital Association (AHA) and the National League for Nursing Education (NLNE). Another example of cooperative planning involved a survey of nursing schools in psychiatric hospitals under the auspices of a joint committee approach by the American Psychiatric Association (APA) and the NLNE. However, it should be noted that these examples are not of individual collaborative relationships, but of organizations, and are tenuous at best (Roberts, 1959).

The ANA code of 1950 spelled out a relationship of nurse to physician as a complex mix of dependent and independent responsibilities. Roberts (1959) stated that "The nurse is obligated to carry out the physician's orders intelligently, to avoid misunderstandings or inaccuracies by verifying orders, and to refuse to participate in unethical procedures. The nurse sustains confidence in the physician and other members of the health team" (p. 563). However, if every nursing decision made must come from within the orders flowing from another profession, the relationship cannot be collaboration but instead becomes supervised delegation. Kinlein (1977) identified the dilemma in nursing as a blockage of the ability of nurses to initiate nursing diagnoses, design nursing care, or establish a distinctive practice when the power of the medical judgment is the prime source of all decision making regarding patient care. Nursing judgments thus become delegated medical judgments because they are aimed at a medical goal and have to agree with that goal. Kinlein describes an example of a physician snatching a chart from her hands while she was teaching a student regarding a treatment regimen. The doctor stated, "What are you doing, talking about that? That's none of your concern. Just teach those students to give bedpans and then to remove them" (1977, p. 30), leaving both nurse faculty and student to conclude that either the nurse has to learn more and become a doctor or learn less so that he or she is prepared merely to carry out orders. In this situation, Kinlein notes, the nurse was expecting the physician to be knowledgeable, the patient expected both physician and nurse to be knowledgeable, and the physician expected the nurse to have no knowledge. This is an unacceptable situation, as well as a clear example of noncollaborative, unidisciplinary practice, with no communication between the two sets of providers except through a hierarchical, supervisory relationship. The current system of care delivery is described as one supporting professional individualism, prerogatives and separatism of roles, defensiveness, lack of continuity, redundancy, excessive costs, little cooperation and teamwork, and grossly inadequate and outdated systems of communication (Fischman, 2002; Norsen, Opladen, & Quinn, 1995; O'Neil & Pew Health Professions Commission, 1998). However, during the last three decades (1972–2002), an emphasis on the need for collaborative practice continued to intensify, requiring physicians and nurses to intently study the issues and begin working through the relationship-building process required to establish a collaborative practice. Pearson (2002) noted that "the irony of our continuing struggle with organized medicine is that, even while we fight against medicine's inappropriate domination over our practice, we must maintain and enhance our working relationship with individual physicians, for patients are best served when providers work together" (p. 22). This requires a team effort within an environment of mutual respect and valuing of each professional role. The 2008 Pearson report on the legal status of advanced practice nursing emphasized that no physician involvement is required for advanced practice nursing in 23 states for diagnosis and treatment and in 12 states for prescribing. However, this movement toward full autonomy of practice does not necessarily equate to "solo practice." As the *American Family Physician* noted, "collaboration improves health care outcomes for patients. APNs and physicians should work together to create new models of integrated education and collaborative care with patients as the focus. . . . The credible evidence showing that collaboration improves health care outcomes for patients entreats the two professions to put cooperation before professional roles" (Phillips, Green, Fryer, & Dovey, 2001, p. 1325). An increasing number of health-care studies continue to affirm the need for and value of collaboration, emphasizing that efficient delivery and quality of care may be very dependent on the level of collaboration among professional care providers (Hojat et al., 2003; Zwarenstein & Bryant, 2000).

Status of Collaborative Practice in Advanced Practice Roles

The growth and acceptance of the APN role has hinged on the willingness of the profession to acknowledge and support the role, provide advanced education and experience, and promote a clarity of role that facilitates development of a sense of self-identity and a clear understanding by other disciplines, the policy makers and legislators, and the public. As each of the four APN practices—certified registered nurse anesthetists (CRNAs), certified nurse-midwives (CNMs), clinical nurse specialists (CNSs), and nurse practitioners (NPs)—has moved toward autonomy in practice, establishing positive relationships with the medical community has been key. Stanley notes that "consumer satisfaction and physician advocacy have proved to be powerful stimuli" for operationalizing the APN role (2005, p. 34). Applying Benner's (1984) competencies and domains of nursing practice from novice to expert levels to advanced practice, Fenton and Brykczynski (1993) identified additional domains and competencies and verified the high level of expertise at the APN level. However, the scope of practice flowing from this model of expertise needs to be clearly identified. It is critical for the practice of all APNs, while maintaining clinical practice distinctions, to be conceptually united, stressing commonalities while acknowledging differences in practice patterns but promoting an interdisciplinary focus in their practice (Stanley, 2005). Once the role is clarified, scopes of practice delineated, common practice elements of APNs made known, and support from professional colleagues and consumers ongoing, the challenges faced in establishing collaborative practice will be greatly minimized. Without these foundational components, the challenges of creating truly functional teams will continue to be significant. This section provides a brief overview of role development challenges and achievements for each of the four APN practices including their approach to collaborative practice.

The Certified Registered Nurse Anesthetist

Clarity of role and a reach for autonomous practice was forged early in the development of nurse anesthetists. Alice Magaw, a pioneer in the field who worked at the Mayo clinic in the early 1900s, supported the separation of nurse anesthesia from nursing service administration, emphasizing its need for recognition and requirements for specialized education. During World War II, the role was identified as a clinical nursing specialty within the military field, and in 1945 a formal national certification process was established. Unfortunately, interdisciplinary struggles have prevailed throughout the history of their role development beginning with unsuccessful attempts in 1911 by the New York State Medical Society to declare that nurse anesthesia was illegal. Challenges have continued up to the present day, and confusion exists relating to the relationship of nurse anesthetists to physicians, whether anesthesiologist or surgeon (Faut-Callahan & Kremer, 1996).

The scope of practice of the CRNA has been described as a practice in collaboration with legally required professional health-care providers (American Association of Nurse Anesthetists [AANA], 2007). This description noting a "legally required collaborator" has led some to regard the legal status of nurse anesthesia as a "dependent function" under physician control and continues to result in considerable challenges in development of a high-level collaborative practice model (Bigbee, 1996; Faut-Callahan & Kramer, 1996). The degree of independence or supervision varies with state law. Some states use the term *collaboration* to define a relationship in which each party is responsible for their field of expertise while maintaining open communication on anesthetic techniques. Other states require the consent or order of a physician or other qualified licensed provider to administer the anesthetic. Currently the Centers for Medicare and Medicaid Services (CMS) require physician supervision as a requisite for nurse anesthetist services to Medicare patients. However, in late 2001, a rule was published in the *Federal Register* that allows a state to be exempt from this physician supervision requirement for nurse anesthetists after appropriate approval by the governor. To date, 14 states have opted out of the federal requirement (Blumenreich, 2007, p. 93).

But challenges remain. One CRNA recently described his practice as a noncollaborative practice but within an "improved" setting resulting from a change of billing directly by the CRNA. Although this improved the working relationship and allowed for a greater sense of autonomy, there often is still exclusion from hospital, departmental, and anesthesia group responsibilities in that only physicians can participate in hospital committees or represent the group. Note that this varies from state to state and from institution to institution.

The Certified Nurse-Midwife

In the colonial and pioneer history of the United States, midwives were respected members of both settler and American Indian communities. However, since the early 1900s the role has had a stormy history caused in no small part by the low status of women, sparse education, religious intolerance, and increased domination of physicians as obstetricians with movement toward birthing in hospitals. In 1921, the Maternity Center Association of New York and the Henry Street Visiting Nurse Association proposed establishing a school of nurse-midwifery. However, strong opposition from medicine, nursing, and the public arose, mainly because of a generally held negative view of the role of midwife as an exemplar of inadequacy, little education, and social incompetence. In 1925, the role was moved to a new level of recognition and respect with the inauguration of the Appalachian clinics of Kentucky by Mary Breckenridge (Dorroh & Norton, 1996).

Still, even today, because of lack of support from physicians and hospitals, CNMs are often unable to practice or their practice is severely limited. However, the number of CNMs practicing in the Unites States has moved from just 275 in 1963 to over 4000 by 1995 (American College of Nurse-Midwives [ACNM], 2007a). CNMs consider interdisciplinary practice as a sine qua non of their practice, and this position has been affirmed in their standards of care and formal definitions of practice. (ACNM, 2007b). In 1971, the American College of Nurse-Midwives (ACNM), the American College of Obstetricians and Gynecologists (ACOG), and the Nurses Association of the ACOG issued a joint statement supporting the concept of obstetrical team practice. However, the teams were to be "directed by a physician," formalizing a hierarchical practice pattern that continues to pose challenges to development of a collaborative approach to practice (Bigbee, 1996). The ACNM statement on collaborative management defines collaboration as "the process whereby a CNM or certified midwife (CM) and physician jointly manage the care of a woman or newborn who has become medically, gynecologically or obstetrically complicated" (ACNM, 1997). The need for collaboration is indicated by the health status of the client rather than by statute or edict. However, the number of viable practices currently differs considerably state by state because of legal and legislative requirements for collaboration and the parameters of required collaborative practice protocols, which vary from state to state. In discussing the extent of collaboration with currently practicing CNMs in Missouri, one CNM noted that of the group of physicians who were in the practice she joined, 50% saw the move to collaboration as obligatory and 50% welcomed it. From the perspective of the CNMs, relationships with the physicians varied from supportive and respectful (60%), to a wonderful team relationship (20%), to an obligatory "we are there so they have to talk to us" scenario (20%).

One major issue affecting role and collaborative functions is the collaboration of CNMs with midwives who are not nurses, a situation that some CNMs and APNs feel "muddies" the meaning of the APN role. However, in examining midwifery practice along a continuum of relationship intensity, it is possible that physician, CNM, and nonnurse-midwife partnerships are "at the cutting edge of developing a transdisciplinary workforce, a legion of people with different backgrounds but the same core set of midwifery competencies" (Dorroh & Norton, 1996, p. 414). Another factor threatening the future of the collaborative relationship is malpractice insurance cost. For example, in one CNM/physician practice group, the CNMs noted the cost of malpractice insurance increased from $18,000 to $40,000 during 1 year, and their practice group could not afford to cover the additional costs. The individual CNMs do not get paid for all the calls they take, nor are they able to perform enough births to cover the cost on their own insurance. This inequity of practice compensation coupled with the lack of 100% support of their practice by the physician group resulted in an interdisciplinary practice in which relationships were too inconsistent to survive. Consequently, these midwives no longer practice midwifery but only provide women's health.

In October 2002, the joint statement between the ACNM and the ACOG was revised for the fifth time in only 30 years. An ongoing concern of many CNMs and physicians was the language and the inferences of previous documents, readily open to multiple interpretations. The leadership of ACNM and ACOG decided to develop an entirely new statement, one that was more reflective of the current status of each profession, as well as contemporary realities within the women's health-care system. The 2002 ACNM/ACOG joint statement was created and has been jointly endorsed by both parties as a document ". . . that promotes respect and collaboration between CNMs/CMs and [medical doctors] and encourages individual practices to work collegially together to meet the needs of individual patients" (Shah, 2002, p. 2). The simplicity of the statement is perhaps its greatest asset. By not dictating specific protocols or responsibilities, professional accountability is placed where it rightfully belongs ". . . on each respective profession and the individual women's health care professional" (p. 3). It is the board of directors' hope and expectation that this new version of the joint statement will be welcomed by the members of ACNM and that it will continue to serve as an impetus to greater mutual understanding and support between CNMs/CMs and physicians for generations to come (Shah, 2002).

The Clinical Nurse Specialist

The CNS role, which originated in the late 1930s, was formalized as a nurse-clinician to be prepared in graduate nursing programs. Its emergence represented a major shift of focus in graduate education from the choice of a functional role of primarily teacher or administrator to the selection of a clinical specialization in practice. Of the multiple specialties represented by the CNS role, psychiatry was the first to move to graduate education and is among the most highly respected. Some have attested that collaborative activities with physicians seemed to come more naturally for this group because of their graduate-level education, which allowed CNSs and physicians to more readily relate to each other as peers (Bigbee, 1996). Key elements of CNS practice identified by American Association of Critical-Care Nurses (AACN, 2007) include "collaborating with other disciplines to provide interdisciplinary best practices" (p. 7). Collaboration is one of the eight CNS competencies considered essential for nurses providing care in the acute care setting. These competencies are part of the AACN synergy model for patient care, recommended as a guide for clinical practice in acute care. The model is predicated on the fact that patient outcomes are optimal when patient characteristics and the nurse competencies are in synch (Kaplow, 2007). One CNS described two different practices she has experienced: one a wonderful, respectful collaborative agreement and one that ended because of severe problems and irreconcilable differences. She could describe nothing more, noting that the situation was "too fresh and painful, much like I'd imagine a divorce." Another CNS described her collaborative practice level as a real partnership, almost perfect, with a great deal of mutual caring and respect between providers. Interactions were grounded in self-confidence and personal mastery by each partner and they planned together "always!" Yet another CNS noted that her collaborating physicians needed some education on what the CNS could and could not do, but they learned as they jointly practiced, and a real comfort level occurred after about 6 months. She commented that "I have to drive him with my vision." These CNSs have experienced a wide variety of practice patterns along the collaboration continuum, but the major attributes of the levels of collaboration they report consistently become more positive, productive, and interactively complex as the relationship becomes more mutually valued and partner driven.

The Nurse Practitioner

The role of the NP has been described as an innovative role in primary care, grown from the role of the public health nurse, and possessing a high degree of autonomy in practice (Bigbee, 1996). Since its inception in the 1960s, a considerable expansion of the concept of the NP role has occurred, as NPs have moved into a multitude of settings that are not necessarily primary care, such as long-term and acute care. Because of the unique and varied ways in which the role has developed, coming from certificate programs, many within medical schools, and gradually moving into graduate nurse programs, the history of collaboration is a patchwork quilt. Support of and opposition to the role has come from both medicine and nursing. Martha Rogers (1972) opposed the role as demeaning to nursing in deference to medical practice, and this view, supported by many other nurse educators at the time, created serious divisions within the nursing profession. Although some NPs found relief and role satisfaction in their practice, others, especially NP educators, worked to enhance the role and move it into graduate-level education. Medical opposition, which existed from the beginning and is mostly related to control and competition in practice, is often couched in terms of *patient safety*. Because of these powerful sources of opposition, the focus on collaboration has been both a boon and a boondoggle to NP practice. Hanna (1996) stresses the importance of the interdisciplinary team and the responsibility of the NP to assist in collaborative team development. However, when the term *collaboration,* often found in state nursing practice acts, conveys a concept of "supervision," there are many who would strike the word from any documents. The evolving acute care NP (ACNP) role requires a very explicit differentiation of medical and nursing domains within a collaborative practice. Strong support from nursing service, and better yet, having the ACNP housed within the nursing department, allows for easier differentiation of role by each partner. This promotes a team in which each partner comes from a solid professional sense of self and can then join with others to fuse into an autonomous, interdependent team of providers. In contrast, when the ACNP is "supervised" by a resident or is employed by a medical specialty department, it becomes more difficult for the practitioner to participate equally in decision making and to consider himself or herself a full partner in the practice (Lott, Polak, Kenyon, & Kenner, 1996).

The role of the NP within managed care systems has evolved into a process of collaboration, coordination, and negotiation, requiring the creation of new relationships among a wide range of personnel. Role negotiation is a key component of this type of practice, in which the required interaction between professionals for the specific purpose of changing the other's expectation of one's role, can result in increased job satisfaction, reduced role conflict, and a more positive team relationship (Miller & Apker, 2002). Way and Jones (1994) describe a family practitioner-NP dyad in which medical guidelines were developed for a shared practice. This practice is one in which care is shared, authority is shared, referrals are bilateral rather than unidirectional, and each partner is very knowledgeable regarding the knowledge, skill, and approaches of the other. A professional partnership promoting collaboration replaces competition with shared responsibilities, in which each partner brings a unique and necessary set of knowledge and skills to the practice, in addition to sharing the load of overlapping skills. The fear of loss of professional uniqueness is met head on by the description of practice models in which the concept of collaboration is grounded on the premise that the expertise and unique abilities of each team member, when combined into a synchronous whole, deliver a high level of care not possible through the efforts of a single provider (Norsen et al., 1995).

A review of two rural Ontario primary care practices between NPs and family physicians (FPs) found comparable involvement of both in health-promotion activities and considerably greater focus of NPs on disease prevention and supportive care. However, they also found NPs underutilized in relation to curative and rehabilitative services, with referral patterns being largely unidirectional, from NP to FP. Authors note that such a one-sided referral process does not reflect collaboration, which demands shared, reciprocal practice patterns (Way, Jones, Baskerville, & Busing, 2001). Rationale offered for these drawbacks to a full collaborative practice included unclear medicolegal issues affecting the ability to "share responsibility," a lack of interdisciplinary education at both undergraduate and graduate levels, and lack of knowledge and practice experience regarding the scope of NP practice. In addition, the regulated drug list required for Ontario NPs does not permit NPs to renew medications for stable chronic illnesses, limiting their scope of practice as well as hampering the ability of the NP to assist patients in management of their chronic illnesses (Way et al., 2001).

In contrast, in a Missouri primary care setting, the NP described her practice as very high on the interdisciplinary scale. She works with seven physicians, two of which she has worked with for more than 8 years. Meetings are consistent, brief, and specific, and communication is described as a professional exchange of facts and perspectives. There is no one-sided power show, and mutual respect is present. The physicians encourage her to do independent clinics 3 days a week, and there is no supervision, but only ready availability for consultation and referral. If the physicians need assistance or consultation, they call the NP. Within this practice can be found a number of the critical indicators and attributes of collaboration, especially the autonomy of role.

A FRAMEWORK FOR COLLABORATION

The Concept

Collaboration is described by Sullivan (1998) as a "dynamic, transforming process of creating a power-sharing partnership" (p. 6). A dynamic process, it includes the flexible distribution of both status and authority and requires both relationship building and shared decision making. A distinctive interpersonal process, it requires that the partners recognize and acknowledge their shared values and commit to interact constructively to solve problems and accomplish identified goals, purposes, or outcomes. Power, a key component within a collaborative practice, requires the active contribution of each participant, respect for and openness to each others' contributions, and use of negotiation in forming new approaches to practice that use the strengths of each participant (Hanson & Spross, 1996; Way et al., 2001).

The Components

A viable and high-level collaborative practice may be readily identified simply by the existence of four essential components: separate and unique practice spheres, common goals, shared power control, and mutual concerns. Table 9-1 presents these components essential for a positive practice, the key attributes of a highly collaborative practice, and practitioner competencies contributing to success.

TABLE 9-1		
Components of Collaborative Practice		
Essential Components	**Key Attributes**	**Competencies**
Separate and unique practice spheres Common goals Shared power control Mutual concerns	Autonomous, trusting relationship Confidence in partner's skill Bidirectional referrals and consultation Consensus-driven decision Equitable reporting lines and evaluators Mutually defined goals of the practice Open, informal communication Parity between providers (physical space, caseload, and support staff) Positive support by colleagues, support staff, and consumers	Assertiveness Communication skills Conflict management Cooperation Coordination Clinical skills Mutual respect Decision-making skills Positive attitude Trust Willingness to dialogue

1. *Separate and unique practice spheres.* Both physician and nurse must identify components of their practice that are separate and unique from the other and identify components that they share. A high-level collaborative practice requires an autonomous, trusting relationship within which bilateral consultation and referrals are the norm. Autonomy exists within each practitioner's skill and competence and allows for confident decision making. It is the *trust* of the team that empowers that person to practice independently within his or her defined scope of practice. As one APN noted, "You must be willing to expand your boundaries but know your limitations and where you feel comfortable in your practice" (Bailey & Armer, 1998, p. 243). The existence of bidirectional referral and consultation reflects a high level of trust between practice partners. In one instance, the physician response to a consultation request was, "Now this is not what you have to do, this is what I'd recommend. But the final decision is yours, because it's your patient" (Bailey & Armer, 1998, p. 243).

2. *Common goals.* When responsibility for practice goals is agreed to by both partners, the partners are well on their way to a synchronous relationship. As one provider in a highly collaborative practice noted, "Care by all providers is based on mutually defined goals of the practice" (Bailey & Armer, 1998, p. 245). All of the participants cited by Bailey and Armer (1998) stressed that responsibility for patient outcomes was the key driving force in their collaborative actions. One APN noted, "If there's a patient [I treated] who calls in and . . . says 'I'm just not better,' she'll [the physician] say things like 'If I had treated you, I would have given you the same thing.' It just sets the patient at ease because they realize that we're working together" (p. 245).

3. *Shared power control.* Each physician and nurse partner assumes individual accountability along with a shared responsibility for actively participating in the decision making as well as supporting the consensus-driven decisions and sharing in their implementation. One physician commented, "[The APN] really enjoys the kids and I do too, but she winds up doing a lot more pediatrics than I do. That's fine because she's more into wellness and preventative things than I am and that's just a reflection of our training" (Bailey & Armer, 1998, p. 245).

Ongoing and consistent communication is key to developing a shared-power practice. Providers must be comfortable in sharing information both about patient care and issues of collaboration and team functioning. One APN participant noted that a collegial relationship is essential for good communication to exist, saying, "There's not room for a hierarchical chain of command because that really inhibits communication. Both partners need to be safe confronting each other and be able to stand up for each other when necessary" (p. 235). Another commented that "He [the physician] respects what I'm saying to him. . . . He is approachable regardless of how bad his day may be going" (p. 245). Without shared decision making, Sullivan (1998) argues that collaboration cannot exist.

4. *Mutual concerns.* To ensure mutual concerns are met, providers need to have skills of assertiveness, cooperation, and coordination. Assertiveness can be described as the ability to express a viewpoint with confidence and with attention to being factually accurate and focused on the patient need. Six of the seven pairs of participants in the study conducted by Bailey and Armer (1998) identified this attribute as key in their practice, noting that all key decisions were made through negotiation and discussion. In a separate study of nurse-physician decision making regarding patient transfers from an intensive care unit (ICU), the majority of the nurses perceived their involvement in collaboration and decision making to be very low; interestingly, they were generally satisfied with this lower level of perceived collaboration. Although transfer decision making was a task nurses noted they were not usually involved in, the level of satisfaction with the current process did correlate positively in relation to the level of perceived collaboration with the physician. It appears that collaboration may be a task-specific phenomenon, interpreted and experienced differently by each provider (Higgins, 1999). Acknowledgment and respect of other opinions and viewpoints while maintaining the willingness to examine and change personal beliefs and perspectives stresses the interdependence of the practitioners on the team. Collegial relationships replace hierarchical authority with equality and shared decision making. Decisions made by compromise are based on the expertise of each member; there are different levels of input, but it is always in the best interest of the patient. For example, in a surgical care situation, the physician is in charge of the operation, the physician and NP or CNS jointly care for the patient postoperatively, the NP or CNS is in charge of discharge planning, and in some settings, the CRNA might also be on the surgical team, assuming full responsibility for anesthesia delivery. The key aspect of team success is the knowledge and use of each member's expertise by the others. Coordination of the necessary components of care usually falls to one member as an effective and efficient manner of handling the details around the total patient care plan. Often the nurse assumes this responsibility, but this is not always the case, nor does it need to be. One APN noted, "There are many times the physician will say to me 'This is a nurse practitioner patient,' and it's somebody that has all kinds of sociological problems. Problems that I could coordinate . . . and that's good; that's a compliment to nursing. He actually has learned what we do" (Bailey & Armer, 1998, p. 243). Trust is the bond that unites all the components of collaboration. "Without the element of trust, cooperation cannot exist, assertiveness becomes threatening, responsibility is avoided, communication is hampered, autonomy is suppressed, and coordination is haphazard" (Norsen et al., 1995, p. 45).

The Intensity Continuum

The level of collaboration within a practice can be found by identifying the intensity of professional relationships (high to low) and the type of collaborative structure found along a complexity continuum of unidisciplinary, multidisciplinary, interdisciplinary, or transdisciplinary practice (**Fig. 9-1**). The

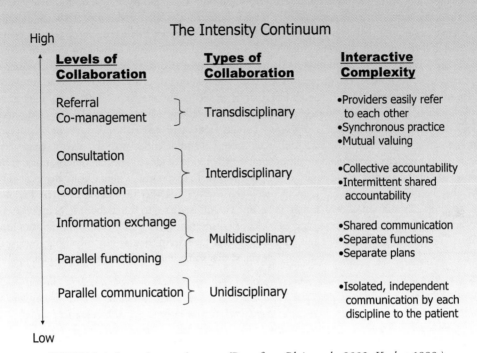

FIGURE 9-1 Intensity continuum. *(Data from Blais et al., 2002; Kuehn, 1998.)*

interactive complexity of the practice will increase as the structure becomes more complex, offering greater challenges to the team but resulting in even more positive and productive outcomes of practice.

Professional staff in any health setting (e.g., licensed practical nurse [LPN], social worker, NP, physician, radiology technician, and so on) are coming from a *unidisciplinary* base. As students, they were prepared for the interactive world of practice within the security of working with students, faculty, and practitioners of their discipline and program. They begin to develop personal mastery of professional knowledge and skill, an essential requirement for functioning effectively at the more complex levels of interactive relationships found in collaborative practice. Educational experiences with students of other professions, however, are generally very limited, usually to clinical encounters with a shared patient experience. As the professionals begin to share responsibilities for the same patient or patient populations, they begin, of necessity, to interact with each other, and a *multidisciplinary* practice model emerges. This is a level of information exchange, with no presumption of shared planning. Each fulfills a discipline-specific role, but communicates with others on an as-needed basis. This level exemplifies the "chimneys of excellence" approach in which work is accomplished not by team effort but by a collection of professionals working for the most part in "isolated splendor" (Kuehn, 1998, p. 27). However, within this multidisciplinary framework, an *interdisciplinary* relationship can begin to develop as two or more members begin to coalesce their roles toward a common vision or goal. There begins to be a sense of shared investment and a desire to plan together for a better outcome. As each professional shares discipline-specific expertise, cross-fertilization of ideas starts to occur and group ownership of the practice begins to emerge. The dynamics that revolve around the emerging practitioner-to-practitioner relationships concern issues of leadership, power control, norms, values, group behavior, and conflicts, and demand skills in communication, collaboration, and conflict resolution. The intensity of relationships is at a peak when a practice moves into a *transdisciplinary* level. It becomes a practice without professional boundaries, a synthesis of knowledge and practice. Here the practitioners are able to rise above fears of being subsumed and the individual visions of each become a shared vision with "laser-beam" intensity. The plan of care is owned by all, including the patient, and the goal of quality patient care transcends any "turf" issues. As the number of participants increases, the resulting diversity, complexity, and intensity of relationship building requires that each feels that he or she "owns" the vision. The critical indicators of collaboration are now a part of each and a visible part of the whole. At this level, communication through dialogue is the key to success. *Discussion,* coming from the same root word as *percussion,* implies a hard exchange of ideas bouncing back and forth, presented and defended with the need to come to a decision. In contrast, the art of *dialogue* allows for free exploration of ideas, issues, and innovations, with no sense of defensiveness and the ability to suspend personal viewpoints. When a team arrives at this point, they become in such close alignment that when working together they enter the "transdisciplinary" stage of collaboration, in which they act as one and do not have to think about it. Senge (1994) offers an example using the Boston Celtics, a basketball team that won 11 world championships in just 13 years. The famed Celtics center Bill Russell described their team play as not friendship, but as a synchronous relationship among the players. He stated that sometimes during a game, it would:

> "... heat up so that it became more than a physical or even mental game ... and would be magical. ... When it happened I could feel my play rise to a new level. ... It would surround not only me and the other Celtics but also the players on the other team, and even the referees. ... At that special level, all sorts of odd things happened. The game would be in the white heat of competition and yet I wouldn't feel competitive, which is a miracle in itself. ... The game would move so fast that every fake, cut and pass would be surprising, and yet nothing could surprise me ... during those spells I could almost sense how the next play would develop and where the next shot would be taken" (p. 234).

Tresolini and Pew-Fetzer Task Force (1994) states, "Practitioner's relationships with their patient, their patients' communities, and with other health care practitioners are central to health care and are the vehicle for putting into action a paradigm of health that integrates caring, healing, and community" (p. 19). To develop positive relationships with other health-care practitioners, comprehensive care requires the collective contributions of many varied professionals with highly developed skills, including self-knowledge and traditions of knowledge in the health professions; team and community building; and work dynamics of groups, teams, and organizations. Practitioners must be familiar with the healing approaches of other professions and cultures, be aware of historic power inequities across professions, identify similarities and differences among traditions of community members, know the value of the work of others, and learn from having had experiences of working with people from other disciplines and healing traditions. The key to team building is the affirmation by all of a shared mission, tasks, goals, and values (Jehn, Northcraft, & Neale, 1999; Senge, 1994).

The "Iceberg" Effect

Where the team of APN and physician falls on the collaboration continuum, as well as the intensity of the relationships, is determined by a number of critical factors. These factors can be visualized as an iceberg, with many visible and quite openly known and others that remain quite invisible or unacknowledged although still extremely significant in their affect on the success or failure of the collaborative effort (Pearson & Jones, 1994; Plant, 1987; **Fig. 9-2**).

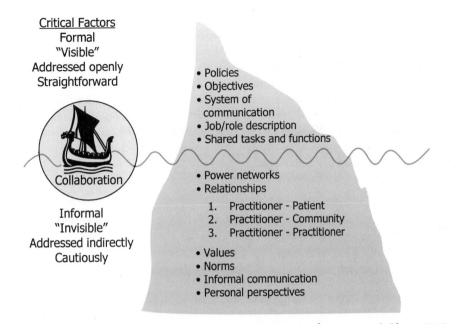

FIGURE 9-2 Iceberg factor. *(Data from Kuehn, 1998; Pearson & Jones, 1994; Plant, 1987.)*

The formal "visible" systems include many common components of practice such as organizational policies, clinic objectives, systems of communications, and role or job descriptions. These are accessible and changeable and are readily addressed in open, rational discussion. In contrast, the "invisible," informal systems, including power networks, values, and norms, are not as accessible but subtly present, difficult to change, and often give a sense of being untouchable. Many of the barriers to collaboration are hidden here. Only through working together can a team become aware of the impact of this invisible system and work to eliminate the barriers. The barriers must first be identified and acknowledged and then strategies applied to remove or neutralize them as the partners in practice work to become a viable team.

BARRIERS TO COLLABORATION

Barriers to collaboration hinder positive change and growth in our health-care system, frustrate the professionals trying to work as a team, and can negatively affect the future of health care. Key barriers that continue to challenge collaborative efforts include educational isolation, professional elitism, organizational hierarchy, unrecognized diversity, role and language confusion, inadequate communication patterns, and professional dissonance. It is important to understand the basis for these barriers and the need for them to be dissolved.

Educational Isolation

Despite an increasing call for an interdisciplinary approach to education in the health professions, many educators continue to use a traditional linear approach with built-in assumptions of bureaucratic organizational structures, standardized sets of relationships and roles, and systematized methods of record keeping, billing, and payment for services. Past studies exploring the status of interdisciplinary education have noted many inherent problems associated with developing interdisciplinary educational programs, citing workload stress, intense workload demands, lack of academic and institutional support, and often seemingly insurmountable complications with clinical arrangements (Kuehn, 1998). In addition, some nurse educators have expressed concerns that the traditional concept of a nursing workforce is challenged by calls for health care to be delivered by interdisciplinary teams, fearing that this focus has the potential of obscuring the unique contribution of nursing to health-care delivery (National League for Nursing [NLN], 1997). However, shared educational experiences can actually help clarify roles because as faculty and students work together, they begin to better understand the contribution each profession makes to the practice (Hojat et al., 2003).

Professional Elitism

Educational isolationalism easily leads to professional elitism as each profession educates "its own" with a sense of importance and unique worth. Although "importance" and "worth" are valued aspects of self-identify, a pervasive sense of professional elitism running through this approach can result in the work of each professional taking priority over helping each other or putting the patient's needs first (O'Neil & Pew Health Professions Commission, 1998). In his classic discourse on medical dominance, Friedson (1970) claimed that the dominant position of the medical profession in the health division of labor "allows it to reinforce and protect itself from outside influence and to claim and maintain jurisdiction and control over many more areas than logic or evidence justifies. . . . It is 'professionalism' itself that seems to transform the ideal responsibility to serve the good of the general public into a limited concrete responsibility to serve the good of one's personal public" (p. 152). Professionalism consists of three components: professional ideals of knowledge and service, the professional occupation and the life career it provides, and the character of the work itself. The life career is the vehicle through which the ideals are put into practice, and the character of professional work is defined by the profession itself. The commitment to healing and to service is thereby limited by the definition of healing and public service crafted by the profession. Friedson (1970) states, "Operative professionalism is thus constituted by commitment to occupationally defined knowledge and technique and occupationally defined public service, to a particular occupation's view of correct knowledge and ethicality" (p. 153), while demanding the freedom to practice using independent individual judgment. Friedson (1970) describes this as "professional imperialism and narrowness . . . A professional who is so qualified as to perform this extraordinary work of medicine . . . must himself be a rather extraordinary, gifted, person . . . as are his colleagues and his profession. . . . This professional pride leads the worker to consider himself to be quite different from, indeed superior to, those of other occupations. When outsiders doing work related to his, support a set of goals flowing from a different set of paradigms than those of his own profession, the professional rather feels that they and their occupation should either be converted and controlled, or if not destroyed, then excluded from any significant interaction. . . . The thrust of professional activity becomes a mission to build barriers that keep the profession and its clientele safe from those beyond the pale while seeking jurisdiction over all that cannot be excluded" (pp. 154–155). A physician attitude of superiority, supported by a hierarchal organization structure, is a major factor in the political battles over practice and reimbursement. Nurses, however, need to acknowledge that nursing has also been guilty of elitism and of exhibiting professional dominance and defensiveness, both in relating to other nurses with different levels of education and expertise, as well as in working with other health-care professionals. Lack of understanding and acceptance of roles and responsibilities of other professionals is the basis for much of the elitism still prevalent today.

Organizational Hierarchy

In a provocative sociological analysis of health services work, Friedson (1970) identified "professional dominance" as the key to what he described as the inadequacy of health services. He described the organizational structure of health services as revolving around professional authority, with a foundational structure of dominance by a single profession over a variety of other "subordinate professions." Professional behaviors and roles are contingent to some degree on the influence of patient preference, colleague groups, formal training, and the trappings of professionalism, including autonomy, expertise, and control. To reconcile the concepts of autonomous expert with hierarchal authority, there needs to be a company of equals with minimal hierarchal differentiation in which advice is delivered rather than orders. The two lines of authority in medicine and health care historically include the administrative authority of the "office" and the medical authority of professional skills and expertise. The medical profession (a) is an occupation with a special form of institutionalized privileges and authority granted by others on a basis of faith and trust because their knowledge and work are considered very complex and nonroutine work, (b) holds a special form of legal "power" based on "expert status," and (c) has a special position of dominance in the set of other occupations providing health care. This results in professional control of information and suspicion of the value of what lies "outside" their domain. Friedson (1970) suggests that this autonomy and dominance need to be and can be controlled by an administrative structure that stresses accountability for effective and humane services and is responsive to the patient.

> For a profession to be true to the ideal of a profession, members must let go of the total authority and control over the terms and content of their work and cease total dominance in favor of a division of labor. The physicians must temper autonomy and dominance with administrative accountability, accountability to the patient, self-regulated peer review and encouragement of other providers to assume responsibilities of health care . . . [However] no service using other providers is possible . . . without the active cooperation of the dominant profession. If the profession does not trust them, or if it resents and fears them, it will not refer patients to them, nor will it graciously receive patients referred from them . . . Mere administrative fiat is not enough . . . Optimal forms of health services require that physicians be positively interested in working with other health professionals . . . [For] without positive encouragement by physicians . . . patients will not make willing and comfortable use of other providers (pp. 231, 234).

Supervision is defined as critically watching and directing activities or a course of action. The basis for supervision of health-care providers has been sometimes cited as a result of documented inadequacy; lack of knowledge, experience, or skills in relation to the person supervised; legal requirements; a lack of trust or confidence despite no legal limits requiring supervision; perceived safety needs of patient or provider; and history, tradition, or local institutional policy. In exploring the difference between "under the supervision of" compared to "ownership of practice decisions," it may be most helpful to view them not as polar opposites but as different levels of collaboration along a continuum of autonomous practice. Supervision may not preclude some level of collaboration, but it seems to severely limit its scope. When "medically delegated functions" are described as diagnosis and management of short-term episodic illnesses and early detection and management of stable chronic ones, the extent of collaboration possible within such a "delegated" mindset is questionable. Is shared decision making even possible within a hierarchical model of supervised practice?

Another aspect to consider is the line of reporting accountability. If different for each practitioner, does that negatively affect the practice? A NP-staffed "fast track" in the emergency department (ED) of Vanderbilt University Medical Center was designed using written protocols created collaboratively by the NPs and the medical director of the ED. Although the NPs reported to the ED nursing director and the physicians to the ED medical director, the collaborating practice was well established within a few months, with a growing sense of confidence and trust between these distinct professional providers. Covington, Erwin, and Sellers (1992) state, "By performing the dual role of physician and nurse, the NP eliminates the fragmentation of care often seen in the ED," where patients see many different physicians, nurses, and staff members, and there is no consistent provider (p. 124). The report made no mention of the effect of the parallel reporting system or the level of collaboration achieved. In addition, the language, "dual role of physician and nurse," leads to a misconception of the nurse role. No nurse can assume the role of a physician, nor can a physician assume the role of a nurse. It is possible that certain responsibilities, functions, and skills are learned and assumed by both providers. When the nurse assumes some of the responsibilities, functions, and skills traditionally assumed by the physician, if they fall within the scope of nursing practice, they are nursing. If they fall outside, then they are considered medically directed acts, and the nurse in that instance is serving as a physician assistant. Kinlein (1977) stressed that if a physician, a member of another profession, determines by his or her orders what actions a nurse, a member of a separate profession, will take, then the practice is no longer the essence of nursing but becomes "medically-directed care" delivered by nurses (p. 30). Supervised or medically directed care seems to fall within the framework of multidisciplinary interactions representing a very limited level of intensity of relationships and collaboration.

Unrecognized Diversity

Diversity in a health-care team can have a powerful impact on its success or failure as a cohesive workgroup. It can bring a wealth of helpful differences but can also be the cause of great conflict within the group. Cultural diversity may be easily recognized and acknowledged, but there are many complex aspects of diversity that may not be recognized and that can undermine team efforts. Three major categories of diversity include informational, social category, and value (Jehn et al., 1999). Informational diversity reflects the differences in knowledge and perspectives of team members, flowing from their education, experiences and levels of expertise. Social category diversity relates to race, gender, and ethnicity and is the aspect we are most familiar with as cultural diversity. Value diversity reflects the differences in member's perspectives of the mission, goals, and values relating to the work at hand. A 1999 study of the impact of diversity on work group performance found that different forms of diversity can result in different levels of performance within the team. Having high information diversity (differences in education and experience) can make a team quite effective because of the many professional perspectives that can be available to the team. However, if it is accompanied by high value diversity, the team will be malfunctional. Over time, age, gender, and race differences in a group become less important but value diversity—differences in understanding of the mission, goals, and values—becomes the more important component as a predictor of conflict or success. The complexity of relationships within a team is heightened by the level and type of diversity. Often unrecognized or unacknowledged, value diversity may be the most critical factor in the success or failure of teamwork and collaboration (Jehn et al., 1999).

Role and Language Confusion

The increasingly expanded scopes of nursing practice being experienced across the United States continues to be hampered by inconsistencies of legal language and titling variations among states. Collaboration, often used in statute, is frequently interpreted in rules and regulations as "supervision," implying a hierarchical relationship and a contradiction to the critical indicators of collaboration. For collaboration to consistently mean an egalitarian, collegial relationship, the legislative language must be more clearly defined. The question becomes whether power sharing can coexist with a supervision requirement in a practice. When collaboration is mandated, or termed *supervision*, then the process of shared practice becomes one of forced negotiation in which the dominant profession, medicine, has the choice of collaboration, with no legal need for a collaborative partner, whereas the subjected profession, nursing, must obtain a collaborative partner to legally practice within the full scope of its practice (Sullivan, Morgan, Heimerichs, & Scott, 1998). In the 20th Annual Legislative Update, Pearson (2008) notes that in relation to diagnosing and treating aspects of NP practice, 23 states now have no statutory or regulatory requirements for physician collaboration, direction, or supervision; four require physician involvement but no requirement for written documentation of relationship, and 24 require physician involvement documented in writing. In regard to the prescribing aspect of practice, although 12 states now have no requirement for any physician involvement, the other 39 (including the District of Columbia) require physician involvement documented in writing. Physician involvement can be termed *collaboration, supervision, direction, delegation,* or *authorization.*

One major issue regarding such statutory and regulatory requirements is the lack of consistency in terminology and the lack of clarity regarding the level of collaboration that exists if it does exist. Even when termed *collaboration,* it may not represent an equal relationship. The expectation of collaboration within a clinical team has long been a distinct focus of nursing practice (ANA, 1998). However, statutory requirements for collaboration for advanced practice nursing couched as "delegated" or "supervised" practice are not acceptable for a number of time-tested reasons. If patterns of practice are legislated, legislative judgment becomes limited by the parameters of the legal definitions, rules, and regulations of the state in which practice is located. The flexibility needed for individual clinical situations may be seriously compromised by these legally defined parameters. The result is that, because of restrictive legislation, rules, regulations, and reimbursement policies, advanced nursing practice often still depends on the willingness of a physician collaborator, whereas the same limitations are not placed on the physician. The ANA (1998) states, "One can only imagine what the reaction of organized medicine would be if a state legislature attempted to delineate when and how internist physicians should refer patients to a specialist" (p. 4). Legislatively mandated collaboration often results in a conflict (Sullivan, 1998). In states where APN practice is controlled by joint board decisions, the negotiation process of joint rule-making can become very hostile because of an unequal balance of power among the parties. Further, when membership of the board of nursing includes representatives of each level of nursing, those members not in advanced practice lack the knowledge base required for debating advanced practice issues such as prescriptive authority. The subsequent rules passed may be far more restrictive than had been imagined from the broader language of the statute. Reasons offered by Sullivan et al. (1998) for the failure of these disparate groups to accomplish an externally imposed power-sharing partnership are not difficult to understand. They state,

> *Because the participants did not share a common purpose or vision, and were forced to meet, it is not surprising that they did not work well together or achieve a satisfactory result—by any standards. Because the representatives were forced to come together and their Boards had their budgets held hostage to the process, it was not unexpected that despite the need to reach some level of agreement there was little commitment to a win-win situation. . . . Instead, representatives of each discipline worked to protect their distinctly different professional agendas. It became not a collaborative process but a legalistic and formalized process of enforced negotiation (p. 350).*

In examining the role of "primary care provider," the essential features of primary care identified by Starfield (1992b) included first contact care, longitudinality, coordination, and comprehensiveness. As a physician, Starfield contended that the role of nonphysician personnel in industrialized nations was not significant to the degree that there is "attainment of all the unique and essential features of primary care" (p. 145). She identified three types of functions performed by nonphysician personnel: (a) supplementary, extending the efficiency of the physician by assuming the technical tasks, usually under the direction of the physician; (b) substitutive, providing services usually provided by physicians; and (c) complementary, extending the effectiveness of physicians by doing things physicians do not do at all, do poorly, or do reluctantly. Noting that the nonphysician role has not been clarified to the extent that the three functions can be differentiated, Starfield concluded that primary care is largely a physician-dominated effort. Although primary care cannot function without some teamwork involving other practitioner providers, she believed that there is little evidence supporting the concept of team practice and little research indicating when and under what conditions a team approach may be more effective than a singular practice approach. In conclusion, Starfield asserted that primary care should be provided by physicians and the concept of *teamwork* in primary care needed to be researched regarding (a) standards for different roles and relationships, (b) identification of which type of delegated function—substitutive, supplementary, or complementary—is most appropriately assumed by what level or type provider, and (c) how well the attributes of primary care are achieved by nonphysicians in comparison with care by physicians. Concerns raised by Starfield's discussion of primary care center on the language used, as well as her consistent adherence to the traditional medical viewpoint of the physician as the "captain of the ship." The use of the term *team* is quite perfunctory and seems to imply only a multidisciplinary collection of individuals gathered by the physician to facilitate his or her practice. The three functional types—supplementary, substitutive, and complementary—are each defined in relation to their ability to enhance physician effectiveness rather than as shared components of a joint practice. In addition, Starfield frames the role of the nonphysician provider by tasks and functions severely limiting the scope of advanced practice (Starfield, 1992a).

An interesting counterpoint is offered by King, Parrinello, and Baggs (1996). They view collaboration as interdependent, interdisciplinary practice in which the "substitutive" APN role is more appropriate in a primary care setting in contrast to the complementary role more applicable in acute care settings. They note that problems arise with this interpretation unless the roles of the partners are clearly understood; with misunderstanding often comes limitations to the scope of practice for the APN. However, there are difficulties with the use of the term *substitutive* because it implies a temporary stopgap until the "regular" practitioner can be provided.

Another language issue relates to the use of protocols. Is a protocol a "red flag," a "red herring," or an excellent tool for clinicians? Protocols are defined as the "detailed plan of a scientific or medical experiment, treatment, or procedure" (Merriam-Webster, 1994). In research, they need to be followed "to the letter" to have accurate, consistent, and comparable sets of data. The concern with protocols comes with their use in statutes, rules, and regulations as a definitive set of boundaries restricting practice to sets of predetermined criteria. If the perception of nursing is as a dependent practice under physician supervision, the mechanisms created for allowing advanced practice often include a system of protocols designed with the approval of the "collaborating" physician. However this "solution" compromises the concept of nursing autonomy, suggests that the nurse is incapable of making accurate choices among treatment options and becomes implicit "standing orders" reinforcing nursing dependency (Baer, 1993). For example, in Arkansas, neither protocols nor a collaborative practice agreement with a physician is required unless the APN has prescriptive authority. If they receive prescriptive authority, they must then have a collaborative practice agreement with a physician, but no protocols are required under law. In contrast, NPs in California must use standardized procedures or protocols developed by the NP and the "supervising" physician; CNMs in California may order Schedules III through V controlled substances only within a patient-specific protocol approved by the "supervising" physician. In Alabama, NPs and CNMs must practice with protocols approved by the board of nursing and board of medicine, and they must include a formulary of drugs, treatments, tests and procedures, a plan for emergency services, a referral process, a mechanism for quality analysis, and a written plan for review of medical records.

In contrast, practice guidelines are systematically developed statements to assist practitioner and patient decisions about appropriate health care for specific clinical circumstances. These can simply be broad statements or can be very detailed based on literature review as well as expert opinion. Typically, clinical guidelines reflect more than local consensus regarding appropriate diagnosis and treatment of a condition. Clinical guidelines also can be developed to describe the indications for procedures and the process of care. The Agency for Healthcare Research and Quality (AHRQ, formerly the Agency for Health Care Policy and Research) uses the term *clinical practice guidelines* to describe systematically developed statements to assist practitioner and patient decisions about appropriate health care for specific clinical conditions. These are written by independent multidisciplinary panels of private-sector clinicians and other experts, supported by AHRQ. Practitioners must have clinical guidelines for reimbursement from Medicare (Newman, 1996), and they are viewed sometimes as an excellent tool for communicating the role to funding agencies (Way & Jones, 1994).

One additional aspect of language confusion is that of "titling" of APNs. Among the many titles found in the different state statutes are advanced nurse practitioner (ANP), APN, advanced practice professional nurse (APPN), advanced practice registered nurse (APRN), advanced registered nurse practitioner (ARNP), certified nurse practitioner (CNP), and registered nurse practitioner (RNP). The latest development in advanced practice, the launching of doctorate of nurse practice programs, has created even more language challenges as the term *Dr. Nurse* is causing many physician groups to challenge not only the terminology but the concept itself (Landro, 2008). With some physician groups still insisting on supervision, the challenge remains to get past the language barriers and clarify roles to foster a collaborative approach to care.

Inadequate and Inappropriate Communication Patterns

When physicians and nurses do not share information or concerns, when communication is a one-way street, or there is an inadequate system of written and verbal communication, quality of patient care will suffer. Poor communication patterns also affect working relationships and seriously hinder any attempts at collaboration, often resulting in separate professional decision making that can create confusion and safety issues (Clarin, 2007; Zwarenstein & Bryant, 2000). Inappropriate communication patterns may reflect a pattern of "physician abuse." In a survey of nurse-physician relationships (Rosenstein, 2002), the level of respect for nurse input and collaboration was rated significantly higher by the physicians than by the nurses, whereas ratings on how important the physician's disruptive behavior was in contributing to nurse dissatisfaction and low morale, were rated significantly lower by the physicians. These findings reflect a dissonance in perception that is often a result of poor communication and lack of trust, creating a defensive, noncollaborative practice environment in which the number of errors rise and patient safety and positive patient outcomes are threatened. Magnet hospitals, emphasizing collaboration between physicians and nurses, have been documented as having better patient outcomes and fewer problems relating to shortages, turnovers, or abuse (Fischman, 2002).

Professional Dissonance

When diversity is not recognized and acknowledged, the result is professional dissonance and a serious negative impact on the capacity for teamwork. Confusion of language, differing communication patterns and ways of interacting, and difficulty respecting each other's skills and roles are inevitable. A recent study of attitudes regarding teamwork by critical care nurses and physicians developed a seven-item "teamwork climate scale," which found nurses and physicians had distinctly different attitudes toward teamwork. They placed the source of the differences in status/authority, responsibilities, gender, training, and professional cultures (Thomas, Sexton & Helmreich, 2003). Baggs and Schmitt (1997) described collaboration as a twofold process of working together and sharing information. In their study of nurses and physicians in a medical ICU, they found that collaboration would occur only if the time and place were appropriate, the physician felt the nurse had the knowledge needed, and trust, respect, and sincere interest in teamwork were present. For example, the physicians felt the general medical unit nurses did not have the same level of knowledge about medical illness as the medical ICU nurses. This perceived knowledge level was a precondition to the physician's willingness to collaborate with the nurses.

Differences and similarities of physicians and nurses in their perceptions related to the four indicators of nurse-physician collaboration were identified in the ANA social policy statement of 1980: mutual power control, mutual safeguarding of provider concerns, responsibility for practice, and practice goals. The findings offer an interesting portrait of the collaborative perspective of the partners. Although nurses and physicians were in agreement on power-control, most affirmed that the physician initiated more communications than the nurse. This chapter identifies this as representing a lack of mutual power control (Jones, 1994). In examining provider concerns, nurses and physicians were rated on the degree to which they achieved both assertiveness and cooperativeness, with high levels of both dimensions indicating collaboration. Nearly half of the responses reflected competition, compromise, or accommodation as the preferred method of safeguarding concerns. They did not agree on where *responsibility for practice* should rest in 10 different areas (e.g., referral, prescription, infection prevention, diagnosis)—on nurse, physician, or both, and they agreed on only 4 of 24 practice goals (e.g., maintain elimination patterns, promote cardiovascular healing). Although it is noted that assuming primary responsibility for a patient goal by a specific provider may be patient specific, the conclusion reached was that nurses and physicians who cannot agree on provider responsibility regarding areas of practice and patient goals, reflecting a lower level of collaboration, will not be able to deliver the same high level of coordinated patient care as those nurse-physician teams who agree on the areas of responsibility (Norsen et al., 1995).

The Bottom Line

Barriers to collaboration hinder positive change and growth in our health-care system but do not need to be perpetuated. Organizational climate and culture is a living, growing aspect of institutional work life that binds the organization together. Professions and professionals are not static. They can and must work to eliminate barriers to collaboration and create a new culture of team practice in health care. The following strategies are offered for creating the necessary climate for collaborative practice.

STRATEGIES FOR SUCCESS

Collaboration is defined as a "dynamic, transforming process of creating a power-sharing partnership . . . for purposeful attention to needs and problems in order to achieve likely successful outcomes" (Sullivan, 1998, p. 6). It is a developmental process that emerges slowly through a series of sensitive and delicate interactions. Members of this newly forged partnership join forces in the belief that the common need they recognize can best be met through their combined efforts. Levels of collaboration achieved depend on context, ability, and the desire of the prospective partners to skillfully develop the practice. Based on the conceptual framework of collaboration described in this chapter, some key strategies are offered for developing a successful collaborative team.

Create an Effective Team

Teamwork is a critical need for today and the reality of tomorrow's practice. Peters and Waterman (1982), focusing on people as the means to achieve productivity, noted that coworkers should be treated as partners. The reality of this shift of power from an authoritarian command structure to one of collegial team work can result in innovation, rapid response, and greater access by the customer. However, it requires a considerable mind shift by participants. The redesign of a health-care delivery model that supports an interdisciplinary team approach requires a radical way of thinking to acknowledge that this new model is not something "out there," but belongs to each of the participants as they confront their learned beliefs and perspectives. In addition, the participants must realize that they must undergo a significant cultural shift in accepting that they become a community of learners, a "learning organization" that never "arrives" but continues to translate a shared vision into an ever-evolving practice (Senge, 1994). The key feature of this learning organization is a realization that the role of the "grand strategist" at the top is no longer possible because of the complexity and dynamic status of work. Instead, they tap each individual participant's commitment and capacity to learn. Unlike a linear approach, the learning organization forges ahead based on shared understandings of interrelationships and patterns of change. The five qualities needed for participants in the learning organization include the following:

1. *Personal mastery.* The practitioner is true to a personal vision while staying committed to the truth of the current reality.
2. *Use of mental models.* Learning is accelerated as we mentally consider alternative scenarios for care delivery. Participants do not become so attached to one scenario because it could freeze them into rigid adherence to outdated approaches to care.
3. *Shared vision.* Shared vision is described by Senge (1994) as the "first step in allowing people who mistrusted each other to begin to work together as it creates a common identity and sense of purpose" (p. 208).
4. *Team learning.* Nurses, physicians, and others on the team learn to think together about complex issues, acknowledging that the whole is truly greater than any of the individuals. They develop what is termed *operational trust* and master the practice of both dialogue and discussion. The apex of "team" is at the transdisciplinary level.
5. *Systems thinking.* Foundational in team work, systems thinking forces a focus on the whole pattern of the collaborative practice, rather than any isolated role. The structure or key interrelationships of the practice pattern influence behavior and decision making and are examined collectively.

Key components of effective teams identified by the Institute of Medicine (2001) in their report "Crossing the Quality Chasm" include the following:

1. *Team makeup:* Appropriate size, composition, and power to reduce or eliminate negative effects of status differences;
2. *Team processes:* Communication pathways, conflict management procedures, and leadership focused on excellence and clarity of goals, roles, and expectations for the team;

3. *Team job:* Matching roles and training to level of complexity of the case, promoting cohesiveness when work is highly interdependent; and

4. *Context and environment of the setting:* A culture of openness, honest admission of abilities and limitations by team members, and support of administration for the team approach, including provision of time, resources and rewards needed (p. 132).

Accept Growth and Development as a Joint Responsibility

For the concept of collaborative practice to grow and flourish, interdisciplinary education must be supported, affirming the values and roles of both physician and nurse. This requires educational institutions to reaffirm the value both of education for and evaluation of the effect of collaboration on outcomes. In practice, bidirectional referrals must be promoted and must include the expanded NP scope of practice and "skill set" in the NP role description. Professionals and the public must be educated regarding the role by both physician and nurse partners. In recent literature reporting on physician abuse, strategies recommended to improve collaboration included physician education, zero tolerance policies, role-playing, and changing the culture of the environment from defensive and hierarchical to supportive and collegial. Nurse responsibility for the problem, in tolerating the behavior, perpetuating the inequalities in the nurse-physician relationship, and sometimes countering with abusiveness, should also be addressed with education, role playing, assumption of accountability, and an assertive sharing of the nursing perspective (Fischman, 2002).

Use Protocols and Guidelines Wisely

In clinical practice, *protocol* is often used synonymously with *clinical guidelines* and is representative of a statement of agreement between an APN and his or her collaborating physician. When the providers agree on a standard of care acceptable to both, the guidelines or protocols stand as their codification of acceptable criteria for diagnosing and managing an illness or condition. Texts such as *Patient Care Guidelines for Nurse Practitioners* (Hoole, Pickard, Ouimette, Lohr, & Powell, 1999) and *Gerontological Protocols for Nurse Practitioners* (Brown, Bedford, & White, 1999) offer excellent resources for practitioners, as well as sometimes serving as the basis for legal documentation to allow for treatment and prescriptive privileges through incorporation into the collaborative agreement as the agreed-to standard of care. This is a positive viewpoint of guideline and protocol use. However, guidelines and protocols can also become very limiting factors to a practice. Physicians, too, sometimes hesitate to support the concept of guidelines in their practice. Historically, guidelines represented collective wisdom gathered over time and were considered no threat to autonomy. In contrast, guidelines today are not as willingly accepted because of the fear that they might influence or "manage" physician behavior. If guidelines or protocols allow room for the exercise of provider judgment, they will support provider autonomy as well. Guideline development needs three aspects to accomplish its goal. Identification of key decisions and their consequences must first be outlined. In the case of the APN, decisions of when to call the physician with questions and refer the patient to outside specialists is one aspect. The process of reviewing charts and prescriptions is another aspect for the APN and physician. Finally, reimbursement from insurance providers must be defined because of strict insurance policies and legislative mandates. Although state and federal statutes may allow for certain billing practices, the viability of the practice may be hampered when NPs are limited to lesser reimbursement amounts or are refused reimbursement. Legislative language in many states must continue to be reworked to clarify the meaning of the terminology, the role and scope allowed, and the affect on practice viability of protocols and clinical guidelines.

Watch Your Language

Language is one of the most significant facets of relationships. In an editorial from *American Family Physician* (Phillips et'al., 2001), a physician professor took aim at the use of the term *health-care provider,* noting that "calling me a 'provider' lumps my physician colleagues and me with individuals who are frankly less qualified and yet aspire to do the same work we do . . . the use of terms . . . although 'politically correct' diminish us as professionals" (p. 1342). That same year an article in the *Annual Review of Medicine* (Cooper, 2001) was titled "Health care workforce for the twenty-first century: The impact of nonphysician clinicians." No APN I have ever known has positively embraced the concept of his or her practice as being that of a "nonphysician clinician." In a forecast study of Missouri nursing (Kuehn & Porter, 1993), the first round of the Delphi brought together both nurse and nonnurse participants. One physician commented that it was the first time he had ever been called a *nonnurse* and found it rather demeaning. When he was reminded of the nurse correlative, being termed a *nonphysician,* we came to a shared understanding of the awkwardness of either term in supporting a sense of collegiality. In stark contrast to Starfield's language of dependency flowing from "delegated medical functions," the nursing language describing role stresses the need to avoid definition by function or tasks (1992a). Orem (1995) stresses that a task orientation for nursing disallows the focus on person. To define oneself as nurse, the following questions must be answered:

> What do I do (scope of practice)?
> How do I do it (methods of practice, tasks)?
> Who do I care for?
> Why do they need or want my care?

The ANA social policy statement identified collaboration as a standard of practice (1995). Although advanced practice nursing texts have consistently addressed the concept of collaborative practice, undergraduate nursing texts on professional practice have not historically addressed collaboration. Often the word is not even found in the index, and if it is, it has nearly always referred to collaboration between nursing practice and education or between types of nurses within a same setting situation. However, this too is changing. A new chapter in the 2002 text *Professional Nursing Practice,* "The Nurse as Colleague and Collaborator," notes in the introduction that "changing models of health care have created a need for modification of traditional roles. Nurses and physicians have been especially affected by these changes and work more collaboratively" (Blais et al., p. 199). The concept of team, proposed by Senge (1994) and Porter-O'Grady (1992) stresses a partnership approach, with partnerships arranged around the patient, clearly defined linkages between providers, and clarity regarding role function and expectations.

In a spring 2001 report, *The health care workforce in ten states: Education, practice and policy* (American Federation of Teachers [AFT] Healthcare, 2001), 10 pilot states were studied regarding the status of their health-care workforce. Aspects compared were data collection status and process, practice issues, influences, and policies. In describing licensure and regulation of practice, the extent of physician supervision varied considerably among states and among types of providers. In this study, the role of the CNS was not addressed. In Illinois, the CRNAs must be under direct supervision of a physician and have a written practice agreement with that physician. NPs and CNMs must also have a written collaborative agreement with a physician; however, this does not require direct supervision nor even an employment relationship. The question becomes: Why would a physician agree to this responsibility on his or her license if no employment need or gain was part of it? Some charge a fee; however, the question lingers regarding how much "liability" one professional will or should assume for another for pay. In Washington state, APN practice calls for both "independent judgment" and "collaborative interaction with other health-care professionals" (AFT Healthcare, 2001, p. 50). However, neither collaborative interaction nor other health-care professionals is defined in the practice act. Although the affect of the enforced collaboration and supervision on APN practice (noted in 9 of 10 states studied) was not addressed, researchers affirmed that:

> . . . the greatest opportunities for influencing the various environments affecting the health workforce lie within state governments. States are the key actors in shaping these environments as they finance and govern health profession education; license and regulate health profession practice and health insurance; purchase service; pay designated providers under Medicaid programs; and often assume responsibility for design and/or subsidy of programs providing incentives for health professionals to choose specialties and practice location (AFT Healthcare, 2001, p. 2).

Socialize Students to Communication Skills Needed for Collaborative Interactions

When education includes the process of establishing an interdisciplinary team, this practice helps create a system for promoting collaborative practice and education, and facilitates the use of essential communication skills. Group dynamics, role theory, organization theory, change theory, negotiation strategies, team interactions, networking, and focus on the need for organizational leadership for supporting interdisciplinary programs are also key factors in preparing students for a collaborative world. One point highly stressed is the insistence that interdisciplinary teams should deliver care and have a solidly positive practice in place before integrating students into the teams (Hanson & Spross, 1996; Norsen et al., 1995; Tresolini & Pew-Fetzer Task Force, 1994).

COLLABORATIVE MODELS

Primary Nursing Model

A national project conducted by the National Joint Practice Commission (NJPC, 1981) required hospitals to demonstrate 100% registered nurse staffing within a primary nursing model of practice, individual clinical decision making by the nurse, a joint practice committee with equal representation of providers, an integrated patient record, and joint evaluation of patient care. The structural elements of integrated records, joint practice committees, and joint care review reflect the common goals, mutual concerns, and shared power control identified as critical indicators of a high-level collaborative practice (see Table 9-1). Primary nursing, "the performance of clinical nursing functions by registered nurses with minimal or no delegation of nursing tasks to others" (NJPC, p. 11), is considered essential for enabling the nurse to better enter into a collegial relationship with the physician. The emphasis on the primary nurse role, coupled with the element of increased nurse responsibility for decision making, relates accountability directly with collegiality and individual clinical decision making by nurses is considered to be a prerequisite for shared decision making— you cannot share what you do not have (Devereux, 1981; Sullivan, 1998). The results from the four participating hospitals were positive in relation to improved doctor-nurse communications, increased mutual respect and trust between physicians and nurses, increased job satisfaction for physicians and nurses, and highly satisfied patients.

Differentiated Practice Model

In more recent years, the cost effectiveness of the primary nurse model has been challenged, with the reality of achieving it amidst a nursing shortage frequently precluding its use as a viable model. However, newly developing models of differentiated practice have converted the "primary nurse" concept into that of patient care coordinator (PCC) who assumes 24-hour accountability for specific patients. The PCC, however, does not deliver all the care personally. Instead, a team of other nurses and ancillary help assume major responsibility for care delivery, each with specific roles and levels of accountability. Each nurse is paired with certain physicians and his or her patients, and trust and collaboration are more readily developed as nurse and physician work together. This collaborative system model of patient care delivery is resulting in higher levels of coordination, cost effectiveness, and patient and provider satisfaction than previously seen in less collaborative models (Devaney, Kuehn & Jones, 2002; Koerner & Karpiuk, 1994).

Collaborative Practice Model in a Clinic

A new collaborative practice model was established in the early part of 2000 in an inner-city clinic in Beirut, Lebanon, and the positive impact on quality of care of patients with diabetes mellitus type 2 after 3 and a half years was nothing less than amazing (Arevian, 2005). The researchers first identified four key elements essential for the model—"collaborative defining of the problems; joint goal setting and planning; providing a continuum of self-management and support services; and maintaining active and sustained follow-up" (p. 446). In developing the model, they determined that thorough preparation of the professional team members would be an essential factor for success. In addition they developed provider support systems, including standardized guidelines for care management, provided for patient education in illness management skills and consistent access to a single team member. The development process was proven to be very effective because teams reported a high level of enthusiasm, cooperation, willingness to share expertise, and acknowledgment of skills of other colleagues. As one physician said "we were treating each other like colleagues, with mutually respectful relationships," and another noted that he gained insights into "how much and how well the other team members contributed to patient care" (p. 449). Outcomes reported included improved documentation, patient recruitment, and glycemic control, as well as decreased cost of care. The most amazing aspect of the clinic was the positive response of team members to each other's skills and expertise in a Middle Eastern culture in which nurses are still considered as "handmaidens" to physicians. Additionally, the positive patient response to active participation in their care was surprising in a Lebanese culture that encourages "passive submission" to the physician authority figure (Arevian, 2005, p. 450). The development process of this collaborative practice model can serve as an excellent template for clinics and provides additional proof of the values of interprofessional collaboration.

Evercare: Collaboration in Long-Term Care

For over 30 years, collaborative practice models have been developing in long-term care (LTC). The positive impact of nurse practitioner-physician partnerships in LTC has been reported in studies of the Nursing Home Demonstration Project and the Teaching Nursing Home Project among others. In the 1980s, two nurse practitioners developed the LTC model of care teams that focused on coordinated care of frail and elderly nursing home residents (Kappas-Larson, 2008). They founded the Evercare company, which now is nationwide, and the model is used in both nursing homes and the community, where nurse/physician teams care for seniors who are still living independently at home. Seven specific practice roles of Evercare NPs include collaborator, clinician, care manager/coordinator, coach/educator, counselor, communicator, and cheerleaders. The collaborator role is described as "being a clinical co-decision maker with the physician, a responsibility that brings with it shared power and risk in managing the medical care of the nursing home resident" (Abdallah, Fawcett, Kane, Dick, & Chen, 2005, p. 24).

The NPs serve as the center of the interprofessional care team in which both physician and nurse are valued partners, and it is required by Evercare that each NP establish a positive relationship with their collaborating physician. As physicians become more aware of and comfortable with the NPs skill and expertise, they grow more supportive of the role. Active participation by physicians in LTC patient care is reported higher in Evercare programs; perhaps their increasing comfort in LTC care participation is due to their confidence in their NP partner. Physicians have said that "one of the most important components of their experience with Evercare is the personalized and coordinated care patients receive, thanks in part to the quality of Evercare's NPs and care managers"(Kappas-Larson, 2008, p. 135).

CREATE THE FUTURE

The call for collaboration continues to accelerate, driven by consumer and insurer demands for high-quality care at low cost; the existence of fragmented, disorganized, impersonal, and inaccessible care; numerous reports and commissions recommending collaboration; and the demands of some accrediting agencies for collaboration (Bodenheimer, 2008; Zwarenstein et al., 1998). The Institute of Medicine Committee in their call for the design of a new health system for the 21st century that better meets patient needs, recommended that health-care processes be redesigned in accordance with 10 new "rules" (Institute of Medicine, 2001). The rules speak to a system of care delivery focused on continuous healing relationships, shared knowledge and decision making with patients, and cooperation among professional providers as reflected by active collaboration and communication, emphasizing cooperation in patient care as more important than professional prerogatives and roles. An emphasis on teamwork stresses good communication, use of expertise and knowledge of each team member, and "where appropriate, sensibly extending roles to meet patient's needs" (Institute of Medicine, 2001, p. 83). Collaboration is considered intrinsic to nursing and the norm for professional practice and has been identified by Sullivan as "a health care imperative" (1998, p. 62). With health care increasingly provided in complex systems of care, the interactions of various providers is not only inevitable but essential for quality holistic care. However, agreement on basic definitions of medical and nursing practice is the sine qua non of collaboration between the sets of providers.

During the tumultuous years of the mid-1990s, amidst national debates regarding comprehensive federal health-care reform, the leaders of the American Medical Association (AMA) and the ANA drafted the following joint definition of collaboration:

Collaboration is the process whereby physicians and nurses plan and practice together as colleagues, working interdependently within the boundaries of their scopes of practice with shared values and mutual acknowledgment and respect for each other's contribution to care for individuals, their families and their communities (ANA, 1998, p. 2).

Although this definition was adopted by the ANA board of Directors in 1994 it has never been adopted by the AMA. In considering strategies for successful collaboration, perhaps revisiting this mutually developed definition with medical and nursing organizations and practice boards on a state by state basis will provide the groundswell for a truly meaningful sense of shared practice relationships (ANA, 1998).

Three shifts of mind are required if we are to create and discover our unfolding, forward moving future:

> *How we see the world of health care*
> The future is not fixed.
> *How we understand relationships*
> Relationships are the organizing principle of the world.
> *How we make commitments*
> The trust is to be willing, to be in a "state of surrender," to know that what we need at the moment to meet our destiny will be available to us. This trust alters our relationship with the future—we create our future rather than react to it when we arrive (Jaworski, 1996, p. 184).

References

Abdallah, L., Fawcett, J., Kane, R., Dick, K., & Chen, J. (2005). Development and psychometric testing of the Evercare Nurse Practitioner Role and Activity Scale (ENPRAS). *Journal of the American Academy of Nurse Practitioners, 17*(1), 21–26.

American Association of Critical-Care Nurses. (2007). *Acute and critical care clinical nurse specialists: synergy for best practice.* Philadelphia: WB Saunders.

American Association of Nurse Anesthetists. (2007). *Scope and standards for nurse anesthesia practice.* Park Ridge, IL: Author. Retrieved April 18, 2007, from the American Association of Nurse Anesthetists Web site: www.aana.com.

American College of Nurse-Midwives. (1997). *Collaborative management in midwifery Practice for medical, gynecological and obstetrical conditions.* (Position Statement). Washington, DC: Author.

American College of Nurse-Midwives. (2007a). *A brief history of nurse midwives in the U.S.* Retrieved May 10, 2007, from the American College of Nurse-Midwives Web site: www.mymidwife.org.

American College of Nurse-Midwives. (2007b). *Core competencies for basic midwifery practice.* Retrieved May 10, 2007, from the American College of Nurse-Midwives Web site: www.midwife.org.

American Federation of Teachers Healthcare. (2001). *The health care workforce in ten states: Education, practice and policy. A report of the state of the healthcare workforce 2001.* Washington, DC: American Federation of Teachers/American Federation of Labor—Congress of Industrial Organizations.

American Nurses Association. (1995). *Nursing's policy statement.* Washington, DC: Author.

American Nurses Association. (1998). Collaboration and independent practice: Ongoing issues for nursing. *Nursing Trends and Issues, 3*(5), 1–12.

Arevian, M. (2005). The significance of a collaborative practice model in delivering care to chronically ill patients: A case study of managing diabetes mellitus in a primary health care center. *Journal of Interprofessional Care, 19*(5), 444–451.

Baer, E. (1993). Philosophical and historical bases of primary care nursing. In M. Mezey & D. McGivern (Eds.), *Nurses, nurse practitioners: Evolution to advanced practice* (pp. 102–110). New York: Springer.

Baggs, J., & Schmitt, M. (1997). Nurses' and resident physicians' perceptions of the process of collaboration in an MICU. *Research in Nursing and Health, 20*(1), 71–80.

Bailey, J., & Armer, J. (1998). Registered nurse–physician collaborative practice: Success stories. In T. J. Sullivan (Ed.), *Collaboration: a health care imperative* (pp. 225–249). New York: McGraw-Hill.

Benner, P. (1984). *From novice to expert.* Menlo Park, CA: Addison-Wesley.

Bigbee, J. L. (1996). History and evolution of advanced nursing practice. In A. B. Hamric J. A. Spross & C. M. Hanson (Eds.), *Advanced nursing practice: an integrative approach* (pp. 3–24). Philadelphia: WB Saunders.

Blais, K. K., Hayes, J. S., Kozier, B., & Erb, G. (2002). *Professional nursing practice: concepts and perspectives.* Upper Saddle River, NJ: Prentice Hall.

Blumenreich, G. (2007). Another article on the surgeon's liability for anesthesia negligence. Legal Briefs. *AANA Journal, 75*(2), 89–93.

Bodenheimer, T. (2008). Coordinating care—A perilous journey through the Health Care System. Health Policy Report. *New England Journal of Medicine, 358*(10), 1064–1071.

Brown, J., Bedford, N., & White, S. (1999). *Gerontological protocols for nurse practitioners.* Philadelphia: Lippincott Williams & Wilkins.

Clarin, O. (2007). Strategies to overcome barriers to effective nurse practitioner and physician collaboration. *Journal for Nurse Practitioners, 3*(8), 536–548.

Cooper, R. A. (2001). Health care workforce for the twenty-first century: the impact of nonphysician clinicians. *Annual Review of Medicine, 52,* 51–61.

Covington, C., Erwin, T., & Sellers, F. (1992). Implementation of a nurse practitioner-staffed fast track. *Journal of Emergency Nursing, 18*(2), 124–131.

Devaney, S., Kuehn, A., & Jones, R. (2002). The Fitzgibbon hospital experience. *The Missouri Nurse, 14,* 29.

Devereux, P. M. (1981). Essential elements of nurse–physician elements. *Journal of Nursing Administration, 11*(5), 19–23.

Dorroh, M., & Norton, S. F. (1996). The certified nurse-midwife. In A. B. Hamric, J. A. Spross, & C. M. Hanson (Eds.), *Advanced nursing practice: an integrative approach* (pp. 395–419). Philadelphia: WB Saunders.

Faut-Callahan, M., & Kremer, M. (1996). The certified registered nurse anesthetist. In A. B. Hamric, J. A. Spross, & C. M. Hanson (Eds.), *Advanced nursing practice: An integrative approach* (pp. 421–444). Philadelphia: WB Saunders.

Fenton, M., & Brykczynski, I. (1993). Qualitative distinctions and similarities in the practice of clinical nurse specialists and nurse practitioners. *Journal of Professional Nursing, 9*(6), 313–326.

Fischman, J. (2002). Nursing wounds. *U.S. News & World Report, 132*(21), 54–55.

Friedson, E. (1970). *Professional dominance: the social structure of medical care.* New York: Atherton Press, Inc.

Hanna, D. (1996). Primary care nurse practitioner. In A. B, Hamric, J. A. Spross, & C. M. Hanson (Eds.), *Advanced nursing practice: An integrative approach* (pp. 337–355). Philadelphia: WB Saunders.

Hanson, C., & Spross, J. (1996). Collaboration. In A. B. Hamric, J. A. Spross, & C. M. Hanson (Eds.), *Advanced nursing practice: An integrative approach* (pp. 229–248). Philadelphia: WB Saunders.

Higgins, L. W. (1999). Nurses' perceptions of collaborative nurse-physician transfer decision making as a predictor of patient outcomes in a medical intensive care unit. *Journal of Advanced Nursing, 29*(6), 1434–1443.

Hojat, M., Gonnella, J. S., Nasca, T. J., Fields, S. K, Cicchetti, A., et al. (2003). Comparisons of American, Israeli, Italian and Mexican physicians and nurses on the total and factor scores of the Jefferson scale of attitudes toward physician-nurse collaborative relationships. *International Journal of Nursing Studies, 40*(4), 427–435.

Hoole, A., Pickard, C., Ouimette, R., Lohr, J., & Powell, W. (1999). *Patient care guidelines for nurse practitioners* (5th ed.). Philadelphia: Lippincott Williams & Wilkins.

Institute of Medicine. (2001). *Crossing the quality chasm: A new health system for the 21st century.* Washington, DC: National Academies Press.

Institute of Medicine. (2004). *Keeping patients safe: Transforming the work environment of nurses.* Washington, DC: National Academies Press.

Jaworski, J. (1996). *Synchronicity: the inner path of leadership.* San Francisco: Berrett-Koehler.

Jehn, K., Northcraft, G., & Neale, M. (1999). Why differences make a difference: A field study of diversity, conflict and performance in workgroups. *Administrative Science Quarterly, 44*(4), 741–763.

Jones, R. A. P. (1994). Nurse–physician collaboration: A descriptive study. *Holistic Nursing Practice, 8*(3), 38–53.

Kaplow, R. (2007). Synergy model: Guiding the practice of the CNS in acute and critical care. In American Association of Critical-Care Nurses, *Acute and critical care clinical nurse specialists: Synergy for best practice.* Philadelphia: WB Saunders.

Kappas-Larson, P. (2008). The Evercare story: Reshaping the health care model, revolutionizing long-term care. *Journal for Nurse Practitioners, 4*(2), 132–136.

King, K. B., Parrinello, K. M., & Baggs, J. G. (1996). Collaboration and advanced practice nursing. In L. Hickey, R. Oimette, & S. Venegoni (Eds.), *Advanced practice nursing: Changing roles and clinical applications* (pp. 146–162). Philadelphia: Lippincott Williams & Wilkins.

Kinlein, L. (1977). *Independent nursing practice with clients.* Philadelphia: JB Lippincott.

Koerner, J., & Karpiuk, K. (1994). *Implementing differentiated nursing practice: Transformation by design.* Gaithersburg, MD: Aspen.

Kuehn, A. F. (1998). Collaborative health professional education: An interdisciplinary mandate for the third millennium. In T. J. Sullivan (Ed.), *Collaboration: A health care imperative* (pp. 419–465). New York: McGraw-Hill.

Kuehn, A. F., & Porter, R. (1993). Study design. In T. J. Sullivan (Ed.), *Missouri nursing 2000: Creating a positive future. A report of the Missouri Nursing 2000 Study Group* (pp. 42–54). Jefferson City, MO: Missouri Nurses Association.

Landro, L. (2008, April 2). Making room for "Dr. Nurse." In The Informed Patient. Retrieved April 8, 2008, from the Wall Street Journal Online Web site: www.online.wsj.com/article.

Lott, J. W., Polak, J. D., Kenyon, T. B., & Kenner, C. A. (1996). Acute care nurse practitioner. In A. B. Hamric, J. A. Spross, & C. M. Hanson (Eds.), *Advanced nursing practice: An integrative approach* (pp. 351–373). Philadelphia: WB Saunders.

Markowitz, G., & Rosner, D. (1979). Doctors in crisis: Medical education and medical reform during the progressive era, 1895–1915. In S. Reverby & D. Rosner (Eds.), *Health care in America* (pp. 185–205). Philadelphia: Temple University.

Merriam-Webster's Collegiate Dictionary (10th ed.). (1994). Springfield, MA: Merriam-Webster.

Miller, K. I., & Apker, J. (2002). On the front lines of managed care: Professional changes and communicative dilemmas of hospitals nurses. *Nursing Outlook, 50*(4), 154–159.

National Joint Practice Commission. (1981). *Guidelines for establishing joint or collaborative practice in hospitals.* Chicago, IL: Neely.

National League for Nursing. (1997). *Commission on a workforce for a restructured health care system.* Part 2. New York: NLN.

Newman, D. (1996). Program practice management for the advanced practice nurse. In A. B. Hamric, J. A. Spross, & C. M. Hanson (Eds.), *Advanced nursing practice: An integrative approach* (pp. 545–568). Philadelphia: WB Saunders.

Norsen, L., Opladen, J., & Quinn, J. (1995). Practice model: collaborative practice. *Critical Care Nursing Clinics of North America, 7*(1), 43–52.

O'Neil, E. H., & Pew Health Professions Commission. (1998). *Recreating health professional practice for a new century. Fourth report.* San Francisco, CA: Pew Health Professions Commission.

Orem, D. (1995). *Nursing: Concepts of practice.* St. Louis: Mosby.

Pearson, L. (2002). 14th annual legislative update. *The Nurse Practitioner, 27*(1), 10–52.

Pearson, L. (2008). A national overview of nurse practitioner legislation and healthcare issues. In The Pearson Report. *American Journal for Nurse Practitioners, 12*(2), 9–15.

Pearson, P., & Jones, K. (1994). The primary health care non-team? *British Medical Journal, 309*(6966), 1387–1388.

Peters, T., & Waterman, R. (1982). *In search of excellence.* New York: Warner Books.

Phillips, R. L., Green, L. A., Fryer, G. E., & Dovey, S. M. (2001). Trumping professional roles: Collaboration of nurse practitioners and physicians for a better US health care system. *American Family Physician, 64*(8), 1325.

Plant, R. (1987). *Managing change and making it stick.* London: Fontana.

Porter-O'Grady, T. (1992). *Implementing shared governance.* St. Louis: Mosby.

Reverby, S. (1979). The search for the hospital yardstick. In S. Reverby & D. Rosner (Eds.), *Health care in America.* Philadelphia: Temple University.

Reverby, S. (1987). *Ordered to care: The dilemma of American nursing, 1850–1945.* New York: Cambridge University.

Roberts, M. M. (1959). *American nursing.* New York: Macmillan.

Rogers, M. (1972). Nursing: To be or not to be. *Nursing Outlook 20*(1), 42–46.

Rosenstein, A. H. (2002). Nurse–physician relationships: Impact on nurse satisfaction and retention. *American Journal of Nursing, 102*(6), 26–34.

Senge, P. (1994). *The fifth discipline.* New York: Currency and Doubleday.

Shah, M. A. (2002). Make way for a new ACNM/ACOG joint statement. The President's pen. Retrieved July 1, 2002, from the American College of Nurse-Midwives Web site: www.midwife.org/prof/display.cm/?id=274.

Stanley, J. (2005). *Advanced practice nursing* (2nd ed.). Philadelphia: F.A. Davis Company.

Starfield, B. (1992a). *Primary care: Concept, evaluation and policy.* New York: Oxford University Press.

Starfield, B. (1992b). The future of primary care in a managed care era. *International Journal of Health Science, 27*(4), 687–696.

Sullivan, T. J. (1998). Concept analysis of collaboration: Part 1. In T. J. Sullivan (Ed.), *Collaboration: A health care imperative* (pp. 3–42). New York: McGraw-Hill.

Sullivan, T. J., Morgan, S., Heimerich, S., & Scott, J. (1998). When collaboration is legislatively mandated. In T. J. Sullivan (Ed.), *Collaboration: A health care imperative* (pp. 325–357). New York: McGraw-Hill.

Thomas, E., Sexton, J. B., & Helmreich, R. (2003). Discrepant attitudes about teamwork among critical care nurses and physicians. *Critical Care Medicine, 31*(3), 956–959.

Toffler, A. (1970). *Future shock.* New York: Random House.

Tresolini, C. P., & Pew-Fetzer Task Force. (1994). *Health professions education and relationship-centered care.* San Francisco, CA: Pew Health Professions Commission.

Way, D., & Jones, L. (1994). The family physician-nurse practitioner dyad: Indications and guidelines. *Canadian Medical Association Journal, 151*(1), 29–34.

Way, D., Jones, L., Baskerville, B., & Busing, N. (2001). Primary health care services provided by nurse practitioners and family physicians in shared practice. *Canadian Medical Association Journal, 165*(9), 1210–1214.

Workman, L. (1986). No free lunches. *Missouri Nurse, 55*(5), 16.

Zwarenstein, M., & Bryant, W. (2000). *Interventions to promote collaboration between nurses and doctors.* Cochrane Database of Systemic Reviews, (2), CD000072.

Zwarenstein, M., Bryant, W., Baillie, R., & Sibthorpe, B. (2000). *Promoting collaboration between nurses and doctors* [Cochrane Review]. The Cochrane Library: Issue 4. Oxford.

10

Participation of the Advanced Practice Nurse in Managed Care and Quality Initiatives

Rita Munley Gallagher

Advanced practice nurses (APNs) have been notably absent from managed care plan provider panels.[1] In addition, their efforts are not fully recognized in national quality activities. Is this because of their predominantly employee status? Are they reticent to take on the full responsibility of a primary care provider, fearful of accepting accountabiity, hesitant to mobilize consumer support on their own behalf? Or, is it a more fundamental issue . . . an issue of respect?

INTRODUCTION

Today's evolving health-care environment has transformed the way many health-care services are provided and paid for. The approach to health-care service delivery has undergone a significant alteration in both its contracting and reimbursement mechanisms. Fee-for-service is no longer the primary source of pricing; prospective payment, global pricing, and capitation are also prominent. Along with these changes comes a significant increase in financial risk to the provider. By taking on liability not only for service delivery costs, but also for level of use, providers have been "forced," under managed care, into assuming roles historically reserved for insurance carriers. In addition, demonstration of practitioner accountability for quality is moving into the forefront of health-care delivery. More than 240,000 APNs (Division of Nursing, U.S. Department of Health and Human Services, 2006)—and their numbers are growing—are carving out a larger role in delivering safe, effective, patient-centered, timely, efficient, equitable health care. This chapter focuses on the' involvement of APNs within managed care plans and within the national quality enterprise and offers suggestions for increasing their visibility within both.

ADVANCED PRACTICE NURSES

APNs possess the education and expert clinical knowledge to enable them to practice in multiple settings. The expertise of APNs enables them to complement other practitioners within the health-care arena. In primary care, meta-analyses indicate that nurse practitioners (NPs) and physicians provide

---

[1]The views expressed in this chapter are those of the author and do not represent official position of the American Nurses Association.

the same level of care in regard to assessment and the accuracy of their diagnoses with similar patient outcomes. In addition, NP care is associated with greater degrees of patient satisfaction, communication, patient education, and quality of care (Bryant-Lukosius, Dicenso, Browne, & Pinelli, 2004). Yet they are often underused by managed care plans (MCPs). State governments have been moving to increase their regulation of MCPs. Many states have passed laws expanding patient rights, guaranteeing access to care, requiring point-of-service options, including whistleblower clauses, and establishing provider due process protections. However, a number of self-insured MCPs have successfully challenged state health insurance regulations under the Employee Retirement Income Security Act (ERISA), based on their contention that they are self-insured employee health benefit plans. As a result, these types of plans are exempt from many state regulations, such as any willing provider and nondiscrimination provisions (American College of Nurse-Midwives [ACNM], 1997). With a background in patient education and certification in a specialty at the master's level, the APN is well equipped to provide quality care in a cost-effective environment (Hylka, 1997). Yet APNs remain largely absent from MCP panels, thereby limiting enrollee access to their services, which gives rise to suspicions of lack of respect for nursing overall.

MANAGED CARE PLANS

MCPs are rapidly becoming the overseers and administrators of health-care services for most U.S. Americans. MCPs have assumed the management and control of the overwhelming majority of health-care services provided throughout the entire United States. Nearly 85% of the U.S. population is currently covered under MCPs; the majority (50.46%) in commercial plans with approximately 35% covered by Medicare or Medicaid (Managed Care Fact Sheets, 2008).

Managed care has been defined as "a comprehensive approach to health care delivery that encompasses planning and coordination of care, enrollee and practitioner education, monitoring of care quality, and cost control" (American Managed Care and Review Association [AMCRA], 1995, p. 10). At least in theory, managed care is designed to foster the effective, appropriate, and efficient monitoring of a specific population's health. Managed care calls for providers to assume responsibility and accountability for the health-care needs of a specifically defined population, while at the same time agreeing to accept the financial risk inherent in taking on that responsibility.

MCPs have been defined as insurance plans in which the insurer determines, under written standards, the medical necessity of medical services and directs care to the most appropriate setting so as to provide quality care in the most cost-efficient manner. These plans typically include the following activities: prior authorization; prospective, concurrent, and retrospective utilization review; discharge planning; quality-assurance activities; and reimbursement (North Shore-Long Island Jewish Health System, 2008). In many MCPs there is said to be some level of restriction on access to practitioners, which are imposed in an effort on behalf of the MCP to improve efficiency in the health-care delivery system (Hicks, Stallmeyer, & Coleman, 1993). In managed care, the burden of risk is shared. Unlike traditional indemnity plans in which the insurance company bears the financial risk and burden of enrollees requiring more complex and costly care, various incentive plans and capitation place the risk (and burden) on the managed care provider—whether that be a plan, APN, physician, mental health-care provider, or other practitioner (Himali, 1995).

In addition to point-of-service (POS) plans, the most common types of MCPs include health maintenance organizations (HMOs) and preferred provider organizations (PPOs), a component of which are exclusive provider organizations. All are grounded in provision of care to a specified cohort of enrollees at an established per member/per month rate (**Box 10-1**).

BOX 10-1
Types of Managed Care Plans

- Health maintenance organizations (HMO) usually only pay for care within the network. The enrollee chooses a primary care provider who coordinates most of the enrollee's care.
- Preferred provider organizations (PPO) usually pay more if the enrollee receives care within the network, but they still pay a portion if the enrollee goes outside the network.
- Point of service (POS) plans let the enrollee choose between an HMO or a PPO each time care is needed.

The historical goal of managed care is to deliver value to the consumer by providing access to quality, cost-effective health care (Stahl, 1995). This mission is not always readily apparent in practice or necessarily shared by all MCPs. However, as systems of managed care continue to develop, the goals are expanding to include, among others, a focus on outcomes analysis, development of practice guidelines, the building of provider panels with a host of practitioners, and the coordination of service provision among providers (May, Schraeder, & Britt, 1996). Managed care has become a way of life for all health-care practitioners and must include APNs.

Competencies Necessary in the Managed Care Environment

Despite naysayers' comments to the contrary (Stires, 2002), managed care is here to stay. However, although the fit between its stated health-care promotion and disease prevention goals is in line with those of the APN, MCPs also place renewed emphasis on the "bottom line" in an often very competitive market. To prosper in such an arena, a number of skills are needed; these include marketing, advertising, and finance, which are generally considered as being beyond those included in the basic nursing curriculum.

Of great relevance to the APN is a process of self-assessment designed to assist in attaining an optimal level of success in the managed care arena (Leider & Bard, 1993). It has been said that to form an optimal system of "managed" care a new paradigm of professional practice is needed. In this "new" system, the practitioner needs to be capable of integrating the traditional curing focus with an ability to manage the health of individual enrollees and the covered cohort, overall. In addition to appropriate credentials, to be successful in managed care APNs must possess the following skills:

- Clinical accountability
- Communication skills
- Leadership skills
- Team-building abilities
- Negotiation and conflict resolution skills
- Ability to engage in quality management activities
- Financial acumen

APNs who see themselves as possessing these competencies can improve chances of successfully negotiating a contract with an MCP by doing the following:

- Highlighting communication; enhancing documentation; becoming familiar with the "ins and outs" of the contract
- Being ready to follow through with commitments

- Educating MCPs on the value—both quality value and efficiency value—of their services
- Improving fiscal and management system capacities
- Being creative, flexible, and willing to work with the MCP to meet mutual goals

To operate successfully in the managed care environment, it is crucial that APNs work collaboratively with case managers, identify gaps in service that they are capable of filling, and hone the skills necessary to succeed in contracting with the MCP as well as in securing needed benefits on behalf of their enrollees (Lachman, 1996).

MCPs are interested in a provider's ability to provide financial and cost data cross-referenced by client characteristics, including clinical complexity, resource utilization, therapy and pharmaceutical use, length of stay, and outcome criteria. In addition, the APN must be able to detail the processes established to ensure quality improvement and outcomes of activities. Administrative expertise, including quality and financial reporting mechanisms, must be in place. Operating standards focused on efficacy and outcome measurement criteria along with practitioner performance evaluations are also closely scrutinized by the MCP (Walker, 1996). At a minimum, it is assumed that all parties preparing to enter into a contract do so voluntarily and knowingly; having read, and understanding fully, the document. Failing to read the contract critically, as well as failure to have it reviewed by an attorney, can result in significant problems at a later date.

Contracting with Managed Care Plans

There are a number of challenges inherent in providing health-care services, which makes the decision to enter into a contractual managed care agreement particularly attractive, and also potentially difficult. For instance, working to move from the employee role by attempting to force MCPs to bill directly for their services is seen by some NPs as counterproductive (Hill, Cohen, & Mason, 1999; Mason et al., 1999). They hold the perspective that, if the MCP is unable to continue billing under the physician's name, the MCP will experience a decrease in overall payment dollars that may result in further APN exclusion from provider panels. Such challenges may also result in a significant number of APNs continuing in the traditional role of employee, albeit with an MCP as employer instead of the traditional hospital or nursing home. According to the American Academy of Nurse Practitioners (AANP) and Goolsby (2004), approximately three-quarters (77.1%) of NPs work as employees, and the rest work under contract (11.9 %), in partnership (6.6%), or independently (0.9 %).

When an APN *does* consider entering into a managed care contract, numerous questions arise that require answers (Butler, 1995): Are there regulatory or legislative constraints or safeguards? Do they apply equally to APNs as well as to other practitioners? Will the MCP require capital outlays to upgrade practitioner skills? How are client care protocols or treatment guidelines adopted in contracting with managed care entities determined? How will the quality of client care be ensured? What are the processes for patient transfer? These and other relevant issues must be clarified by the APN before contractual integration into any managed care system. Clearly, prospective planning is a critical choice in the decision-making process preparatory to contracting with an MCP **(Box 10-2).**

APNs must know whether the MCP with which they are negotiating does the following:

- Confronts the realities of providing adequate care to clients
- Supports strong research and development programs
- Promotes health education and disease prevention
- Strongly integrates the perspectives of relevant enrollee groups
- Promotes collaborative care

BOX 10-2
Tips for Contracting with Managed Care Plans

Following are six tips for successful contracting with an managed care plan (MCP):

1. Do your homework! Know as much about the MCP plan as you can before you start to negotiate a contract. If you can, talk with other practitioners already in the plan.

2. Be a tough but fair negotiator up front and then a team player once you have signed on. If you want to make changes in the contract, do it before signing, not afterward.

3. Evaluate the "attitude" of the plan and cultivate a relationship with its officials. Do not expect plans to improve after you have signed on.

4. Work diligently at clarifying ambiguous language. Much of a contract's improvement comes from clarifying items prospectively rather than negotiating substantive changes. Start with the less important issues when negotiating. It is important to know what you want and to know your limits. Before you go plunging into the most important or serious issues, start with the smaller ones (Caesar, 1995).

5. Particular attention should be paid to any specific processes required by the MCP in relationship to the transfer of a patient (Buppert, 2008).

6. Seek competent legal advice to avoid contracting pitfalls. The MCP does.

- Collects and disseminates accurate data
- Advocates for financing reforms that better fund primary care
- Does a thorough job of attending to psychosocial factors
- Promotes palliative care, when appropriate
- Educates the public on the benefits of a healthy lifestyle
- Incentivizes APNs commensurate with the risks they accept

Reimbursement

When Medicare and Medicaid were first enacted in 1965 by amendment of the Social Security Act, few nurses were practicing independently; thus, no provisions were made for direct payment to them. Enactment of the Omnibus Budget Reconciliation Act (OBRA) of 1989 allowed for Medicaid coverage of services by family NPs and pediatric NPs and extended Medicare Part B coverage to NPs in skilled nursing facilities only (with no provision for coverage of services provided by clinical nurse specialists [CNSs]) and with the payment going to the facility, not directly to the NP. Medicare Part B coverage was extended to services provided by both NPs and CNSs in nonmetropolitan statistical areas (i.e., rural areas) by OBRA '90, establishing NPs and CNSs as Medicare providers. The 1990s saw a number of attempts by the American Nurses Association (ANA) and others to expand coverage for APN services (Abood & Keepnews, 2000), culminating with the signing of the Balanced Budget Act (BBA) of 1997 by President Bill Clinton. The BBA extended reimbursement opportunities for APNs by removing geographical and practice site restrictions. However, significant barriers to full and autonomous practice for APNs remain firmly entrenched in the health-care delivery system. Federal (and many state) laws do not provide adequate support for the removal of barriers to practice for APNs that are created by policy makers, health-care institutions, insurance payors, or MCPs. These barriers include denial of claims from third-party payors; failure to include APNs on preferred provider panels; institutional and provider policies that inhibit the objective and accurate assessment of the quality of care and benefits provided by use of APNs; and institutional and provider limitations on APN scope of practice, including contracting with MCPs. Although the BBA did allow for direct Medicare reimbursement for services provided by NPs and CNSs regardless of geographical location or practice setting, it was at only 85% (80% for CNSs) of the amount Medicare reimbursed physicians. This inequity has resulted in continued billing for APN services as *"incident to"* the physician (i.e., allowing a service provided by an APN to be billed at 100% of the fee schedule when the physician is on site and available for consultation, if necessary) adding to the *"invisibility"* of APNs.

Of interest to APNs are strategies related to the recently restated Centers for Medicare and Medicaid Services (CMS) vision of the right care for the right person, every time (CMS, 2008). To achieve this vision, CMS, too, is committed to covering care that is safe, effective, timely, patient centered, efficient, and equitable. Historically, Medicare's payment system has rewarded quantity, rather than quality of care, and provides neither incentive nor support to improve health-care quality. Value-based purchasing (VBP), which links payment more directly to the quality of care provided, is a strategy that can help transform the current payment system by rewarding providers for delivering high-quality, efficient clinical care. Through a number of public reporting programs, demonstration projects, pilot programs, and voluntary efforts, CMS has launched VBP initiatives in hospitals, physician offices, nursing homes, home health services, and dialysis facilities.

There is administrative as well as evidentiary support for VBP. Higher spending does not equate with higher quality, and VBP has the potential to improve quality and avoid unnecessary costs. In 2006, Congress passed Public Law 109-171, the Deficit Reduction Act of 2005 (DRA), which under Section 5001(b) authorized CMS to develop a plan for VBP for Medicare hospital services commencing with fiscal year 2009. The VBP plan defined in the DRA applies only to subsection (d) hospitals, and does not apply to critical access hospitals or to other hospital types that are not paid under the Inpatient Prospective Payment System (IPPS). The hospital-acquired conditions provision (DRA Section 5001(c)) is a step toward VBP for hospitals. For implementation on October 1, 2008 (i.e., fiscal year 2009') CMS is adding additional conditions to the provision: serious preventable events, catheter-associated urinary tract infection, surgical site infection—mediastinitis after coronary artery bypass graft (CABG) surgery, falls and trauma fractures—dislocations, intracranial injuries, crushing injuries, and burns among them. As a result, CMS (and an increasing number of other third-party payors) will no longer make higher payments for selected conditions, such as those detailed in the previous sentence, that were not present at the time of hospital admission (CMS, 2007, p. 1).

While many VBP strategies are focused solely on hospitals, there are aspects directed to practitioners including those related to resource use, a voluntary reporting program and the physician quality reporting initiative (PQRI) that should be particularly relevant to APNs. On December 20, 2006, Public Law 109-432, the Tax Relief and Health Care Act of 2006 (TRHCA) was signed. Division B, Title I, Section 101 of the law authorized the establishment of a physician quality reporting system by CMS. CMS has titled the statutory program the PQRI. PQRI establishes a financial incentive for eligible professionals to participate in a voluntary quality reporting program. On December 29, 2007, the president authorized PQRI's continuation.

For fiscal year 2008, PQRI consisted of 119 quality measures, including two structural measures related to the use of technology. Under PQRI, covered professional services are those paid based on the Medicare physician fee schedule. To the extent that eligible professionals are providing services that get paid under the Medicare physician fee schedule, those services are eligible for PQRI. Included among the professionals eligible to participate in PQRI are physicians and physician assistants, NPs, CNSs certified registered nurse anesthetists (CRNAs; and anesthesiologist assistants); certified nurse-midwives (CNMs); therapists; and others.

The financial incentive for eligible professionals who successfully reported the designated set of quality measures during 2008 was 1.5% of total allowed charges for covered services payable under the physician fee schedule. Financial incentives earned for reporting were paid from the federal supplementary medical insurance (part b) trust fund and to a host of health-care professionals, APNs included.

Advanced Practice Nurse Participation in Managed Care Plans

Great strides have been made in recent years to establish APNs as independent practitioners providing health-care services. APNs' practices are more widely accepted by health-care consumers than in previous years. During the past three decades, research has continued to demonstrate that APNs have established and built on a record of delivering quality health care. Despite that fact, there are continuing indications that APNs face significant barriers in the health-care marketplace, including the absence of full access to MCP provider panels. APNs also experience significant barriers in the credentialing process of MCPs, to inclusion on MCP provider panels, and to being listed in MCP provider directories. The result of these barriers is that consumers' choice of providers is limited. Furthermore, the APN's role is relegated to employee in many cases, as opposed to that of independent contractor as is the case of most other classes of practitioners. In addition to barriers to inclusion on MCP panels, insurers and employers have also added arbitrary restrictions to APNs' practices such as adding physician supervision or needless patient record cosignatory requirements. These requirements are not necessarily in adherence with state practice laws and increase the cost of APNs' services, thereby creating disincentives to employers and consumers to use APNs.

A secondary issue is that there is little, if any, data collection regarding the role of APNs in MCPs. Most HMOs do not have formal methods for estimating and reporting nonphysician provider care, thus making it difficult to track APN use, efficiency, quality, and credentialing. With disparities in prescription labeling, it is equally hard to track APN prescribing patterns. These impediments make APNs the invisible providers, caring for many patients and generating revenue without recognition of their efforts (O'Grady, 2008).

The practice environment in the states in which they are chartered influences the policies of MCPs. The legal definition of APN scope of practice, the type of physician collaboration required (or not required), prescription writing authority, and state insurance laws may all affect the reimbursement and use of APNs. As health-care delivery systems evolve into increasing numbers of multistate MCPs, the procedures and policies affecting APNs are not always clear. In some cases, the multistate corporations may elect to establish their own sets of rules instead of following state law. Multistate policies tend to diminish use of the separate states' APN scopes of practice, sometimes substituting stricter physician collaboration policies, or limiting nurses' prescriptive writing authority to MCP formularies. "Managed care plans operating in more than one state must comply with the regulations of each jusisdiction . . . States may also require that out-of-state HMOs register to do business . . . Multi-state operations can become expensive if plans are subject to numerous financial examinations and other regulatory requirements . . . Historically, group insurance policies have generally been subject to the laws of the state of issuance . . . This general rule has been eroded by extraterritorial application of state insurance law" (Kongstvedt, 2000, p. 1330). Inconsistent application and interpretation of state insurance law can adversely affect reimbursement and MCP plan inclusion of APNs. To lend conformity and simplify regulatory compliance, MCPs have generally resorted to application of the most rigorous (and hence, most restrictive) rules promulgated among the states in which they provide services.

Unfortunately, only a small (but growing) number of states require MCPs to include NPs in provider panels and list them in directories provided to enrollees (Abood & Keepnews, 2002). APNs must now direct their efforts toward ensuring that additional states enact such legislation and that MCPs allow them the recognition they so richly deserve. Whether the APN intends to work as an employee of an MCP or to seek inclusion on an MCP's provider panel by contracting with one, there is a need to develop a base of consumer support.

The issue is not one of APN competence or of the quality of the care they provide. Decades of reports have documented the quality of NP practice (AANP, 2008). The Office of Technology Assessment (OTA) reported NPs as being especially valuable in improving access to primary care and supplementary care in rural areas and in health programs for the poor, minorities, and people without health insurance (OTA, 1986). OTA found the quality of NP care to be as good as or better than care provided by physicians and found NPs superior at counseling, communications, and interviewing (OTA, 1986). Having an NP manage uncomplicated patients hospitalized for decompensated heart failure was associated with a significant decrease in total hospital costs, a trend toward decreased length of stay, and no significant change in the 30-day readmission rate (Dahle, Smith, & Wilson, 1998). The Gallup Organization has also noted the public's willingness to accept APNs as everyday health-care providers (Gallup Organization, 1993). Yet it has been said that nurses—not just APNs, but all nurses—are invisible in health care (Hazzard, 2002). However, that perspective is changing. A 2002 poll commissioned by Johnson and Johnson found only 25% of those polled had ever heard of a nurse practitioner (Poll, 2002, p. 14). Conversely, most respondents (90%) to a later survey knew about NPs, and the majority had seen an NP for their care. Eighty-two percent of NP users were satisfied or very satisfied with the care they had received compared to a 70% satisfaction rate for current providers (Brown, 2007). Nevertheless, the skills of many APNs remain underused.

As ANA and the state nurses associations continue to advocate for the right of APNs to fully practice within their scope without arbitrary barriers, physicians have stepped up efforts to confine the practice of APNs. For over a decade, organized medicine has fostered comprehensive grassroots and media campaigns to promote supervised, collaborative practice between physicians and APNs and has increased its public opposition to the expanded scope and independent practice of APNs (Japsen, 2006).

Yet another strategy that has been put forth by organized medicine is advocation for the relaxation of antitrust laws as they apply to health-care professionals. Legislation has also been introduced on both the federal and state levels to provide collective bargaining rights for health-care professionals. Only those employees deemed nonsupervisory under the National Labor Relations Act are accorded the rights to collectively bargain; however, these legislative proposals would provide physicians the right to enter into joint negotiations with insurance companies to work out payment arrangements, clinical practice conditions, and more. Such activity is currently forbidden under state and federal antitrust laws and is considered anticompetitive collaboration among competitors. In some instances, the courts have held that such collaboration on prices and market access are illegal boycotts. Changes in law being advocated by physician organizations would not onl allow negotiation, but also would weaken the ability of the APN to prove antitrust violations by physician competitors, thereby ignoring their ability to take part equally in the competitive managed care arena, regardless of the quality of the care they provide.

In response to efforts by the American Medical Association (AMA) and other physician groups to limit the ability of licensed health-care professionals to provide care to millions of patients, the Coalition for Patients' Rights (CPR) was formed to ensure that the growing needs of the U.S. health system can be met and that patients have access to quality health-care providers of their choice. CPR urges all health-care professionals to work together to counter the AMA's actions. The coalition represents more than three million licensed professionals who provide a diverse array of safe, effective, and affordable health-care services.

CPR has expressed concern about the negative impact on patients if their ability to seek care from APNs, psychologists, CNMs, chiropractors, and many other licensed, qualified health-care providers is limited. The coalition has called on the AMA and other physician groups aligned with the AMA to cease their divisive efforts to oppose the established practice rights of CPR members. The coalition also seeks an end to legislation at the state level that would reduce provider options for patients (CPR, 2006). Among successful state initiatives are those in Colorado, which improve access to care, minimize the barriers to completing the paperwork associated with health status, and increase the number of available providers for Colorado Medicaid recipients. In Oklahoma, a bill placing the regulatory authority of APNs within purview of the board of medicine was defeated. Not so in Georgia and Alabama, where limits have been imposed via the regulatory process that call for APNs to include a written practice agreement and fee with the application to practice. As a result, only a fraction of eligible APNs have registered. Similar regulatory barriers are being faced by APNs in Pennsylvania. Examples of barriers include limitations on prescriptive authority such as the ability to prescribe only a 30-day supply of Schedule II drugs, and opposition to removal of the APN to physician ratio. "This high degree of variation across the States for APN regulation has spotlighted the need to ensure that regulation serves the public, promotes public safety, and does not present unnecessary barriers to patients' access to care" (O'Grady, 2008, p. 8).

Alignment of all aspects of regulation is the goal of the Consensus Model for *APRNAPN* Regulation developed by the APRN Consensus Workgroup and the National Council of State Boards of Nursing APRN Advisory Committee (2008). The APN model of the future defines APNs as being a CRNA, CNM, CNS, or certified nurse practitioner (CNP), all of whom will be educationally prepared to provide care to patients across the health wellness-illness continuum. Population foci will include: psych/mental health; gender-specific; adult-gerontology; pediatrics, neonatal; and individual/family across the life span. The model calls for specialty practice, while optional, to build on the APN role and population-focused competencies with a target date for implementation of this regulatory model and all recommendations by the year 2015.

NATIONAL QUALITY EFFORTS

The public concern for error and patient safety together with the continuing "quest for quality" has created renewed responsibility and accountability for the outcomes of patient care. The National Quality Forum (NQF), a private, nonprofit, voluntary, consensus standard setting organization comprised of approximately 400 organizations from federal and state governments and private sector entities, including a number of nursing organizations, the first of which was the ANA, is prominent in the national quality arena.

The mission of the NQF is to improve the quality of U.S. health care by setting national priorities and goals for performance improvement, endorsing national consensus standards for measuring and publicly reporting on performance, and promoting the attainment of national goals through education and outreach programs (NQF, 2008). Nursing is active in all aspects of NQF activity on: steering committees and their technical advisory panels; the National Priorities Partners Committee, the Consensus Standards Advisory Committee (CSAC); and the NQF Board of Directors. The central activity of NQF is the endorsement of performance measures as "voluntary" consensus standards, and the identification of gaps in health-care quality research.

Voluntary consensus standards, although relatively new in the health-care arena, are not new to other industries. And since passage of the National Technology Transfer and Advancement Act of 1995 (Public Law 104-113) voluntary consensus standards have legal standing. The voluntary consensus process, even in the face of strict requirements as to time frames and transparency, is more timely than is the federal rule-making process. One key component of the act is its obligation of the federal government to use voluntary existing consensus standards, thus encouraging the federal government to take part in the NQF process. Federal agency involvement in NQF serves to encourage both public and private purchasers, accrediting bodies, practitioners and providers, and the pubic to also take part. NQF is governed by a board of directors representing health-care consumers, purchasers, providers, health plans, and experts in health services research. The NQF board also includes representatives from two federal agencies, the CMS and the Agency for Healthcare Research and Quality (AHRQ).

The NQF recognizes the value of nursing to health-care quality. The NQF nursing care performance measures project established consensus on a set of evidence-based measures for evaluating the performance of nursing in acute care hospitals. It also addressed the implementation of those measures within health-care organizations to improve nursing care and patient outcomes; in addition it designated a subset of measures that are appropriate for public reporting (such as on the Web site, Hospital Compare, that was developed by the Hospital Quality Alliance [HQA] of which the ANA is a principal).

HQA developed and launched Hospital Compare to provide information to the public on hospital quality. Since its inception, HQA has worked to increase hospitals' voluntary participation in public reporting and expand the set of quality measures being reported. The information on Hospital Compare helps patients compare how often individual hospitals provide specific types of care most patients should always get for certain conditions, such as giving heart attack patients an aspirin on arrival at a hospital. Nursing is integral to patient care and is delivered in many and varied settings. The sheer number of nurses and their primacy in caregiving are compelling reasons for measuring their contribution to patients' experiences and the outcomes that are attained (NQF, 2007). However, nursing measures are not, as yet, included in Hospital Compare **(Box 10-3)**.

The Joint Commission is engaged in a "comprehensive test of the NQF nursing-focused performance measures to determine whether they can be used nationally to identify opportunities to improve the quality of patient care provided by nurses. The project is being funded by a grant from the Robert Wood Johnson Foundation. Testing of the integrated set of measures is expected to yield a set of refined technical specifications that can be used by hospitals nationwide and included in quality initiatives used by the Hospital Quality Alliance, Centers for Medicare and Medicaid Services (CMS) and The Joint Commission" (Hill, 2007). The information available to assist consumer decision-making (such as is provided on Hospital Compare) would be greatly enhanced by the inclusion of NQF-endorsed nursing-sensitive measures **(Box 10-4)**.

Advanced Practice Nurse Participation in Quality Initiatives

In addition to the NQF-endorsed nursing-sensitive measures, other clinician-level quality measures are of relevance to APNs, including those developed by the AMA-Physician Consortium for Performance Improvement (AMA-PCPI/Consortium), whose goal is to improve patient health and safety by:

- Identifying and developing evidence-based clinical performance measures
- Promoting the implementation of clinical performance improvement activities
- Advancing the science of clinical performance measurement and improvement

BOX 10-3
The Value of Measuring Nursing Care

To increase the value of information provided to consumers regarding the quality of nursing care by nursing-sensitive measures, interested parties should focus on the following points:

1. Nurses represent the largest, single group of health-care professionals.

■ Of the total licensed registered nurse (RN) population in March 2004, 83.2% (an estimated 2,421,461) were employed in nursing (Health Resources and Services Administration [HRSA], 2004).

■ By endorsing 15 voluntary consensus standards for nursing-sensitive care, the National Quality Forum (NQF) noted "nurses, as the principal frontline caregivers in the U.S. healthcare system, have tremendous influence over a patient's healthcare experience" (NQF, 2004).

2. Evidence substantiates nursing's influence on inpatient outcomes.

■ A growing body of evidence demonstrates nursing's impact on the provision of care that is safe, effective, patient centered, timely, efficient, and equitable:

  ■ The adequacy of nursing staffing and proportion of RNs is inversely related to the death rate of acute medical patients within 30 days of hospital admission (Tourangeau et al., 2005).

  ■ Increasing RN staffing could reduce costs and improve patient care by reducing unnecessary deaths and reducing days in the hospital (Stone et al., 2007).

  ■ Patients hospitalized for heart attacks, congestive heart failure and pneumonia . . . are more likely to receive high-quality care in hospitals with higher registered nurse staffing ratios (Landon et al., 2006).

  ■ Higher fall rates were associated with fewer nursing hours per patient day and a lower percentage of registered nurses . . . (Dunton, Gajewski, Taunton, & Moore 2004).

  ■ Nurses can accurately differentiate pressure ulcers from other ulcerous wounds in Web-based photographs, reliably stage pressure ulcers, and reliably identify community versus nosocomial pressure ulcers (Hart, Bergquist, Gajewski, & Dunton, 2006).

  ■ A 10% increase in the number of patients assigned to a nurse leads to a 28% increase in adverse events such as infections, medication errors, and other injuries (Weisman, 2007).

  ■ Understaffing of registered nurses in hospital intensive care units increases the risk for serious infections for patients, specifically pneumonia (Hugonnet, Uçkay, & Pittet, 2007).

  ■ According to The Joint Commission (2005), "quantifying the effect that nurses and nursing interventions have on the quality of care processes, and on patient outcomes, has become increasingly important to support evidence-based staffing plans, understand the impact of nursing shortages and optimize care outcomes."

3. Measures have been fully developed, are in use, and have been previously vetted.

The endorsement of the 15 nursing-sensitive measures by NQF was an initial (albeit significant) step toward standardized measurement of nursing care; detailing its relationship to the quality (and efficiency) of health care.

■ Scientific acceptability is a component of the NQF endorsement process and hence, NQF-endorsed nursing-sensitive measures are valid and reliable (NQF, 2002).

■ This initial measure set complements and extends existing hospital care measures of relevance to nursing care in the NQF *national voluntary consensus standards for hospital care: an initial performance measure set* (NQF, 2003). For this reason, their implementation can be viewed as a natural, next step.

BOX 10-3
The Value of Measuring Nursing Care—cont'd

■ Collectively, the measures "provide consumers a way to assess the quality of nurses' contribution to inpatient hospital care, and they enable providers to identify critical out-comes and processes of care for continuous improvement that are directly influenced by nursing personnel" (NQF, 2004).

4. There has been a public call for information about nursing care quality.

■ Enhancing the initial nursing-sensitive measure set through the inclusion of additional measures will increase the overall value of the set.

■ Consumers will benefit from information regarding the impact of nursing care as they make decisions regarding care.

5. Evidence exists that the public reporting stimulates quality improvement and choice.

■ Making performance data public results in improvements in the clinical area reported upon (Hibbard, Stockard, & Tusler, 2005).

■ Making performance information public appears to stimulate quality improvement activi-ties in areas where performance is reported to be low. The findings . . . indicate that there is added value to making this information public (Hibbard, Stockard, & Tusler, 2003).

6. There is agreement among diverse health care stakeholders that the NQF-endorsed nursing-sensitive measures should be incorporated into national and state hospital performance measurement and reporting activities.

■ In 2007, interviews were conducted with nearly three dozen national health-care, hospital, and nursing leaders, principles of nursing performance measurement efforts, and hospital representatives to determine their interest in and use of the NQF15. Recommendations derived from the data gathered from these interviews and published by NQF (2007) point to several complementary and incremental actions that can be collectively undertaken by health-care stakeholders to advance hospital performance measurement and accelerate our collective understanding of nursing's key role in quality. Among these recommendations is a "call" to health-care leaders to fully integrate the NQF15 into national and state hospital performance measurement and reporting initiatives, including, but limited to, Hospital Quality Alliance (HQA; NQF, 2007).

7. Significant operational lag times exist.

To make viable information available to consumers on Hospital Compare, the following must be considered:

■ The CMS/Joint Commission aligned manual is updated twice a year, effective with April and October discharges.

■ The manual must be posted for measurement systems approximately 120 days or 4 months before these dates.

■ Potential time frames following the project coming to an end and recommendations possibly to NQF in early 2009 which include:

  ■ Manual posted on respective Web sites June 1, 2009/Data Collection begins October 1, 2009.

  ■ Manual posted on respective Web sites December 1, 2009/Data Collection begins April 1, 2010.

BOX 10-4
National Quality Forum-Endorsed National Voluntary Consensus Standards for Nursing-Sensitive Care

Patient-centered outcome measures:
1. Death among surgical inpatients with treatable serious complications (failure to rescue): The percentage of major surgical inpatients who experience a hospital-acquired complication and die.
2. Pressure ulcer prevalence: Percentage of inpatients who have a hospital acquired pressure ulcer, stage 2 or greater.
3. Falls prevalence: Number of inpatient falls per inpatient days.
4. Falls with injury: Number of inpatient falls with injuries per inpatient days.
5. Restraint prevalence: Percentage of inpatients who have a vest or limb restraint.
6. Urinary catheter-associated urinary tract infection for intensive care unit (ICU) patients: Rate of urinary tract infections associated with use of urinary catheters for ICU patients.
7. Central line catheter-associated blood stream infection rate for ICU and high-risk nursery patients: Rate of blood stream infections associated with use of central line catheters for ICU and high-risk nursery patients.
8. Ventilator-associated pneumonia for ICU and high-risk nursery patients: Rate of pneumonia associated with use of ventilators for ICU and high-risk nursery patients.

Nursing-centered intervention measures:
9. Smoking cessation counseling for acute myocardial infarction.
10. Smoking cessation counseling for heart failure.
11. Smoking cessation counseling for pneumonia.
Each measures the percentage of patients with a history of smoking within the past year who received smoking cessation advice or counseling during hospitalization.

System-centered measures:
12. Skill mix: Percentage of registered nurse, licensed vocational/practical nurse, unlicensed assistive personnel, and contracted nurse care hours to total nursing care hours.
13. Nursing care hours per patient day: Number of registered nurses per patient day and number of nursing staff hours (registered nurse [RN], licensed vocational/practical nurse [LVN, LPN], and unlicensed assistive personnel) per patient day.
14. Practice environment scale-nursing work index: Composite score and scores for five subscales: (a) nurse participation in hospital affairs; (b) nursing foundations for quality of care; (c) nurse manager ability, leadership, and support of nurses; (d) staffing and resource adequacy; and (e) collegiality of nurse-physician relations.
15. Voluntary turnover: Number of voluntary uncontrolled separations during the month by category (RNs, APNs, LVN/LPNs, and nurse anesthetists [NAs]).

Consortium activities are carried out through cross-specialty work groups established to develop performance measures from evidence-based clinical guidelines for select clinical conditions. Membership is open to any organization or individual committed to health-care quality improvement or patient safety and who participates in the development, review, dissemination, or implementation of performance measures and measurement resources. More than 200 performance measure descriptions and specifications for selected clinical topics and conditions are available for implementation (AMA, 2008). The Consortium's approach to measure development includes the following steps:

1. Identifying opportunities for improvement
2. Involving representatives from all medical specialties and other relevant health-care disciplines in the process
3. Linking measures to an evidence base
4. Supporting clinical judgment and patient preferences
5. Testing measures
6. Promoting a single set of measures for widespread use and multiple purposes

Practitioners of all relevant disciplines of medicine—as well as other health-care professionals for whom the care topic is within their scope of practice—are involved in each measure work group, APNs included (Kmetik, 2007; **Box 10-5).**

BOX 10-5
American Medical Association—Physician Consortium for Performance Improvement Measures

Descriptions and specifications for American Medical Association-Physician Consortium for Performance Improvement (AMA-PCPI) performance measures are available for 31 clinical topics or conditions:

- Acute otitis externa/otitis media with effusion
- Adult diabetes
- Anesthesiology and critical care
- Asthma
- Chronic kidney disease
- Chronic obstructive pulmonary disease
- Chronic stable coronary artery disease
- Community-acquired bacterial pneumonia
- Emergency medicine
- End-stage renal disease
- Eye care
- Gastroesophageal reflux disease
- Geriatrics
- Heart failure
- Hematology
- Hepatitis C
- Hypertension
- Major depressive disorder
- Melanoma
- Oncology

Continued

BOX 10-5
American Medical Association—Physician Consortium for Performance Improvement Measures—cont'd

- Osteoarthritis
- Osteoporosis
- Outpatient parenteral antimicrobial therapy
- Pathology
- Pediatric acute gastroenteritis
- Perioperative care
- Prenatal testing
- Preventive care and screening
  - Adult influenza immunization*
  - Colorectal cancer screening*
  - Problem drinking*
  - Screening mammography*
  - Tobacco use
  - Prostate cancer
- Radiology
- Stroke and stroke rehabilitation

*Indicates performance measures included in the preventive care and screening measures collection.

Nurses are the primary caregivers in all health-care settings. As such, they are critical to the provision of quality care. "Gaining a more in-depth understanding of the role that nurses play in quality improvement and the challenges nurses face can provide important insights about how hospitals can optimize resources to improve patient care quality" (Draper, Felland, Liebhaber & Melichar, 2008). All nurses must have thorough evidence-based knowledge of the impact of the care they provide on the outcomes patients experience. Measurement must be integrated into professional nursing practice at all levels, including the practice of APNs, and not simply considered to be a separate activity.

RECOGNITION AND CONSUMER SUPPORT

APNs are health-care professionals who do the following:

- provide high-quality health-care services
- diagnose and treat a wide range of health problems
- stress both care and cure using a unique approach
- focus on health promotion, disease prevention, health education, and counseling
- assist patients to make wise health and lifestyle choices (AANP, 2008, p. 1)

Simply put, APNs engage in many of the practices that patients are seeking. Why, then, are MCPs not clamoring to engage their services? How can APNs increase MCPs' demand for their services? In short, how can APNs market themselves (and their advanced practice roles) to both the MCP and its enrollees? APNs focus primarily on health promotion and disease prevention—factors frequently overlooked by traditional primary care providers. They have significant experience in both the acute and ambulatory care arenas. These abilities coupled with APN's possession of case management skills make them ideal for involvement in MCPs not merely as employees but as fully credentialed members of the MCP's provider panel. Although continuing emphasis is placed on quality, managed care's focus on reduction of costs has often resulted in a type of "managed competition" in which enrollees' benefits are restricted through limitation of their access to a variety of providers. It is within this trap that APNs frequently find themselves. To flourish in the managed care environment, APNs must market themselves to the MCP and to enrollees.

Marketing begins with a survey of the desires, needs, and expectations of the "customer," which in managed care is the enrollee. Armed with that information, APNs should then structure a plan to meet those needs. Because most APNs practice in a specialty area, the marketing plan should focus on the provision of related services, known as a *market segment.* An APN can choose to focus on a population with a single condition (e.g., individuals with insulin-dependent diabetes), a specific enrollee need (e.g., rehabilitation following amputation), or a particular population (e.g., older adults). A primary decision centers on whether to engage in provision of services to a single population, a variety of populations, or to all plan enrollees.

Marketing principles are sometimes referred to as the four Ps: product, price, promotion, and place (NetMBA, 2008). The first "P," product, encompasses the specialty practice services APNs provide, amplified by health promotion and disease prevention skills. The APN's product is self-evident. Thorough understanding of the second "P," price, is essential to the success of the APN, be it within an MCP or in independent practice. Although the marketplace, itself, has significant impact on demand for an APN's services as well as on how much it is willing to pay, the APN is the final arbiter as to price. It is critical that the APN has full knowledge of the costs of *all* of the components of the services delivered, not just personal compensation. The most difficult "P" for many nurses, not just APNs, to engage in is promotion. Nurses do not usually excel at "tooting their own horns." Self-promotion, or marketing, is unfamiliar to most nurses. Nurses generally operate from a mindset that views all health-care providers as doing their utmost to provide high-quality care. To increase recognition as well as consumer, or enrollee, support, APNs must be willing to call attention to the positive aspects of the safe, effective, patient-centered, timely, efficient, equitable care they provide. Finally, APNs must make an informed decision as to the last "P," place; that is, whether or not to engage in providing care as an employee, an independent practitioner, or as a contractual partner in an MCP.

CONCLUSION

Today's health-care delivery system, with increased merger activity between insurance companies and health systems and the biased policies of providers and MCPs, has created an environment in which APNs experience significant barriers to their ability to practice. Strategies are needed to unite the collaborative efforts of ANA, constituent member associations, other national APN organizations, and individual APNs to identify trends related to exclusionary behavior and to develop an effective multipronged approach to address anticompetitive policies and practices, such as that proposed by CPR.

Nurses have looked to antitrust protections for relief from practices that block their full participation in the health-care market. CNMs and CRNAs used federal antitrust laws to limit boycotts and expand their market share. The Federal Trade Commission (FTC) has rendered opinions that provide the foundation for anticompetitive action by registered nurses. The Department of Justice and the FTC have issued joint guidelines for antitrust enforcement in the health-care industry that offer general direction about those practices that are (and that are not) likely to trigger action by these enforcement agencies.

Restrictive policies at the state level must be addressed by a comprehensive state-based strategy to better define and combat state-based anitcompetitive behavior. Such strategies should include use of agencies such as state insurance commissions, state boards of nursing, and consumer and regulatory entities to enforce the law and to challenge anticompetitive activities.

It is crucial that nurses in general, and APNs in particular, work to gain recognition for the high-quality, cost-effective care they provide. ANA remains committed to monitoring state and federal activities of organized medicine to counteract their effectiveness. To the extent that organized medical societies focus their efforts on opposing or supporting legislation, even through the use of exaggerated arguments and legislative strategies, the major option available to nursing is to oppose those efforts and to respond to them by ensuring that legislators and the public hear the facts about APN practice.

APNs continue to be notably absent from MCP provider panels and from the national quality enterprise. This is likely due, in part, to their predominately employee status. In moving to contract independently with MCPs, APNs can take on full responsibility as managed care providers. In addition, APNs can engage in the collection and reporting of data using measures related to the quality of care they provide. Those data, in addition to informing nursing practice, can help purchasers and consumers decide where to look for high-quality, effective, efficient care. Using data, APNs can mobilize consumer support for their services thereby increasing respect for themselves and on behalf of nursing overall. It is up to individual APNs to professional nursing, to NQF, and to all who have interest in the provision (or receipt) of quality health care to advance quality in a collaborative, coordinated way. For after all, healthcare quality really is an art . . . "more like ballet, than hockey" (Crosby, 1979, p. 20).

References

Abood, S., & Keepnews, D. (2000). *Understanding payment for advanced practice nursing services, Volume one: Medicare reimbursement.* Washington, D.C.: American Nurses Association.

Abood, S., & Keepnews, D. (2002). *Understanding payment for advanced practice nursing services, Volume two: Fraud and abuse.* Washington, DC: American Nurses Association.

American Academy of Nurse Practitioners. (2008). *Why choose a Nurse Practitioner as your healthcare provider?* Retrieved April 6, 2008, from the American Academy of Nurse Practitioners Web site: http://npfinder.com/faq.pdf.

American College of Nurse-Midwives. (1997). Tip sheet for ACNM state legislative contacts. *ACC Certified Midwives.* Retrieved April 19, 2008, from the American College of Nurse-Midwives Web site: www.midwife.org/display.cfm?id=503.

American Managed Care and Review Association Foundation. (1995). Managed care overview. Washington, DC: Author.

American Medical Association. (2008). *Physician consortium for performance improvement.* Retrieved February 4, 2008, from the American Medical Association Web site: www.ama-assn.org/ama/pub/category/2946.html.

APRN Consensus Workgroup and the National Council of State Boards of Nursing APRN Advisory Committee. (2008). *Consensus model for APRN regulation: Licensure, accreditation, certification and education.* Washington, DC: Author.

Brown, D. J. (2007) "Consumer perspectives on nurse practitioners and independent practice." *Journal of the American Academy of Nurse Practitioners, 19*(10), 523–529.

Bryant-Lukosius, D., Dicenso, A., Browne, G., & Pinelli, J. (2004). Advanced practice nursing roles: Development, implementation and evaluation. *Journal of Advanced Nursing, 48*(5), 519–529.

Buppert, C. (2008). How to fire a patient. *Journal for Nurse Practitioners, 4*(2), 97–99.

Butler, R. N. (1995). Ten geriatric messages for managed care. *Managed Care and Aging, 2*(2), 1.

Caesar, N. B. (1995). How to negotiate before you sign the dotted line. *Physician's Managed Care Report, 3*(12), 142.

Centers for Medicare and Medicaid Services. (2007). Hospital-acquired conditions (HAC) in acute inpatient prospective payment system (IPPS) hospitals. Retrieved May 8, 2008, from the Centers for Medicare and Medicaid Services Web site: www.cms.hhs.gov/HospitalAcqCond/Downloads/hac.fact.sheet.pdf.

Centers for Medicare and Medicaid Services. (2008) *Quality improvement work.* Retrieved February 4, 2008, from the Centers for Medicare and Medicaid Services Web site: www.cms.hhs.gov/QualityImprovementOrgs/.

Coalition for Patients' Rights. (2006). *Coalition for patients' rights (CPR) calls on AMA to cease divisive efforts to limit patients' choice of providers.* Retrieved February 23, 2008, from the Coalition for Patients' Rights Web site: www.patientsrightscoalition.org/news/.

Crosby, P. B. (1979). *Quality is free.* New York: New American Library.

Dahle, K. L., Smith, J. S., & Wilson, J. R. (1998). Impact of a nurse practitioner on the cost of managing inpatients with heart failure. *American Journal of Cardiology, 82*(5), 686.

Division of Nursing, U.S. Department of Health and Human Services. (2006). *The registered nurse population. Finding from the March 2004 national sample survey of registered nurses. June, 2006.* Rockville, MD: U.S. Department of Health and Human Services, Health Resources and Services Administration, Bureau of Health Professions.

Draper, D. A., Felland, L. E., Liebhaber, A., & Melichar, L. (2008). *The role of nurses in hospital quality improvement.* Retrieved April 20, 2008, from the Center for Health System Change Web site: www.hschange.org/CONTENT/972/.

Dunton, N., Gajewski, B., Taunton, R.L., & Moore, J. (2004). Nurse staffing and patient falls on acute care hospital units. *Nursing Outlook, 52*(1):53–59.

Gallup Organization. (1993). *ANA-commissioned survey.* Princeton, NJ: Author.

Goolsby, M. J. (2004). *2004 National NP sample survey comparisons over 15-year period.* Retrieved April 11, 2008, from the American Academy of Nurse Practitioners Web site: www.aanp.org/NR/rdonlyres/ewz24bs6jt72aeldxgvk3woyo4dhasuc5hvwpt65bs2iyej2edd3723ri3ggbwiptvoym2x7o37rwridsnb2tf3gfxh/2004NatlNPSampleSurveyWeb.pdf.

Hart, S., Bergquist, S., Gajewski, B., & Dunton, N. (2006). Reliability testing of the National Database of Nursing Quality Indicators' pressure ulcer indicator. *Journal of Nursing Care Quality, 21*(3), 256–265.

Hazzard, J. P. (2002). The invisible people. *Advance for Nurse Practitioners, 10*(7), 80.

Health Resources and Services Administration (HRSA). (2004). *National sample survey of registered nurses.* Retrieved May 10, 2008, from the Bureau of Health Professions Web site: http://bhpr.hrsa.gov/healthworkforce/rnsurvey04/.

Hibbard, J. H., Stockard, J., & Tusler, M. (2003). Does publicizing hospital performance stimulate quality improvement efforts? *Health Affairs, 22*(2), 84–94.

Hibbard, J. H., Stockard, J., & Tusler, M. (2005). Hospital performance reports: Impact on quality, market share, and reputation. *Health Affairs, 24*(4), 1150–1160.

Hicks, L. L, Stallmeyer, J. M., & Coleman, J. R. (1993). *Role of the nurse in managed care.* Washington, DC: American Nurses Association.

Hill, C. (2007). *The Joint Commission awarded Robert Wood Johnson Foundation grant to test nursing-focused quality of care measures.* Oakbrook Terrace, IL: The Joint Commission.

Hill, D. T., Cohen, S. S., & Mason, D. J. (1999). Managed care for NPs: Focus groups reveal perils and promises of managed care for nurse practitioners. *Nurse Practitioner, 24*(2), 15–16.

Himali, U. (1995). Managed care: Does the promise meet the potential? *The American Nurse, 27*(4), 14, 16.

Hugonnet, S., Uçkay, I., & Pittet, D. (2007). "Staffing level: A determinant of late-onset ventilator-associated pneumonia." *Critical Care, 11*(4), R80.

Hylka, S. C. (1997). Managing under managed care: The role of the advanced practice nurse in surgery. *Today's Surgical Nurse, 19*(1), 29–32.

Japsen, B. (2006, June 12). Rise of retail clinics giving doctors a chill AMA to make push for more scrutiny of sites staffed by nurse practitioners. *The Chicago Tribune.* Retrieved April 7, 2008, from the *Chicago Tribune* Web site: www.acnpweb.org/files/public/ChicagoTrib_Retail_Clinics_AMA_June_2006.pdf.

Kmetik, K. (2007). PCPI: What you should know about Consortium performance measures. *Journal of Family Practice, 56*(10 suppl A): 8A–12A.

Kongstvedt, P. R. (2000). *The managed health care handbook.* Sudbury, MA: Jones and Bartlett Publishers.

Lachman, V. D. (1996). Positioning your business in the marketplace. *Advanced Practice Nursing Quarterly, 2*(1), 27–32.

Landon, B. E., Normand, S. L., Lessler, A., O'Malley, A. J., Schmaltz, S., Loeb, J. M., et al. (2006). Quality of care for the treatment of acute medical conditions in U.S. hospitals. *Archives of Internal Medicine, 166*(22): 2511–2517.

Leider, H. L., & Bard, M. A. (1993). Self-assessment and managed care. In D. B. Nash, *The physician's guide to managed care.* Gaithersburg, MD: Aspen.

Managed Care Fact Sheets. (2008). *Managed care national statistics.* Retrieved April 11, 2008, from Mycol Web site: www.mcareol.com/factshts/factnati.htm.

Mason, D. J., Alexander, J. M., Huffaker, J., Reilly, P. A., Sigmund, E. C., & Cohen, S. S. (1999). Nurse practitioners' experiences with managed care organizations in New York and Connecticut. *Nursing Outlook, 47*(5), 201–208.

May, C. A., Schraeder, C., & Britt, T. (1996). *Managed care and case management: roles for professional nursing.* Washington, DC: American Nurses Association.

National Quality Forum. (2002). *A comprehensive framework for hospital care performance evaluation.* Washington, DC: Author.

National Quality Forum. (2003). *National voluntary consensus standards for hospital care: An initial performance measure set.* Washington, DC: Author.

National Quality Forum. (2004). *National voluntary consensus standards for nursing-sensitive care: An initial performance measure set.* Washington, DC: Author.

National Quality Forum. (2007). *Tracking NQF-endorsed consensus standards for nursing-sensitive care: A 15-month study.* Washington, DC: Author.

National Quality Forum. (2008). *Mission.* Retrieved February 2, 2008, from the National Quality Forum Web site: www.qualityforum.org/about/mission.asp.

NetMBA. (2008). *Marketing mix: The 4Ps of marketing.* Retrieved April 6, 2008, from NetMBA Web site: www.netmba.com/marketing/mix/.

North Shore-Long Island Jewish Health System. *Insurance and managed care glossary.* Retrieved April 9, 2008, from the North Shore-Long Island Jewish Health System Web site: www.nslij.com/body.cfm?id=568.

Office of Technology Assessment, Congress of the United States. (1986). *Nurse practitioners, physician assistants, and certified nurse-midwives: A policy analysis.* (HCS 37). Washington, D.C.: U.S. Printing Office.

O'Grady, E. T. (2008). Advanced practice registered nurses: The impact on patient safety and quality. In *Patient safety and quality: An evidence-based handbook for nurses.* (AHRQ Publication No. 08-0043). Rockville, MD: Agency for Healthcare Research and Quality. Retrieved April 20, 2008, from the Agency for Healthcare Research and Quality Web site: www.ahrq.gov/qual/nurseshdbk/.

Poll. (2002). 3 of 4 Americans never heard of NPs. *Advance for Nurse Practitioners, 10*(7), 14.

Stahl, D. A. (1995). Managed care and subacute care: A partnership of choice. *Nursing Management, 26*(1), 17–19.

Stires, D. (2002, October 14). The coming crash in health care. *Fortune,* 205–212.

Stone, P. W., Mooney-Kane, C., Larson, E. L., Horan, T., Glance, L. G., Zwanziger, J., et al. (2007). Nurse working conditions and patient safety outcomes. *Medical Care, 45*(6): 571–578.

The Joint Commission. (2005). *Implementation guide for the NQF endorsed nursing-sensitive care performance measures.* Oakbrook Terrace, IL: Author.

Tourangeau, A. E., Doran, D. M., McGillis Hall, L., O'Brien Pallas, L., Pringle, D., Tu, J. V., et al. (2005). Impact of hospital mursing care on 30-day mortality for acute medical patients. *Cancer, 104*(5), 975–984.

Walker, C. (1996). Opening the door to managed care. *Subacute Care, 3*(2), 33.

Weisman, J. S. (2007). Hospital workload and adverse events. *Medical Care, 45*(5), 448–454.

Resource Management

11

Christina M. Graf
Eileen D. Flaherty

INTRODUCTION

In any setting, the advanced practice nurse (APN) pursuing clinical practice objectives influences and is affected by the environment of an organization—whether the organization is as large as a multiple entity system or as small as a single-person practice. The organization provides the structure in which the goal of the APN will be pursued.

The underlying assumption for any organization is that its reason for existing—and continuing to exist—is to produce some product or service (output) that is of value. The corollary assumptions are that because the output is of value it will generate revenue and that the revenue generated will both cover the costs of the resources expended (input) and provide some level of profit. Profit is necessary to ensure the continued viability of the organization, for example, to upgrade existing facilities, to replace outdated equipment, to expand services, or to add new programs, and in for-profit organizations, to provide a return for investors or owners and encourage continued investment. If this does not occur, the organization will not survive. Prudent management dictates that to succeed in its mission, the organization ensures its financial viability through appropriate prioritization of outcomes and effective use of resources.

Organizational decisions about programs and process can affect both the content and direction of the APN's practice or in fact determine to what extent, if any, APNs are able to practice within the organization. The absence of effective input from clinicians can result in inappropriate or ineffective expectations of the clinician. Similarly, clinicians' decisions can generate unintended consequences that undermine the health and strength of the organization. Therefore, the APN needs to understand the business structure and systems of the organization and the extent to which his or her clinical practice affects and is affected by these systems. How does the APN's practice affect revenue generation and expenditure of resources? To what extent do business and fiscal policies enhance or constrain clinical practice? The APN must be able to articulate these interactions in the language of business to influence appropriate decision making. This requires an understanding of the business and financial aspects of the organization.

STRUCTURE

In accomplishing its mission, an organization engages in a series of transactions that it tracks and manages through its financial system. These transactions are categorized according to the chart of accounts, which is a matrix structure that organizes the transactions. One axis of the matrix, the account codes, aggregates transactions according to type (e.g., patient care revenue, salaries, office supplies, and maintenance contracts). The other axis, the cost center, revenue center, or responsibility center, aggregates transactions according to function and may be identified by product line (e.g., cardiac center, cancer care center), physical location (e.g., patient care unit, outpatient clinic), or activity (e.g., blood bank, hemodialysis). The detailed designations in the chart of accounts are specific to each organization, and as such, not only aggregate transactions for better information and management but also provide a picture of the organization and its internal structure. The aggregated transactions are summarized in a statement of operations called the profit and loss (P & L) or income and expense (I & E) statement that also quantifies the operating margin or the gain or loss (income minus expense) from operations. See **Table 11-1.**

Most health-care organizations use accrual accounting in preparing financial statements. Accrual accounting specifies that revenues are recognized when services are provided and expenses are reported as resources are used. Thus revenues reported for activities within a particular cost center are

TABLE 11-1

Sample Profit and Loss Statement

Profit and Loss Statement Fiscal Year 2008 (in Thousands of Dollars)

	Actual	Budget	Variance	Variance Percent (%)
Patient services revenue				
Inpatient	$515,994	$496,843	$19,151	3.9
Outpatient	$341,769	$332,764	$9,005	2.7
GPSR	$857,763	$829,607	$28,156	3.4
Deductions from revenue				
Contractual allowances	$498,732	$479,560	–$19,172	–4.0
Charity care	$23,760	$22,230	–$1,531	–6.9
Net patient services revenue	$335,272	$327,818	$7,454	2.3
Indirect research revenue	$31,555	$30,951	$605	2.0
Other operating revenue	$16,089	$15,126	$964	6.4
Total operating revenue	$382,916	$373,894	$9,022	2.4
Expenses				
Salaries and wages	$152,628	$151,908	–$720	–0.5
Employee benefits	$26,517	$26,726	$209	0.8
Supplies	$58,682	$56,421	–$2,261	–4.0
Utilities	$9,503	$10,187	$685	6.7
Other	$81,249	$77,487	–$3,762	–4.9
Depreciation	$27,300	$27,468	$168	0.6
Provision for bad debt	$8,758	$10,126	$1,368	13.5
Interest	$4,956	$5,485	$529	9.6
Total operating expense	$369,592	$365,806	–$3,786	–1.0
Income (loss) from operations	$13,324	$8,088	$5,237	—
Percent of total revenue	3.5%	2.2%	—	—

NOTE: Positive variances are favorable to budget; negative variances are unfavorable to budget.
  GPSR, Gross patient services revenue.

matched to the expenses generated in producing those revenues, and they reflect the activity and resource use that occurred in that reporting period, regardless of when actual monies for services are received or bills for resources are paid.

REVENUE

Revenue or income refers to the monies received for services provided and reflects the volume of output of the organization. Revenue is based on the price or charge allocated to each specific service, activity, or item. The organization's charge master is a list of the prices charged, which are intended to reflect the related costs plus some margin of profit. However, charges are usually discounted or bundled under a global fee for most payors, entirely waived for charitable care, or not collected from those who are expected to pay. Therefore, charges are not necessarily an accurate reflection of actual income from the service, activity, or item.

Revenue is generated primarily from the day-to-day activities of the organization and is termed operating revenue. In health-care organizations, the majority of the operating revenue is related to patient or client services rendered and may come from a variety of payors: the federal government (e.g., Medicare, military and veterans benefit programs), state governments (e.g., Medicaid and other state programs), other third-party payors (e.g., Blue Cross/Blue Shield, health maintenance organizations [HMOs], indemnity insurance plans), or the recipient of the service (self-pay).

Medicare revenues are determined not by charges or specific services but by a prospective payment system that allocates a fixed payment based on an episode of care. The payment is determined for inpatient episodes of care by the discharge diagnosis (diagnosis related group [DRG]) and is adjusted for variations in regional cost of living, urban versus rural setting, and organizational involvement in medical education. Except for some small amount of adjustment for cost or length of stay outliers, the payment to an organization for each DRG is constant regardless of costs incurred. This prospective payment system is not applicable to psychiatric and rehabilitation units or hospitals, children's and cancer hospitals, or long-term care facilities, which are reimbursed on a reasonable cost basis, with some limits, for patients eligible for Medicare. For outpatients, Medicare has developed a similar prospective payment system using ambulatory payment classification (APC) groups, aggregating services that are similar clinically and with respect to resource requirements. Medicare reimburses providers for services based on prior fixed rates for the APCs.

Medicaid and other state-sponsored payment programs reflect not only the intent of the program, but also the economic and political environment of the state, and thus vary widely from state to state. The state determines what will be covered and the level of reimbursement and may limit payments through global or flat rate fees for episodes of care, exclusion of certain services from coverage, discounting of specific charges or targeted spending caps.

Many nongovernmental third-party payors negotiate contracts with health-care organizations, which may include DRG-like prospective payment systems, discounted or adjusted rates, risk-sharing agreements such as flat rate payments per person, per month for all defied care needs, prior authorization requirements, or other mechanisms that minimize the cost to the payor and distance the revenue from the charge. These payors, primarily managed care organizations (MCOs), also include in their reimbursement systems copays, specified dollar amounts per episode of care, deductibles, and identified annual dollar amounts or deductibles that are paid directly by the consumer. Indemnity insurance payors typically reimburse based on charges, or more commonly on a negotiated percent of charges, but here also there may be copays, deductibles, payment ceilings, or service exclusions that shift the burden to the insured. In any case, indemnity insurance provides only a small percentage of the income of health-care organizations. Even smaller is the proportion of self-pay patients who are able to afford health care. The growing number of uninsured, who have no access to federal, state, or private coverage, generates a significant level of charitable care and bad debt for many health-care organizations.

In addition to the many reimbursement methods that exist, new payment mechanisms continue to emerge. For example, many payors have begun to link quality measures and outcomes with reimbursement incentives, also referred to as pay-for-performance programs. The intention of such programs is to encourage continuous improvement in the quality of care delivered in all health-care settings. In these arrangements, health-care organizations and their providers are held accountable to achieving defined quality standards to receive full payment for services.

The sum of the charges appears on the financial statement as gross patient services revenue (GPSR). Deductions from revenue include contractual allowances, which is the difference between the charge and the actual payment negotiated with third-party payors, and charitable care, for which services are not billed. (Note that bad debt is not considered a deduction from revenue. It is in fact an expense incurred because anticipated income for billed services is determined to be uncollectible.) Net patient services revenue (NPSR) equals GPSR minus contractual allowances and charitable care.

In addition to patient services revenue, organizations may generate other operating revenue, income from other day-to-day activities in areas such as the parking garage or the cafeteria, or indirect research revenue, such as the overhead received from research sponsors for providing facilities and administrative support for research projects. Total operating revenue is NPSR plus other operating and research revenue, and it reflects the total reimbursement in actual monies that the organization expects to receive from operations.

The organization may also generate nonoperating revenue that is not tied directly to the services or products provided and is managed and reported separately from operating revenue. Interest income may be generated on cash or investments. Gifts or donations may be given to a not-for-profit organization for a specific purpose or for the general purposes of the organization. If they are specific-purpose gifts, they may not be used for any alternative purpose without the express consent of the donor. If the gift is in the form of an endowment, then the principle (the original amount of the gift) is invested and only the interest income on the investment may be used.

EXPENSE

Expenses are costs incurred in providing services or producing products. Wage and salary expenses are the costs of personnel, which are the labor costs required for production. Salaries are determined by the organization, subject to regulation regarding minimum wage and fair labor practices, and in some organizations, union contracts. They include base wages plus any differentials, premiums, bonuses, or other monetary rewards. Fringe benefits fall into two categories, those mandated by law, such as unemployment insurance and worker's compensation, and those specific to the organization, such as health insurance and pension benefits. Other benefits that incur costs are related to the organizations' personnel policies regarding sick, vacation, holiday, and other paid time off. In addition to the obvious salary cost for the worker on paid time off, there is an additional expense in the form of replacement cost (the cost to ensure that another worker is available) or the productivity cost (the cost of the output or associated revenue that is not realized). In a practice, for example, if practitioners are functioning at efficient levels, the absence of one practitioner on a paid leave will result either in loss of revenue for patients not seen or increased costs for a temporary replacement for the practitioner. Note that this relates to paid absence. Unpaid absence leaves unspent wages available to support a temporary replacement or provides a cost offset to unrealized volume and associated revenue.

Nonsalary expenses are those nonpersonnel costs for consumable supplies, minor equipment, and related activities used in the delivery of service. Some are directly related to patient care activities, such as medical supplies, drugs, and blood products. Others are related to supports for the care process (e.g., office supplies, telephone charges), the environment (e.g., maintenance contracts, utilities), personnel (e.g., seminar registration, consultation fees), and interest on loans or bad debt.

Another type of expense is depreciation or the loss in value of capital assets. Capital expense refers to major investments in durable assets, such as facilities, equipment, and machinery. Capital assets are expected to have a value and useful life significantly greater than that of minor equipment. The threshold for determining what is capitalized is set by the organization and usually describes both a monetary value and an expected life span. For example, the threshold for capital might be equipment that costs more than $500 and has a useful life greater than 3 years. Under these guidelines, neither a $100 intravenous pole (monetary threshold) nor $1000 worth of instructional videotapes (life span threshold), would be considered capital, whereas a portable ultrasound or a computerized medical record system, would be capitalized. Because capital assets are expected to be used over an extended period of time, their full purchase price does not appear as an operational expense at the time of purchase. Rather, in each reporting period for the duration of its useful life, the income and expense report reflects the capital depreciation or the loss in value of the capital asset as a result of use during the period. For example, if a capital purchase of $12,000 is expected to have a useful life of 10 years, then one-tenth of its value is estimated to be used each year. Therefore, the financial statement would report depreciation of $1200 per year or $100 per month.

COST CONCEPTS

There are a variety of cost concepts that are relevant in understanding resource management.

Variable Versus Fixed Costs

Variable costs are those related to the volume of activity and fluctuate based on changes in volume. Fixed costs are those that remain constant regardless of fluctuations in volume. In personnel, the staff nurses may be considered variable—more are needed when the unit is at 90% occupancy than when it is at 75% occupancy—whereas the clinical specialist and nurse manager are fixed—one allocated to the unit regardless of the number of patients. Similarly, medical supply expense is variable based on patient volume and acuity, whereas maintenance contract expenses may be fixed based on the terms of the contract and not driven by volume. Some expenses may be step-variable, that is, fixed over a short range and variable over a longer range. For example, one secretary may be sufficient for a practice with up to four clinicians, but a second secretary may be required if an additional clinician enters the practice. In that case, the number of secretaries is fixed at two unless the number of clinicians increases beyond eight. In general, all costs that are fixed in the short run are variable in the longer run (**Fig. 11-1**).

Direct Versus Indirect Costs

Direct costs are those related to the process of producing a product or service. Indirect costs are those incurred in supporting that process. In practice, the identification of expenses as direct or indirect depends on the context. In addressing an individual patient, caregivers—nurses, therapists, practitioners—would be considered direct, whereas the leadership and support staff—secretaries, clinical specialist, or nurse manager—would be considered indirect. In considering

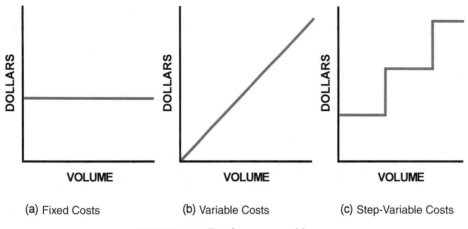

(a) Fixed Costs   (b) Variable Costs   (c) Step-Variable Costs

FIGURE 11-1 Fixed versus variable costs.

patient populations aggregated by clinical care unit or practice, the entire staff of that unit or practice could be considered direct whereas support departments—human resources, environmental services, fiscal affairs—are identified as indirect.

Total Versus Unit Costs

Total cost is the aggregate cost incurred within a given time period for all volume of activity in that same time period. Unit cost is the cost of one unit of volume, calculated as the total cost divided by the total units of volume. Marginal cost is the additional cost required to produce one more unit of volume. Because the total cost includes both variable and fixed costs, it is possible to achieve economies of scale by increasing volume—and variable costs—on the unchanged fixed cost base. In that case, total cost increases, but the cost per unit of volume goes down. The marginal cost of the added volume is equal to the variable cost. If a clinical care unit can increase its occupancy, it will expend more in variable direct care staff, but the cost per patient day will decrease because the fixed costs are spread over more patient days. Marginal cost for each additional patient day is equal to the cost of the variable staff and supplies for that patient day. However, if the patient day volume increases to the point where it is necessary to open another unit, then additional fixed costs and additional variable costs will be incurred. Cost per patient day across both units will escalate because of the added fixed costs, until additional volume reduces the unit cost. The marginal cost for the first additional patient day beyond those on the original unit is both the variable cost for that patient day and the fixed cost for the new unit. Therefore, opening the second unit for an increase of one patient per day could be prohibitively expensive unless there is expectation of a relatively rapid volume increase.

Incremental Versus Opportunity Costs

Incremental cost is the added cost incurred for an activity that would not be expensed if that activity did not occur. As such, it differs from marginal costs, which refers to the cost of adding one more unit of output, if the activity or program or project adds multiple or different units and looks at all additional volume together with all additional related costs. These costs may be variable or fixed, but they are essentially new costs and do not include current costs that may be redirected to the new activity. For example, if a clinical nurse specialist (CNS) proposes to teach a new series of classes on pediatric cardiac life support, incremental costs could include items such as demonstration mannequins, audiovisual aids, books, or other informational material and supplies for practical application. These would all be incremental costs because they would be incurred specifically for the purpose of the program. The participants' salaries are incremental if they are paid beyond their usual or regular hours to attend the program. If the program is to be given within the participants' regular working hours and it will be necessary to provide additional staff hours to cover those in class, then these replacement costs are also included in the incremental costs. The CNS's time in preparation and teaching and the facilities or space in which the classes are taught would not be considered incremental costs because—if the classes were not given—the CNS's salary and the cost of maintaining the facilities would still be incurred. The incremental costs would be calculated for the number of students and programs presented over a given period of time.

Opportunity cost measures the loss of the effect of the next best alternative use of the resources allocated to a particular use. If the program described is approved for implementation, what activity will the CNS forego to implement the program? If the facilities are not used for this purpose, how will they be used? If the participants are taking the course during their regular working hours and replacement is not required, what will they not be doing that might otherwise have been done? If the incremental resources were not allocated to this program, what would they be used for? The answers to these questions describe the opportunity costs. Identification and quantification of opportunity costs can provide important information in setting priorities and analyzing alternatives.

BUDGETING

Effective management presumes that an organization, in planning for its continuing existence, is able to describe and project the level of activity or production of services or products it will experience and anticipate the resources that will be required for that level of activity. The budget is the translation of that plan into quantities and dollars. The conceptual plan on which the budget is based may describe the projections for the entire organization or for some particular sector or activity and will determine the scope of the budget, including the time frame and the level of detail.

Types of Budget

Strategic planning is likely to be translated into a long-range budget that addresses the direction of the organization over the next 3 to 5 years or more. For this type of budget, the projections of volume and resources will be at a high level, with estimations of revenue and expense totals but not at an extremely detailed level. The major drivers of volume and resources will be described and quantified, for example, anticipated changes in the patient mix, Medicare reimbursement rates, treatment protocols, or pharmaceutical expenditures. Other factors will be estimated in the aggregate based on current experience. The strategic plan and long-range budget are schematic representations of the direction of the organization rather than detailed blueprints. They need to be reviewed and refreshed at regular intervals to ensure that the organization continues to move in its preferred direction and to respond to significant changes in the health-care environment.

The operational budget, on the other hand, addresses the detailed, day-to-day activity of the organization. This type of budget looks in extensive detail at the projected volume and resources and the associated revenue and expense over a prescribed period of time. Usually the operating budget is constructed for the fiscal year, the organization's 12-month accounting cycle. The budget describes anticipated activity based on the specific operational goals and plans of the organization for that period of time and incorporates assumptions that will affect revenue and expense, for example, changes in reimbursement or inflationary increases in the cost of utilities or supplies. The budget is prepared at the detailed level of account within cost center. Actual experience is reported against the budget for each accounting cycle or month and cumulatively for the fiscal year to date and is reported for each cost center and account code. However, each fiscal year's operating budget is independent of other years, that is, the positive or negative variance and the unspent budgeted monies from one fiscal year are not carried over into the next. The operating budget as a plan is valuable at the detailed level, the level at which the work occurs, and at which the activity and resources must be managed. Aggregation of the budgeted and actual revenue and expense at the organizational level is also useful in providing overall direction and evaluation for the organization as a whole.

The capital budget reflects the projected expense for necessary facility improvement or acquisition of major durable equipment. Funding for the capital budget comes from the profit generated from operations, or from loans, which are also dependent on the organization's ability to generate a profit from operations. Although the capital budget may be prepared in yearly cycles, unlike the operating budget it is contained by the time frame of the project rather than of the budget year. Thus, capital funds may be allocated over several budget years for a particular remodeling project or equipment replacement proposal, and unlike the operating budget, the funds will carry over from year to year until the project is completed. The capital budget is based on the plans and projections of the organization and will address the facilities and equipment needed to expand or upgrade services. These can generate the need for new or added clinical equipment such as cardiac monitors and ultrasound equipment; computer hardware (computers, monitors, printers) and major software (electronic medical record, provider order entry system); and facilities improvement (renovation and remodeling). The capital budget also needs to address the maintenance needs of the organization, and therefore will also include such things as replacement of existing equipment, for example, beds or ventilators that have reached the end of their useful life or facilities maintenance, such as the heating, ventilation, air conditioning (HVAC) system. Finally, in preparing the capital budget, it is important to consider any additional nonsalary costs that will be incurred because of the use of the capital asset. For example, purchase of a monitoring system, clearly a capital expense, can also generate operating costs in the form of replacement leads or probes, batteries, or electrocardiogram tracing paper, and potentially salary costs if additional personnel hours are required to monitor the monitors or file the tracings. These expenses must be identified and incorporated in the appropriate operating budget.

Frequently, organizations will consider initiating new activities or expanding or changing existing ones. The program budget is useful for this purpose. This type of budget isolates one activity or program from all other organizational activities to evaluate its effectiveness. The basis for the program budget is the conceptual plan of the program or the program proposal, which also determines the time frame for the budget as well as the types of expenses to be included (e.g., total costs, incremental costs, opportunity costs). A plan to expand the hours of service for a medical urgent care clinic, using existing facilities, and equipment may be adequately described in a program budget that looks only at incremental volume, resources, revenue, and expense for the current fiscal year. Evaluation of the fiscal viability of the plan would consider the extent to which incremental revenue exceeds incremental expense. A plan to add a neonatal intensive care unit in a service that previously provided only routine and intermediate care would require a more extensive program budget. The quantification of activity would need to address potential volume—both numbers of neonates and clinical conditions—and probable income based on payor mix and reimbursement rates. Resource requirements would include both capital expenditures for facilities and major equipment and operational expenses for personnel, supplies, minor equipment, utilities, and overhead. Because of the time required to set up the program and the anticipated ramp up from opening to full occupancy and use, the program plan would cover an extended period of time. Fiscal estimates would then need to be adjusted for the effect of inflation and reimbursement changes. Evaluation of the program would include a calculation of breakeven, that is, the point at which the average total revenue for an admission is equal to the average total cost. Before breakeven, the program generates a loss for each admission. After breakeven, the program generates net revenue for each admission **(Fig. 11-2).** Determination of the value of a program considers more than the fiscal benefit, (e.g., opportunity costs, social benefits, and costs or public relations value). These factors are difficult to quantify and are therefore not part of the program budget, although they would be contained in the program proposal. When a program budget is approved and implemented, it becomes part of the operating budget for the implementation period and for all subsequent years. However, it is also useful to evaluate actual experience against the original program budget.

The projection of the cash budget is critical in the life of the organization. In the other types of budget, one of the guiding principles is matching revenue to expenses (i.e., identifying the income for the activity that occurred in a particular time period and the expenses related to that activity that were incurred in that time period). Typically, however, the actual receipt of the revenue and the payment of the expenses do not occur in the same time period. Services are billed to third-party payors, but the actual revenue is received weeks or even months later. Supplies are ordered, delivered, and used, but the organization may be billed days or weeks later and the bills may be paid on a 30-, 60-, or 90-day payment cycle. Thus, the revenue and expense projections for a particular accounting cycle in the operational budget, for example, do not reflect that cycle's cash flow, the actual cash coming into, and going out of the organization. The cash budget projects this flow over

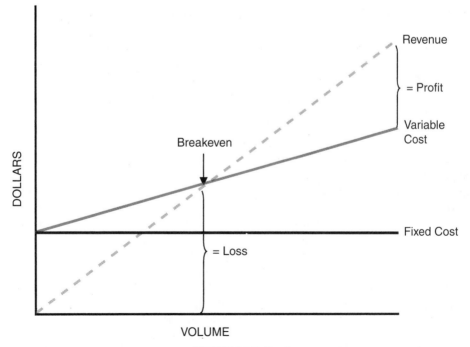

FIGURE 11-2 Breakeven.

the course of the fiscal year to ensure that there will be sufficient money in the organization to meet its obligations to its employees for payment of salaries, to its suppliers for paying of bills, and to its lenders for repayment of loans.

Budgeting Process

The budget process is based on the conceptual plan, goals, and objectives of the organization. The process will translate these into quantifiable units of service and required resources. The first step in this process is the identification of the activity that generates revenue and drives resource use. Within the health-care system, there are typical volume statistics that are used to quantify activity: admissions, discharges, patient days, patient visits, procedures, and tests. In the aggregate, however, these measures do not have the level of precision needed for accurate prediction of revenue and expenses. For purposes of predicting revenue, the volume needs to be further defined to reflect the basis of payment—by payor, by service, by product line, by DRG, or by test or procedure code.

For the purposes of predicting resource use, however, these categories may need to be further refined. DRG payments, for example, reflect medical condition and interventions but do not as clearly reflect nursing care needs of patients. As a result, patients in the same DRG—and generating the same revenue—may have different nursing care needs based on age, functional capabilities, communication issues or learning needs, and thus generate different levels of resource use. Payment systems may be based on global fees (e.g., for normal pregnancy and delivery) or on panels of patients (with the practice or organization receiving a per patient per month payment regardless of use of services) that are not reflective of the individual variability in care needs and resource requirements. It is necessary, therefore, to develop workload measures that identify both the resource drivers, that is, the significant activities that generate resource use, and the elements that account for individual variation within those drivers. For example, in the cancer infusion unit, the primary measure may be the patient visit or the therapeutic protocol. However, resource use may vary based on whether this is a new or returning patient, the length of the treatment, the patient's response to the therapy, or other issues or concerns that the patient raises in the course of the visit. Although it may not be possible to implement a workload measure that addresses this variability in minute detail, it is possible to develop measures that differentiate among patients and aggregate those with similar resource requirements. For patients with the same medical condition or undergoing the same therapeutic protocol, it may be possible to identify variations in resource use based on age, stage of treatment, functional level of activity, or other indicators. Using these indicators and the primary volume indicator of visit or protocol to describe patient populations can then be used to generate a more accurate projection of required personnel and materiel resources. The patients can be aggregated into groups with similar resource requirements and the groups can be weighted based on their average use relative to one another. For example, in a particular practice, patients receiving a specific intervention may require 15 minutes of the clinician's time. However, a follow-up patient may only require 10 minutes and a new patient may require 40 minutes. All patients, however, may require 5 minutes for documentation and 5 minutes for follow-up. The intervention patient, therefore, will consume 25 minutes of time and the others 20 minutes and 50 minutes, respectively. If the intervention patient is the benchmark and weighted at 1, then the follow-up patient is weighted at 0.8 ($20/25 \times 1.0$), and the new patient at 2 ($50/25 \times 1.0$). Projecting visits by patient type and applying the appropriate weights will give a more accurate representation of the anticipated workload than projecting the visits alone.

Variable personnel and material resource requirements are based on the projected workload volume. Using historical and current data, it is possible to construct a ratio of resources to volume—personnel hours per unit of work or supplies per unit of work. The personnel hours will include more than the direct care hours because there is indirect time in the form of orientation for new staff, continuing education for current staff, practice or departmental meetings, teaching or precepting, or other organizational activities that are a necessary part of the working year. In addition, the personnel hours must reflect the impact of benefit time because the individual on sick, holiday, or vacation time is not available to attend to the workload. Therefore, the personnel budget should be constructed first on the ratio of direct care hours to workload, that is, projected workload multiplied by the required hours per unit of work. Indirect time is added to this, based either on a specific identification of the hours in the year that will be allocated to these activities or on a current ratio of indirect to direct care hours. For example, if clinicians are currently spending an average of 36 hours per week in direct patient activities and 4 hours per week in other organizational activities, the 11% (4/36) needs to be added to the calculated direct care hours to project the total worked time. In the same way, paid time off must be added, calculated as the number of paid absent days projected, or if there is variability, current paid absent days as a percentage of total worked days.

Variable supplies can also be projected using a ratio of current use to workload and projecting that same ratio into the future. This approach assumes that future use rates will mirror current ones. Changes in procedures, practices, or products could affect this, however, and to the extent that those changes can be quantified, it is possible to adjust the ratio. Current use relevant to the change can be replaced with the anticipated use and the ratio recalculated. Personnel and materials that are not volume driven are projected based on function and analysis of current use. It is important to remember that all fixed resources become variable over the long range, so it is important to look at the overall growth of volume and workload to determine whether the level of fixed resources continues to be sufficient.

When the projections of activity and resources have been completed, they are translated into dollars. The simple definition of total revenue is volume multiplied by price. However, this must be adjusted for the payor and contractual variations previously noted. Personnel expenses are based on the salaries for the positions identified, including the cost of differentials, premiums, and fringe benefits. Nonsalary expenses will incorporate the existing cost for projected materials and supplies adjusted for anticipated price increases and general inflation. The revenues and expenses are totaled for the organization and the profit identified. If there is no profit—if the projected expense exceeds the projected revenue—or if the level of profit is not at the level needed to achieve its fiscal goals, the organization moves into negotiation phase of the budget process. This is the most difficult phase of the process as the organization reviews its objectives and identifies steps to be taken to resolve the issue. If the conceptual plan, goals, and objectives for the budget were well thought out and clearly stated at the outset, and the activity and resources projected and quantified in relation to the plan, the negotiation phase is more likely to produce the budget plan that is most beneficial for the organization and its mission. Individual participants need to speak to the priorities and requirements of specific departments or programs but also evaluate them in relation to the requirements of other areas and of the total organization.

The final stage of budgeting, and the most important one, is implementation with evaluation. The plans developed and refined through the rest of the process—initiatives, practice changes, productivity improvements, and new or expanded programs—now move into the operational life of the organization.

Ongoing analysis identifies the extent to which actual experience matches budget projections. The organization can thus adjust as needed to unanticipated events that may affect overall outcomes. The analysis of actual to projected experience can be either fixed or flexible. Fixed budget analysis compares actual revenue and expense to the calculated budget. Variances may be favorable to budget—better than anticipated (i.e., more revenue or less expense)—or unfavorable to budget—not as good as anticipated (i.e., less revenue or more expense). The limitation of this type of analysis is that it assumes that the budget is static, unaffected by events or activities that differ from budget assumptions related to outputs and inputs. Flexible budget analysis assumes a more dynamic budget, one in which the outputs and inputs can change, but the relationship between the two remains constant. Thus, if a particular level of output drives an identified level of input, changes in the level of output will drive corresponding changes in the level of input.

If six intensive care patients require four nurses to care for them, a 3:2 patient-to-nurse ratio, then nine patients will require six nurses. On a fixed budget analysis, the output—patients served—is favorable to budget because there are more patients served and presumably more revenue than projected. The input, however, is unfavorable to budget because there are more staff and presumably more expense than projected. On a flexible budget analysis, however, the 3:2 ratio of output to input remains constant and the experience mirrors the budget. If the nine patients require only five staff, then the ratio is 3:1.8, and the actual experience is favorable to budget on a flexible budget analysis, even though the output and expense is unfavorable to budget on a fixed analysis.

Clearly, there is a place for both types of analysis in evaluating actual performance against projected. As noted in the previous discussion on cost concepts, although in the long run all costs are variable, in the short run some costs are variable and some are fixed. It is appropriate, therefore, to use a fixed budget analysis to evaluate fixed costs, and a flexible budget analysis to evaluate variable costs.

MANAGING RESOURCES

The objective of financial management is to ensure that the organization generates a profit that is sufficient to maintain viability. The purpose of ongoing budget analysis is to determine the extent to which the organization is meeting its targets over a given period of time or for a particular program or activity and to correct or improve its performance. Prudent management demands that the organization maximize revenue and contain costs to generate profit. Because both revenue and expenses are initially generated primarily by the clinicians who are providing services, it is important that all clinicians, including APNs, understand and appreciate their contribution to the fiscal soundness of the organization. In this context, it is necessary to emphasize that fiscal considerations do not drive the activities of the organization. It is the mission, vision, and goals that determine direction and activities. However, the financial structure provides the framework for these activities and identifies at least one level of constraint and of opportunity. In this respect, it is not unlike managing personal finances. An individual may have a personal objective of obtaining an advanced degree in a particular field. The possibility of achieving that objective will be influenced by the individual's own intelligence, knowledge, experience, and persistence, as well as by the availability and quality of academic programs. It will also be constrained or made possible to the extent that the individual can use current earnings and savings, access scholarships or awards, or incur debt to achieve this goal.

Maximizing Revenue

Revenues are a composite of volume (the number of services provided) and price (income received for each service provided). Effective organizations ensure that they are generating as much income as possible. Fraudulent or deceptive practices such as billing for services not provided or providing unnecessary, expensive services clearly must be avoided. However, ethical strategies for maximizing revenues can be employed and can relate either to volume issues or price issues.

Once an organizational activity passes the breakeven point—that is, the point at which revenue equals expense—any additional volume will generate profit, all else being equal. It is not surprising, therefore, that there is so much emphasis, especially in practices, on how much volume and revenue the individual practitioner generates. In fact, in incentive practices within larger organizations, financial rewards to practitioners are based on volume and productivity. The measurement for identifying the individual practitioner's contribution to the organization most frequently is based on services billed. There is a desire, and in many situations even a demand, to demonstrate that the individual clinician is generating enough revenue to cover salary and to contribute to profit. This has driven the appropriate efforts of nurse practitioners (NPs) to secure billing privileges. (See Chapter 6 for an extensive discussion of reimbursement issues.) However, this direct billing is not available in all settings or through all payors. Even where it is available, it may not be advantageous to the practice for the NP to bill directly. For example, under certain payor regulations or contractual agreements, it may be possible for a particular NP visit to be billed either directly by the NP or indirectly through the physician. If the billing option is legitimate, and the revenue for the indirectly billed visit is greater, then the practice will bill through the physician to maximize their revenue. However, the imperative to demonstrate the NP's contribution to the practice remains. Therefore, it is important to develop other measures of volume and activity that can be used to evaluate the extent to which the NP is generating revenue. These measures will be internal to the organization, but they need to be regularly reported and evaluated in relation to the overall success of the practice. Such measures will be required as well, in other circumstances, in which capitated or managed care payment systems do not accurately reflect through the billing system, the volume of activity generated for the practice by the NP.

In other organizational settings, volume may be measured by charges generated for particular procedures, tests, or services. This often leads clinicians to look for new ways of charging for various activities, assuming that this will maximize revenue, and at the same time, demonstrate their impact on revenue enhancement. With the decline of fee-for-service payment systems, however, increasing charges results in increased revenue potential from only the relatively small percentage of payors who have fee-for-service insurance or are self-pay. Even this potential may not be realized because of exclusions or payment maximums set by the insurer or because of the inability of the self-pay patient to pay all of the expenses for an episode of care. Unless there is significant revenue potential for an isolated activity, the income realized may not offset the cost of implementing and processing the charge.

Rather than focusing on charges, therefore, it is more effective for APNs to address issues with systems or practices that affect the volume of activity that is the basis for payment. Under Medicare's prospective payment system, for example, payment is based on the number of patients discharged within specific DRGs. If the length of stay per discharge can be reduced, then a greater volume of patients can be admitted. What are the systems or practice issues that increase the length of stay, without adding therapeutic value for the patient? What processes could occur before admission or subsequent to discharge that would reduce the length of stay? What services need to be provided that will attract patients to the facility? Consideration of these questions has led to a variety of approaches that ultimately result in increased volume, for example, preadmission testing and evaluation with same-day admission for surgical patients; telephone triage and follow-up or home visit programs for patients with early discharge; clinical pathways, case management, and early discharge planning programs; protocols to prevent or promote early identification and treatment of complications of hospitalization, such as nosocomial infections or decubitus ulcers; or enhancing and expanding specific services such as cardiology or oncology. APNs in the inpatient setting are uniquely positioned to influence the efforts that affect volume. The APNs can identify approaches through study and analysis of existing systems and research on best practices. They can have significant input into the development of programs or protocols as part of the multidisciplinary team. They may support the implementation of changes through clinical evaluation, consultation, and education. Finally, the APNs may be the most appropriate clinicians to manage the particular program or activity.

In addition to adding volume, revenue can be increased by increasing reimbursement rates, the amount that the organization is actually paid for each product or service. However, this deceptively simple strategy is constrained by regulatory, contractual, and economic considerations. Actual reimbursement is determined by government regulation, contract negotiation, or organizational definition. Government regulated reimbursement, such as for Medicare or Medicaid, is not organization specific, and although concerted lobbying efforts may have some impact, the potential for change is limited. Organizations may present evidence that they qualify for certain levels of reimbursement (e.g., for direct medical education benefits) but otherwise will have little opportunity to affect payment levels. Reimbursement rates set through contract negotiations have greater potential for change, but only during the period of open contract negotiations. Because the negotiation outcome needs to be satisfactory to both parties, and because both parties as business organizations are interested in maximizing their profit, rate increases preferred by the one party may need to be tempered to be acceptable to the other party. Charges defined by the organization can easily be increased, but the associated reimbursement rates cannot for many payors, and even with fee-for-service payors, may result in lower rather than increased revenue if the price increases result in a loss of volume to organizations with more competitive prices.

Strategies relating to the impact of price issues on maximizing revenue more successfully address systems to ensure that the organization receives all the revenue to which it is entitled under the existing regulations, contractual obligations, and pricing structure. Payment for services is contingent on the organization's demonstrating that it has in fact provided the relevant service or product. Different payors have varying requirements in the way that claims are processed, the forms that are used, and the specific data that are included. It is important, therefore, to understand what is required, where it needs to be recorded, and how it is presented to the payor.

All payors will require some level of detail on the services provided. This may be in the form of an itemized statement of all billable charges for an episode of care or an itemization of relevant codes. Current procedural terminology (CPT) is a coding system developed by the American Medical Association that identifies procedures and services provided by clinicians. CPT codes are commonly required for billing outpatient, emergency, and perioperative procedures. International classification of diseases, ninth modification (ICD-9) is developed by the World Health Organization and adapted for use in the United States by the federal government. It classifies diseases by system or category (e.g., blood disorders, neoplasms, and infectious diseases) and may be used alone or in conjunction with other classification systems. DRGs and APCs as previously discussed are used for Medicare claims and for selected nongovernmental payors. Certain payors may also require evidence of preauthorization for specific procedures or treatments or referral authorization for specialty evaluation and management. Clinicians in many practices or in ambulatory settings may be more directly involved in identifying the appropriate code for the services rendered and must have a thorough understanding of the coding system and the relationship of codes to services provided. In other settings, coding may not be done by the clinicians, but the codes are determined based on information that the clinicians provide. The source document for information for coding and billing is the patient's medical record. Documentation in the medical record validates to the payor that the billed services were provided and justifies the organization's claim for payment. Inaccurate or incomplete documentation can lead to lost revenue opportunities if the coders are unable to identify all of the services that can appropriately be charged.

Reimbursement is negatively affected by payor denials and delays. Payors may deny reimbursement for services not covered (excluded from reimbursement based on the patient's policy or the contractual agreement with the organization) or for services not authorized (lacking required prior approval from the payor or from a designated clinician). Payment may also be denied for services deemed by the payor to be incompatible with the diagnosis, medically unnecessary, or not adequately validated. Payors who reimburse for hospital care on a per diem basis may carve out days for payment denial, if delays in scheduling tests or consultations or in initiating discharge planning and referrals result in additional, otherwise avoidable inpatient days. Billing challenges by payors may also result in payment denials if supporting documentation does not appear in the medical record that the billed services were in fact rendered. Payors will audit records to validate that billed services have been provided even after payments have been made. If there is not adequate supporting documentation, the organization is at risk not only for repayments, but also for additional financial penalties.

Inadequate documentation can lead to delays in billing, if additional information needs to be accumulated before coding determinations can be made. Lack of compliance with payors' filing requirements may also result in denial of payment. Claims that are questioned initially may be resubmitted with additional evidence of the validity of the claim, but this involves rework and delays. In addition, most payors have a filing limit, a defined period of time in which a "clean" bill is presented for the organization to be reimbursed at all. Delays in processing and submitting bills and generating reimbursement, whether related to incomplete documentation or because of other systems issues, also result in lost opportunities for interest income. Money that the organization has received can earn significant investment interest even in the short term. Money in accounts receivable—that is, income that is anticipated but not yet received—does not generate any additional revenue for the organization.

The APN in a practice setting that bills directly or indirectly for the practitioner's clinical activity needs a clear understanding of the requirements and systems for billing—what can be billed, how it is processed, what documentation is required, and time frames for billing. By following through on these requirements, the APN is able to contribute directly to the timely and accurate generation of income. In other settings, the APN with an understanding of the systems for reimbursement to the organization contributes indirectly by providing and promoting accurate and complete clinical documentation, identifying systems issues that can generate delays in the billing cycle, and supporting practices that enhance the potential for maximizing revenue.

Containing Costs

The volume of products or services produced drives the total expenses of an organization. These costs are a function both of intensity, which is the extent of resources required for each unit of volume, and of price, which is the cost to the organization of individual resource units. Cost containment focuses on identifying the least costly alternatives for supplying the personnel and materials to produce these services or products. In addressing cost containment, the organization evaluates the alternatives not only in terms of total expenditures but also in relation to potential impact on other aspects of the organization. It is less costly to pay lower salaries, but if salaries are not competitive in the market then costly vacancies and turnover are likely to result. Inferior products that are less costly to purchase may generate additional expense in replacement, rework, decreased customer satisfaction, and loss of business. The desired alternative, therefore, is the least costly alternative that is consistent with the mission and goals of the organization.

Wage and salary expenses constitute a significant proportion of the costs in health-care organizations. Market forces, regulatory requirements, and ethical personnel management practices provide a framework for personnel expenditures. Within this framework, however, the organization has flexibility in controlling expenses related both to intensity and price of personnel resources used. Intensity addresses the number of personnel or staff hours required to manage a given patient population. The volume and type of patients and their particular care needs—the workload generated by that patient population—drive the personnel resources required. Measuring and managing workload variability can provide opportunities for cost containment. For example, scheduling staff in consideration of daily, weekly, or seasonal volume variations can minimize expensive "down time" as well as the staff frustration resulting from inadequate staffing at busy times. This requires an ongoing analysis of workload patterns and trends to identify recurring variations. Unexpected variations may be addressed with the use of overtime or outside agency personnel. Both of these alternatives are more expensive than the normal personnel costs for the workload involved, but they are justifiable for unpredictable workload variations. A consistent increase in activity, however, requires a consistent plan for managing the workload. If a practice is increasingly seeing patients later than the usual scheduled hours and incurring overtime and other increased costs as a result, it is worthwhile to analyze the cause of the variation. System inefficiencies may be delaying patient throughput, and thus generating additional unnecessary expenses that can be eliminated by addressing the inefficiencies. Patterns of patient scheduling may be changing, resulting in fewer visits scheduled earlier in the day with more down time, suggesting that scheduled staff hours need to be adjusted to accommodate patient preferences. However, the variation may be the result of a net increase in numbers of patients and visits. If this is so, then an analysis of the fiscal impact of the increased revenue and increased expense may demonstrate that adding regular staff to cover the increased activity will be more cost effective than continuing to use overtime.

Intensity of personnel resource use may also be related to inefficient clinical practices. Routines, procedures, and protocols that are based on tradition ("we've always done it this way") rather than on analysis or research-based evidence may include unnecessary and time-consuming activities that do not add value for desired outcomes. How are medication administration times determined? What are the indicators that determine the level of support for activities of daily living that each patient requires? How frequently is it necessary to monitor vital signs on postoperative patients? In what circumstances are isolation precautions instituted and under what circumstances can they be discontinued? How effective are the standard protocols for preparation for tests? Do the standard patient teaching tools and programs result in patient learning? Does the timing of drawing blood for laboratory tests make sense in relation to the timing of meals or medication administration or other treatments? It may be instructive to evaluate the care that patients with the same condition receive from different caregivers or in different settings to determine whether differences in practices result in differences in outcomes. In some circumstances it may become evident that practices in one setting are more resource intensive but do not add value and can be adapted or eliminated.

For personnel resources, price is generally equated with the cost of salaries and benefits. Containing costs by reducing salaries or benefits is not often possible given market conditions and the mobility of today's work force. It is possible, however, to ensure that the least costly resources are used in any given situation. Overtime, for example is an expensive way to staff. It can be used effectively for the occasional unanticipated increase in workload, but extensive, continuous use of overtime requires identification of causes and alternative approaches, as noted in the preceding example of a practice experiencing consistent overtime. In addition to volume increases, variability in workload practices, or system inefficiencies, overtime may be related to the capabilities of the staff involved. For example, inexperienced staff may need assistance with particular patient issues or with development of organizational skills, or experienced staff may be struggling with unfamiliar procedures or patient conditions. For these staff, education and mentoring can promote developing competencies that also increase efficiency and ultimately reduce the overtime. The mix of staff may not be appropriate or the total numbers of staff may not be sufficient for the workload experienced. In these circumstances, it can be less costly to provide more skilled staff or more total staff at regular salaries than to continue with overtime.

One approach addresses the mix of personnel and the perceived advantages of reducing the numbers of professional staff and substituting less expensive unlicensed assistive personnel (UAPs). In some circumstances, this may be effective, but given the increasing acuity of patients, such substitution may be counterproductive. In acute care settings, for example, patients are requiring more and more complex care, most of which cannot be delegated to unlicensed staff. In addition, unlicensed staff increases the workload of the professional staff because they assume the added responsibility of directing and supervising the UAPs. For direct care, it may be less costly to have a higher percentage of licensed staff and fewer total numbers than to have a lower percentage of licensed staff and greater total numbers. However, if the professional staff are responsible for clerical or environmental tasks that can appropriately be delegated to less costly personnel, providing those supports can be an effective cost management approach.

Cost containment efforts can also address some of the hidden costs in personnel management. Turnover generates significant costs in recruiting, hiring, and orienting new personnel. Additional costs may be incurred before the new employee is available if vacancies need to be covered with overtime or more expensive outside agency personnel. Programs to promote staff retention can therefore be valuable in reducing turnover and its associated costs. Absenteeism can also be costly. Some level of unanticipated absenteeism due to illness is anticipated. However, staff dissatisfaction, unmanageable workloads, frequent excessive overtime requirements, or on-the-job injuries can also contribute to high levels of absenteeism. The cost is increased by the need for replacements, again often with overtime or agency personnel. In addition, costs to the organization for worker's compensation are directly related to the number of claims filed out of the organization. Cost can be lowered—and potentially, staff satisfaction and efficiency increased—by identifying and addressing the factors contributing to absenteeism and on-the-job injuries.

Like wages and salaries, the costs for supplies and equipment are affected by market issues and regulatory requirements, as well as by the volume and type of services provided. Intensity in this context refers to the number and kind of materials used for these services. Cost containment looks at the least costly alternative to providing the services. This can be addressed on two levels. What are the specific supplies and equipment required for a particular procedure, protocol, or service? Additionally, given that a specific item is required, which is the best product to select among the alternatives available? In relation to the first question, it is important to look at the work and how it is accomplished. Materials assumed to be necessary for the service provided may incorporate items that are no longer necessary, do not add value, or are useful only to a subset of the patients receiving the service.

With the materials necessary for a service identified, the focus moves to selection of specific items among those available. Product evaluation requires the involvement of clinicians and others in the organization. Inherent in the identification of an item as necessary for a particular service is the description of its purpose and how it is to be used. The primary concern in product evaluation is how well the different products under review meet these criteria. Other criteria also need to be considered, such as availability from the manufacturer and storage and maintenance requirements. A product that meets all clinical criteria, but cannot be produced and delivered on a timely basis, or has high maintenance (and associated down time) potential, may not be preferable to a less exotic but more available and reliable product.

Prices for materials and supplies are negotiated with vendors. Organizations may identify cost containment opportunities in the course of these negotiations through volume discounts or as part of purchasing groups. This raises the issue of managing the tension between standardization and customization. Frequently, standardizing supplies and equipment across service areas has significant benefits in reducing the expense for purchasing, storing, distributing, and using specific products. Although this limits the range of products available to the clinician, it also limits the time needed to become familiar with the product, to develop ease in working with it, and to use it in a variety of settings. It may, however, generate some level of waste if, for example, a standardized pack of supplies for a particular procedure contains items that are used in most but not all situations. Customization, on the other hand, matches the products specifically to the individual patient, clinician, or situation. It can have advantages in being more effective in achieving the desired outcome or in reducing the potential for waste. However, customization sometimes is more a matter of individual clinicians' preferences than of value added for the patient. It is important then to evaluate the pros and cons of standardization or customization in specific circumstances to identify the least costly alternative. In general, for products and processes that are used in a variety of settings, standardization is preferable not only because of the cost and productivity benefits but also because it promotes consistency in providing services. Alternatives to standardization should be undertaken only after careful evaluation to ensure that the marginal benefit of customization—that is, the greater value that accrues from the alternative—outweighs the fiscal and operational benefits of standardization.

As the previous discussions suggest, the appropriateness of measures to contain costs cannot be evaluated in isolation from outcomes. Cost efficiency identifies the minimum expenditure necessary to achieve an outcome. Cost effectiveness identifies the minimum expenditure necessary to achieve the outcome that is consistent with the organization's mission and goals. Cost effectiveness, therefore, incorporates an element of quality that is not inherent in cost efficiency. Vacuum-assisted dressing for postsurgical wound healing is significantly more expensive than traditional dressings and would not be considered cost efficient in a simple analysis that addressed only the expense incurred for dressings until wound healing is achieved. However, because it accelerates wound healing, this intervention reduces the necessary length of hospitalization and extent of postsurgical follow-up. As such, it is certainly cost effective, with benefits for both the patient and the provider organization. In some circumstances quality measures are not sufficiently developed to allow precise measurement of cost effectiveness, but to the extent that such measures are available or can be approximated, they should be incorporated into analysis.

Cost effectiveness and efficiency are typically analyzed using productivity measures or cost-benefit analysis. Productivity is the relationship of inputs and outputs, of resources used, and products or services produced. Productivity relationships are expressed as ratios and can focus either on the output or on the input. Focus on the output addresses the question, "what does it take to produce the output?" and is the ratio of input to output or resources divided by products or services. Examples of productivity measures focusing on output include hours per patient day, cost per procedure, and visits per episode of care. Focus on input addresses the question, "how well are resources being used?" and is the ratio of output to input or products or services divided by resources. Examples of productivity measures focusing on input include visits per full-time equivalent worker (FTE), tests per staff hour, and case hours per available room hour. Productivity improves when output remains constant and input decreases or when output increases and input stays constant. Productivity declines when output remains constant and input increases or when output decreases and input stays constant. Productivity ratios are of little value in isolation. Comparisons of productivity ratios to targets set during the budgeting process, to historical experience and trends, and to other internal or external benchmarks are valuable for analysis and identification of opportunities for increasing efficiency and effectiveness.

Cost-benefit analysis is frequently used to evaluate a particular program or project or to compare programs, approaches, or activities competing for resource allocation. The analysis compares the revenues and expenses generated by the program to determine the net benefit (income minus expense) or the ratio of benefits to costs (income divided by expense). Determination of the value of the program to the organization, however, is not determined exclusively by analysis of the financial benefit. Benefits and costs that are difficult to quantify, such as social benefits and costs, opportunity costs, public relations value, and loss leader opportunities, may be of considerable importance to the organization, and influence decisions to implement or continue specific projects and programs.

Productivity is often focused on personnel resource use, but the concept also applies to material resources and to the overall use of services. Length of stay or number of days per inpatient stay, for example, can be considered to be a productivity measurement that identifies the relationship between the episode of care (output) and the patient days, representing the aggregated resources required to provide for that episode (input). Comparisons are made among patients or groups of patients for a given time period or across multiple time periods and against internal and external benchmarks. Productivity improves if the length of stay (and associated expense) decreases for the same level of activity.

Cost-benefit analysis can identify the impact of productivity improvements for the organization. Baseline analysis of the net benefit (revenue minus expense) identifies the profit margin. Productivity improvements are designed to increase the profit margin by reducing the cost (but maintaining consistent income) for each episode of care. Moreover, decreasing length of stay has the added opportunity of creating capacity for additional volume. That volume will generate additional income and additional expense. Assuming a consistent patient population, if the cost per episode of care remains the same, the total profit (income minus expense) will increase although the profit per case remains the same. However, the cost per episode of care may well decrease (as fixed costs are spread over more cases) and enhance both the total profit and the profit per case. Cost-benefit analysis can also identify potential negative aspects of productivity improvement efforts. Length of stay reductions must be consistent with good clinical practice. Early discharge of patients may be clinically premature and result in readmission of the patient for continuation of care. Obviously, for the patient this is an undesirable outcome, and therefore could not be considered cost effective. It cannot even be considered cost efficient because many payors, particularly those who reimburse on a cost per case, identify a time period after discharge during which a readmission (for a condition related to the original hospital stay) will be bridged to the original admission. Additional expense will be incurred, but the merged admissions will be considered as one episode for the purposes of reimbursement, and additional payment will be denied.

Implications

Reimbursement levels and the associated incentives to contain costs are to a large extent payor driven. Reimbursement systems structured as fee-for-service include little incentive for the provider organization to contain costs. Because reimbursement is generated by charges that are paid either in full or at some negotiated percentage, increased use results in increased revenue, so long as costs do not exceed the level of reimbursement. The majority of payors, however, have built into their reimbursement systems some incentives for containing costs. Reimbursement at the per diem or per visit rate is an incentive to reduce resource use and increase efficiency for that day or visit. Reimbursements based on cases (e.g., DRG based) build in incentives to reduce the length of stay and the resource use during the stay. Capitated reimbursement systems create the additional incentive to reduce the number of episodes of care—admissions or visits. Individual payor variations on the systems add complexity for providers and consumers. Some, for example, may offer additional payments for achieving specific clinical quality outcomes with defined patient populations such as pediatric asthma patients or patients with adult-onset diabetes. Others may have payment tiers for certain benefits, with different consumer copays for different levels of services (e.g., generic versus brand pharmaceuticals).

Clinicians, however, generally are not attuned to incorporating reimbursement variables into clinical decision making for individual patients and prefer to provide care that is "payor-blind." They do have a responsibility, however, to promote efficiency in the allocation and use of health-care resources and not only for the viability of the organization within which they practice. As health-care costs escalate, insured patients increasingly are at risk for higher out-of-pocket costs, including deductibles into the thousands instead of the hundreds of dollars before the insurer assumes liability, and they are entitled to value for their expenditure. In addition, social justice demands that constrained resources be used judiciously to ensure the maximum availability of health care to all members of society. The most appropriate approach for clinicians, therefore, is to provide cost-efficient and effective care for all patients, regardless of payor.

Fortunately, in many circumstances, cost containment efforts developed to accommodate a given payment modality can be designed to benefit—or at least not disadvantage—patients of other payors as well. Programs to reduce length of stay, efforts to improve productivity, analyses to identify most cost-effective products, and benchmarking to identify best practices may be initiated because of the structure of one payment methodology, but their beneficial effects need not be limited to patients of that insurer type. However, because resources are not unlimited, in different circumstances difficult choices need to be made. Organizations rarely can respond to all requests for resources and often are in the position of needing to select among competing priorities that may all be necessary and worthwhile. Should the organization expand the cardiac program or the pediatric program? Upgrade the provider order entry system or the patient registration system or the payroll system? Authorize additional FTEs for nurses or dietitians or secretaries or translators? Purchase software programs for patient teaching or for staff education? Replace the ventilators in the critical care units or the ultrasounds in the echo lab? Add intravenous pumps or wheelchairs or computers or employee lockers? Renovate existing space for a conference room or an office or a family waiting room? Construct additional ambulatory facilities or additional inpatient facilities? The decisions will require compromise and consensus and a clear understanding of the benefits not only for the organization but also for the staff, and most importantly, for the patient. Therefore, fiscal decisions that have significant clinical implications, as well as clinical decisions that have significant fiscal implications, need to be made at the organizational level and represent both the clinical and fiscal issues. APNs have the knowledge and expertise to provide the clinical input and advocate for the patient. To have a credible voice in this decision-making process, they must also have a clear understanding of the business and fiscal issues that affect resource allocation and management.

Mediated Roles: Working Through Other People

12

Thomas D. Smith

Maria L. Vezina

Mary E. Samost

ADVANCED PRACTICE AND PARTNERSHIPS

The four established advanced practice roles, specifically nurse practitioners (NPs), clinical nurse specialist (CNS), certified nurse-midwife (CNM), and certified registered nurse anesthetist (CRNA), reflect significant professional and educational development.[1] According to Nursing's Social Policy Statement (American Nurses Association [ANA], 2003), these roles include specialization, expansion, advancement, and autonomy, suggesting the necessary skills of managing people, the organization, and the environment of care. For example, the CNS (advanced practice nurse [APN]) role centers on the synthesis, integration, transformation, and translation of best practices as articulated in the literature (National Association of Clinical Nurse Specialist [NACNS], 2007). Davies and Hughes (1995) note "The term advanced nursing practice extends beyond roles. It is a way of thinking and viewing the world based on clinical knowledge, rather than a composition of roles" (p. 157). This view of the world is an interactive process that emphasizes direct and indirect partnerships with both patients and a diverse group of health-care providers. In addition to clinical competency, the varied aspects of advanced practice also require socialization skills to form the foundation for collaboration, consultation, and clinical leadership. Although advanced practice roles require autonomy and authority to be fully enacted, the ability to achieve patient and system outcomes is dependent on partnerships with others to manage interdependent and interdisciplinary relationships. National Association of Clinical Nurse Specialist (NACNS) (2007) remarked "the synergy of working with and leading/coordinating teams of professionals in a highly communicative, focused care environment regardless of setting will continue to be the hallmark of practice into the future" (p. 8).

CORE COMPETENCIES

APNs function as providers using evidence-based knowledge to minister direct care, diagnose and manage health-care problems, coordinate services, educate patients and families, advocate for patients, and manage the health-care system in all its dimensions. This care approach supports the

[1]The authors wish to acknowledge the following APNs who contributed to the exemplars in Boxes 1 through 5: Arlene Butler MS, ANP, GNP; Kathleen Capitulo DNSc, RN, FACCE; Lisa DesJardins MS, FNP; Susan Frost MS, CRNA; Patricia Tang Leung MS, ANP, GNP; Cynthia McKie-Addy MS, RN; Susan Nevins MA, ACNP, CNRN, CCRN; Christine Obremski MS, CNM; Eileen O'Connor MS, FNP; Janet Van Cleave MS, ACNP; and Li-Chen Wann MS, ANP.

continued focus on prevention of disease, maintenance of function, and resolution of functional problems (Institute of Medicine [IOM], 2004).

Accordingly, six core competencies further define advanced nursing practice **(Fig. 12-1)**. These competencies have repeatedly been identified as essential features of advanced practice (American Association of College of Nursing, 1996; ANA, 2003; Davies & Hughes, 1995; NACNS, 2004; National Council of State Boards of Nursing, 2006). These core competencies include:

1. Expert guidance and coaching of patients, families, and other care providers
2. Consultation
3. Research skills, including use, evaluation, and conduct
3. Clinical and professional leadership, which includes competence as a change agent
5. Collaboration
6. Ethical decision-making skills

Given this overview of core competencies, the theme of relationships within the health-care arena is evident. The ability to work with and through others is inherent within these competencies and consequently indicates a strong foundation for practice. Although not explicitly stated in definitions of advanced practice, there is a growing understanding that APNs must be skillful and cognizant of the key elements of their partnerships with patients and other health team members. Managing the interpersonal strategies of providing care is critical to success as an independent care provider in a competitive health-care marketplace. The traditional care provided by APNs was in the complex, acute setting; care is now moving into the community and is increasing the need for the APN to

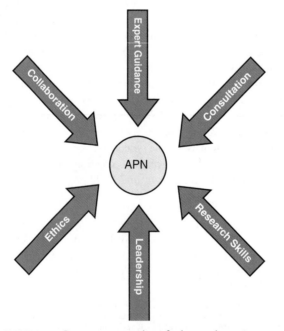

FIGURE 12-1 Core competencies of advanced nursing practice.

assess his or her strengths to provide accountable practice while working successfully with other people. According to the Institute of Medicine (IOM, 2004), the opportunities presented by the current practice environment can be met through a strong foundation of clinical practice, specialty expertise, and a rigorous graduate education.

With reference to the six core competencies, several interpersonal themes emerge. For example:

1. Expert guidance and coaching of patients, families, and other care providers reflect a mentor role, with expectations of others to either take the lead or share the pathway of care.

2. Consultation is the direct involvement of another practitioner, which denotes the need to confirm findings, diagnosis, or plan of care. The responsibility for care, however, rests with the primary practitioner. It can require an overlap within the same specialty for an added opinion or a discussion with a specialist for another view or preference of treatment. In either situation, the partnership is necessary for optimal patient care and a deliberate approach in the management of practice.

3. Research skills, including use, evaluation, and conduct, support the professional obligation to improve practice, often involving APNs with other practitioners to evaluate methods of delivering care. Innovative change is possible when health-care professionals come together to redesign clinical practices. Efforts such as interdisciplinary education, research, and evaluation initiatives can have a potent effect on optimizing the system of health care.

4. Clinical and professional leadership can be powerful when approached in an interdisciplinary manner. Although the unique roles of distinct professions are useful within the framework of individual competencies, in patient care, the leadership of a team can be a supportive experience for patients, especially for those with limited access to a health system. A focus on the specific patient and not on professional turf conflicts requires skill in leadership and change agency. In this realm, the blurring of roles is often helpful and not hurtful.

5. Collaboration means to "work together, especially in a joint intellectual effort." The American Nurses Association (ANA, 2003) Nursing's Social Policy Statement cites qualities such as a common focus, a recognition of another's expertise, and a collegial exchange of ideas and knowledge. Hamric, Spross, and Hanson (2005) refer to collaboration as a "dynamic, interpersonal process in which two or more individuals make a commitment to each other to interact authentically and constructively to solve problems and to learn from each other in order to accomplish identified goals, purposes or outcomes" (p. 318). By definition, then, collaboration identifies relationships and while involving an interpersonal process, it cannot be ordered or required. The focus of the relationship needs to be positive and grounded in a problem-solving approach, creating interdependence as a mutually saisfying experience between the involved parties. Although collaboration is a cornerstone of many APN roles, it eludes some clinicians. Consequently, models of collaboration have emerged to assist in structuring relationships and guiding the process of working partnerships.

6. Ethical decision-makings skills are a central component of effective advanced practice. "To be professional is to be ethical, and to practice ethically requires an understanding of ethics, values and oneself" (Thompson & Thompson, 1985). The goal of ethical practice is to do the right thing for the right reason (Thompson, Kershbaumer, & Krisman-Scott, 2001). Although grounded in one's values and presentation of self, the inclusion of the team in ethical decision making is key to the holistic care of patients. Ethical clinical practice requires an atmosphere of trust, mutual respect, and commitment to critical thinking and reasoning.

To create this atmosphere, APNs, as the managers of care, need to work with others in an inclusive manner, so as to build a team whereby the ability to express values, feelings, beliefs, and knowledge can be encouraged and ensured as the ethical dimension of practice emerges.

MODELS OF COLLABORATION

The basis of collaboration is the belief that quality patient care is achieved by including the contributions of all care providers. Collaboration is often cited as the "key to success" for any initiative that extends beyond an individual's scope of activity. Collaboration is therefore the foundation of effective patient care. True collaborative practice has no hierarchy. The contribution of each participant is based on the knowledge or expertise brought to the situation rather than a traditional employer/employee relationship (Kraus, 1980). According to Arcongelo, Fitzgerald, Carroll, and Plumb (1996), there are a variety of interpersonal attributes that are necessary for successful collaboration. These include trust, knowledge, shared responsibility, mutual respect, positive communication, cooperation, coordination, and optimism (p. 107) **(Fig. 12-2)**. The authors define these attributes as follows:

- *Trust* among all parties establishes a quality working relationship; it develops over time as the parties become more acquainted.
- *Knowledge* is a necessary component for the development of trust. Knowledge and trust remove the need for supervision.
- *Shared responsibility* suggests joint decision making for patient care and outcomes, as well as practice issues, within the organization.
- *Mutual respect* for the expertise of all members of the team is the norm. This respect is communicated to the patient.
- *Communication* that is not hierarchical but rather two way ensures the sharing of patient information and knowledge. Questioning of the approach to care of either partner cannot be delivered in a manner that is construed as criticism, but as a method to enhance knowledge and improve patient care.

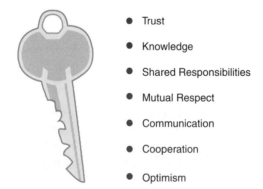

Collaboration Is the Key to Success

- Trust
- Knowledge
- Shared Responsibilities
- Mutual Respect
- Communication
- Cooperation
- Optimism

FIGURE 12-2 Collaboration attributes.

- *Cooperation* and *coordination* promote the use of the skills of all team members, prevent duplication, and enhance productivity of practice.
- *Optimism* promotes success when the involved parties believe that collaboration is the more effective means of promoting quality care.

Although these attributes are key in any collaborative relationship, it is primarily the unique contribution of each member of the team that determines a successful outcome.

Although there are several models of collaborative practice, they often are distinguished by two factors:

1. How is the expertise of each member of the team used to the fullest?
2. Who is responsible for decision making and patient care?

Strumpf and Whitney (1994) describes three practice models commonly used in primary care:

1. the parallel model
2. the sequential model
3. the shared model

In the parallel model, a NP (or APN) manages stable patients, and the physician cares for those who are more medically complex. In the sequential model, the NP performs the intake assessment and the physician assumes responsibility for differential diagnosis and management, or the pattern may be reversed, with the physician screening all patients and delegating the care of patients identified as less complex to the NP (APN). In the shared model, the NP and the physician care for an individual patient on an alternating schedule **(Table 12-1)**.

Arcongelo et al. (1996) identify a fourth model, the collaborative model, which involves the NP as the primary care provider without regard for the complexity of the problem. The NP collaborates as needed to provide safe, high-quality care but practices autonomously and independently. The communication in this model is ongoing, may transition to a comanagement arrangement during an unstable or complex period, but always involves the input of the two professionals in establishing the plan of care. One outcome of this style is the ability for the APN to expand his or her knowledge and skills within the complex realm of patient care and establish closer contacts with consulting team members while managing the complexity.

TABLE 12-1			
Model of Collaborative Practice			
	Parallel Model	**Sequential Model**	**Shared Model**
Advanced practice nurse role in patient care	Manage stable patients	Perform intake assessment	Manage patients who are determined by the physician to be less complex
Physician role in patient care	Manage medically complex patients	Diagnose and manage patients	Perform initial screening of patients Manage more complex patients

Regardless of the model of collaborative practice, the elements of trust and a positive working relationship are vital. Collaborative relationships are a "work in progress," not facilitated by inflexible expectations or boundaries. Over time, mutual expressions of expertise become grounded in an invisible pattern that is the glue of the successful relationship, reflective of growing skill, trust, and confidence among partners.

The advantages of collaboration often begin with negotiation by the involved roles regarding which patients and conditions are best managed by the APN or the physician. This process may seem to be a hurdle to competent and successful APNs, but armed with data, performance indicators (both financial and clinical), and the maturation of one's practice, the process of collaborative decision making promotes effectiveness of care. For example, in the management of chronic illness, NPs tend to prescribe fewer drugs, order fewer tests, choose less expensive treatments, and spend more time with patients (Fitzgerald, Jones, Lazar, McHugh, & Wang, 1995). According to hospital salary surveys, the cost of a NP is often 50% of the physician's or less. Subsequently, an effective collaborative NP/physician practice would enable physicians to spend more time with patients with more complex health needs while NPs focus on the care of more stable patients.

In all health-care settings, it is becoming an increasing challenge to provide the ongoing surveillance and case management that can support the sick patients to function at their highest level possible. Naylor et al. (1994) found in a study of elders that APNs were able to reduce posthospital complications and readmissions. The management of acute illness of established patients has also demonstrated a minimization of complications and cost while maximizing the quality of life for patients. Physicians are then available to deal with those situations that require the clinical decision making and intervention of the doctor. It is becoming increasingly apparent that future trends in health care will require greater collaboration and role recognition among all health-care providers as a strategy to relate effectively to all patients.

Barriers to collaboration can be rooted to the many traditions of the "Doctor-Nurse Game," which range from sex-role stereotypes to incongruent expectations of knowledge and skill acquisition. Intertwined within these concepts are those related to cultural, social, psychological, and financial complexities of the health-care system. Nonetheless, when patient-focused approaches to health care are endorsed, the critical aspects of collaborative relationships, skills, and practices are uncovered. The opportunities that patient-focused approaches fully engage among various health-care disciplines become self-evident over time. In other words, the dimensions of the physician-nurse relationship are fundamentally tied to the quality of patient care (Brandt, 2001). This observation alone provides the health-care system and clinicians with primary motivation to encourage effective relationships between professionals to identify opportunities for working through and with one other.

CLINCIAL RELATIONSHIPS

The nature of advanced practice is such that the most patient care can be managed because of the skill and knowledge of the practitioner within the role. However, each practitioner acknowledges the critical significance of consultation and referral when used in a timely and effective manner. Imbedded in these partnerships are the issues of relationships within the health-care team, communication styles, trust, and the ability to interact within these clinical relationships without a hierarchical framework. Although many APNs have formal consultative relationships within their scope of practice, others do not. In addition, these formal structures vary among states and health-care institutions, with a range of directives from state boards, often from different disciplines. Legislation and statute aside, the ability to work within a model of consultation and referral is necessary. Each member of the health-care team has knowledge and skill to offer the other and a partnership can often effect changes in practice and influence patient care outcomes that would not be possible if managed alone. Many consultative practices are also influenced by the environment whereby specialty and primary care is clearly differentiated. In these situations, consultative relationships are vital to care processes.

Often, consultation and referral activities are confused with supervision, comanagement (the working together to manage a complex case), and direct oversight. In these situations, the accountability for practice may become lost, and roles are blurred. The limits of one's practice expertise or the need to receive advice should be viewed as complementary, not as a deficiency or "take over" approach. The professional interactions inherent in consultation and referral expand the APN's ability to work with and through others, while maintaining autonomy over the situation until there is a mutually identified decision that a change in care is necessary. Although comanagement and referral (the relinquishing of care temporarily or permanently) may have different themes, the goal of care is still accomplished within a partnership mode. Hamric, Spross, and Hanson (2005) state that APNs themselves are often confused about the differences. They refer to a more thoughtful definition of collaboration described as "a dynamic, interpersonal process in which two or more individuals make a commitment to each other to interact authentically and constructively to solve problems and to learn from each other in order to accomplish identified goals, purposes, or outcomes. The individuals recognize and articulate the shared values that make this commitment possible" (p. 318). Within this framework of collaboration, the varying processes of consultation, referral, or comanagement may assume the added dimension of a therapeutic, professional relationship acknowledging the role each member plays while supporting the complexities inherent in the delivery of quality patient care. Although knowledge, skill, and clinical expertise are all key factors in day-to-day practice, the elements of working with each other in this collaborative manner will determine and distinguish the best practices.

INTERDISCIPLINARY TEAMING

The importance of integrated health-care teams is fueled by a number of factors, including the increasing complexity of patient needs, especially among the growing population of elders; expansion in the continuum of care in various health-care delivery models; the sophistication of telecommunications and information networks; and changes in methods of health-care financing. It is also evident that members of the health-care team—physicians, APNs, registered nurses (RNs), social workers, and other clinicians—often practice independently of one another, rendering care as if services for the same patient or groups of patients were unrelated. This multidisciplinary approach to care has been compared to the parallel play of children—noninteractive and nonintersecting activity (Clark, 1994) **(Fig. 12-3)**.

In an effort to improve on this approach, interdisciplinary teaming was proposed as an alternative model of care (Pfeiffer, 1998). Interdisciplinary teaming requires that the members of the health-care team integrate their discipline's work and create plans of care together, centering this plan on the patients' needs. This form of teamwork, interdisciplinary care, has been defined as a "special form of interactional interdependence between health care providers who merge different but complementary skills in the service of patients and in the solution of their health problems" (Tsukuda, 1990, p. 670) **(Fig. 12-4)**. The term *complementary* defines the team approach. However, a collection of like-minded individuals does not result in an interdisciplinary team. Because of the nature of

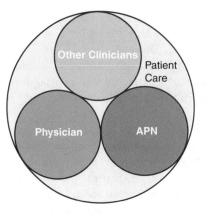

FIGURE 12-3 Multidisciplinary approach to patient care: noninteractive and nonintersecting activity.

this teaming, there must be a clearly defined purpose, goal, and approaches to team activity, as well as the value and understanding that mutual accountability of each team member is crucial to the team's overall performance. The primary purpose of this type of team is collaborative decision making for patients. Decision making, in this model, occurs in a unified timeline. Often, in a multidisciplinary team approach, a sequential timeline is experienced as a dependent process in which the final decision is made by the "lead" member who pulls everything together. This type of decision making is limited, and potentially ineffective, when complementary activity is desired.

For the APN, the influence of interdisciplinary teams is powerful. Creative teamwork can be achieved between at least two disciplines or expanded to include additional disciplines as well. Changing the norms of practice, however, may be necessary. Interdisciplinary teams are the epitome of working with and through others, while recognizing the importance of an individual's clinical expertise.

There are a number of dimensions to consider when implementing interdisciplinary team relationships. According to Howe, Cassel, and Vezina (1998), these dimensions include:

Skills
■ Conflict resolution
■ Team interaction
■ Communication
■ Leadership

Attitudes
■ Respect for other disciplines
■ Respect for patient and family input
■ Respect for patient management and patient-focused care
■ Awareness of outcome-based practice

Knowledge
■ Roles, responsibilities, and scope of practice for each discipline
■ Role of the extended team

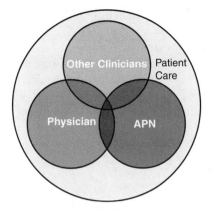

FIGURE 12-4 Interdisciplinary approach to patient care: health-care providers integrate their work, focusing on their patients' needs.

- Group dynamics
- Application of clinical concepts among disciplines
- Up-to-date knowledge of the health-care environment

Inherent within this interdisciplinary framework, collaboration underpins the field of day-to-day practice within a team concept. According to Tsukuda and Stahelski (1990), collaboration takes on the dimension of cooperation with others, adding trust as an essential component of this interactional style, because patient outcomes are consistently dependent on the efforts of others. As a team member, one may ask:

- Are my own goals consistent with team goals?
- Do I advocate solutions for problems that will benefit all team members?
- Do I work for consensus?
- Do I cooperate with other team member's activities?
- Do I do an equitable share of the group workload?
- Do I feel individual responsibility for the joint outcomes of the group members?
- Do I support the team in dealing with larger organizational issues?
- Do I view my contributions as belonging to the group—to be used or not—as the group decides?
- Do I listen to team members in a positive and respectful manner?
- Do I actively participate in team meetings and assignments?

Advocates of interdisciplinary team approaches to care realize that there are many psychosocial influences on health and disease. This underscores the importance of relationship-centered care (Tresolini & the Pew-Fetzer Task Force, 1994) and patient-centered care (Coles, 1995), which are based on interpersonal communication techniques and a collaborative care model. A paradigm shift for all members of the health-care team may be necessary because new core competencies are required and need to be role modeled for the successful transition to occur. APNs are often members of these teams and are positioned to initiate the transition to a more collaborative and patient-focused approach in their practice. APNs often assume a mediated role to introduce these changes in the delivery of patient care and to assist the team in its growth and development in the core competencies of interdisciplinary team approaches.

APNs may take a leadership role in influencing stages of team development. Their role is easily linked to the various members of the health-care team, allowing APNs the advantage of connecting with each discipline, clearly expressing the similarities and the differences of each member's role and contribution. With this common ground set, the formation and development of a team can occur.

According to Tuckman (1965), four stages of team development are discussed:

- Forming
- Storming
- Norming
- Performing

As implied by the stages, the creation and maintenance of teams is personnel intensive, with professional adjustments required by every member of the team. Roles and relationships may be challenged, but they may also move to a new level whereby extraordinary achievements can occur. In this context, interdisciplinary teaming with its strong emphasis on relationship-centered care may be a "best practice" for the 21st century.

PROFESSIONAL NURSING CONNECTIONS

Expanded roles for nurses span a century of growth and development, with the earliest days of clinical specialization in anesthesia, operating room, and obstetrical nursing. However, the knowledge and skills required in a basic nursing education lay the foundation for the advanced practice platform. Common ground skills and competencies include patient assessment, health promotion and maintenance, health education, advocacy, caring, accountability, continuity, and collaboration with other health team members. This overlap and sharing of skills create a bond of practice between RNs and APNs—forming professional nursing connections. How do these two groups move together in partnership? Hopefully, they join together with respect for the value of each role, intending to effectively use the expertise of each professional, while avoiding duplication of effort and promoting true collaborative relationships. Such connections can broaden the scope of health care and achieve professional satisfaction for both RNs and APNs.

Regardless of the common ground, however, each advanced practice specialty has dealt with resistance from other nurses because advanced roles have often represented innovations in practice that shook the status quo of the nursing establishment and the overall health-care system (Bigbee & Amidi-Nouri, 2000). Rigid boundaries were often created and the struggle for recognition and acceptance followed. However, through organized and focused educational and political efforts, tensions were lessened and improved relationships flourished.

The roles of the RN and the APN sometimes clash within the context of leadership for the delivery of patient care. Once an understanding of expertise and specialization is clearly reached and communicated, the contribution of each role can be qualified, recognized, and a complementary approach to health care defined. Evaluative research can also assist in this recognition and educational process—providing data to understand the effect of advanced practice nursing care on quality patient outcomes. Together, professional connections between the RN and APN can be fortified and not diluted by professional conflict.

The common ground between RNs and APNs create a powerful force in health-care delivery. The professional bonding that exists between both groups can reinforce the image of the RN as caregiver and the APN as the leader of care. By practicing together, the RN-APN team can design approaches to care that recognize each other's strengths and expertise respectively—resulting in a dynamic practice arena free of hierarchy, rather a community of nurses leading care.

EXEMPLARS: ENACTING ADVANCED PRACTICE ROLES

The enactment of the advanced practice roles of the acute care NP, the CNS, CNM, the primary care NP, and the CRNA are best detailed through the narratives set forth by the following exemplars. Using a standard set of interview questions listed, these enactments are related to existing practice settings. See **Boxes 12-1** through **12-5**.

Advanced Practice Nurse Interview Questions

To guide the interview process for chosen groups of APNs, the following questions were used consistently for each group with the intent of assessing roles, expectations, and influences on practice.

1. How would you describe your role?
2. How would you describe your working relationship with physicians, other nurses, and other members of the health-care team?
3. What does *referral* mean to you?
4. What does *consultation* mean to you?
5. How open are members of other disciplines in taking direct referrals or consultation from you?
6. What degree of authority do you experience in these situations and in your role?
7. Do you observe that you bring about change and a higher order of knowledge to your practice area?
8. Can you discuss a situation that may exemplify your role, especially regarding your work through other people?

BOX 12-1
The Acute Care Nurse Practitioner

This group of nurse practitioners (NPs), situated within an oncology inpatient practice, describes their role as geared to management of their patient's experience of illness. The patient's diagnostic work-up is often completed before admission in the community setting. Therefore, the patient's in-hospital experience becomes the focus, with management of the acute phase of illness and treatment options as primary goals of care. They describe their perspective as multidimensional. Using their registered nurse (RN) background, they always view the patient in a holistic manner. Advanced practice clinical competencies engage their ability to case manage and guide patients and families through the complexity of health care. Within this framework, the NP's relationships with the health-care team are key because they do spend significant amounts of time discussing medical management and locating resources, integrating feedback from other disciplines, and identifying alternatives to the health-care system when challenged by the limitations of third-party payers. Given their range of activities, this group of acute practice nurses (APNs) consistently relate to a variety of other disciplines, primarily medicine, nursing, and social work.

    This group describes their autonomy as follows. "We feel that our common ground is the care of the patient. Working with our team of physicians allows us many choices and flexibility.

Continued

BOX 12-1
The Acute Care Nurse Practitioner—cont'd

We decide the day-to-day care for our patients, and in acute or critical episodes, we often inde-pendently manage the process. Although critical incidents may be a time when the physician takes a more active role, this does not necessarily translate into the need to 'take over'. The goal is to work together—not to work around each other or without each other." The NP is usually the leader of care because of a number of factors including the close relationship to the patient and family members, the advantages of consistency of care by the NP, and well-defined collaboration between physician and NP.

Regarding their relationships with RNs, the NPs state: "There is nothing better than work-ing with a competent nurse. When this relationship occurs, there is such a strong bond, that you firmly believe that there is absolutely nothing that can stand in the way of quality." On the other hand, NPs state that some nurses can become more passive about patient care when relating to a NP. Because the RN recognizes the "nurse" in the NP role, the RN may relinquish aspects of their responsibility for patient management or assessment to the NP. This transfer rarely occurs within the RN-physician relationship. NPs must therefore carefully assess the nature of the NP-RN relationship to avoid jeopardizing their ability to work through others while facilitating the advanced practice perspective.

Within the acute care NP role, referrals are commonplace—NP to nutritionist, social worker, physical therapist, and home care services. Physicians often refer their patients to NPs, acknowledging their specialization, expertise, and consistency of care. Consultations are more informal within the inpatient setting. When acute patient situations occur, however, clinical consultation is common. NPs state: "Not a day goes by that I am not involved in a clinical consultation primarily focused on symptom management, such as pain control, the side effects of chemotherapy, nausea, vomiting, constipation or palliative care." This type of consultation is almost always verbal for it seems "physicians want to maintain control of the written consulta-tion process within the hospital experience." NPs consult other NPs as well, often involving clinical specialization expertise—usually within a verbal, face-to-face framework.

The degree of authority within the discipline of nursing is explained by acute care NPs in a variety of ways. NPs are integral in the decision making about their patients and have significant influence on the nursing care being delivered. Using a specialization approach, acute care NPs take advantage of opportunities to teach about clinical sequelae and implica-tions. One NP states: "I often teach at the bedside about what is going on with the patient and I am watchful for the types of questions the nurses have. This helps me observe the growth of the staff and assess their advancing competency. It is really a very rewarding experience for me." Through rounding with staff nurses, NPs also have the opportunity to clarify the patient story and often act as a facilitator of communication about patients among team members. NPs state their role as "performing the editing role"—distinguishing the critical elements of the patient story and routing the necessary data in a more concise and relevant way to obtain what is necessary for their patients. As one NP stated, "Our role within the interdisciplinary team is one of monitor of the communication patterns and the perspective at hand. We often translate what is going on into a relevant, concise language that evokes a rapid, clear understanding by those team members who need to hear the information."

According to this group, the design of the acute care NP embraces many relationships within the health-care team and consists of these major components:

■ gatekeeper
■ decoder of the complexity of the situation

BOX 12-1
The Acute Care Nurse Practitioner—cont'd

- director of care, delineating roles and responses
- problem solver, often suggesting alternatives when barriers arise
- provider of a secure environment for staff nurses to ask questions and learn
- guide for directing the patient care experience, providing the driving force behind what needs to be done, when, and why

Integral to the these components is the ability to work with others, to recognize the many roles inherent within the heath-care team, to value the team's input and contribution, and to recognize that influencing others should be always focused on the unified goal of quality patient care.

BOX 12-2
The Clinical Nurse Specialist

The clinical nurse specialists (CNSs) describe their role as multifunctional, defining their framework of practice as more focused within a nursing model rather than medicine. CNSs categorize their role into two primary domains: clinical and professional. Clinically, this CNS group describes their role as including a major teaching component and direct clinical practice to facilitate and influence care of complex patients. These functions are often intertwined because they routinely bring about change and a higher order of knowledge by role modeling, mentoring, and coaching staff to perform at "the next level." CNSs also intervene within the health-care team to make clinical recommendations to change the course of action or resolve conflicts for optimal patient care. Professionally, the CNS also assumes major responsibilities for the development of policies, procedures, protocols, and standards of care. Within this context, the education of patients in health promotion and maintenance is key. Standards of care are holistic in nature, spanning the physical, psychosocial, and spiritual needs of patients. The needs of nurses are also critical. The CNS encourages the professional growth of staff, often provides career counseling, and directs the building of expertise among nurses in a specific, individualized manner.

The CNSs describe their role with physicians as collegial with a defined focus on specialty patient care management, often receiving referrals for a specific patient population (i.e., diabetes) or an occurrence such as death/dying and bereavement. CNSs are consistent in their view of the "big picture" not just focusing on disease and pathophysiology but the patient's response to the disease. With other nurses, CNSs describe their role as an enabler—one of camaraderie focused on patient care. CNSs also provide clinical, professional, and legal clarification regarding issues of care to ensure a safe patient environment.

When asked about autonomy, this CNS group cited self-direction and motivation as key elements in working with others. Several strategies are used to engage others in change and ultimately provide state-of-the-art, valid, and effective approaches to care:

- Use benchmark data and national standards to energize staff to change or modify practices.
- Develop and educate staff so they can question their patient care environment and relate to a higher level of performance.

Continued

BOX 12-2
The Clinical Nurse Specialist—cont'd

■ Involve staff in various levels of patient care projects, moving forward together in change.

■ Ground all projects in the literature and best practices so as to base decisions on evidence and promote confidence in the process.

The CNS role engages an inclusive approach within these strategies, which guarantees a successful and lasting outcome over time.

Referrals are routine in complex cases. The CNS is often the originator of referrals to other members of the health-care team, but integral to bringing team members together to problem solve. Inclusiveness is again a key element of the CNS practice domain and a hallmark of their effectiveness in patient care through their ability to relate to others.

Consultation, on the other hand, is associated with the level of the CNS's clinical expertise and is often initiated by other members of the health-care team—physicians, nurses, and social workers. As an inductive thinker, the CNS has a clearly articulated interest in the patient experience of care. Using these tenets of practice and change—standards, safety, and ethics—the CNS is able to define a plan for care, engaging caregivers to undertake the plan and empowering others to assume an appropriate trajectory for the patient.

As the integrator of care, the CNS exemplifies how positive interdisciplinary relationships ensure positive outcomes for patients. CNSs are teachers, clinical experts, care providers, case finders, role models, mentors, patient advocates, coaches, team members, policy makers, project leaders, innovators, case managers, career counselors, and change agents. With a vision of best practices as their foundation for care, the CNS holds the value of expertise and dynamic working relationships within the health-care team as critical elements to the success of their role.

BOX 12-3
Nurse-Midwife

Nurse-midwives in a combined ambulatory and inpatient setting describe their advanced practice role as primary caregiver of women along the life cycle with a focus on low-risk obstetrical and gynecological care, health promotion, wellness, family-centered care, risk assessment, and management of common illnesses and acute conditions. Clinically, this group views their role as centered on direct care with a strong emphasis on patient education and health promotion. Their relationships with other members of the health-care team revolve around this focus. Midwives independently care for a patient caseload, often comanaging more acute conditions with physicians or employing the physician as consultant.

Regarding referral, midwives in this practice describe the process as formalized and often interchangeable with consultation. They define many of their referrals as transfers to the care of a physician because of a specialized need of the patient over time. Ongoing referrals to other disciplines are also common, usually engaging the services of social work and home care. In these instances, the midwife maintains the primary care responsibility for the patient. With consultation, the process is also formal. Using written communication, consultations are often provided through the required practice protocols that identify the consulting physician and the decision guidelines for the consultation. Within this collaborative relationship, the midwife is able to transition the care of the patient when a condition warrants. This can be accomplished in a comanaged arrangement or by a referral of the care responsibility to

BOX 12-3
Nurse-Midwife—cont'd

another caregiver. However, the midwife has an expectation to be involved in the communication of the plan of care and the ultimate follow-up of the patient being referred. The midwife explains that the "relationships with physicians in my practice are necessary and denote many shared responsibilities. I find this relationship to be within an interdependent framework since we both need to work together to manage the patient safely in given situations. I have a consulting agreement with a primary physician for immediate feedback and intervention as well as with other physicians who are colleagues and can be employed for a less acute need. But I also have the need to maintain my primary care role for my patients."

Working with the nursing staff involves interdependence. The need for the registered nurse (RN) to facilitate a plan of care and become integral to the education of patients is key. One midwife states, "I find that once my role is accepted and understood, positive relationships follow and communication about patients is facilitated. I admit that I need nurses to ultimately deliver good patient care. I cannot do everything myself." Nurses and other health team members who seek out the midwife as primary caregiver ultimately affect an improved patient experience because the model of working together and understanding the role is achieved. One midwife states that over the past decade this recognition of the midwife role has improved tremendously, especially because of updated scope of practice legislation and changes in third-party reimbursement.

When asked about autonomy and authority over practice, nurse-midwives strongly identify that their influence over care processes is recognized by others. The primary reason for this influence is the public respect, acceptance, and demand for their roles and services. They add that this authority is stronger and more flexible in an ambulatory setting and can be less autonomous in a hospital-based birthing unit, especially when associated with a medical residency program. Interdisciplinary competition in these settings can affect the perceived authority and working relationships of the midwife with other clinicians as well as patients.

When discussing their relationships with nurses, midwives were clear that within the specialty of women's health, RNs do not abdicate components of their roles to midwives. RNs often question an approach to care, exchange ideas to complement care, and practice as team members. The specialty of women's health is often not characterized as illness-focused but within a health promotion/health maintenance framework, enabling the team approach to flourish. Respect for the team's contribution to the varied aspects of the needs of patients enables the nurse-midwives to work effectively with and through others. As one nurse-midwife summarized her role: "Being on the same page in our plans for care is easily delineated within this advanced practice role. Thus collaboration is a natural outcome. Respect is key, and once earned, paves the way to collaborative practice."

BOX 12-4
The Primary Care Nurse Practitioner

This group of primary care nurse practitioners (NPs) view their role as provider of a comprehensive holistic health-care experience for their patients. With independence and autonomy, the primary care NP has a threefold responsibility to assess, diagnose, and manage a variety of common illnesses within all the dimensions of the physical, psychosocial, and financial elements of care. "My caseload of patients" is a common reference point, delineating the

Continued

BOX 12-4
The Primary Care Nurse Practitioner—cont'd

accountability of this group of NPs for their patients over time—not limited to a hospital experience but to the continuum of care. In primary care, the NP possesses a leadership role in the practice generally by providing a surveillance function—a "third eye"—always watchful of the effectiveness of day-to-day patient care delivery. The need to evaluate systems and clinical outcomes are essential to the role.

The team approach in this type of practice is fundamental and involves a strong interdisciplinary, participative approach to care. Patients are independently managed, comanaged with physicians, or referred within their continuum of care. The need to relate effectively with all members of the health-care team is constant. Multidisciplinary options coexist within an interdisciplinary framework—creating many opportunities for therapeutic relationships among staff, patients, and family members.

Within the primary care practice, RNs are the "heart" of any clinical operation. The RN complements the APN role, especially in the areas of patient teaching, patient monitoring, and data gathering. Although roles are often strongly delineated, sharing clinical activity among health-care team members is consistent and necessary.

As a result of the primary care focus, referrals to specialists are commonplace. But as one NP explained, "Losing the primary relationship with a patient to a specialist is a concern." The information and insight the specialist provides will enhance the care the patient receives from their primary care provider. There are also instances when a specialist and primary care provider work collaboratively on the health-care management of a patient over the longer term. Feedback on the means to best manage the patient is the expected outcome. One NP stated: "We expect to have our patients return to us for their care and to benefit from the expertise and evaluation by the specialist."

Consultations, on the other hand, are frequently engaged by other caregivers. Within a mature primary care practice, a multidisciplinary team approach is often developed. Formal consults usually occur within the practice. The opportunity to have "curbside" or "hallway" consults with these same specialists or experts exists as well. This type of consultation is often informal. The NPs from this practice cited that the key criteria for successful and effective consultations of any type include the development of positive relationships, a clear direction of the plan of care and a model of inclusivity among team members.

Primary care NPs describe their authority as an essential part of their potential for success in their role, while maintaining autonomy and a knowledge base to provide sufficient holistic primary care to patients. Practicing side-by-side with other physicians and other NPs create opportunities for sharing advice or consultation. Leading patient care in this practice setting is very satisfying and empowering to this group of advanced practice nurses (APNs). At the same time, however, this sense of control and satisfaction occurs only when interdisciplinary teamwork is achieved by:

- listening to others
- teaching others
- demonstrating the APN role in positive, creative ways
- communicating openly
- demonstrating expertise

Respect from other members of the team enables the primary care NP to facilitate and lead care effectively. When sharing the same mission, within this framework of practice, advancement of learning and change occurs. By empowering and educating staff at all levels,

BOX 12-4
The Primary Care Nurse Practitioner—cont'd

the barrier of the "task" is removed and has been replaced with a "connection" to the patient's illness experience. Assisting staff to understand the rationale for care is a definitive way to initiate change and a higher level of performance. In addition, the primary care NP often exhibits his or her own clinical specialization and expertise, which may provide a different perspective of care, adding to the knowledge base of the staff. As educator, the NP is capable of working through other people, engaging the staff's interest in the mission and work at hand. For knowledge is power, and this power translates into effective practice.

BOX 12-5
Nurse Anesthetist

The role of the certified registered nurse anesthetist (CRNA), within a hospital practice, is described as an advanced practice specialty with a strong and eventful history that has provided many benchmarks for nurses seeking expanded roles. As an anesthesia provider, the goal of the CRNA is to provide safe and comfortable anesthesia for all types of surgical procedures in multiple settings across the care continuum for patients of all ages spanning the American Society of Anesthesiologists (ASA) classifications of "healthy" to "gravely ill/impending death." In discussing this broad role definition, the concept of independence is also clearly expressed especially because the CRNA often is able to administer anesthesia without the direct supervision of a physician, depending on state regulations and the requirements of the employing health-care institution. For example, this CRNA stated that in her practice an anesthesiologist is required to practice in specified ratios with the CRNA and that an anesthesiologist must be present in the room at the start of general anesthesia induction.

The clinical relationship between the CRNA and the anesthesiologist is clearly described as one of a collegial and trusting nature, with open communication. However, outside of the clinical arena, the political tension between the two disciplines is present and with a long history of debate and interprofessional struggle and competition. With the demonstration of expertise, however, positive communication patterns and relationships have developed around the patient and quality care in institutional settings. The day-to-day operational framework has thereby demonstrated advancement over time in terms of professional acceptance and colleagueship.

Within the operating room, the surgical team assumes a vibrant interdependent structure. This CRNA stated: "Teamwork is the expectation in the operating room setting. The involvement with RNs, surgeons, and surgical technologists is intense and very focused on the individual patient and the procedure at hand and can sometimes be described as somewhat of an isolating relationship because of this directed focus." Regarding the relationship between the CRNA and RN, it is described as important but less influential in affecting the role of the CRNA when compared with the other team members like the surgeon or technologist. The relationship with surgeons is described as one of respect for the specialization of anesthesia and sometimes dependent during the course of surgery because the CRNA often leads patient stabilization efforts when a critical change in condition occurs.

In the specialty of anesthesia, the CRNA usually does not make referrals but is the recipient of referrals from other providers. With the exception of some specialized services such as pain management, CRNAs do not have their own patient caseload because the patients have

Continued

BOX 12-5
Nurse Anesthetist—cont'd

a primary relationship with their surgeon. Consultations, on the other hand, comprise a major component of anesthesia practice. Consultations reflect clinical, legal, and medical aspects of the plan of care. Surgeons frequently request a consult from a CRNA, respecting the expertise of this specialization to assess the risks of surgery. In this endeavor, the surgeon is dependent on the expertise of the anesthesia specialist. Within this activity, the CRNA attains primary patient and family contact, subsequently establishing the patient-family relationship.

Authority in practice is significant within the specialty of anesthesia. "Many other disciplines do not share a common ground in this specialty: thus my role is unique within patient care." The CRNA in this practice comments that she also identifies that through her unique expertise, the independence and influence of her role takes hold. "Other members of the health care team recognize my competence, which directly affects my sense of autonomy and authority. I am called upon to assist others in their clinical assessment of patients as well as the advancement of professional knowledge and skills of residents and nurse anesthesia students. With this broad range of influence, my sense of authority is promoted."

The ability of the CRNA to influence change and a higher order of knowledge in the arenas of perioperative and perianesthesia practice is strongly affected by teaching by example, demonstrating competence, and role-modeling professional behaviors to all members of the health-care team. Using this framework, the CRNA in this practice identifies that she is able to influence change and advance knowledge by relying on a clinical approach rather than with an academic approach. In many practices, however, CRNAs also assume formal faculty roles within various levels of educational programs throughout the country.

Although working through other people is an expectation of any health-care professional role, interdisciplinary exposure is often more limited for CRNAs and can potentially contribute to isolation. Interdisciplinary relationships are strongest within the perioperative team of the surgeon, anesthesiologist, nurse, and technologist. Extending this relationship to other clinical staff and family members is challenging. In addition, CRNAs are often placed within a separate administrative structure within the health-care facility or practice, contributing to the isolation, especially from other professional nurse colleagues.

Within the context of advanced practice, the goal of the CRNA is to promote nursing, advance health care, and ensure a safe and quality patient care experience. As the earliest advanced practice role, CRNAs have successfully built a strong presence in health care.

SUMMARY

The dynamic interplay of partnerships and interdependence between advanced practice and other team roles in health care is a professional challenge. Working with and through others is the cornerstone of the successful engagement of the health-care team and endorses the presence of advanced practice over time.

References

American Association of Colleges of Nursing. (1996). *The essentials of master's education for advanced practice nursing.* Washington, DC: Author.

American Nurses Association. (2003). *Nursing's social policy statement.* Washington, DC: Author.

Arcongelo, V., Fitzgerald, M., Carroll, D., & Plumb, J. (1996). Collaborative care between nurse practitioners and primary care physicians. *Primary Care, 23*(1), 103–113.

Brandt, A. (2001). The nurse physician relationship in historical context. In M. Hager (Ed), *Enhancing interactions between nursing and medicine*. New York: Josiah Macy Jr. Foundation.

Bigbee, J., & Amidi-Nouri, A. (2000). History and evolution of advanced nursing practice. In A. B. Hamric, J. A. Spross, & C. M. Hanson (Eds.), *Advanced nursing practice: An integrative approach* (2nd ed.). Philadelphia: WB Saunders.

Clark, P. (1994). Learning on interdisciplinary gerontological teams: Instructional concepts and methods. *Educational Gerontology, 20*(2), 349–364.

Coles, C. (1995). Educating the health care team. *Patient Education and Counseling 26*(5), 239–244.

Davies, B., & Hughes, A. M. (1995). Clarification of advanced nursing practice: Characteristics and competencies. *Clinical Nurse Specialist, 9*(3), 156–160.

Fitzgerald, M. A., Jones, P. E., Lazar, B., McHugh, M., & Wang, C. (1995). The midlevel provider: Colleague or competitor. *Patient Care, 29*(1), 20–37.

Hamric, A. B., Spross, J. A., & Hanson, C. M. (2005). *Advanced nursing practice: An integrative approach* (3rd ed.). Philadelphia: WB Saunders Company.

Howe, J., Cassel, C., & Vezina, M. (1998). Structuring the GITT didactic experience. In E. Siegler, K. Hyer, T. Fulmer, & M. Mezey (Eds.), *Geriatric interdisciplinary team training* (p. 90). New York: Springer Publishing Company.

Institute of Medicine. (2004). *Quality chasm series: Patient safety—Achieving a new standard for care.* Washington, DC: National Academy Press.

Kraus, W. A. (1980). *Collaboration in organizations: Alternatives to hierarchy.* New York: Homan Sciences Press.

National Association of Clinical Nurse Specialists. (2004). *Statement on clinical nurse specialist practice and education* (2nd ed.). Harrisburg, PA: Author.

National Association of Clinical Nurse Specialists. (2007). *Competency validation survey.* Harrisburg, PA: The Association.

National Council of State Boards of Nursing Advanced Practice Registered Nurses Task Force. (2006). *Draft: A vision of the future of advanced practice regulation.* Chicago: Author.

Naylor, M., Brooten, D., Jones, R., Lavizzo-Mourey, R., Mezey, M., & Pauly, M. (1994). Comprehensive discharge planning for the hospitalized elderly: A randomized clinical trial. *Annals of Internal Medicine, 120*(12), 999–1006.

Pfeiffer, E. (1998). Why teams? In E. Siegler, K. Hyer, T. Fulmer, & M. Mezey, (Eds.), *Geriatric interdisciplinary team training* (p. 16). New York: Springer Publishing Company.

Spross, J. A., & Baggerly, J. (1989). Models of advanced practice. In A. B, Hamric & J. A. Spross, (Eds.), *The clinical nurse specialist in theory and practice* (2nd ed., 19–40). Philadelphia: WB Saunders.

Strumpf, N., & Whitney, F. (1994). Teaching collaborative skills to nurse practitioner students. In E. Siegler & F. Whitney (Eds.), *Nurse-physician collaboration.* New York: Springer Publishing Company.

Thompson, J. E. & Thompson, H. O. (1985). *Bioethical decision making for nurses.* Norwalk, CT: Appleton Century Fox.

Thompson, J. E., Kershbaumer, R., & Krisman-Scott, M. (2001). *Educating advanced practice nurses and midwives: From practice to teaching.* New York. Springer Publishing Company.

Tsukada, R. A. (1990). Interdisciplinary collaboration: Teamwork in geriatrics. In C. K. Cassel, D. E. Riesenberg, L. B. Sorenson, & J. R. Walsh (Eds,), *Geriatric medicine* (2nd ed., 668–675). New York: Springer-Verlag.

Tsukuda, R. A., & Stahelski, A. J. (1990). Guide to team skills: Predictors of cooperation in health care teams. *Small Group Research, 21*(2) 220–233.

Tresolini, C. P., & The Pew-Fetzer Task Force (1994). *Health professional education and relationship-centered care.* San Francisco: Pew Health Professions Commission.

Tuckman, B. W. (1965). Developmental sequences in small groups. *Psychological Bulletin, 63*(1), 384–399.

13

Reporting Relationships: Follow the Money

Mary Lou S. Etheredge

INTRODUCTION

Collaboration, partnerships, team work, joint problem solving, and *teaming across boundaries*—are some of the words and phrases used to describe expectations and performance of today's highly effective work teams. This language represents a change in philosophy, thinking, and approach from "vertical hierarchies" to "horizontal networks," linking traditional functions through interfunctional teams (Hirschhorn & Gilmore, 1992). In the context of "breaking down traditional boundaries," the phrase *reporting relationships* seems oddly out of place and outdated.

In daily work life, advanced practice nurses (APNs) may find themselves in a place between the traditional boundaries of hierarchy created by financial structures and more nontraditional alignments that extend far beyond structural hierarchies. There is wide variation of opinion among the four APN groups (clinical nurse specialist [CNS], certified nurse-midwife [CNM], certified registered nurse anesthetist [CRNA], and nurse practitioner [NP]) regarding the preferred types of organizational alignments. In large measure this is attributable to differences in practice styles and role implementation among the APNs within each group and within the specialties themselves. It is difficult to find common ground, yet some preferences and common themes recur among the four APN groups. This chapter identifies two recurrent themes and outlines related issues as they are described by APNs in practice and by their professional organizations.

RECURRENT THEMES

The first and most prevailing theme is that finances dictate the structure for reporting alignments. Like all other employees, APNs are subject to those who "hold the purse strings." However, APNs are creating and participating in more fluid employment arrangements (i.e., private or group practice, contracted employees, or joint administrative and clinical positions) that realign finances, roles, and relationships. Such arrangements are more prevalent for CRNAs and CNMs, who are historically less likely to be in traditional employer/employee relationships. Ongoing changes in state and federal reimbursement regulations have also increased options for NPs and CNSs who are forming private practices or group practices in varied geographical and more mainstream locations.

The second theme is that APNs prefer a reporting structure that enables the clinical work, provides for ongoing knowledge and skill development, and allows for their full scope of practice in a manner that differentiates their advanced practice from that of other colleagues (physician and nonphysician). For some APNs, this is best expressed in a line position budgeted in the specialty area. For others, the best alignment comes from a position budgeted in nursing service. Still others prefer a private practice, solo, or contract arrangement. The specific specialty area—including the practice setting itself; the type and complexity of the patient population; the compatibility of values and beliefs among providers, including the "match" in provider practice styles and personality—directly affects the nature and quality of interdisciplinary alignments. An organizational structure can be designed that eliminates competition for dollars and frees the interdisciplinary group from the "hierarchy of organizational titles" and roles to "figure out what kind of roles they need to play, and what kind of relationships they need to maintain, in order to use their differences effectively in productive work" (Hirschhorn & Gilmore, 1992, p. 105). This capitalizes on the contributions each member of the interdisciplinary team brings to the table and renders the language of "reporting" relationships passe.

THE BUSINESS OF RELATIONSHIPS

Simply defined, a business is any activity that seeks profit by providing goods or services to others. Although the goals of a nonprofit business do not include making a personal profit for its owner, these businesses do strive for gains that are used to meet the stated social and organization goals (Nickels, McHugh, & McHugh, 1999). "Not for profit" goes hand in hand with "not for loss." Which services generate revenue, which services incur loss, how much "gain" remains after the income and expenses are tallied, how risk is distributed, and how the revenue and expenses are accounted for are universal considerations for all profit and nonprofit businesses from the cottage industry to the largest corporation. According to this basic definition, health care is and always has been a service business.

So what has changed? The most obvious change is the steadily decreasing flow of dollars coming into the business for the services provided. In the presence of limited resources from declining revenue, difficult decisions about the business are forced. Whoever oversees the source(s) of revenue becomes the authority for decision making that affects services, roles, personnel, relationships, values, and future direction. Competition for the resources intensifies. Synergy around roles and relationships is replaced with battles around turf and territory. Competition for scarce resources evokes a "not enough" mentality. Surviving in the midst of scarcity is perceived as a matter of job and self-preservation. Literally experienced as a matter of survival ("I need this job to feed my family"), protecting boundaries becomes the symbol for protecting livelihood or the viability of the business itself.

Following the money is especially telling for APNs in employee positions because it crafts and dictates the design of the vertical, horizontal, lateral, administrative, and clinical relationships. "Reporting" relationships are born between those who pay the salaries for positions (or their representatives) and those who are paid. Following this salary trail exposes the reporting/organizational relationships that yield important information about the "how" and the "why" of the position.

FOLLOWING THE MONEY

Nationally, there are more than 180,000 APNs found in a variety of geographical and practice settings (**Table 13-1**). They practice in a myriad of settings, including community health centers, correctional institutions, school-based clinics, long-term care facilities, nursing homes, employee health centers, community birthing centers, primary care practices, physician offices, and hospital-based inpatient and outpatient departments. In each of these settings, there are different reporting arrangements that reflect a variety of financial models and philosophies.

TABLE 13-1		
Numbers of Advanced Practice Nurses and Their Practice Settings		
APN	**Number**	**Practice Setting**
CRNA*	>37,000	Every practice setting in which anesthesia is delivered: hospitals, surgical suites, critical access ambulatory surgical centers, obstetrical delivery rooms, and U.S. military and physician offices
CNM† (includes CM)	>11,000	Hospitals, health centers, birth centers, and private practice with physicians
CNS‡	>15,344	Private practice, homes, offices, HMOs, and universities
NP§	>120,000	Hospitals, private practice, private office with physicians, clinics, correctional institutions, universities and colleges, and HMOs

*American Association of Nurse Anesthetists as of March, 2008.
†American College of Nurse-Midwives as of 2007.
‡Pearson, 2008.
§American Academy of Nurse Practitioners as of 2007.

   APN, advanced practice nurse; CRNA, certified registered nurse anesthetist; CNM, certified nurse-midwife; CNS, clinical nurse specialist; HMO, health maintenance organization; NP, nurse practitioner.

Within each of these geographical and practice settings, APNs are solo practitioners, employees of physician groups, employees of hospitals and clinics, and contracted employees. There is not necessarily one reporting alignment that is correct for all APNs in all settings. The most satisfying, as described by APNs, are those that are patient focused, that allow practice within the full extent of the APN's scope while fostering positive relationships among colleagues from other disciplines (especially physicians), and that provide equitable compensation for services. As an employee in a hospital or clinic setting, the cost center in which the APN position is placed depends on who contributes the dollars that pay for the position. Where the dollars come from in large measure determines where and how the accountability for practice, performance, and role are defined, developed, and implemented. When the department of anesthesia pays for the CRNA's salary (and receives any associated revenues), the CRNA reports to anesthesia. If CNMs are placed in the nursing service cost center, their primary reporting relationship is through nursing. When a group of physicians hire an NP, CNM, CNS, or CRNA, they have identified needs within the setting that they believe can be met by hiring an APN, who ultimately reports to those physicians.

Heavy workloads of the hiring person, group, or discipline usually precipitate initial inquiry about the introduction of APN positions. When volume, demand, or need is greater than can be accommodated, discussions begin around how to increase provider capacity. The costs and benefits of adding another position and the exact type of position (physician or nonphysician) are part of the discussion and decision-making process. Because an APN's salary is less than that of a physician, adding an advanced practice position is one attractive option. If viewed as "a physician substitute," the boundaries of the APN role, lines of reporting, expectations for performance and often the work itself, is based on meeting the identified needs of the physician stakeholders and in need of clarification from the outset.

The needs that are identified in advance by the stakeholders are declared with varying degrees of clarity and urgency to remedy specific, immediate, and often temporary circumscribed situations.

A "quick and dirty" solution or interim stop-gap measure may be the goal. Stakeholders often comment, "we have more demand than capacity," or "we need someone to handle the high volume of patient calls." An added attraction to the comparatively low salary of the APN (when compared to physician counterparts) is that she or he can do the work of both a physician and a nurse as needed. In addition, some of the APN services can be billed and reimbursed. For those holding the purse strings, this is the ultimate in efficient use of personnel—an appealing option. Analysis of the appropriate type of role (APN, medical doctor, or RN) to meet the needs, often does not occur in advance, beyond "running the numbers." Decisions to hire an APN are often made in the absence of nursing counsel, especially if this is the first role of its kind in the particular setting, nursing is not subsidizing the position or contributing to its subsidy, or there is not a nursing presence within the practice or group to offer guidance. Design flaws are often embedded in these APN roles that are created either in the absence of accurate information or through faulty interpretation of scope of practice, state regulations, and prescriptive authority. Driven solely by stakeholder needs, "filler roles" are created that are not necessarily APN roles. Blending components of advanced practice with general nursing practice creates a role that is not rewarding, effective, or clear. Although some APNs may accept these roles as an entry into a setting, if the role is to evolve, part of their work must be to inform and educate managers and colleagues about scope of practice, prescriptive authority, reimbursement regulations, and their proper application. Simply put, they will need to advocate for their importance on many levels.

The primary intent then, based on the setting's identified needs, is to "download" or delegate to the APN some of the work of the hiring persons. Each contributor (investor) to the APN's salary has a personal stake (measured by the monetary contribution to salary) to define "what" is done. Of course each investor looks for a positive "return on investment." (Patient outcomes and patient satisfaction are excellent objective measurement indicators of good returns on investment.) However, the personal desires, opinions, and expectations of the investors may be the primary gauge by which the return on investment is measured when any of the following apply to each investor or member of a group practice:

- The investors are working financial contributors to the practice setting.
- The investors are downloading some of their own work.
- The investors are referring "their patients."
- The investors are contributing to the APN's salary.

This subjectivity provokes feelings of entitlement and possessiveness that are interpreted as broad license to dictate not only how the work gets done, but also the scope of the APN role itself. (Comments include, "These are my patients. I pay, therefore I have a say.") Renditions of this theme to control the methods to control the results vary based on the setting. If there is variation or lack of consensus among the vested members about what the work is, adding personal preferences about how the work gets done further confuses the message and the expectations for the position. For some who provide or manage the dollars, the responsibility to manage includes authority to control risk. This hierarchical approach defines and shapes the relationship. The urgency to reframe this relationship is heightened, as is the skill required to do so. If not anticipated, recognized, and discussed (and in some situations avoided), the APN can be personally frustrated and severely constricted in practicing to the full extent of his or her authority, capacity, and capability.

Following the money leads us through a maze of complexity and interdependencies to the decision makers and the issues that contribute to developing or maintaining these relationships that can severely constrict the APN role. Realigning these vertical hierarchies can and does occur on the local level, one relationship at a time.

INTERNAL AND EXTERNAL FORCES

Reporting relationships are further influenced by a multitude of internal and external forces. These include, but are not limited to, history; policies based on interpretation and application of state and federal regulations and reimbursement practices; the dynamics of existing roles, including status; power; and availability of basic information about the advanced practice role itself. The interplay among these forces creates layers of entanglements that challenge the APN's ability to influence decisions that are made by those who control the cash. For example, *supervision, consultation, collaboration,* and *independent practice* are terms to describe scope of practice for APNs that are defined differently from state to state in each of the regulatory arenas. These same terms are frequently used interchangeably to describe reimbursement criteria for nonphysician providers. In the reimbursement arena these words have different meanings than in the practice arena. Because of the disparate and often contradictory definitions and interpretations, some APNs and their representative professional organizations contend that collaboration and consultation are code for supervision; supervision means tight control; cooperation means acquiescence; and partnership is veiled subservience. The lack of clarity and consistency around the nuances of definition naturally leads to skepticism from APNs. This skepticism is fueled by the inaccuracies (intended or otherwise) found in specific practice policies. Billing policies spawned from inaccuracies in interpretation of scope of practice, prescriptive privilege, or reimbursement regulations create a mass of confusion and bureaucracy that may result in reductions in revenue for a practice setting and a narrowing of scope of practice for the APN. This revenue loss puts the APN role at risk. (See Reimbursement: Can the Position Pay for Itself? in this chapter).

A consequence of inaccuracies in interpretation, application, or interchangeability of reimbursement and scope of practice language is the creation or perpetuation of a hierarchy of "coordinating work activities" that function as a strict chain of command. In many practice settings, history places physicians at the top of this chain, but today's individualistic and educated workforce is less tolerant of rigid structures and formal hierarchy (McShane & Von Glinow, 2000, p. 562). The chain-of-command approach does not encourage thoughtful analysis of the intricacies of interdependent roles and relationships. "Interdependence (is) the principle that each part needs the help of the other parts . . . in order to survive" (Handy, 1989, p. 125). The chain-of-command approach contributes to top-down alignments that serve to maintain the "silos" of functional departments, creating barriers rather than breaking them down. These challenges and opportunities present themselves regularly to APN employees in practice.

When a physician takes on the role of "manager" in addition to the role's legitimate rights and authority, additional dynamics are introduced. The power (im)balance that is inherent in any relationship in which a particular person holds the purse strings, and hence the authority to "cut the position," is magnified by the history of interprofessional role relationships between doctor and nurse. Each participant brings past history and experiences of the doctor/nurse dyad into the new relationship. This combination of roles (physician and manager), entangled with past experiences and preferences (previous physician/nurse relationships) and the lack of basic information about the scope of APN practice or role in the presence of limited resources, can exhume the "traditional unilateral line of authority from physician to nurse" (Benner, Tanner, & Chesla, 1996, pp. 280–306). Reenacting hierarchical interactions can be a familiar frame of reference for one or both participants. Reframing this relationship within the context of the advanced practice role takes concerted and deliberate effort. In a relationship based on such a hierarchical view of the world, the implication is of superiority and submissiveness (Satir, Banmen, Gerber, & Gomori, 1991). The monetary contributions accompanied by legitimate decision-making authority and responsibility promotes in some the development and maintenance of traditional hierarchical relationships. This hierarchy may be reinforced by the overlay of the traditional doctor/nurse hierarchy. Virginia Satir notes the following:

> *In the hierarchical model, relationships exist in only one variety: somebody is on top, and somebody is on the bottom. It is a dominant/submissive arrangement, sometimes called the threat-and-reward model. This type of relationship has been considered normal for centuries. Often the only question is: "Is it malevolent or benevolent?" Dominant/submissive relationships fall along a continuum from having uncaring tyrants to having kind ones, and from having unhappy victims to compliant ones (Satir et al., 1991, p. 7).*

The "overarching theme is one of authority" (Handy, 1989, pp. 123–124). This approach no longer works well in situations in which there is a need for cooperative efforts among clinicians from different professional disciplines.

SPECIALTY ALIGNMENTS

Patient-focused practice and opportunities for ongoing development of clinical expertise within the specialty area are held in high value for and by all APNs. In all employment arrangements, clinical competence is the foundational skill of all APNs, and as such, is a universal expectation of practice. For both these reasons, many APNs prefer that the position be placed in the specialty cost center rather than in the nursing service cost center. APNs contend that placement in the specialty cost center builds stronger alliances with colleagues from other disciplines (especially physicians) who share the same clinical focus. These colleagues understand the constraints and demands of the specialty. They share common interests in knowledge and skill development and quality-of-care issues. This commonality of purpose and experience connects, is sought out, is valued, and is appreciated by APNs.

This alignment has its pressure points. Positioned in specialty cost centers, APNs must continuously orient physicians and administrators (often there are dual reporting relationships) to the similarities and differences in their role as compared with the roles of other providers. It is a constant challenge to clearly articulate and demonstrate how these differences add value and revenue. Controlling expenses and generating revenue are ever-present components of the work, whether overtly or subliminally. Charting and staying the course in these financial waters requires that APNs demonstrate nonclinical skills of advanced practice. Nonclinical skills—including negotiation and interpersonal skills; the ability to articulate and clarify the issues surrounding scope of practice, prescriptive authority, and reimbursement; financial acumen; skills in change management and leadership; along with relationship-building skills—complement and enhance the clinical skill set of all APNs (Hamric, Spross, & Hanson, 2005; Hickey, Ouimette, & Venegoni, 2000). Credibility is established through clinical competence. Mason, Leavitt, and Chaffee (2002) state, "Once clinical competence has been achieved, then interdependence and collegiality with peer groups is the next level to achieve" (p. 375). Given equal clinical competence, nonclinical skills begin to differentiate one APN's practice from another. Developing and using this repertoire of clinical and nonclinical skills is not optional. In many practice settings, one APN is the symbol for all APNs. This is why positive working relationships with physician colleagues at the local practice level are so powerful. Effective individual working relationships on the local level create an "epiphany" for physicians that make them informed, vocal, and enthusiastic supporters of APN practice with their physician colleagues.

ADVANCED PRACTICE NURSE CLINICAL AND FUDUCIARY LEADERSHIP

Despite these forces and role dynamics, the APN is not a passive player. In fact, as previously stated, the APN occupies the most pivotal position for informing and influencing colleagues about scope of practice, role, and interdisciplinary relationships. By modeling the behaviors of competent APN practice, by actively participating in initially designing the role, and by building relationships with individual physicians, administrators, and colleagues from both nursing and other clinical disciplines, the APN embodies a truly "value-added" role.

The APN must think and act like a leader. As Handy (1989) states, "A leader shapes and shares a vision which gives point to the work of others" (p. 134). By this, Hardy means that the APN must demonstrate qualities of a leader by influencing ideas and building consensus. Within this definition, all APNs are leaders and lead by living the vision. The following example from an experienced, masters' prepared CNM employed by the obstetrical/gynecological department of an academic medical center demonstrates these principles:

> *CNM: The "nurse midwife product" is shaped by the midwifery philosophy of care and the discipline of nursing. We believe pregnancy and childbirth is a normal process; in starting with lower intensity interventions progressing to higher intensity interventions if needed; including the family in care, and in educating and working with the patient so that the patient makes well-informed choices. Barring changes in condition or safety we abide by the patient's choices. This philosophy makes the nurse midwife a patient "advisor." We are in a "co-charge" role with the patient. This is a very different approach from the medical model. The question becomes "Is there a place for the nurse midwifery philosophy of care in the OB practice?" There may be verbal support for the midwifery role and the diversity of service it represents to the community at large, but there may be a lot of ambivalence about a place for midwifery in the OB practice.*
>
> *INTERVIEWER: How does this ambivalence present itself?*
>
> *CNM: . . . . as value equated and measured by technical skill (the number of procedures), as standards of productivity that are measured by the procedures that CNMs do not do, and practicing within someone else's philosophy is expected. The patients are the physicians' patients not the group's patients (physicians and CNMs). I call it "hamburger helper." This happens in primary care too. You step in for certain visits, do specific tasks as requested. There is no room for "independence of thought," anybody can do the tasks (messaging a belly, interpreting blood work, etc.). The tasks are the "overlapping spheres between disciplines." It is the context: what's included in the conversation, what's emphasized that distinguishes providers. These are complementary philosophies. It's the "philosophical compatibility" that enriches care for patients. Rather than a physician substitute, nurse midwives are "an alternative." We fight for our existence every day.*

This CNM is clear in her articulation of what a CNM brings to an obstetrician practice that is different from other providers. She is accepted and recognized by physician colleagues as a superb CNM and as a leader among other CNMs. In addition to her clinical skills, she brings skills in assessing the system of care within which the CNMs function and is thoughtful and purposeful about the interventions to influence the system to change. She is educated about the expectations and ingredients that add value and revenue. In addition she challenges the system by posing the question regarding a place for providers who approach care from a different point of view, rather than as "fillers" or "substitutes" for physicians.

Despite these pressure points, this CNM believes her obstetrician practice is suited to a CNM given the specialty focus and because the revenues and expenses are going into the same cost center. When the CNM reports to nursing there is frequently a disconnect between revenues and expenses. There is no idea about what revenues are being generated by the CNM. Expenses are usually in the nursing cost center and revenues in the obstetrician practice cost center. The CNMs are viewed primarily as an expense. Tracking expenses and revenues is an important activity for all APNs because it better enables measuring financial contributions and makes these contributions more visible. This obstetrician group experienced a steady reduction in its practice sites. Despite the reduction, CNMs maintained the same number of deliveries over an 8-year period, a notable accomplishment. However, in a financially driven practice, maintaining the revenue when there is pressure to increase the gain nullifies the achievement. Hence, "we fight for our existence every day."

For this CNM, the ultimate relationship alignment is to be positioned in a CNM cost center, separate from medicine or nursing. According to the American College of Nurse-Midwives, CNMs are less likely to be in employer/employee relationships and more likely to be in group practices.

Filling in the gaps, noted in the previous excerpt as "hamburger helpers," is a theme that is echoed when APNs are positioned in the nursing service cost center. Some APNs (especially hospital-based CNSs and NPs) prefer this placement because of the clearer connection to the clinical discipline of nursing. APNs can reap the benefits of a clear and unified nursing voice from a nurse executive who is modeling effective working relationships with physician leadership and is visible throughout the organization.

Steeped in the pressures of organizational work, nurse executives, managers, and colleagues may also not have accurate information about the role. Differences in scope of practice, constraints, and demands of the specialty, including time and clinical practice challenges of each specific specialty area, require constant reorientation. The potential gain in visibility and voice that is achieved by being part of a larger community of nursing colleagues can be diminished when these colleagues and the nursing executive leadership and management have limited understanding of the role and the pressing issues facing APNs in practice. Consider the following example:

> *A masters' prepared CNS with a specialty in oncology and ethics was hired into an inpatient unit-based position by the nurse manager of the unit. The position was budgeted for 20 hours per week. Of the 20 hours that were budgeted, 10 hours were allocated to the unit and 10 hours were approved by the nurse manager and those in authority to be distributed throughout the hospital for ethics education and consultation. This arrangement was satisfactory for all parties until the nurse manager resigned from the position. The new nurse manager was displeased with the previously agreed-on arrangement. Why was she paying for 20 hours of CNS time and only receiving the benefits of 10 hours? Where was the CNS spending her time? What was the value added to the unit paying her wage? Why was the 10 hours not being distributed among the beneficiaries instead of coming solely from her unit's budget? Wouldn't she and the unit be better served if the CNS conducted chart reviews or helped to reduce the nurse manager's burden in some way? Renegotiating the role, instructing the nurse manager about the role and where the added value lies for her, and working to legitimize the hours that were spent off the unit became the priority work of this CNS.*

This nurse manager is asking and seeking answers to questions well within her legitimate role and authority. The CNS's relationship to this nurse manager's cost center is clear. In our current fiscal environment, nurse managers are more clearly and strictly instructed to "hold the line" on budgets. Scrutinizing positions and providing justifications for them are expected behaviors in the manager role. These factors combined to create a possessiveness and a feeling of ownership of the CNS's time by the nurse manager. Past agreements were void and in need of renegotiation with this current nurse manager. In the meantime, the CNS felt her position was in jeopardy of elimination at worst and quite possibly "marginalized" at best.

Often APNs in line positions in nursing service feel that nurse managers are no better informed about the nuances of the APN role than nonnurse managers and for that reason do not use the role to its full potential. Lack of clarity about the components of the role prompt many managers to use the APN to do "scut" work or as "filler." This is another opportunity for an APN to reduce the risk factors associated with lack of fundamental accurate information about the role. Each APN has the ability and the responsibility to directly influence the thinking of managers from any discipline, including nursing, if they accept the accountability for doing so as an inherent part of the role.

REIMBURSEMENT: CAN THE POSITION PAY FOR ITSELF?

The source of funding for an APN position provides important information for reporting structures and the corresponding accountability. How much of the cost of the APN is "reimbursed" is a question that runs parallel in importance to the funding for the position. (Some would argue that reimbursement is the first question that is raised before budgeting for an APN role is undertaken.) The issues surrounding reimbursement for APNs are discussed within other chapters in this text. The need for continued change in the reimbursement and regulations governing APN practice is well documented elsewhere in this work and in others (Mason et al., 2002; Safriet, 1992). The importance of reimbursement to this discussion rests in examining the language that is currently in use and how that language is interpreted in the practice setting. How much of the APN's work can be reimbursed? Translated, this ultimately becomes "Can the position pay for itself?"

The federal government was the first to reimburse CNMs and NPs in 1978 under the Civilian Health and Medical Program of the Uniformed Services (CHAMPUS) program. Currently, all categories of NPs and CNSs are reimbursable under CHAMPUS. Medicaid first reimbursed CNMs in 1980 and deemed NP services reimbursable in 1982. The Omnibus Budget and Reconciliation Act (OBRA) of 1989 specifically provided for direct reimbursement by Medicaid of services provided by certified pediatric NPs and certified family NPs (Sellards & Mills, 1995). OBRA '89 also allows an employer of an NP to submit claims to Medicare for NP services rendered to nursing homes or skilled nursing facilities. OBRA '90 contained a provision granting reimbursement to NPs and CNSs who deliver services in rural areas.

Implementation of the Balanced Budget Act of 1997 established reimbursement to NPs and CNSs under Medicare Part B in all geographical areas. For the first time, these APNs were recognized Medicare providers with their own provider numbers under which to bill for services provided, regardless of geographical area. The reimbursement rate for NPs who bill under their own provider number is 80% of the lesser of the actual charge, or 85% of the physician fee schedule. The reimbursement rate for NP services billed and submitted under the "incident to" physician provision remains at 100%. Although it was expected that the incident to provision would be eliminated as a result of this legislation, which went into effect January 1, 1998, to date it is still in place in the outpatient setting. (In the hospital setting, the "shared visit rule" is used when the service is split or shared between a physician and nonphysician provider from the same group practice and the physician provides any face to face portion of the evaluation or management of the patient).

Economically, the incident to provision remains appealing even though it carries with it two mandatory provisions that restrict the NPs scope of practice and dictates the APN/physician relationship.

The first provision states that the physician under whose number the bill is submitted must be on site at the time the service is rendered. The second provision states that the APN cannot initiate a plan of care, but he or she can follow the plan of care as dictated by the physician. Some settings have developed policies that require a physician signature of the NP's progress note to "prove" that the physician was on site at the time the service was rendered. Such policies were developed and implemented as a response to interpretations of reimbursement regulations to prove physician involvement that justified the additional 15% fee. Requiring physician signatures on NPs' progress notes was interpreted by many physicians and administrators as a supervision requirement of NP practice, when in fact it was strictly a billing policy. This interpretation reinforces the traditional hierarchical model. Such financial policies designed, developed, and implemented to comply with the "supervision" requirement for reimbursement regulations imposed restrictions that went well beyond those promulgated by some state nurse practice acts. The result is an unnecessary narrowing of the scope of NP practice.

Policies based on misinterpretations such as these create confusion and needless oversight of NP practice on the part of physicians and administrators. Clarifying the differences between the reimbursement definition of supervision and the particular state's scope of practice definition of supervision becomes the work of every NP in practice. This is arduous and often frustrating work; however, it is work that can be done only at the grassroots level and is every bit as important as providing competent clinical care. If it is not attended to in practice, the NP's role is in financial jeopardy. This poses a direct threat to the viability of the position.

Billing incident to makes it more tedious (although not impossible) to track the APN's volume (i.e., financial contribution) to a practice because bills are submitted under the physician's provider number rather than the NP's provider number. Some practices separate the "service provider" (the NP) from the "billing provider" (the physician) to track who gets credit for the visit and for generating the revenue.

Creating opportunities to improve cash flow is life sustaining for any business. Translated to dollars, the hard-won success of NPs and CNSs to bill for services using their own provider number (represented by the Balanced Budget Act) means a decrease of revenue to the practice of 15% per patient. Annualized, this may mean too significant a reduction in revenues for many settings. For the decision makers holding the purse strings, these are clear and straightforward financial decisions: use both options for as long as allowed, that is, bill using the incident to provision when a physician is on site and bill under the NP's own provider number when the physician is not on site. When the incident to provision is eliminated, as many predict, there will be a point of choice for the decision makers in practice settings. If economics is the primary driving force behind practice management decisions, many APN positions may be in jeopardy.

Many believe that "as Medicare goes, so go the other insurers." Viewed as the pacesetters for other third-party carriers, it has been predicted that more of the other insurers will follow Medicare's lead. Medicaid, although partially funded on the federal level, is managed with fund disbursement on the state level. Therefore, even if federal regulations have allowed for 100% reimbursement of APN services, the state law must recognize the APN as a provider of service for reimbursement to occur. And reimbursement varies from state to state as to which category of APN and which services provided by the APN are covered by Medicaid (Meredith & Horan, 2000). Decisions made by managed care companies, private indemnity insurance companies (fee-for-service companies), health maintenance organizations, and other insurers also vary from state to state in scope and in the amounts reimbursed. Reimbursement continues to expand for NP services in most states (Pearson, 2008). In the meantime, APNs are held hostage to those who pay their salaries as they interpret each state's reimbursement and practice regulations.

Implementing on the local level the hard-won gains made in the political and legislative arenas is a challenge for every APN. Financially driven decisions and billing policies like the one noted previously serve as prompts for some APNs to seek other employment options. In these options, APNs seek greater influence, decision-making authority, and accountability regarding finances, schedules, and inter- and intradisciplinary clinical relationships. Increasingly more varied for each specialty, options are limited by the regulations for direct reimbursement in each state. Freedom to make these choices allows the realignment from the singular bottom line of economics to the "triple bottom line" of economics, patient care, and accountability for results. These arrangements are described by some APNs as the ones that allow for the closest patient-centered interrelationships among clinical disciplines. APNs have long been the sole providers of care in many underserved rural areas, nursing homes, and long-term care facilities. The APNs in these settings are recruited, given incentives, and reimbursed without challenge. Only recently because of changes in reimbursement has this movement spread to more populated locations. As reimbursement options expand (e.g., through Medicare Part B, Medicaid, and commercial insurance), more and more NPs in primary care are joining their CRNA and CNS colleagues and forming practices with other NPs in mainstream locations. Although this is a much smaller and more recent movement, these NP practices are offering service options to patients. In 1997 the Department of Veterans' Affairs began to reimburse NPs in solo practice (Warshaw, 1998). The highly publicized NP practice (the Columbia Advanced Practice Nurse Associates), affiliated with Columbia University School of Nursing and Columbia Presbyterian Medical Center in New York City, measured and compared outcomes of NP and physician care in the primary care setting. The direct comparison of outcomes was comparable for patients with NPs and physicians as providers with the same authority, responsibilities, productivity, administrative requirements, and patient populations (Mundinger et al., 2000).

CRNAs were the first nursing specialty to be accorded direct reimbursement rights under the Medicare program in 1986 (American Association of Nurse Anesthetists [AANA], 2008). Consider the following from a conversation with a CRNA who has been in private solo practice for 18 years:

CRNA: The advantages of private practice (for me) is that of being my own boss. There is more financial freedom and more freedom to practice. As sole owner of the corporation, contracts are made with surgeons and surgical centers. If necessary I subcontract to other CRNAs. Reimbursement for services allows this to happen. I set my own fees, do my own billing through a billing service, bill the patient or the insurance company directly (with a 98% collection rate), and maintain my own malpractice insurance. I work very closely with the surgeons and centers that contract for my services. There's a strong sense of comradery. The primary goal is to meet the needs of the patients. We are most interested in patient care rather than economics because we are all getting paid for our services. There is no competition to keep you out, though it is harder to get a contract in a fairly large hospital.

INTERVIEWER: What are the disadvantages to private practice?

CRNA: The downside is when there is no work, there is no salary. For example, one of the surgeons I contract with is taking a month off. It's been a busy month prior so it should work out fine. I always have the option of marketing to others. I started by advertising and marketing to office surgery centers primarily. The relationships developed over time with two or three centers.

INTERVIEWER: What is the patient response?

CRNA: Generally it's fine. Every once in a while a patient will request an anesthesiologist and that's their right. Most patients like the idea that the surgeon and I work together regularly, so we are very familiar with each other's practice. We have a familiarity with each other that instills a comfort level in patients.

This CRNA, like many of her APN colleagues, speaks of the advantages and the freedom that private practice brings. The disadvantages noted are few. For these APNs, the work of marketing and financing their own practice offers the most personal and professional rewards and the highest degree of choice for the patients and providers.

Other arrangements find APNs in dual clinical and administrative roles in a variety of settings (e.g., operating rooms, student health services, primary care, and ambulatory clinic settings). In these positions, APNs are in administrative leadership roles, developing and managing budgets, and influencing practice and organizational policies while continuing clinical work in the APN role. In these arrangements, physicians, and members of other clinical disciplines administratively are accountable to the APN. The role reversal of physicians reporting to APNs introduces dynamics that are variations on the themes previously discussed. In these arrangements, the clinical alliances around patient care must be developed and maintained, although the administrative relationships are reversed from the traditional hierarchical alignment. In some settings this works well. In others, problems surface. This is reportedly as much related to the nature of the people involved as it is to the roles. This multifaceted role requires multifaceted skills. In a legitimate and more visible leadership role, with corresponding organizational responsibilities, these APNs balance the clinical role behaviors of APN with the role behaviors of administrator/manager/leader. As organization leaders, these APNs are in highly visible positions to inform, educate, and influence thinking about APN roles and practice. These positions afford APNs a more public forum to educate to the APN role.

CONCLUSION

There is wide variation of opinion regarding the preferred reporting arrangements among the four categories of APNs. In fact there may not be any specific arrangement that would be agreed on by the majority. There is little difference of opinion on the characteristics of preferred alignments, including enabling the clinical work, providing for ongoing knowledge and skill development within the specialty, functioning within the full scope of practice allowed by law and regulation, differentiating advance practice from the practice of other colleagues (physician and non-physician), and fair and equitable compensation for services. APNs seek out these characteristics in the preferred arrangements, whether located in traditional employee/employer arrangements or in private, solo, or group practice settings.

There is little variation in the opinion that finances dictate the alignments. Along with the finances comes the authority to make decisions and exercise options. Implementation of an accurate interpretation of reimbursement regulations is imperative at the practice level.

Although crucial political and legislative battles continue on the national level between organized nursing and medicine, individual APNs and groups of APNs in every practice setting carry on the work of care while continuing to develop and maintain effective working relationships with individual physician and nonphysician colleagues. They model the behaviors of advanced practice, including collegiality, joint problem solving, stewardship of scarce resources, and leadership. The general lack of understanding and accurate information regarding APN roles by nurses, physicians, administrators, and colleagues from other disciplines can lead to intradisciplinary and interdisciplinary role conflicts. It then becomes imperative that each APN accept accountability to educate and accurately inform colleagues of the salience of the role to practice management issues. Each individual APN is a symbol of all APNs and as such is in an incredibly powerful position to influence thinking and change perceptions one relationship at a time. This cannot be underestimated nor should it be underused.

Our society recognizes value in terms of money. When all is said and done, the most powerful predictor of reporting arrangements comes down to finances. Whoever pays the APN's salary has the ultimate authority in any setting to create, define, influence, and position the advanced practice role.

References

American Association of Nurse Anesthetists. (2008). *Nurse anesthetists at a glance.* Retrieved October 4, 2008, from the American Association of Nurse Anesthetists Web site: www.aana.com/crna/ataglance.asp.

Benner, P. A., Tanner, C. A., & Chesla, C. A. (1996). *Expertise in nursing practice.* New York: Springer.

Hamric, A. B., Spross, J. A., & Hanson, C. M. (2005). *Advanced nursing practice: An integrative approach* (3rd ed.). Philadelphia: WB Saunders.

Handy, C. (1989). *The age of unreason.* Boston: Harvard Business School.

Hickey, J. V., Ouimette, R. M., & Venegoni, S. L. (2000). *Advanced practice nursing.* Baltimore: Lippincott Williams & Wilkins.

Hirschhorn, L., & Gilmore, T. (1992). The new boundaries of the boundaryless company. *Harvard Business Review, 92*(304), 104–115.

Mason, D. J., Leavitt, J. K., & Chaffee, M. W. (2002). *Policy and politics in nursing and healthcare.* Philadelphia: WB Saunders.

Meredith, P. V., & Horan, N. M. (2000). *Adult primary care.* Philadelphia: WB Saunders.

McShane, S. L., & Von Glinow, M. A. (2000). *Organizational behavior.* Boston: Irwin McGraw-Hill.

Mundinger, M. O., Kane, R. L., Lenz, E. R., Totten, A. M., Tsai, W. Y., Cleary, P. D., et al. (2000). Primary care outcomes in patients treated by nurse practitioners. *Journal of the American Medical Association, 283*(1), 59–68.

Nickels, W. G., McHugh, J. M., & McHugh, S. M. (1999). *Understanding business.* Boston: Irwin McGraw-Hill.

Pearson, L. (2008). Twentieth annual legislative update. *The Nurse Practitioner, 33*(1), 10–34.

Safriet, B. J. (1992). Health care dollars and regulatory sense: The role of advanced practice nursing. *Yale Journal on Regulation, 9*(2), 417–488.

Satir, V., Banmen, J., Gerber, J., & Gomori, M. (1991). *The Satir model family therapy and beyond.* Palo Alto, CA: Science and Behavior Books.

Sellards, S., & Mills, M. E. (1995). Administrative issues for use of nurse practitioners. *Journal of Nursing Administration, 25*(5), 64–70.

Warshaw, R. (1998). Too much independence for NPs? *American College of Physicians Observer.* Retrieved June 3, 2003 from the American College of Physicians Web site: www.acponline.org/journals/news/Jan98/toomuch.htm.

Competency in Advanced Practice

14

Evidence-Based Practice

Deborah C. Messecar
Christine A. Tanner

INTRODUCTION

Translating evidence into practice is a key skill for advanced practice nurses (APNs). Evidence-based practice builds on the process of using knowledge gleaned from systematic reviews and the results of individual studies, but includes much more, such as evidence from opinion leaders, the products of reasoning, and patient preferences, to name a few (Melnyk & Fineout-Overholt, 2005). With nursing's long history of efforts to increase use of research in practice, the movement to teach evidence-based methods for clinical decision making has intensified in APN programs. A second major impetus for the movement to evidence-based practice is the growth of scientific evidence supporting health care and the development of methods for integrating the available evidence expeditiously into guidelines for practice. Information technology has greatly augmented our abilities to access this information. A third factor is that media dissemination of information has made patients increasingly savvy about different available treatments, enabling them to ask more informed questions about their illnesses and care. Fourth, the urgency of using evidence to improve clinical care has been highlighted by new Institute of Medicine (IOM) reports on knowing what works in health care (IOM, 2008) as well as prior reports on quality and safety (IOM, 2001, 2004).

The objective of this chapter is to present an updated review of clinical judgement and the different patterns of clinical reasoning and their relationship to evidence-based practice. New conclusions from research on clinical judgment are presented to illustrate how nurses use reasoning patterns as they assess patients, selectively attend to clinical cues, interpret these data, and respond or intervene. The role of context, the knowledge and experience background of the nurse, and the effect of knowing the patient on these reasoning processes is described. A research-based model of clinical judgment (Tanner, 2006) is presented to provide a framework for understanding how the APN can draw on clinical decision-making skills developed over time in practice along with new skills in accessing and evaluating evidence to continuously improve the methods of care he or she is employing. In addition, tips on how to access and evaluate research evidence to improve the quality of the APN's clinical judgments are provided.

EVIDENCE-BASED PRACTICE: DEFINED

Historically there has not been uniform agreement about what is included in evidence-based health care (Tanner, 1999). Evidenced-based practice was initially presented as a new paradigm in health professions practice. This approach devalued intuition, the use of clinical opinion based on experience, and basic scientific rationale as sufficient grounds for clinical decision making, and instead stressed the examination of evidence solely from clinical research (Bergus & Hamm, 1995). The aim of evidence-based practice defined in this manner is to reduce wider variations in individual clinician's practices, eliminating worst practices and enhancing best practices, thereby reducing costs and improving quality. This goal and the assumptions underlying what counts as evidence were troubling to many clinicians (Dearlove, Rogers, & Sharples, 1996; Mitchell, 1999; Smith, 1996). Their concern was that expert clinical judgment would be replaced by a cookbook approach to decision making. In response to this criticism, Sackett, Rosenberg, Gray, Haynes, and Richardson (1996) revised their definition of evidence-based medicine to be more comprehensive in its view of what counts as evidence and what should figure into decisions regarding patient care:

> *Evidence based medicine is the conscientious, explicit, and judicious use of current best evidence in making decisions about the care of individual patients. The practice of evidence based medicine means integrating individual clinical expertise with the best available external clinical evidence from systematic research (p. 71).*

This view recognized individual clinical expertise, which is defined as the proficiency and judgment that individual clinicians acquire through clinical experience and clinical practice, as a valid source of evidence. Increased expertise not only includes more effective and efficient diagnosis, but also more thoughtful identification and compassionate use of individual patients' predicaments, rights, and preferences in making clinical decisions about their care (Sackett et al., 1996). Best available external clinical evidence was defined as clinically relevant research, which may include basic sciences research, but was preferentially from patient-centered clinical research that focuses on the accuracy and precision of diagnostic tests (including the clinical examination), the power of prognostic markers, and the efficacy and safety of interventions. Use of external clinical evidence should invalidate previously accepted diagnostic tests and treatments and replace them with new ones that are more powerful, more accurate, more efficacious, and safer. External clinical evidence can inform, but can never replace, individual clinical expertise, and it is this expertise that decides whether the external evidence applies to the individual patient at all, and if so, how it should be integrated into a clinical decision.

RESEARCH ON CLINCIAL JUDGMENT AND THE RELATIONSHIP TO EVIDENCE-BASED PRACTICE

What is clinical judgment? Almost all health professionals view clinical judgment as an essential skill. In nursing, the terms clinical *decision making* or *problem solving*, and more recently *critical thinking* have been used interchangeably to refer to the same phenomenon, which has been viewed as a disengaged, analytical, and objective process, directed toward resolution of problems and achievement of clearly defined ends. However, recent research on expert practice suggests that clinical judgment is far more complex (Tanner, 2006) and incorporates skills that look more like engaged practical reasoning. Engaged practical reasoning occurs when the nurse recognizes a pattern by being attuned to subtle changes in the patient's clinical state and other salient information and then forms an intuitive clinical grasp of the situation without evident forethought (Tanner, Benner, Chesla, & Gordon, 1993). This flexible and nuanced ability to read the clinical situation is key to interpreting what is going on and responding appropriately. Knowledge of the illness experience for both the patient and the family as well as their physical, social, and emotional strengths and weaknesses are just as important as clinical features of the disease.

Clinical judgment is thus defined as an understanding or inference about a patient's needs, concerns, or health problems, followed by the decision to act (or not act), to use or modify standard approaches, or to improvise new ones as deemed appropriate by the patient's response (Tanner, 2006).

Clinical reasoning, in contrast to clinical judgement, is the thinking process by which clinicians make their judgments and includes both the process of generating alternatives, weighing them against the evidence, and choosing the most appropriate course of action (Tanner, 2006).

Clinical judgment has been studied from different theoretical perspectives (Benner, Tanner, & Chesla, 1996; Brannon & Carson, 2003; Kosowski & Roberts, 2003; Ritter, 2003; Simmons, Lanuza, Fonteyn, Hicks, & Holm, 2003; White, 2003), clinical foci (McCarthy, 2003) and with different research methods (Benner et al., 1996, Kosowski & Roberts, 2003; McDonald, Frakes, Apostolidis, Armstrong, Goldblatt, & Bernardo, 2003; Ritter, 2003; Simmons et al., 2003; White, 2003). From this growing body of literature on clinical judgement, several general conclusions can be drawn.

The Clinician's Background Is More Influential on Clinical Judgment Than Objective Data

The clinician's background influences his or her clinical judgment in a given clinical situation more than the objective data at hand. Clinical judgment requires knowledge, which is abstract, generalizable, and applicable in many situations. Knowledge required for clinical judgment is derived from science and theory and grows with experience as scientific abstractions are filled out in practice. This knowledge is often tacit and is an important factor in aiding clinicians to recognize clinical states instantaneously.

The clinician's background includes experiential learning, particularly that gleaned from personal clinical experience. Three types of knowledge play a part in how the clinician perceives a given situation. Theoretical knowledge, which is acquired through understanding of scientifically derived knowledge and theory, is used in a particular situation as a specific application of an abstract rule or principle. The description of techniques of examination of the thorax and lungs in a physical assessment text is an example of theoretical knowledge that may be applied by the clinician to individual patients. Practical knowledge is acquired through working with many patients. So, adapting or revising one's examination of the thorax and lung techniques for a patient that cannot sit up based on one's past experience or the experience of others is an example of practical knowledge. Knowledge, both theoretical and practical, often determines what stands out as important in a particular situation. Research-based knowledge can contribute to the clinician's overall knowledge base for assessing risks. Knowledge helps the clinician selectively observe. Research directed toward describing phenomena of concern to the nurse helps provide information about what cues are highly associated with particular problems. This allows the nurse, using this knowledge base, to select data relevant to determining the problems the patient may be experiencing. Knowledge also guides action and contributes the clinician's repertoire of interventions.

An additional essential component of the knowledge required for clinical judgment is the importance of knowing the individual patient and being able to draw on this understanding to better predict and anticipate individual patient responses (Benner et al., 1996, Peden-McAlpine & Clark, 2002). Clinicians come to clinical situations with their own perspectives on what is good and right, and these values profoundly influence what they attend to, the options they consider using, and ultimately what they decide to do (Benner et al., 1996; Ellefsen, 2004). The clinician's outlook is not determined by individual notions of right and wrong, but rather is developed through interaction with others in the practice discipline. For example, the ethic for disclosure to patients and families or the importance of comfort in the face of impending death sets up what will be noticed in a given clinical exchange and will shape the way in which the clinician responds. Stereotypes and biases also affect perception.

Good Clinical Judgment Requires Knowing the Patient and Responding to Their Concerns

In addition to theoretical and practical knowledge, knowledge of the particular patient, both knowing their typical responses and knowing the patient as a person are central to good clinical judgment (Sackett, Haynes, Guyatt, & Tugwell, 1991; Tanner et al., 1993). When the clinician knows the typical patterns of responses, certain aspects of the situation stand out as salient and others recede in importance. Comparing the current picture to the patient's typical picture allows the clinician to make important qualitative distinctions about how a patient's condition has or has not changed. Knowing the patient facilitates the provision of individualized care.

Knowing patients is defined as a taken-for-granted understanding of patients that come from working with them, listening to their accounts of their experiences with illness, watching them closely, and understanding how they typically respond (Tanner et al., 1993). This tacit knowledge, which the clinician may not be able to fully describe to an outside observer, is more than what can be obtained in formal assessments. Knowing the typical pattern of responses, certain aspects of a patient's situation stand out as salient, and other aspects of that same patient situation may recede in importance. Understanding how this patient responds under these circumstances forms the basis for the individualized care called for by the 'IOM's report (2001) on quality.

The level of involvement with the patient influences the way the clinician engages in problem solving, the outcome of the process, and the sense of satisfaction on the part of the clinician (Benner et al., 1996). Central to sound clinical decision making is a concern for revealing and responding to patients as persons, respecting their dignity, and caring for them in ways that preserve their personhood. Developing a sense about the right level of involvement is a skill learned through experience. The skilled clinician has a good clinical grasp, recognizing both familiar and individual patterns. The patient's responses to the nurse's actions are observed, and the nurse's reactions are then modified according to how the patient is responding (Tanner, 2006). Clinical grasp and clinical response are therefore inextricably linked.

Clinical Judgment Is Influenced by the Context in Which Care Occurs

Neither context nor emotions have typically been accounted for in most models of rational decision making. Models of decision making that ignore context, emotion, and the individual's experience eliminate the possibility of seeing these as important in clinical judgment. However, from the work of Benner et al. (1996), we know that judgment occurs in the context of a particular situation, when the nurse is emotionally attuned to the situation, and meaningful aspects simply stand out as important and the choice of responses is guided by the nurse's interpretation of the particular situation. The context for practice that influences decisions to test and treat can include political and social milieu (Tanner, 2006), as well as patient factors like socioeconomic status (Scott, Schiell, & King, 1996). Another view is that social judgment or moral evaluation of patients is socially embedded, independent of patient characteristics, and as much a function of the pervasive norms and attitudes of the clinicians in a given setting (McDonald et al., 2003).

For clinician providers, health care is increasingly practiced in a context of heightened accountability (Klardie, Johnson, McNaughton, & Meyers, 2004). APNs are expected to demonstrate that they can provide care that is both clinically and cost effective (DeBourgh, 2001; Younglut &

Brooten, 2001). The struggle for the APN in this environment is to deliver quality cost-effective care while still incorporating the needs and preferences of the individual patient (Klardie et al., 2004).

Clinicians Use a Variety of Clinical Reasoning Patterns Alone or in Combination

Work in the art of medical decision making has illustrated that the essence of clinical reasoning continues to elude understanding (Sox, Blatt, Higgins, & Marton, 1991). In studies conducted with nurses during the past 20 years, evidence suggests that nurses use a variety of reasoning patterns alone or in combination (Tanner, 2006). The pattern of reasoning that the clinician uses depends on the demands of the situation, the goals of the practice, the clinician's experience with similar situations, and the perception of what makes excellent practice. The reasoning patterns used are influenced by the nurse's knowledge, biases, and values; the relationship with the patient; and other factors in the clinical situation.

Analytic Processes

An analytic reasoning pattern is characteristic of a beginner's performance or a more experienced clinician when stumped. Analytic reasoning is characterized by deliberate, rational thought that includes the generation of alternatives, weighing against evidence, and evaluating possible courses of action. Analytic reasoning can be influenced by biases and stereotypes. Diagnostic reasoning is an example of analytic thinking. This is a process in which the clinician attends to presenting signs and symptoms (cues), generates alternative explanations for the cues (diagnostic hypotheses), collects additional data to help rule in or rule out possible explanations, systematically evaluates each explanation in light of the data, and arrives at a diagnosis, or inference, about the patient's health status. Once sufficient data are gathered, the process of evaluating hypotheses begins.

Intuition

Intuition is characterized by immediate grasping of a clinical situation and is a function of familiarity with similar experiences (Benner et al., 1996). Intuition is a judgment without a rationale. Researchers speculate that intuition is a form of pattern recognition in which the practitioner picks up on cues that are perceived as a whole and are not arrived at through conscious, linear analytic processes. Experienced clinicians develop a sense of salience, in which important aspects of a given clinical situation stand out because of past experience with similar situations. Rational calculation is not required to make use of this form of reasoning; however, deliberative rationality may be used to check out the soundness of conclusions derived from intuition. The role and desirability of intuitive reasoning patterns continues to be controversial within the nursing literature. Intuition has been decried as a poor substitute for science. In this view, intuition is minimized as nothing more than a special case of inference, drawing on rational processes that are unconscious and inaccessible (Crow & Spicer, 1995; English, 1993).

Narrative Thinking

Evidence suggests that narratives are an important part of clinical reasoning (Bruner, 1986; Kleinman, 1988). Patient narratives provide us with access to understanding the experience of health and illness. Bruner claims that human motives, intents, and meanings are understood through narrative thinking, which he contrasts with paradigmatic thinking that conforms to the rules of logic. Paradigmatic thinking is thinking through propositional argument. Narrative thinking is thinking through telling and interpreting stories. The difference between these two types of thinking involves how humans make sense of and explain what they see. Propositional argument is making sense of a particular by seeing it as an instance of a general type. Narrative thinking is trying to understand the particular case. Kleinman has identified the importance of understanding the narrative component of illness, claiming that patient narratives may help clinicians direct their attention not only to the biological world of disease, but also to the human world of meanings, values, and concerns.

Hence, patient narratives help clinicians to focus their attention not only on the patient's disease problems, but also on the meaning of that illness for that particular patient and on the affect that disease will have on the patient's lifestyle and ways of coping. Hearing the account of an experience with an illness not only improves the understanding of the patient's overall situation, it helps identify problem-solving priorities that cannot be made explicit through disengaged analytical reasoning. Studies of physicians (Borges & Waitzkin, 1995; Hunter, 1991) and nurses (Benner et al., 1996; Zerwekh, 1992) suggest that narrative reasoning creates deep background understanding of the patient as a person; consequently, clinicians' judgments can only be understood against this background.

Clinical narratives are a way of teaching and learning from other care providers and a way of reflecting on and understanding one's own practice. By dialoguing with others who may have different vantage points, knowledge about clinical situations is produced that helps to limit tunnel vision and snap judgments. Using narrative as a way of communicating with other health providers leads to learning how to better identify signs and symptoms in particular patient populations, knowing particular patients and learning to recognize how those patients respond, and identifying clinical experts with whom you can consult (Benner et al., 1996). Discussing your observations and data with more experienced clinicians enhances clinical judgment. Even as an experienced nurse, you consult with colleagues, draw on others' perspectives, and benefit from the pooled experience of other clinicians. Clinical narratives and the multiple perspectives of skilled clinicians work together with science and technology to create knowledge that is both cumulative and reliable.

Clinical reasoning can also include processes, which might be characterized as engaged practical reasoning. Engaged practical reasoning includes recognition of a pattern, an intuitive clinical grasp, or a response without evident forethought. Conditions of uncertainty are what prompt the seeking, appraising, and implementation of new knowledge by clinicians. Uncertainty occurs when the best course of action to take, or best decision, is not readily apparent. The openness to accept that there may be different, and possibly more effective, methods of care than those that are currently employed acts as the impetus to weighing evidence against expectations, norms, or standards.

Reflection on Practice Is Often Triggered by a Breakdown in Clinical Judgment

Reflection is defined as a process of thinking about and exploring an issue of concern triggered by an experience. For example, clinicians are often troubled by a patient encounter that did not go well. Reflecting on the meaning of an experience, making sense of it, and incorporating it into one's view of self and the world is part of everyday life. Reflection prompts the clinician to identify new information or alternative perspectives that can be helpful in future encounters. To engage in reflection, the clinician has to be able to connect the patient's response and outcomes with specific clinical actions. Narrative is an important tool of reflection; having and telling stories of one's experience as a clinician helps turn experience into practical knowledge (Aström, Norberg, Hallberg, & Jansson, 1995; Benner et al., 1996). Use of reflection is a habit and a skill that can be cultivated and developed over time. Through the introspective process of connecting one's actions to patient outcomes, reflection has the potential for generating new knowledge (Kuiper & Pesut, 2004; Ruth-Sahd, 2003).

Model of Clinical Judgment

A research-based model of clinical judgment developed by Tanner in 1998 and revised in 2006 is presented in **Figure 14-1.** There are four key phases in the model. The first is "noticing" in which the clinician develops a perceptual grasp of the situation at hand. In this phase, the clinician's expectations of the situation are formed as a result of his or her knowledge of the patient; clinical or practical knowledge of similar patients; and textbook, and hopefully, research-based knowledge. The context of the clinical situation will further influence the initial grasp of the situation. The second phase depicted in the model is "interpreting." In this phase the clinician forms their understanding of the situation by using one or more reasoning patterns. Assessments and additional data collection may be conducted to rule out hypotheses until the clinician reaches an interpretation that supports an appropriate response. During the "responding"' phase, the clinician may act or chose not to act depending on the situation. "Reflecting" occurs when the clinician observes the patient's responses to the action taken. Reflection-in-action refers to the clinician's ability to see how he or she is responding to the action—and adjust the treatment based on that assessment. Much of this reflection-in-action is tacit and not obvious. Reflection-on-action with its subsequent clinical learning completes the cycle, showing what clinicians gain from their experience contributes to their ongoing clinical knowledge development and their capacity for clinical judgment in future situations.

Summary

The model of clinical judgment presented provides a framework for improving the quality of the clinical judgment used by the APN. First, the model illustrates where in the process of clinical reasoning the knowledge that might be obtained by external evidence can be applied. Second, the model recognizes the value of clinical expertise initially not accounted for by proponents of evidence-based practice. Third, because the model recognizes a broader range of contextual factors that could affect the patient's responses, it is more inclusive in the types of research that are viewed as valid. Fourth, because the model incorporates the value of knowing the patient in the clinical reasoning process, it supports a model of patient-centered care (IOM, 2001).

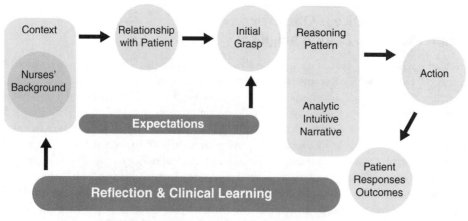

FIGURE 14-1 A model of clinical judgment.

ACCESSING AND EVALUATING RESEARCH EVIDENCE TO IMPROVE CLINICAL JUDGMENTS

Clinicians are under increasing pressure to keep up to date and to base their practice more firmly on evidence (DeBourgh, 2001), but few have the necessary time or skills to do this (Melnyk & Fineout-Overhold, 2005; Rosswurm & Larrabee, 1999; Youngblut & Brooten, 2001). Clinicians may see an overwhelming number of patients during the week, and during each encounter several questions may arise concerning diagnosis, prognosis, treatment, and general care. When asked, clinicians reported that they generate a number of unanswered questions in their patient encounters, a median of one question for every 10 patients they see (Covell, Uman, & Manning, 1985; Gorman, 1993, 2001). Only one-third of these questions are answered at the time of the clinical contact or the point of care (Gorman, 1993), and only little better than half are pursued after the clinical contact (Gorman, 2001).

Yet several problems exist with using the research literature for evidence-based primary care and hospital practice, especially in rural settings (Gorman, 1993, 2001; Melynyk & Fineout-Overhold, 2005; Shapiro, 2007). First, historically only a small fraction of the total research literature included efficacy studies of clinical practice that form the basis for evidence-based medicine (Haynes, 1993). This clinical research literature has been beset for decades with study design and reporting problems (Fletcher & Fletcher, 1979; Schor & Karten, 1966)—problems that continued to exist in the randomized trial (Moher, Jadad, Nichol, Penman, Tugwell, & Walsh, 1995), systematic review (Moher, Cook, Eastwood, Olkin, Rennie, & Stroup, 1999; Sacks, Reitman, Pagano, & Kupelnick, 1996), and guidelines (Shaneyfelt, Mayo-Smith, & Rothwangl, 1999) literature. In the past, it was not surprising that most clinicians considered the research literature to be unmanageable (Gorman, 2001; Melynyk & Fineout-Overhold, 2005; Shapiro, 2007; Williamson, German, Weiss, Skinner, & Bowes III, 1989) and of limited applicability to clinical practice (Greer, 1988; McAlister, Graham, Karr, & Laupacis, 1999). On top of this difficulty, many clinicians do not know how to interpret the statistical results of the studies they do locate (Windish, Huot, & Green, 2007). If clinical research is to improve clinical care, it must be relevant, of high quality, and accessible, and clinicians must have the skills they need to use it.

To access the best possible evidence at the point of clinical contact, the clinician should work on the development of several competencies that support evidence-based practice.

Competencies That Support Evidence-Based Practice

Focusing on Outcomes

Evidence-based medicine has been widely promoted as a means of improving clinical outcomes. To focus on outcomes in medical decision making, Bergus and Hamm (1995) suggest that clinicians use the following four-step process. First, the clinician forms an internal mental framework for the decision task, sketching out the potential treatment options and outcomes. Next, the changes in the different outcomes are estimated. In collaboration with the patient and family, the values of the potential outcomes are considered. The course of action that, on average, will result in the best outcome is then chosen. The scientific evidence—base rate information, sensitivity, specificity, positive predictive value of a positive test results, and proportion of the population positively affected by certain interventions—is the information needed for estimating the likelihood of achieving different outcomes with different courses of action.

Sackett, Straus, Richardson, Rosenberg, and Haynes (2000) and Straus, Richardson, Glasziou, and Haynes (2005) in their guidebooks on the practice and teaching of evidence-based medicine, define the best research evidence as patient-centered clinical research into the accuracy and precision of diagnostic tests, prognostic markers, and interventions. These elements of evidence used for predicting outcomes are defined and described in **Table 14-1.** Several practical implications can be drawn from review of the definitions of the core concepts in the table. For example, to determine the predictive value of a test, clinicians need good estimates of the prevalence or probability of disease in a patient. A limitation of this approach to best evidence is nursing's interest in questions beyond diagnostic tests and interventions (Jennings, 2000). Although evidence from qualitative exploratory studies is not usually included in texts on evidence-based medicine, these studies are also helpful for guiding advanced practice decision making. These studies inform our decision making by helping us better understand patient responses. Understanding patient responses is a critical condition for using reflection to engage in clinical learning.

Asking Answerable Questions

The inability to ask a focused and precise clinical question can be a major impediment to evidence-based practice. To build skill in asking focused clinical questions, it helps to categorize questions according to their level of specificity and according to whom the question applies, the intervention being considered, and the outcomes of interest.

Clinical questions can be categorized into needs for background and foreground knowledge (Sackett et al., 2000; Straus et al., 2005). Background knowledge is needed when our experience with a condition or problem is limited. Background questions ask *who, what, for whom, why, where, when,* and *how well?* Framing a background question is relatively easy because the question is usually asking in general about a disorder. Finding information to answer background questions is also relatively easy. Sources of information likely to provide answers to these questions include textbooks, drug guides or other reference books, and narrative review articles—summaries of an area or topic written by an expert in the field (McKibbon & Marks, 2001).

As clinicians grow in experience, they have increasing numbers of questions about the foreground of managing patients. Foreground questions are prompted by a precise need for information about a specific clinical situation. This skill of framing foreground questions can be improved by breaking the question down into its component parts. Think about the subjects or groups involved, what intervention is being used, and what the outcomes of interest are. The four key elements of foreground questions are: the patient or problem, the intervention or treatment, the comparison intervention or treatment, and the outcome of interest (Sackett et al., 2000; Straus et al., 2005). Foreground questions typically require more information sources to adequately supply the answers (McKibbon & Marks, 2001). For example, questions about treatment effectiveness are best addressed by evidence from a randomized controlled trial (RCT) design, whereas questions about patients' feelings and perceptions about their illness experiences are better addressed in studies that use a qualitative design.

Using the Clinical Literature

The clinical literature can be used for regular surveillance or keeping up to date and for problem-oriented searches. To conduct searchers on a regular basis, clinicians need effective searching skills and easy access to bibliographic databases. After the answerable question has been identified, use the population/problem, intervention, comparison, outcome, time (PICOT) format to help frame the literature search **(Box 14-1).** The PICOT format is a particularly useful framework to help novice searchers organize their electronic database searchers (Craig & Smyth, 2007; Melnyk & Fineout-Overhold, 2005; Shapiro, 2007).

TABLE 14-1		
Information Needed for Estimating the Likelihood of Achieving Different Outcomes with Different Courses of Action		
Core Concept	**Definition**	**Features**
Base rate information: prevalence	The proportion of persons in a given population who have a particular disease at a point or interval of time	Useful for health services planning. May be the only rates available. Prevalence studies are particularly useful in guiding decisions about diagnosis and treatment. Knowing that a patient has a given probability of having a disease influences the use and interpretation of diagnostic tests.
Base rate information: incidence	New cases in a specified period	Use incidence rates when (a) you are comparing the development of disease in different population groups; (b) you are attempting to determine whether a relationship exists between a possible causal factor and a disease. Allows you to determine whether the probability of developing a disease differs in different populations or periods in relationship to specific causal factors.
Sensitivity	Proportion of people with the disease who have a positive test	Determines the ability of the test to identify correctly those who have the disease. The more sensitive a test, the more certain you can be that a negative test rules out disease.
Specificity	Proportion of people without the disease who have a negative test	Determines the ability of the test to identify correctly those who do not have the disease. The more specific a test, the more certain you can be that a positive test rules in disease.
Positive predictive value of positive tests	Probability of disease, given the results of a positive test	Sensitivity and specificity are characteristics of test itself; however, predictive values influenced by how common the disease is. For diseases of low prevalence, the predictive value of a positive test goes down sharply.
Absolute risk reduction	Difference in adverse event rates between the control and experimental group	Is used to help determine the clinical significance of a treatment—needed to calculate NNT.
Number needed to treat	Number of patients needed to treat to prevent one additional bad outcome	Calculated by dividing 1 by the absolute risk reduction. NNT indicates clinical impact of a treatment.
Confidence interval	Range of values on either side of an estimate	A 99% confidence interval is interpreted as the range of values within which one can be 99% sure that the population value lies.
P value	Measure of statistical significance	Specifies the strength of the evidence.

NNT, number needed to treat.

> **BOX 14-1**
> **PICOT Format**
>
> P   Population or problem of interest
> I   Intervention or practice of interest
> C   Comparison intervention or practice—usually what is currently done
> O   Outcome of the intervention or practice
> T   Time frame in which outcome is expected

Two types of electronic databases are available. The first type is bibliographic and permits users to identify relevant citations in the clinical literature. MEDLINE and the *Cumulative Index to Nursing and Allied Health Literature* are examples of this first sort of database. Google Scholar (http://scholar.google.com) is a new database that is also becoming more popular. The second type of database takes the user directly to primary or secondary publications of the relevant clinical evidence. Examples of this second type of database include the *Cochrane Database of Systematic Reviews* and the American College of Physicians (ACP) Journal Club, a publication of the American College of Physicians-American Society of Internal Medicine, which abstracts articles on diagnosis, prognosis, treatment, quality of care, and medical economics. The ACP database has recently been "repurposed" and formatted to make clinician searching for answers to clinical questions easier (Haynes, 2008). These databases are available online from libraries and from the organizations themselves via the Internet.

Appraising Evidence from Studies

After evidence has been retrieved, the next step is to evaluate, or appraise, the evidence for its validity and clinical usefulness. Appraisal is crucial because it lets the clinician decide whether the retrieved research literature is reliable enough to give useful guidance. Because a number of published reports lack sufficient methodological rigor to be reliable enough for answering clinical questions, guidelines for evaluating literature have been developed to assist clinicians without extensive research expertise to evaluate clinical articles (Badenoch & Heneghan 2006).

Box 14-2 shows a typical set of critical appraisal questions for evaluating articles about therapy. These questions were synthesized from a number of sources (Badenoch & Heneghan, 2006; Sackett et al., 1991, 2000; Straus et al., 2005). Although the questions seem to reflect common sense, they are not entirely self-explanatory. Some assistance is required to help clinicians apply them to specific articles and individual patients. The *Evidence-Based Medicine Toolkit* (Badenoch & Heneghan, 2006) provides guidance on how to answer the appraisal questions that they specifically recommend. For example, on the question, "Were research participants 'blinded'?" the text gives the clinician a definition of the term *blinding,* and then might provide an example that would help clinicians decide whether the studies they were evaluating met this criteria. In addition to providing a guide for evaluating therapy articles, the *Evidence-Based Medicine Toolkit* has questions for appraising articles on diagnosis, prognosis, and harm (risks for certain diseases or conditions). As with any other skill, expertise and speed come with practice. The evidence does not automatically dictate patient care, but it does provide the factual basis on which decisions can be made.

BOX 14-2
Appraising Therapy Articles

CRITICAL APPRAISAL QUESTIONS USED TO EVALUATE A THERAPY ARTICLE

Is the study valid?

Was there a clearly defined research question?

Was the assignment of patients to treatments randomized and was the randomization list concealed?

Were all patients accounted for at its conclusion? Was there an "intention-to-treat" analysis?

Were research participants "blinded"?

Were the groups treated equally throughout?

Did randomization produce comparable groups at the start of the trial?

Are the results important?

How large is the treatment effect?

How precise is the finding from the trial?

Sources of Primary Clinical and Research Literature

MEDLINE is provided free on the Internet from many sites, and at least one of these, PubMed (www.ncbi.nlm.nih.gov/PubMed/clinical.html), also includes prestored search strategies that are designed to select studies most likely to be relevant and valid for clinical practice. MEDLINE is produced by the National Library of Medicine in Bethesda, Maryland, and is the best-known bibliographic database of indexed medical literature. MEDLINE is searchable by medical subject heading subheadings, as well as by author, journal, title, and keyword. The journals covered by MEDLINE are noted for their overall reliability and quality; however, the articles still must be scrutinized carefully for their validity and quality as evidence. A hand search of current journals is still one of the best ways to find newly published information. However, this is one of the most time-consuming and labor-intensive approaches to retrieving evidence.

Using Appraising Summaries

Meta-analysis uses statistical techniques to combine results across studies. Integrative reviews rely on summaries, logical synthesis, and narrative to characterize findings. Research-based guidelines center on care of a particular patient population and specify processes of care associated with good outcomes.

Meta-Analysis

Meta-analysis requires enough studies with sufficient commonality to provide a valid conclusion. In other words, studies have to be looking more or less at the same outcome and the same intervention. Meta-analysis is often used when several studies have been conducted but findings were inconclusive. Meta-analyses combine the statistical results from several studies into one statistic that can be used to gauge the size of the treatment's impact on the outcome of interest. To do this, first an effect size is calculated for each finding of interest in the studies being reviewed. Then a pooled effect size is calculated for all findings together.

There is controversy about the statistical techniques and assumptions of meta-analysis. Bias in the combined analysis is possible if the selection of studies was flawed or the elimination of methodologically poor studies was not done using an objective process. There are also inherent problems with data pooling, especially if the studies are not similar enough in design, sample size, outcome types, and forms of the independent variables used. Identifying weaknesses in this kind of systematic review can be done by using the guidelines in the *Evidence-Based Medicine Toolkit* (Badenoch & Heneghan, 2006) or by using a similar guide. Once you have examined the major components of the review, you can make a judgment about whether you think it is a high-quality review and whether the findings are valid.

Integrative Research Review

Integrative research reviews do not use statistical result combining techniques to summarize results across studies. Rather, they rely on logical comparison and synthesis of the reviewer. The integrative research review method is the research synthesis approach that most review articles in clinical care journals use. The quality of these reviews and their resulting conclusions are even more dependent on the reviewer's skill in critical appraisal. High-quality reviews make explicit how studies were selected for review and the rules that were used to judge the overall evidence. The reviewer should state whether some studies were weighted more heavily than others and should provide a rationale for doing so. If some studies were discounted, this also should be described. At present, integrative research review is the only mechanism available for looking at qualitative studies that address the same topic.

Practice Guidelines

Practice guidelines can include formal clinical protocols put forth by a professional organization, clinical paths formed by a practice group, and research-based recommendations that translate conclusions of a meta-analysis or an integrative research review into clinical practice conclusions. A practice guideline should clearly state what the guideline does and does not cover, what patient group it was designed for, the options at each decision point, the actions recommended, and the outcomes associated with each course of action. There should be a clear description of the supporting evidence and how it was gathered and evaluated. Because the literature is always evolving, practice guidelines should be explicit about how current they are. The comprehensiveness of the guideline should also be described.

Locating Sources of Summaries

Ovid (www.ovid.com) has released an integrated literature service called Evidence-Based Medicine Reviews (EBMR). This Web-based service includes the Cochrane Database of Systematic Reviews, Best Evidence, MEDLINE, and full-text journals. This resource contains full-text reviews of clinically relevant articles from throughout the medical literature published in EBMR and ACP Journal Club, and full text topic overviews published in the Cochrane Database of Systemic Reviews, published by the Cochrane Collaboration. Links between the Ovid databases and EBMR allow users to link from a citation to a review to the full text of that reviewed article, and then to other readings referenced in the article.

British Medical Journal (BMJ) publishing group and the American College of Physicians–American Society of Internal Medicine have created *Clinical Evidence,* the first major attempt to provide an up-to-date, evidence-based textbook (www.clinicalevidence.com). Subscribers can choose between receiving the service online, via a handbook titled the *Clinical Evidence Handbook,* or a combination of the handbook plus online, as well as via PDA resources. A free trial is permitted to allow potential users the opportunity to explore the usefulness of the service.

The Agency for Healthcare Research and Quality (AHRQ) National Guidelines Clearinghouse provides evidence-based information on health-care outcomes; quality; and cost, use, and access. In examining what works and does not work in health care, AHRQ's mission includes both translating research findings into better patient care and providing policy makers and other health-care leaders with information needed to make critical health-care decisions. Reports compiled by evidence-based practice centers are available on a range of topics and can cover a number of therapies for a given condition. By using your browser's "Find" feature, you can quickly locate a given topic.

The Cochrane Collaboration produces a structured database of high-quality systematic reviews of RCTs. Originally established in Britain, it is presently composed of numerous centers in several countries. Reviews involve exhaustive searches for all RCTs, both published and unpublished, on a particular topic. One limitation of the database is that the reviews focus mainly on therapies, although an increasing number of reviews on diagnostic topics are being developed. The studies are analyzed using standardized methodology and meta-analysis. The Cochrane Library, now managed by Wiley, contains high-quality, independent evidence to inform health-care decision making. It includes reliable evidence from Cochrane and other systematic reviews, clinical trials, and more. Cochrane reviews bring you the combined results of the world's best medical research studies and are recognized as the gold standard in evidence-based health care.

Nursing-specific resources for evidence reviews have also been developed. The Joanna Briggs Institute (JBI; at www.joannabriggs.edu.au), based in Australia, is committed to evidence translation and use worldwide. They produce evidence summaries and provide guidelines on evidence application to practice. The *Online Journal of Knowledge Synthesis for Nursing* is a peer-reviewed online journal dedicated to the scientific advancement of evidence-based practice in health care. The journal presents current scientific evidence to inform clinical decisions and ongoing discussions on issues, methods, clinical practice, and teaching strategies for evidenced-based practice. Each article is written as a synthesis of research studies on a single topic and concludes with practice implications.

Clinical Significance and Appraisal Process

Having identified evidence that is both valid and relevant, the next step in using the evidence is to make a judgment about applying the evidence with your patient, in your setting. **Box 14-3** provides a list of questions that clinicians can use to make a judgment about the clinical application of the research findings. You must determine whether your patient is sufficiently similar to the study or study participants for the results to be applicable. Critical factors that can affect generalizability include demographics such as race, age, and gender. Other factors to consider relate to the feasibility of implementation of the proposed intervention, diagnostic test, and so on. Once the clinician has weighed the clinical use of the evidence and determined that implementation is feasible or desirable, he or she can either implement it directly in a patient's care or use it to develop protocols and guidelines.

EVIDENCE-BASED PRACTICE AND ATTITUDE

This chapter has not been developed as a stand-alone resource for learning the principles of evidence-based practice. It is almost impossible to learn how to search effectively and appraise efficiently without the help of others and without good resources. Working in groups is the best method to master these skills. Share the task of searching and appraising with others. Use secondary publications such as

---

BOX 14-3
Clinical Significance Appraisal Process

QUESTIONS TO GUIDE THINKING

In terms of applicability to practice, answer the following questions:

Were the subjects similar to patients for whom you might provide care now or in the future?

Could you base an intervention on the findings of this external evidence?

Would any intervention you might identify be within your scope of practice?

What does the body of evidence say about the general question that motivated the inquiry?

What actions does the body of evidence warrant?

---

the *Best Evidence* text developed by BMJ publishing group. Develop a system for storing work and sharing it with others. Electronic information storage and retrieval systems are evolving rapidly, so continued updates in the available technology are necessary. When evidence is used to inform clinical judgment, the APN can take advantage of new knowledge developments so that care can be more individualized, effective, streamlined, and dynamic.

References

Aström, G., Norberg, A., Hallberg, I. R., & Jansson, J. (1995). Experienced and skilled nurses' narratives of situations where caring action made a difference to the patient. *Scholarly Inquiry for Nursing Practice, 7*(3), 183–193.

Badenoch, D., & Heneghan, C. (2006). *Evidence-based medicine toolkit* (2nd ed.). London: BMJ Books.

Benner, P., Tanner, C. A., & Chesla, C. A. (1996). *Expertise in nursing practice: Caring, clinical judgment, and ethics.* New York: Springer.

Bergus, G. R., & Hamm, R. M. (1995). Clinical practice. How physicians make medical decisions and why medical decision making can help. *Primary Care: Clinics in Office Practice, 22*(2), 167–180.

Borges, S., & Waitzkin, H. (1995). Women's narratives in primary care medical encounters. *Women & Health, 23*(1), 29–56.

Brannon, L. A., & Carson, K. L. (2003). The representativeness heuristic: Influence on nurses' decision making. *Applied Nursing Research, 16*(3), 201–204.

Bruner, J. (1986). *Actual minds, possible worlds.* Cambridge, MA: Harvard University.

Covell, D. G., Uman, G. C., & Manning, P. R. (1985). Information needs in office practice: Are they being met? *Annals of Internal Medicine, 103*(4), 596–599.

Craig, J. V., & Smyth, R. L. (2007). *The evidence-based practice manual for nurses* (2nd ed.). Edinburgh: Churchill Livingston Elsevier.

Crow, R., & Spicer, J. (1995). Categorisation of the patient's medical condition—An analysis of nursing judgment. *International Journal of Nursing Studies, 32*(5), 413–422.

Dearlove, O. R., Rogers, J., & Sharples, A. (1996). Evidence based medicine. Authors' redefinition is better but not perfect [letter; comment]. *BMJ, 313,* 170–171.

DeBourgh, G. A. (2001). Champions for evidence-based practice: A critical role for advanced practice nurses. *AACN Clinical Issues: Advanced Practice in Acute and Critical Care, 12*(4), 491–508.

Ellefsen, B. (2004). Frames and perspectives in clinical nursing practice: A study of Norwegian nurses in acute care settings. *Research and Theory in Nursing Practice, 18*(1), 95–109.

English, I. (1993). Intuition as a function of the expert nurse: A critique of Benner's novice to expert model. *Journal of Advanced Nursing, 18*(3), 387–393.

Fletcher, R. H., & Fletcher, S. W. (1979). Clinical research in general medical journals: A 30-year perspective. *New England Journal of Medicine, 301*(4), 180–183.

Gorman, P. (1993). Does the medical literature contain the evidence to answer the questions of primary care physicians? Preliminary findings of a study. *Proceedings—The Annual Symposium on Computer Applications in Medical Care,* 571–575.

Gorman, P. (2001). Information needs in primary care: A survey of rural and nonrural primary care physicians. *Medinfo, 10*(Pt 1), 338–342.

Greer, A. L. (1988). The state of the art versus the state of the science. The diffusion of new medical technologies into practice. *International Journal of Technology Assessment in Health Care, 4*(1), 5–26.

Haynes, R. B. (1993). Where's the meat in clinical journals? *ACP Journal Club, 119,* A16.

Haynes, R. B. (2008). ACP Journal Club is dead . . . long live ACP Journal Club. *ACP Journal Club, 148*(2), A8.

Hunter, K. M. (1991). *Doctor's stories: The narrative structure of medical knowledge.* Princeton, NJ: Princeton University.

Institute of Medicine. (2001). *Crossing the quality chasm: A new health system for the 21st century.* Committee on Quality of Health Care in America. Washington, DC: Author.

Institute of Medicine. (2004). *Keeping patients safe: Transforming the work environment of nurses.* Washington, DC: The National Academies Press.

Institute of Medicine. (2008). *Knowing what works in health care: A roadmap for the nation.* Washington, DC: The National Academies Press.

Jennings, B. M. (2000). Evidence-based practice: The road best traveled? *Research in Nursing and Health, 23*(5), 343–345.

Klardie, K. A., Johnson, J., McNaughton, M., & Meyers, W. (2004). Integrating the principles of evidence-based practice into clinical practice. *Journal of the American Academy of Nurse Practitioners, 16*(3), 98–105.

Kleinman, A. (1988). *Illness narratives: Suffering, healing and the human condition.* New York: Basic Books.

Kosowski, M. M., & Roberts, V. W. (2003). When protocols are not enough: Intuitive decision making by novice nurse practitioners. *Journal of Holistic Nursing, 21*(1), 52–72.

Kuiper, R. A., & Pesut, D. J. (2004). Promoting cognitive and metacognitive reflective reasoning skills in nursing practice: Self-regulated learning theory. *Journal of Advanced Nursing, 45*(4), 381–391.

McAlister, F. A., Graham, I., Karr, G. W., & Laupacis, A. (1999). Evidence-based medicine and the practicing clinician. *Journal of General Internal Medicine, 14*(4), 236–242.

McCarthy, M. C. (2003). Situated clinical reasoning: Distinguishing acute confusion from dementia in hospitalized older adults. *Research in Nursing and Health, 26*(2), 90–101.

McDonald, D. D., Frakes, M., Apostolidis, B., Armstrong, B., Goldblatt, S., & Bernardo, D. (2003). Effect of a psychiatric diagnosis on nursing care for nonpsychiatric problems. *Research in Nursing and Health, 26*(2), 225–232.

McKibbon, K. A., & Marks, S. (2001). Posing clinical questions: Framing the question for scientific inquiry. *AACN Clinical Issues, 12*(4), 477–481.

Melnyk, B. M., & Fineout-Overhold, E. (2005). *Evidence-based practice in nursing and healthcare.* Lippincott, Williams, & Wilkins: Philadelphia.

Mitchell, G. J. (1999). Practice applications. Evidence-based practice: Critique and alternative view. *Nursing Science Quarterly, 12*(1), 30–35.

Moher, D., Cook, D. J., Eastwood, S., Olkin, I., Rennie, D., & Stroup, D. F. (1999). Improving the quality of reports of meta-analyses of randomised controlled trials: The QUOROM statement. Quality of reporting of meta-analyses. *Lancet, 354*(9193), 1896–1900.

Moher, D., Jadad, A. R., Nichol, G., Penman, M., Tugwell, P., & Walsh, S. (1995). Assessing the quality of randomized controlled trials: An annotated bibliography of scales and checklists. *Controlled Clinical Trials, 16*(1), 62–73.

Peden-McAlpine, C., & Clark, N. (2002). Early recognition of client status changes: The importance of time. *Dimensions of Critical Care Nursing, 21*(4), 144–151.

Ritter, B. J. (2003). An analysis of expert nurse practitioners' diagnostic reasoning. *Journal of the American Academy of Nurse Practitioners, 15*(3), 137–141.

Rosswurm, M. A., & Larrabee, J. H. (1999). Clinical scholarship. A model for change to evidence-based practice. *IMAGE: The Journal of Nursing Scholarship, 31*(4), 317–322.

Ruth-Sahd, L. A. (2003). Reflective practice: A critical analysis of data-based studies and implications for nursing education. *Journal of Nursing Education, 42*(11), 488–497.

Sackett, D. L., Haynes, R. B., Guyatt, G. H., & Tugwell, P. (1991). *Clinical epidemiology: A basic science for clinical medicine* (2nd ed.). Boston, MA: Little, Brown and Company.

Sackett, D. L., Rosenberg, W. M., Gray, J. A., Haynes, R. B., & Richardson, W. S. (1996). Evidence based medicine: What it is and what it isn't. *British Medical Journal, 312*(7023), 71–72.

Sackett, D. L., Straus, S. E., Richardson, W. S., Rosenberg, W., & Haynes, R. B. (2000). *Evidence-based medicine* (2nd ed.). Edinburgh: Churchill Livingstone.

Sacks, H. S., Reitman, D., Pagano, D., & Kupelnick, B. (1996). Meta-analysis: An update. *Mount Sinai Journal of Medicine, 63*(3–4), 216–224.

Schor, S., & Karten, I. (1966). Statistical evaluation of medical journal manuscripts. *Journal of the American Medical Association, 195*(13), 1123–1128.

Scott, P., Shiell, A., & King, M. (1996). Is general practitioner decision-making associated with patient socio-economic status? *Social Science & Medicine, 42*(1), 35–46.

Shaneyfelt, T. M., Mayo-Smith, M. F., & Rothwangl, J. (1999). Are guidelines following guidelines? The methodological quality of clinical practice guidelines in the peer-reviewed medical literature. *Journal of the American Medical Association, 281*(20), 1900–1905.

Shapiro, S. E. (2007). Evidence-based practice for advanced practice emergency nurses. *Advanced Emergency Nursing Journal, 29*(4), 331–338.

Simmons, B., Lanuza, D., Fonteyn, M., Hicks, F., & Holm, K. (2003). Clinical reasoning in experienced nurses. *Western Journal of Nursing Research, 25*(6), 701–719; [discussion] 720–724.

Smith, B. H. (1996). Evidence based medicine. Rich sources of evidence are ignored. *British Medical Journal, 313*(7050), 169–171.

Sox, H. C., Blatt, M. A., Higgins, M. C., & Marton, K. I. (1991). *Medical decision making.* Boston, MA: Butterworth-Heinemann.

Straus, S. E., Richardson, W. S., Glasziou, P., & Haynes, R. B. (2005). *Evidence-based Medicine: How to Practice and Teach EBM* (3rd ed.). Churchill Livingstone: Edinburgh.

Tanner, C. A. (1998). Clinical judgment and evidence-based practice: Conclusions and controversies. *Communicating Nursing Research, 31*(2), 19–35.

Tanner, C. A. (1999). Evidence-based practice: Research and critical thinking. *Journal of Nursing Education, 38*(3), 99.

Tanner, C. A. (2006). Thinking like a nurse: A research-based model of clinical judgment in nursing. *The Journal of Nursing Education, 45*(6), 204–211.

Tanner, C. A., Benner, P., Chesla, C., & Gordon, D. R. (1993). The phenomenology of knowing the patient. *IMAGE: The Journal of Nursing Scholarship, 25*(4), 273–280.

White, A. H. (2003). Clinical decision making among fourth-year nursing students: An interpretive study. *Journal of Nursing Education, 42*(3), 113–120.

Williamson, J. W., German, P. S., Weiss, R., Skinner, E. A., & Bowes III, F. (1989). Health science information management and continuing education of physicians. A survey of U.S. primary care practitioners and their opinion leaders. *Annals of Internal Medicine, 110*(2), 151–160.

Windish, D. M., Huot, S. J., & Green, M. L. (2007). Medicine residents' understanding of the biostatistics and results in the medical literature. *Journal of the American Medical Association, 298*(9), 1010–1022.

Youngblut, J. M., & Brooten, D. (2001). Evidence-based nursing practice: Why is it important? *AACN Clinical Issues: Advanced Practice in Acute & Critical Care, 12*(4), 468–476.

Zerwekh, J. V. (1992). The practice of empowerment and coercion by expert public health nurses. *IMAGE: The Journal of Nursing Scholarship, 24*(2), 101–105.

Advocacy and the Advanced Practice Nurse

Karen Piren

Susan C. Reinhard

15

INTRODUCTION

The health-care delivery system is a complicated maze of services with many gates and gatekeepers. Not surprisingly, many consumers need help navigating their way through this intimidating maze. The advanced practice nurse (APN) is in a good position to advocate for individual consumers and families who confront barriers to getting the health-care services that they need. Nurses can also advocate for system changes to remove the barriers. It takes education, sophistication, and determination to advocate at both of these levels. This chapter examines the roots of advocacy in nursing and the skills needed for this practice role. Through case examples, we highlight several opportunities and issues to stimulate dialogue and action.

ROOTS OF ADVOCACY IN NURSING

Nursing leaders like Florence Nightingale, Sojourner Truth, Lillian Wald, and Margaret Sanger are testaments to the nursing profession's historic roots in championing improved health care, especially for the most vulnerable among us (Mason, Leavitt, & Chafee, 2002). These pioneers advanced human rights, compassionate care, and lasting societal changes. Given this impressive legacy, it is interesting that the patient advocate role is seen as an innovation in nursing in the past 25 years, and it is still only in the early stages of acceptance (Mallik & Rafferty, 2000).

Nurse scholars provide support that patient advocacy is an important part of the practice of expert nurses (Segesten, 1993). Indeed, the American Nurses Association (ANA) Code of Ethics for Nurses calls on nurses to collaborate with other health professionals and consumers to promote community and national efforts to meet the health needs of the public. (ANA, 2001). Given the complexities of today's health-care environment, nurse advocates are needed more than ever. The International Council of Nurses (ICN) also includes advocacy as an essential nursing activity. However, the presumption that nurses advocate for patients in all practice settings is based on little evidence (Milette, 1993), and there is scant literature describing how nurses learn how to advocate (Foley, Minick, & Kee, 2002a). It appears that nurses value advocacy, know that they should advocate, and often do so in their daily work. However, the profession does not consistently address advocacy in its body of knowledge and methods for transferring that body of knowledge to entrants in the discipline. In many ways, advocacy is an ambiguous role component for APNs.

Evidence Base for Advocacy

One reason for this ambiguity is that advocacy means many things to many people, and there is no well-accepted, evidenced-based advocacy model for nursing practice. That does not mean that patient advocacy is lacking. It means that it is not well articulated, researched, and taught. Mitchell and Bournes (2000) suggest that "advocacy is a concept that conceals more than it reveals," (p. 209) and that an explicit theoretical foundation for this activity would enhance its value to the nursing profession. Because the profession purports that advocacy is a social mandate for nurses, the need for theoretical explication and nursing research is compelling.

The evidence base for the advocacy role or effectiveness of advocacy interventions is limited. Mallick and Rafferty (2000) examined the growth and diffusion of nurses' claim to patient advocacy in the nursing literature of the United States and the United Kingdom over 20 years (1976–1995). Most of the published manuscripts have come out of the United States and their focus on specialty areas in nursing; other than that, there are few studies. Given the early stages of the empirical exploration in this area, most of the work is exploratory, the methodology is qualitative, and samples are small. However, five studies explored the concept of advocacy in relation to nursing.

Millette (1993) studied the nurse's view of client advocacy and how this concept might affect practice. Surveying 222 nurses and interviewing a subset of 24 of these subjects, this investigator found that the concept of client advocacy has much appeal to practicing nurses, but that they need a high level of moral development to implement this advocacy role in bureaucratic settings. Geoffrey's (1998) study of nine nurses caring for dying patients also addresses the environments in which nurses practice. Using grounded theory to explore advocacy as a means of empowering these dying patients, Geoffrey describes the effects of rituals on the practice of advocacy. Adhering to routines like getting morning care for assigned patients completed before noon keeps the nurse busy enough to avoid talking to patients, determining barriers to recovery, and acting to remove those barriers. Advocacy requires an individualized approach and an openness to challenge power structures. The focus on completing tasks can distance the nurse from patients and lead to poor advocacy skills.

Two other studies explore advocacy among practicing nurses. In a British study, Snowball (1996) used a semistructured interview with 15 medical-surgical nurses to explore their understanding of advocacy. These nurses viewed the therapeutic relationship as the key to advocacy at both the proactive and reactive levels. Foley, Minick, and Kee (2002b) used hermeneutic interpretive methods of stories to study the development of skills in advocating for patients in Army nurses in Bosnia. They found that developing advocacy skills was largely haphazard, not based on what these nurses were taught. But when the nurses found themselves in situations that called for advocacy, they often rose to the occasion, and they developed skills along the way.

These studies document that despite the limited empirical basis for advocacy in nursing, the concept and the practice are evolving in ways that are consistent with the values of the nursing profession. Nurse leaders, researchers, and educators elucidate philosophical foundations for advocacy (Curtain, 1979), required skills (Connolly, 1999), and curricula (Jones, 1982). Advocacy is not always included in descriptions of the advanced practice nursing role (Hamric & Sposs, 1989; Mezey & McGivern, 1999). However, several authors suggest that advocacy is highly desirable, an indicator of excellence in practice, a domain in advanced practice nursing, and an essential component of the primary mental health-care and community support system models (Benner, 1984; Gadow, 1980; Haber & Billings, 1995; Millette, 1993; U.S. Department of Health and Human Services [DHHS], 1987).

Nurses occupy a middle ground between the consumer and the health-care system, an optimal place to mediate (Bishop & Scudder, 1990; Stein, Watts, & Howell, 1990). Although there is a critical need for research and development of the advocacy role, there is some guidance for APNs.

Definitions of Advocacy

What is advocacy? Snowball (1996) suggests that advocacy suffers from conceptual ambiguity. Advocacy is derived from the Latin *advocatus,* which means one who summons to give evidence (Gates, 1995). *Advocate* is a noun and a verb—to act for, speak for, plead for, or defend. *Advocacy* is the function of these verbs and has been described as informing, advising, or counseling (Curtain, 1979; Gadow, 1980, 1989; Kohnke, 1982; Mitchell & Bornes, 2000).

Historically, advocacy has been linked to the potential powerlessness of a patient, although the rising power of the consumer affects our definitions of advocacy (Hewitt, 2002). Shroeder and Gadow (2000) distinguish advocacy from paternalism and consumerism. Paternalism is the commitment to making decisions for the client because the professional is obligated to impose expertise on behalf of the person in need; a person in need is presumed to be incapable of rational judgment. In contrast, consumerism is the commitment to remain uninvolved in client decisions; persons in need are nonetheless capable of rational judgment, and their right to self-determination must be respected. These authors provide a view of advocacy as a practical partnership between a professional who has expertise to offer the client who is experiencing the inherent ambiguity associated with significant health concerns.

Most people confronting a serious health problem require "reorientation" so that they can define the situation, reflect on their values, and make decisions. In this view, advocacy is a partnership in which the person confronting a health issue and the professional offering assistance develop a mutually satisfying interpretation of the situation. In the partnership, they reach a meaning they can both affirm. The meaning can be considered a narrative or interpretation that coherently connects all the elements of the situation. Essentially, "advocacy becomes participation with clients in co-authorship of a health narrative" (Schroeder & Gadow, 2000, p. 85).

Levels of Advocacy

Definitions of advocacy tend to be client- or systems-focused, suggesting two levels of advocacy for APNs. Client-focused definitions of advocacy emphasize enhancing client autonomy and assisting clients in voicing their values (Connolly, 1999). At this individual/family client level, the APN uses a set of skills to help people identify their needs and obtain services and provides support to meet those needs. Systems-focused definitions of advocacy refer to influencing providers to improve existing services and develop new ones (Stuart & Laraia, 2001). At this systems level of advocacy, the APN uses many of the same skills needed at the individual/family level—and some new ones—to advocate for changes in the health-care delivery system itself.

Advocacy at the Individual and Family Levels

The client-focused definition of advocacy speaks to patient advocacy, the most common type of advocacy in nursing practiced at both the individual and family levels. The most dominant model for patient advocacy comes from the counseling paradigm. Arising from the ethico-legal framework of human rights in the 1970s and 1980s, nurses advanced patient advocacy as advising, informing, or counseling (Curtain, 1979). Consistent with the civil rights and women's movements, nurses were moving past previous modes of subservience to physicians and institutions to a direct relationship with the patient. Inherent in that relationship is the recognition that the nurse has the authority that comes with claim to a scientific body of knowledge that is not fully accessible to the lay person (Abbott, 1988). The nurse's ethical responsibility is to transfer as much of that knowledge as possible to the patient and support that person in making informed choices. Patient advocacy becomes teaching, nonjudgmental support of the person's decisions, and assistance in acting on those choices.

This counseling model is the mainstay of advanced practice nursing at the individual and family levels. The more contemporary "consumer empowerment" model reminds us that people do not want or need continual counseling by professionals; they may not be seeking professionals' "noninvolvement," but consumers would prefer consultation rather than counseling. They seek a reduction in the medical model orientation that health professionals know what is best to "protect" patients. Nurses who define advocacy primarily as protecting patients (Foley et al., 2002a) may have difficulty with the contemporary principles of consumer self-advocacy. Consumer advocates do not seek paternalistic protection. They do seek professionals who can help them navigate the system, a high priority for consumers and families who define advocacy as "a go between who knows the system and will advise you" (Connolly, 1999, p. 390).

There are many ways that APNs can advocate at the individual and family level. The following case example provides one exemplar.

Advocacy Exemplar: Individual and Family Level

The complex issues of removing children from their families and placing them with adoption services while negotiating a difficult, fragmented child protection system provides fertile ground and many opportunities for APNs to demonstrate their role as advocates. The overburdened, disjointed systems make it difficult for members of a care team to understand the complexities of an individual seeking to regain custody of his or her children. In many ways, the individual is alone, pitted against a group of professionals representing the children—professionals who barely have time to communicate. Negotiating the system is a complex, difficult endeavor.

Individual and family advocacy can be valuable to individuals attempting to navigate these systems. Vulnerable populations, such as the poor and uninsured, victims of abuse, single mothers, and individuals with developmental disabilities and mental illness are in particular need of advocacy services. Schroeder and Gadow (2000) describe a tradition of service delivery in the United States that effectively prohibits many of these individuals from participating in decisions regarding health care. They describe a system in which professionals identify themselves as the expert authority, thereby disempowering the needs of individuals and destroying the possibility of an equal (or mutual) relationship between an individual and professional. Nurse advocates can counter the effects of this paternalistic system by enhancing personal autonomy and participating with individuals in determining their needs (Shroeder & Gadow, 2000).

The Case of Maria

This case describes Maria and her involvement in the family court system. It illustrates how an APN can identify barriers within a multifaceted system, plan, coordinate, and monitor services and follow up with other advocates within the system.

Maria is a 30-year-old single, bilingual mother of four who was born in the United States to parents of Hispanic origin. Her involvement with the court began several years ago when her estranged husband abused their oldest daughter. Maria herself had also been the victim of his abuse. Although she left her husband shortly after her daughter's abuse, three of her four children were placed in foster care. The fourth resided with Maria's mother, and Maria participated fully in this daughter's daily life. Maria enjoyed a close and loving relationship with her intact family, which included a sister.

Maria was referred to an APN in psychiatric mental health nursing for case management services. She was referred by an urban family court as part of a child welfare mediation process of planning for the future of the three children in foster care. Concurrently, the APN collaborated with a university law school, a court-appointed mediator, various child protection case managers, and Maria's attorney. The nurse provided strength-based case management services (Sullivan, 1991), counseling, and support to Maria during court-mediated meetings, as well as links to services identified by the client and nurse.

In addition to attending monthly mediation hearings over a 6-month period, the APN met with Maria weekly. Maria was a quiet, shy young woman who exhibited developmental and speech delays. Her affect was depressed, and she expressed feelings of hopelessness and despair. The legal system had, in fact, determined that three children would be placed for adoption. Maria, on the other hand, expressed a strong desire to be reunited with her family. In particular, Maria wanted to regain custody of her oldest daughter.

The APN made an initial assessment based on the strengths-based case management model (Sullivan, 1991). Maria had several strengths. She was young, relatively healthy, and able to identify solid family supports. She expressed a fervent desire to care for her children and demonstrated a willingness to discuss difficult, painful issues. She expressed a strong desire to follow the recommendations of the court, although she sometimes found it difficult to do so. In addition to reuniting her family, her personal goals were to obtain a high school diploma and get a driver's license and a car. The ocean was less than an hour away, and she dreamed of driving to the beach with her children to see the ocean for the first time.

Initially, Maria did not make eye contact with the APN, and answered questions only after careful thought. The nurse construed this to mean that Maria was searching for the answer she thought the nurse wanted to hear. Her feelings of powerlessness and hopelessness were highlighted during the first mediation meeting, when the nurse noted that no one in the room spoke to her. They spoke about and around her. For her part, Maria sat quietly listening to the discussion about the future of her family.

Shea, Mahoney, and Lacey (1997) describe the importance of empowerment and advocacy to victims of abuse. According to these authors, creating and sustaining a therapeutic caring relationship, encouraging self-determination, and supporting patient decisions promote empowerment and advocacy. The APN needs to communicate a sense of hope while establishing realistic expectations for success to promote empowerment and independence.

In addition, Shea et al. (1997) recognize that to break the coercive control that abusers have over their victims, nurses need to avoid using interventions that represent further control of the victim, thereby perpetuating the cycle of abuse. Advocates must be wary and avoid paternalistic relationships, exercising care in understanding the needs and desires of those in need of their services (Mitchell & Bournes, 2000).

The primary issue preventing Maria from regaining custody of her children was their safety. Maria's estranged husband had continued to contact her, despite the fact that there was a restraining order against all contact with her or the children. Maria felt powerless and clearly did not know how to react when this occurred. The nurse and university law school advocates readily discovered that Maria had never been provided with a copy of the restraining order. The university law school advocates obtained a copy of the order and gave Maria clear, concise instructions regarding implementation. In addition, they arranged for Maria to receive a free cell phone from a battered woman's shelter, enabling her to call 911 in the event of an emergency. For additional security, the nurse and Maria located a safe house and developed an escape plan.

Continued

There were several other issues apparent to the nurse and university law school advocates in this case. A few are discussed here. First, before the nurse and law school involvement, Maria's only advocate throughout the process had been a very caring but overburdened court-appointed attorney. Although he did everything he could to assist Maria, time constraints and the inability to assess Maria's cognitive deficits limited his ability to assist her. On the other hand, the children had individual case managers, the Department of Youth and Family Services, the Assistant Attorney General, child advocates, individual therapists, and numerous others working on their behalf. It was easy to understand why the court and mediation process were intimidating to Maria and how they contributed to her feelings of hopelessness and powerlessness. A second issue that affected Maria's need for advocacy was that many individuals involved in her case scheduled her appointments at overlapping times without consideration for the time or money required to keep them. In addition, Maria had difficulty reading, a fact that was unknown to any of the individuals involved in her case.

The APN needed to help overcome all of these barriers. Reinforcing her strengths, she helped Maria find hope tempered with realistic expectations. In addition to arming her with the restraining order, cell phone, and escape plan, the APN helped her obtain a city bus pass and a color-coded calendar she could read to help her keep her appointments. She also helped her enroll in high school general equivalency diploma classes. This set of advocacy interventions helped set in motion immediate and long-term forces of self-empowerment for Maria.

In the end, the court changed its position and granted Maria custody of her oldest daughter. The two younger children were placed for adoption in the foster home they had resided in for a number of years. Although Maria was distraught over the loss, she was able to meet the family, who invited her to remain involved in the children's lives.

ISSUES AND DISCUSSION

In this case example, the APN used Sullivan's strength-based case management model to guide her advocacy efforts. She identified strengths, as well as gaps in the system, and applied practical solutions to overlooked troubles. The interventions built on Maria's strengths, supported her autonomy, and ultimately enhanced her self-esteem. Collaborating with child protective services and others involved in the case created an environment wherein the advocates identified an opportunity to propose meaningful interventions and broaden the range of options to Maria, which had long been overlooked by the team.

Connolly (1999) describes skills and competencies needed by the APN patient advocate. These skills include empathetic listening, self-confidence, assertiveness, negotiation, collaboration, communication, physical assessment, mental status assessment, crisis intervention, case management, change agency, and teaching. Snowball (1996) found the therapeutic relationship "key to advocacy," (p. 73). Clearly, all of these skills are within the scope and education of APNs. However, paramount to the success of the patient advocate is a philosophical foundation that individuals, particularly those who are vulnerable and suffer from any disease or impairment, are unique human beings who deserve and require respect, dignity, and the right to make decisions concerning their lives. Curtain (1979) describes nursing as "a moral art," (p. 2). Application of the science that nurses learn, coupled with a desire to improve the lives of other human beings combine to make "human advocacy" a fundamental part of the nursing process.

Systems-Level Advocacy

Systems-level advocacy is nursing practice at the community level. Public health nurses think of it as "upstream thinking." For example, one can treat the child with lead poisoning and help navigate the child and his family through the clinics and lead abatement programs case by case. However, a more upstream advocacy approach would be to prevent lead poisoning through strict preventive policies and programs for abating all houses with lead paint, especially in cities. Consumers need both levels of advocacy. APNs can be engaged in both levels, with different intensity. Although not all APNs desire a policy-level advocacy role, they can support policies and programs that their nursing colleagues are advancing on behalf of consumers.

The advocacy skills that APNs need to successfully advocate for individuals and families are foundational for systems-level advocacy. Advocacy at this level usually involves developing new policies and programs, or at least changing the old way of doing things enough to make a difference for the people that nurses serve. Communication skills are crucial. Active listening skills are as important as verbal skills; indeed more insight is gained from listening than from speaking. Insight into the problem leads to more creative problem solving and ideas for negotiating system solutions. Negotiation is more complex at the systems level than at the individual and family levels because generally there are more stake holders involved when advocating policies and programs. The APN needs to be assertive enough to overcome resistance to change, and collaborative enough to create or join with others who can help advance the advocacy goal.

To be most effective at the systems level, APNs need to understand program and policy development. Hanley (2002) describes several models regarding public policy that can guide APNs. For example, the stage-sequential model details a series of stages, beginning with identifying a policy problem and getting that problem placed on the policy discussion and action agendas in the appropriate forum (i.e., state or federal legislature, administrative agencies, funding organizations, and the like). Developing policy options with supporting budgets and infrastructures for implementation (i.e., staffing, regulations, and so on) follows. Program implementation and evaluation are the final stages. Moving through these stages requires an understanding of the change process in general, with skill development in creating and sustaining a vision for change, anticipating and dealing with resistance to change, developing a broad base of support, and understanding the art of compromise.

Advocacy Exemplar: Freeing People from Nursing Homes

Americans are fiercely proud of their freedom to live their lives as they choose. Many older adults and people with disabilities are in danger of losing that freedom when they have difficulty managing daily living tasks and the challenges of chronic health conditions. The forces driving frail elders and the disabled into institutional care are well documented (Kane, Kane, & Ladd, 1998). Once placed in a nursing home, institutionalized people often find it difficult to return home or to another community-based setting such as assisted living. The "system" works against it. The institutional bias in our federal and state long-term care payment policies is a serious impediment to consumers who want to leave nursing homes. Many states invest most of their dollars in nursing home care as opposed to home care. Professionals often assume that people who enter a nursing home really need that level of care and cannot be returned to their communities. The idea that the older adult's condition might improve, or that there may be other alternatives outside of a nursing home, are foreign concepts to many professionals and state policy makers. Even some who consider themselves to be advocates for the elderly believe that a nursing home is the "safest place" for those who have crossed the institutional threshold. Crossing back seems unthinkable. Navigating the crossing is extremely difficult.

Systems advocacy is needed to change this thinking that is embedded in our policies and programs. We can offer institutionalized elders and people with disabilities more choices, and they can return to the community with help from nurses and others to navigate the way back home.

The Case of Community Choice Counseling

One example of systems advocacy led by an APN is a state program developed as part of a set of "senior initiatives" in New Jersey to offer older adults independence, dignity, and choice (Reinhard, 1999). Known as "Community Choice Counseling," this program has been evaluated by researchers at Rutgers Center for State Health Policy (Howell-White, 2003). The goals and social change strategies used to create this program are offered as an exemplar for systems advocacy.

In 1994, an APN in community health nursing was appointed to serve the New Jersey Commissioner of Health as the Director of Policy and Research. Interested in developing policies and programs to support people with chronic conditions who want to live in their communities, this nurse director investigated the range of community-based options for long-term care available for older adults and people with disabilities. Like most states at the time, New Jersey had few options, and 97% of the public dollars in long-term care were spent on nursing home care (Reinhard, 1999). Despite this dismal record, New Jersey was approximately average among the states (Ladd, 1999). National data document that institutional bias is rampant in this country.

At least three things are needed to change this institutionalization bias. First, more long-term care alternatives must be created by developing programs and obtaining the funding to support them. Second, ways to inform consumers and professionals about these alternatives before people are unnecessarily institutionalized must be developed. Third, strategies to continually assess those who enter nursing homes to see if they still need and prefer that residential care option must be created. The overall goal is to help consumers and professionals understand that people can move in and out of these various long-term care options—it is not a unidirectional, linear movement. People can and should be able to move from nursing homes to their homes, and any other long-term care option.

The most important way to begin this systems advocacy is to develop and communicate a shared vision for change. Indeed, an advocate's most critical driving force for change is the strength and integrity of the vision energizing the goals for change. In this case, it was the vision of "freeing people" from unnecessary and unwanted institutionalization. It is advancing nursing's view that aging is not a period of inevitable decline. The nursing model holds that people of all ages can enter periods of disability, and they can regain health. The assumption that an older adult or a person with a disability can never attain or regain function is an anathema to the nursing paradigm. Independence, dignity, choice: these principles helped the new director to bring together a coalition of advocates and policy makers interested in seeking the policy changes needed to fuel the evolution to the nonlinear, noninstitutional thinking that is consistent with the nursing philosophy of attaining, maintaining, and regaining health and independence.

To achieve this vision, several system changes were needed. First, the governor consolidated all senior programs into one department and appointed the nurse advocate as the deputy commissioner in charge of redesigning long-term care in the state. After considerable negotiation with the governor's office, the state budgeted $60 million in state and federal dollars to develop more consumer-directed home-care options and more respite care for family caregivers (Reinhard, 1999). The state also created a locally based information and assistance system so older adults and their families could learn about their options and navigate the system (Reinhard & Scala, 2001). The state also initiated a counseling program to make sure that people in nursing homes are also able to find out about these choices. That program was named "Community Choice Counseling (CCC)" (Lagnado, 2001).

This program began with energetic nurses in the new New Jersey Department of Health and Senior Services (NJDHSS). Starting with two registered nurses, 300 nursing home residents were helped to return to their homes and communities within 4 months. Telephone follow-up of 10% of these former nursing home residents found positive outcomes, including high consumer satisfaction, few rehospitalizations, and low costs to the consumer and state for community placement. Staff found that many of these older adults and persons with disabilities had "gotten stuck." For some, the admission to the nursing home was intended to be for a few months for recovery from an illness or accident. However, without help from a person outside of the nursing home who could provide specific help to get back to the community, their length of stay turned into 6 months, a year, or more. Based on these initial findings, the nurse leaders obtained the support of the governor to continue and expand the program.

Armed with pilot data, the nurse advocate began to develop a coalition to advocate for change. As nurses learn in their study of the change process, analyzing the driving and restraining forces to change is the starting point. In this case, the restraining forces to changing the institutional bias of long-term care are those who would be most threatened by altering the status quo. Nursing homes worry about the state emptying out their residents. The state's Office of Management and Budget worries about *not* emptying out the nursing homes but about hiring 40 nurses and social workers in the effort to do so. The directors of the county Office on Aging worry that they will have more resource-intense people living in the community if the state "deinstitutionalizes" older adults. Senior advocates who do want more home-care options also worry that the state will not deliver on the home-care side but will simply try to save money by taking people out of nursing homes. All of these concerns are legitimate. Resistance to change can be an advocate's greatest strategy for change because it helps sharpen one's thinking and adjust policies and programs to respond to the concerns raised.

Empirical evidence to support a vision is a strong driving force for change. Skills in conducting research and translating it in a meaningful way are crucial in systems advocacy. In this case, the pilot data were quite helpful in exploding the myth that people who leave nursing homes require an intensive level of care that will "suck the community dry." The evidence shed light on the reality that many people in nursing homes do not need a lot of care. They need supportive services in the community, not necessarily intensive care. The $120 per day spent in a nursing home can go far in the community for many institutionalized persons. For example, some people in the pilot only needed meals on wheels.

Advocates also need to advance a plan for change that addresses the concerns of the resistors. For example, the nurse advocate worked with her department's nurse leaders to initially target particular people in nursing homes to approach for counseling about their choices in the community. The CCC protocol calls for a state-employed nurse to talk with people who have been in the nursing home for approximately 3 to 6 months, a time when they might have recovered from their initial health problems that led to the nursing home admission. These people have exhausted their Medicare benefits and are well on their way to becoming Medicaid beneficiaries. If they are not helped at this point, they will begin to lose their homes and informal supports. Return to the community becomes even more difficult later.

Continued

Resistance to change will continue, especially during the early stages of implementation. Systems advocacy is needed most during this stage because one failure will make it harder to initiate a similar change in the future. The attitude often becomes, "We tried that once and it failed." In this case, CCC staff members reported initial resistance from nursing home staff. In more than one case, nursing home discharge planners stated that they feared dismissal from their jobs if they cooperated with the CCC counselors (Lagnado, 2001). Most felt they needed constantly updated information about community resources and materials to help them explain various nursing home alternatives. The nurse advocate and her staff sought and obtained a grant from the Centers for Medicare and Medicaid Services to help develop those materials.

ISSUES AND DISCUSSION

Advocacy can help move an idea into action. Stabilizing that new policy or program is the only way to make systems advocacy a success. Legislation is one way to make sure that the idea will continue because it becomes illegal to return to the old way of doing things. Another way is to provide evidence that the new way is working and incorporate the new way into the culture of the organization (in this case the state).

To obtain an objective, formative evaluation of this expanded program, NJDHSS contracted with the Rutgers Center for State Health Policy (CSHP) in 1999 to design and implement an evaluation of the CCC program. Initial findings were encouraging (Silberberg & Howell-White, 2000). The most recent findings continue to support a continuation of the program (Howell-White, 2003). What began with a group of spirited nurses in New Jersey has resulted in critical change for the delivery of services to senior citizens. New Jersey has more than doubled the percent of long-term care funds spent on home- and community-based care for older adults. In fact, from its initiation in 1998 to 2004, more than 5000 persons have been transferred from nursing homes to community living (Medstat, 2005).

The CCC program is based on the belief that people want to exercise their choice. No one would be forced to leave a nursing home but would be given information and help to move to their preferred living situation. The CSHP evaluation focused on how satisfied people are with their choice to leave the nursing home and their quality of life in their current living situation. They also examined the dependency needs of these former nursing home residents and the extent to which those needs are being met. The CCC program evaluation resulted in several salient research findings (Howell-White, 2003). Most former nursing home residents are now living in a home-based setting and are very satisfied with their current living situation. Their quality of life improved. Most are able to do things that make life more enjoyable, like visiting with family and friends.

Most are able to perform almost all activities of daily living (i.e., bathing, dressing, eating) and about half of the instrumental activities of daily living (i.e., shopping, cooking, taking prescribed medications). Although former nursing home residents are living fairly independently, receiving only a little help with activities of daily living, many are receiving assistance with the instrumental activities of daily living.

These findings indicate that most former nursing home residents are very satisfied when they are helped to leave a nursing home and return to the community. For the most part, they are receiving the services they need and have an improved quality of life. Moreover, the CCC counselors (and the program, in general) seem to support and help in the nursing home residents' return to the community. Based in part on these findings, the state is continuing the program with the staffing and budget needed to continue it.

This case study exemplifies several simultaneous systems changes. It emphasizes change-agent skills as the most critical advocacy skills needed by the nurses who created and advanced these ideas. Few APNs will choose to lead this kind of systems advocacy. But many will choose to support or resist it. At a minimum, APNs need to understand systems advocacy. Systems advocacy involves citizenship and a call for participation in the decisions that affect our lives and the lives of those we serve (Joel, 1998).

Consumer-Driven Systems-Level Advocacy

Nurses can lead systems advocacy efforts both as professionals and as consumers. One case example comes from the mental health arena. The consumer movement in mental health is a strong model for the influence of consumers. Consumers provide the unique perspective of their experience with mental illness (Solomon, 2001). There is no consumer health-care group more powerful than the National Alliance for the Mentally Ill (NAMI). The consumer movement in mental health and the work of NAMI is reflected in the landmark report, *Mental Health: A Report of the Surgeon General* (U.S. DHHS, 1999). Following this report, The Presidents New Freedom Commission Report *Achieving the Promise: Transforming Mental Health Care in America* (U.S. DHHS, 2003) calls for a transformation of the mental health system with consumer involvement in shifting the mental health system to a system of individually defined recovery. The following describes another exemplar of systems advocacy; this exemplar is driven by consumers, particularly a nurse.

Advocacy Exemplar: A Nurse Consumer in Suicide Prevention

Advocacy is one role consumers may assume. Many health professionals are family member consumers affected by suicide. In fact, the National Strategy for Suicide Prevention (U.S. DHHS, 2001) is directly related to a grassroots movement started by a couple, Elsie and Jerry Weyrauch, who are parent survivors of suicide. Suicide survivors are family members, significant others, or acquaintances who have experienced the loss of a loved one as a result of suicide.

The Case of Elsie

Elsie Weyrauch is a retired psychiatric nurse. Her husband Jerry is a retired navy officer. Elsie and Jerry lost their daughter Terri Ann, a physician, to suicide 15 years ago. Since then, they have worked tirelessly for suicide prevention. They founded Suicide Prevention Advocacy Network, Inc. (SPAN), a grassroots advocacy organization, in 1996 in Marietta, Georgia.

SPAN links the energy of those bereaved by suicide with the expertise of leaders in education, religion, science, business, government, and public service to significantly reduce suicide. It is a nonprofit organization dedicated to the creation and implementation of national, state, and local suicide prevention strategies (SPAN, 2002). SPAN USA includes suicide survivors, suicide attempt survivors, and community activists. SPAN activities have included holding awareness events, visiting and writing letters to legislators, advocating for the passage of congressional resolutions related to suicide, participating in public hearings, hosting suicide awareness events in Washington, DC, cosponsoring a national strategy meeting, and sitting on federal advisory groups.

Continued

The story of SPAN (as described in the national strategy) over 6 years is an inspiring testimonial to the role of consumers as advocates and the nurse-consumer as an advocate. SPAN championed guidelines developed by the United Nations and the World Health Organization (1996) as a way to encourage development of a national suicide prevention strategy for the United States. Their work to marshal social will for suicide prevention generated congressional resolutions recognizing suicide as a national problem and suicide prevention as a national priority. These resolutions provided further impetus to develop a national suicide prevention strategy (DHHS, 2001).

SPAN propelled the creation of an innovative public-private partnership to jointly sponsor a National Suicide Prevention Conference, convened in Reno, Nevada, in October 1998 (also known as the Reno Conference). Participating agencies within the U.S. Department of Health and Human Services (DHHS) were the Centers for Disease Control and Prevention (CDC), the National Institutes of Health (NIH), the Office of the Surgeon General, the Substance Abuse and Mental Health Services Administration, the Health Resources and Service Administration, the Indian Health Service, and the Public Health Service Regional Health Administrators. Conference participants, including researchers, mental health and substance abuse clinicians, policy makers, suicide survivors, consumers of mental health services, school staff, and community activists and leaders discussed eight background papers that were commissioned to summarize the evidence base for suicide prevention (Silverman, Davidson, & Potter, 2001). Working in interdisciplinary groups, participants at the Reno conference offered many recommendations for action that were shaped into a list of 81 by an expert panel.

Surgeon General David Satcher then issued the Call to Action to Prevent Suicide, a blueprint for addressing suicide that succeeded through awareness, intervention and methodology based on the highest-ranked 81 Reno Conference recommendations (U.S. Public Health Service [PHS], 1999). A National Strategy Leadership Consultants Group was formed and four public hearings were held. A federal steering group drafted the national strategy. The surgeon general released the *National Strategy for Suicide Prevention: Goals and Objectives for Action* 2 years after the Reno Conference (U.S. DHHS, 2001). The national strategy is now informing funding priorities, research, and state and local plans. Despite this tremendous progress in suicide prevention, the Weyrauchs continue to urge local, state, federal, and international communities to never let up. Now in their 70s, they exclaim, "We can't wait. We're too old."

ISSUES AND DISCUSSION

Often consumers serve not only as advocates but also as activists who assertively and unrelentingly assault the barriers to their cause. The Weyrauchs have been able to dialogue with every level of government and industry and with mental health professionals and researchers, survivors, and suicidal individuals. For example, legislators who are themselves survivors have come forward as spokespersons for the survivor experience and the need for suicide prevention. From what started in a small operation in their own home, the Weyrauchs have inspired a movement that has spurred increased awareness, legislative activity, partnerships, funding, and collaboration on a state, national, and international level. In fact they have accomplished what mental health professionals and suicidologists only dreamed about. They have served as a bridge for groups to begin dialogue and to take assertive action.

They have also pushed the barrier of stigma. The stigma associated with mental illness, substance abuse, and suicide is the most formidable obstacle to future progress in the arena of mental health, contributing to failure to seek help, low reimbursement for mental health services, and inadequate funding for prevention (U.S. DHHS, 1999). In a SPAN-sponsored event, quilts from many states were displayed on the Capitol steps to bring the faces to the stories of the survivors. Elsie and Jerry always have time to comfort a new survivor at an event and welcome them to the community embrace of survivors, and when they are ready, give them a task.

Clearly one of the contributing factors to their success, in addition to their determination, commitment to their daughter's memory, and tremendous family talent, is combining the forces of their training and experience in military and nursing leadership. They have collaborated with willing partners, such as legislators, who are also suicide survivors and probably most importantly, with the former Surgeon General Satcher. Surgeon General Satcher was the first surgeon general to focus on mental health and suicide prevention.

APNs, including Virginia Trotter Betts and Beverly Malone, past presidents of the American Nurses Association, and Janet Grossman (one of the authors of this chapter), have collaborated with the Weyrauchs in activities such as fundraising, leading the national strategy meeting, serving on conference planning committees, and preparing the national strategy. Nurses have much to learn by listening to the consumer perspective and trying unconventional ways to address critical public health issues such as suicide. Through partnerships, APNs can learn to join forces with consumers and work under their leadership.

To borrow from the view described by Schroeder and Gadow (2000), the Weyrauchs established a partnership in which consumers, professionals, and politicians composed a mutually satisfying interpretation of the urgency of suicide prevention. In the partnership they reached a meaning ("suicide prevention can't wait," and "we don't have much time") that they all affirmed. The meaning was an interpretation that coherently connected all the elements of the situation in coauthorship of a health narrative (Schroeder & Gadow, 2000). The National Strategy for Suicide Prevention is that health narrative.

This exemplar illustrates several of the themes in the literature on advocacy, including the following:

- Advocacy is an activity that is not owned by one sector of health care.
- The consumer is an expert.
- Advocacy is a partnership between consumers and professionals.
- Advocacy calls for the development of creative strategies.

HOW NURSES LEARN ADVOCACY

Whether advocating for individuals and families, or advocating for system changes that will support them better, APNs need to develop many skills. We emphasize those skills in the case examples. Developing these skills takes practice. Benner (1991) emphasizes that the expert nurse learns the advocacy role through regular dialogue with other members of the nursing community, the patient, the patient's family, and other clinicians. Foley et al. (2002a) suggest nurses new to the field need nurturing and administrative support to take on this role.

Curtain (1979) proposes a "philosophical foundation and ideal of nursing is the nurse as *advocate*" (p. 2). Fundamental to nursing is the understanding of each individual as a unique human being and of the needs created by their illness or condition. This knowledge is acquired through the nurse-patient relationship, and therefore is distinctly nursing knowledge. Recognition that it is the individual, not the professional, who can make decisions for himself or herself calls for a synthesis of this knowledge and an understanding that "freedom, respect and integrity are essential to our full development as a person," (p. 3).

Application of this philosophy may be more deeply rooted in a value system than in a learning process (Foley et al., 2002a). In their study, Foley et al. found that advocating for others was a natural and important aspect of practice rather than a learned experience. The value of advocacy stems from family and community experience and is integral to their (nurses) being as persons. Although the value of advocacy cannot be taught, faculty "may need to define advocacy in relationship to patient care," (Foley et al., 2002a, p. 185).

Some nurses learn how to advocate by watching other nurses interact with patients and working with mentors (Foley et al., 2002a). Role modeling and dialogue provide opportunities for positive learning experiences. Expert nurses and clinicians are positioned to provide examples and dialogue necessary to developing advocacy. This finding corresponds to Benner's (1991) belief that advocating is learned as part of the nursing community when the notion of good is enacted and discussed daily. Foley et al. (2002a) state, "Dialogue is essential in a practice such as nursing, in which knowledge is both scientific and historical, and therefore is dependent upon shared understandings among clinicians, patients, and families," (p. 181). However, nurses must experience the concepts of caring, suffering, hope, and recovery to internalize them (Benner, 1991).

Throughout the process of role modeling and mentoring, validation and a supportive environment are necessary if nurses are to gain the confidence required to advocate for patients (Foley et al., 2002a). Experienced nurses who recognize the risk that new nurses take in revealing their knowledge deficits create positive learning experiences and support a foundation for the development of advocacy practice. New nurses require corroboration that their practice and judgment are correct. Foley et al. (2002a) found that "experienced nurses can consciously help new nurses learn advocacy through preceptorships or one-to-one-mentoring," (p. 185).

Graduate programs in advanced practice nursing do not typically prepare graduates in the advocacy role. Sarah Lawrence College offers the only master's degree in the growing field of health advocacy, describing the role as promoting patients' rights in an increasingly complex health-care system. Resources available to the APN include Web sites (such as www.ana.org) and documents such as the *Guide to Grassroots Activism,* available on the American Association of Colleges of Nursing Web site (www.aacn.nche.edu). These references can provide information on important issues that need nurses' advocacy and guidance in preparing correspondence or approaching legislators.

CONCLUSION

Advocacy is not an evidenced-based role, but it is a historic role. APNs need to develop practice skills to advocate at both the individual/family and systems levels. The profession needs to conduct more empirical studies to guide this practice, and we need to strengthen our education and diffusion strategies to advance this practice role. APNs can contribute to all of these efforts. Nurses need to make visible stories of advocacy practice for their colleagues. Advocacy activities of nurses need to be more systematically analyzed and the effect of the activities documented.

References

Abbot, A. (1988). *The system of professions: Essays on the division of expert labor.* Chicago: University Press of Chicago.

American Nurses Association. (2001). *Code for nurses with interpretative statements.* Silver Springs, Md: American Nurses Publishing.

Benner, P. (1984). *From novice to expert: Excellence and power in clinical nursing practice.* Menlo Park, CA: Addison-Wesley.

Benner, P. (1991). The role of experience, narrative and community in skilled ethical comportment. *Advances in Nursing Science, 14*(2), 1.

Bishop, A., & Scudder, J. (1990). *The practical and moral and personal sense of nursing: A phenomenological philosophy of practice.* Albany: State University of New York.

Connolly, P. M. (1999). Consumer advocacy. In C. A. Shea, L. R. Pelletier, E. C. Poster, G. W. Stuart, & M. P. Verhey (Eds.), *Advanced practice nursing in psychiatric and mental health care* (p. 387). St. Louis: Mosby.

Curtain, I. H. (1979). The nurse as advocate: A philosophical foundation for nursing. *Advances in Nursing Science, 1*(3), 1–10.

Diekelmann, N. (1991). The emancipatory power of the narrative. In *Curriculum revolution: Community building and activism* (p. 41). New York: National League for Nursing Press.

Foley, B. J., Minick, M. P., & Kee C. C. (2002a). How nurses learn advocacy. *Journal of Nursing Scholarship, 34*(2), 181–187.

Foley, B. J., Minick, M. P., & Kee, C. C. (2002b). Nursing advocacy during a military operation. *Western Journal of Nursing Research, 22*(4), 492–498.

Gadow, S. (1980). Existential advocacy: Philosophical foundation of nursing. In S. F. Spicker, & S. Gadow, (Eds.), *Nursing: Images and ideals* (p. 79). New York: Springer.

Gadow, S. (1989). Clinical subjectivity. Advocacy for silent patients. *Nursing Clinics of North America, 24*(2), 535–541.

Gates, B. (1995). Whose best interest? *Nursing Times, 91*(4), 31–32.

Geoffrey, M. (1998). Ritual action and its effect on the role of the nurse as advocate. *Journal of Advanced Nursing, 27*(1), 189–194.

Haber, J., & Billings, C. (1995). Primary mental health care: A model of psychiatric-mental health nursing. *Journal of the American Psychiatric Nurses Association, 1*(5), 154.

Hamric, A., & Sposs, J. (Eds.). (1989). *The clinical nurse specialist in theory and practice* (2nd ed.). Philadelphia: WB Saunders.

Hanley, B. (2002). Policy development and analysis. In D. J. Mason, J. K. Leavitt, & M. W. Chafee (Eds.), *Policy and politics in nursing and health care* (4th ed.). Philadelphia: WB Saunders.

Hewitt, J. A. (2002). Critical review of the arguments debating the role of the nurse advocate. *Journal of Advanced Nursing, 37*(5), 439–445.

Howell-White, S. (2003). *Current living situation and service needs of former nursing home residents: An evaluation of New Jersey's nursing home transition program.* New Brunswick, NJ: Rutgers Center for State Health Policy.

Joel, L. (1998). On citizenship in a great profession. *American Journal of Nursing, 98*(4), 7.

Jones, E. (1982). Advocacy—A tool for radical nursing curriculum planners. *Journal of Nurse Education, 21*(1), 40–45.

Kane, R., Kane, R., & Ladd, R. (1998). *The heart of long-term care.* New York: Oxford University Press.

Kohnke, M. F. (1982). *Advocacy: Risk and reality.* St. Louis: Mosby.

Ladd, R. (1999). *State LTC profiles report, 1996. Balancing long-term care.* Minneapolis, MN: Division of Health Services Research and Policy, School of Public Health.

Lagnado, L. (2001, February 21). Living and dying: An innovative New Jersey program offers what may be a more humane alternative to nursing homes. *Wall Street Journal,* p. R11.

Mallik, M., & Rafferty, A. M. (2000). Diffusion of the concept of patient advocacy. *Journal of Nursing Scholarship, 32*(4), 399–404.

Mason, D. J., Leavitt, J. K., & Chafee, M, W. (2002). Policy and politics: A framework for action. In D. J. Mason, J. K. Leavitt, & M. W. Chafee (Eds.), *Policy and politics in nursing and health care* (4th ed., p. 1). Philadelphia: WB Saunders.

Medstat. (2005). *New Jersey—Community choice initiative.* Washington, DC: Promising Practices in Home and Community-Based Services.

Mezey, M., & McGivern, D. (Eds.). (1999). *Nurses, nurse, and practitioners: Evolution to advanced practice.* New York: Springer.

Milette, B. (1993). Client advocacy and the moral orientation of nurses. *Western Journal of Nursing Research, 15*(5), 607–618.

Mitchell, G., & Bournes, D. (2000). Nurse as patient advocate? In search of straight thinking. *Nursing Science Quarterly, 13*(3), 204–209.

Reinhard, S. (1999, April 27). Testimony before the Senate Appropriations Committee. Trenton, New Jersey.

Reinhard, S., & Scala, M. (2001). *Navigating the long-term care maze: New approaches to information and assistance in three states.* Washington, DC: AARP Public Policy Institute.

Schroeder, C., & Gadow, G. (2000). An advocacy approach to ethics and community health. In E. Anderson, & J. McFarlane (Eds.), *Community as partner: Theory and practice in nursing* (3rd ed., p. 78). Philadelphia: Lippincott Williams & Wilkins.

Segesten, K. (1993). Patient advocacy: An important part of the daily work of the expert nurse. *Scholarly Inquiry for Nursing Practice, 7*(2), 129–135.

Shea, C., Mahoney, M., & Lacey, J. (1997). Breaking through the barriers to domestic violence intervention. *American Journal of Nursing, 97*(6), 26–33.

Silberberg, M., & Howell-White, S. (2000). *Transitions to the community: A survey of former nursing home residents discharged after community choice counseling.* New Brunswick, NJ: Rutgers Center for State Health Policy.

Silverman, M., Davidson, L., & Potter, L. (Eds). (2001). National suicide prevention conference background papers. *Suicide & Life-threatening Behavior, 31*(1, Suppl).

Snowball, J. (1996). Asking nurses about advocating for patients: "Reactive" and "proactive" accounts. *Journal of Advanced Nursing, 24*(1), 67–75.

Solomon, A. (2001). *The noonday demon: An atlas of depression.* New York: Scribner.

Suicide Prevention Advocacy Network USA. (March 2002). Newsletter.

Stein, L., Watts, D., & Howell, T. (1990). The doctor-nurse game revisited. *New England Journal of Medicine, 322*(8), 546–549.

Stuart, G. W., & Laraia, M. T. (2001). *Principles and practice of psychiatric nursing* (7th ed.). St. Louis: Mosby.

Sullivan, W. P. (1991). *Case management in alcohol and drug treatment: Conceptual issues and practical applications.* Springfield, MO: Southwest Missouri Center for Social Research.

World Health Organization. (1996). *Prevention of suicide: Guidelines for the formulation and implementation of national strategies (ST/ESA/245).* Geneva: World Health Organization.

U.S. Department of Health and Human Services. (1987). *Toward a model plan for a comprehensive community-based mental health system.* Rockville, MD: Author.

U.S. Department of Health and Human Services. (1999). *Mental health: A report of the Surgeon General.* Rockville, MD: US Department of Health and Human Services, Substance Abuse and Mental Health Services Administration, Center for Mental Health Services, National Institutes of Health, National Institute of Mental Health.

U.S. Department of Health and Human Services. (2001). *National strategy for suicide prevention: Goals and objectives for action.* Rockville, MD: U.S. Department of Health and Human Services, Public Health Service.

U.S. Department of Health and Human Services. (2003). *Achieving the promise: Transforming mental health care in America.* Rockville, MD: US Department of Health and Human Services, New Freedom Commission on Mental Health.

U.S. Public Health Service. (1999). *The Surgeon General's call to action to prevent suicide.* Washington, DC: U.S. Public Health Service.

Case Management and Advanced Practice Nursing

16

Patricia M. Haynor

Denise Fessler

Irene McEachen

Marylou Yam

HISTORICAL BACKGROUND

Case management and advanced practice nursing share a long history in the United States. Although both of these concepts have been coined in nursing literature by these terms only within the last two decades (Tahan, 1998), their roots can be found in nursing history as early as the 1860s (Kersbergen, 1996). Reading between the lines of health-care and nursing history, it is possible to witness the evolution of the process of nurses with expert clinical knowledge who manage care.

The case management process was used in the 1860s in early settlement houses for immigrants and the poor. Information was collected on family needs, required services were determined and delivered, and a system of follow-up was designed to ensure their appropriateness (Reynolds & Smeltzer, 1997). The first board of charities was established in Massachusetts in 1863 to coordinate public services and conserve public funds. Social workers coordinated most of these services for immigrants and the poor under the auspices of charity boards until the late 1800s. Their emphasis at this time was on the management and allocation of funds. In 1877, interagency cooperation and coordination of voluntary and public services to the poor became a reality under the Charity Organization Societies (Tahan, 1998). In 1901, Mary Richmond, a social services pioneer, published a model of case coordination with the client as the core concern among the social-service agencies. Richmond's concern for her clients revolved around the lack of communication and coordination that frequently resulted in the duplication of services as clients moved through the system (Weil & Karls, 1985).

U.S. public health nursing was founded toward the end of the 19th century by Lillian Wald (Dock, 1937). The work of the public health nurse was to respond to the needs of the populations at greatest risk in our society (i.e., new immigrants living in tenement housing) and to provide ways to reduce illness and promote health (Wald, 1915). Wald was considered a visionary not only for the invention of public health nursing, but for the establishment of a nationwide system of insurance payments for home-based care and the recognition of the independence and accomplishments of the public health nurses. Interestingly, the public health nurses in the early 1900s were not subject to physician orders and established themselves as health educators and promoters (Frachel, 1988). The following quote from an editorial in *The Public Health Nurse,* although written in 1919 about the public health nurses, could easily appear in today's literature referring to the advanced practice nurse (APN).

277

Why not come boldly forth, one and all, and claim the right to exercise the promotion of health as a profession? The best educated nurses spend as many years in training to exercise their profession as physicians to prepare themselves for the care and scientific prevention of disease ("The Profession of Promoting Health," 1919, p. 12).

These public health nurses were perceived as the elite in nursing because they practiced autonomously and creatively (Reverby, 1987). The clinical expertise of these nurses is explained historically through the interpretation of practice stories using an approach that seeks to understand the narrative without preconceived expectations or categories (Palmer, 1969). Several competencies of the public health nurse were readily elicited from historical anecdotes: public health nurses' activities included "making inquiries, shrewd identification of evidence, steady plodding, helping others to help themselves, teaching, explanation and demonstration, and organizing a household to knit the family" (Zerwekh, 1992, p. 85). In short, we are looking at a description of the APN! Wald's (1915) early experiments in community-based care left a rich legacy that is still pertinent in today's health-care environment. Her work suggested that we (a) create a mix of public and private programs that link effectively with health-care institutions as "value-added" or complementary to client needs, (b) use evidence-based practice as a counterbalance to document cost versus effectiveness, (c) institute sufficient control over practice to produce desired outcomes, and (d) have expert practitioners with sufficient education and abilities to manage complex care (Buhler-Wilkerson, 1993).

Wald's legacy is similar to the interdisciplinary definition of case management that was developed by the Case Management Society of America (CMSA) in 1995, which defined case management as "a collaborative process which assesses, plans, implements, coordinates, monitors and evaluates options and services to meet an individual's health needs through communication and available resources to promote quality, cost-effective outcomes" (p. 8). It is also similar to the definition proposed by the American Nurses Credentialing Center (ANCC, 1998), which defined nursing case management as:

a dynamic and systemic collaborative approach to providing and coordinating health care services to a defined population. It is a participative process to identify and facilitate options and services for meeting individuals' health needs, while decreasing fragmentation and duplication of care and enhancing quality, cost-effective clinical outcomes (p. 3).

The historical anecdotes of Wald's public health nurses demonstrated the work of an expert nurse who managed care for individuals and populations. These nurses practiced the core functions of case management: assessment, planning, linking, monitoring, advocacy, and outreach.

In the early 1900s, as an expansion of the role of the community-based public health nurse caring for individuals, the federal government mandated the United States Public Health Services to develop a system of case management with the community as the client. Their initial charge was to coordinate larger environmental problems such as sanitation and the prevention and control of epidemics. The thrust to address individual needs through the United States Public Health Services did not occur until passage of the Social Security Act in 1935, which provided funds to support these activities (Shonick, 1988).

The 1920s saw the development of the Community Chest Movement and other social planning agencies (excluding nursing) to deal with coordinating care for families in distress and abused children. Within this same period, child guidance centers were created that experimented with multidisciplinary team planning (including nursing) to avoid duplication or fragmentation of services (Kersbergen, 1996).

After World War II, the Veterans Administration established a center in Los Angeles for veteran's benefits, which was its first model for "one-stop" health care. This was the inception of its ongoing model for a continuum of care (Weil & Karls, 1985).

The 1960s and 1970s witnessed a proliferation of human services as a result of the Civil Rights Movement and President Johnson's "War on Poverty" (Weil & Karls, 1985). This proliferation of newly developed programs resulted in fragmented, duplicative, and uncoordinated services that were difficult for the public to navigate. Case management enabled the consumer to become an active participant in services required. Additional programs for the mentally ill and retarded and legislation for military services health care continued to encourage integration of services and the development of a continuum of care. Demonstration projects in the 1970s created the role of "systems agent," a person charged with coordinating system resources for clients and accountability for this successful movement (Intagliata, 1982). Continuing legislation in the late 1970s (the Developmentally Disabled Assistance Act and the Bill of Rights Act, 1978) mandated that service coordination be accomplished through case-managed services (Intagliata, 1982).

In the 1980s, case management services moved beyond public health and the mentally ill and veteran's administration services into the acute-care hospitals with the initiation of the prospective payment system. The implementation of diagnostic-related groups for the Medicare population created a reimbursement system that rewarded shorter lengths of stay by paying for hospital care by case, rather than by costs or services delivered. Case management, discharge planning, and use review committees were some of the initial tools implemented to facilitate the timely discharge of patients. During the 1980s, health insurance companies also initiated case management to coordinate and allocate services for participants with high costs or catastrophic illnesses (Brault & Kissinger, 1991). The entrance of health maintenance organizations (HMOs) and preferred provider organizations (PPOs) as another insurance product for prepaid health-care delivery added to the frenzy to control costs while delivering quality care. The efforts to coordinate services and control costs affected the majority of health-care consumers as prepaid or per case (Medicare/Medicaid) payment systems became the norm by the late 1980s. At the start of the 21st century, controlling costs remains the mainstay for fiscal viability and nurse case management continues to play a pivotal role in this arena. One of the driving factors for this fiscal effort to control costs is related to the changing demographics of the U.S. public, which shows the number of elderly growing faster than any other segment of the population. As health care continues to become more complex, fragmented, and costly, the nature of case management grows in complexity as well.

CASE MANAGER ROLE COMPETITORS

Case managers may be registered nurses (RNs), social workers, physical therapists, psychologists, physicians, mental health workers, pharmacists, school nurses, or teachers. Although there is consensus about the core functions of case managers (ANCC, 1998; CMSA, 1995; Daniels & Ramey, 2005), the activities within different disciplines are highly variable based on the background of the individual. The type of professional chosen often depends on the setting of care delivery, the type of care coordination required, the payer's preference, federal and state program mandates, or the cost of a particular professional.

In the 1980s and early 1990s, debate in the literature focused on whether nurses were better suited than other health professionals, such as social workers and physicians, to be case managers. Several authors effectively argued that nurses' clinical knowledge and skills, as well as their holistic perspective of client care, made them the ideal case managers (Cohen & Cesta, 1993; Mundinger, 1984; Zander, 1990). Multiple disciplines provide case management services in an ever-expanding array of settings, making standardization of the process and measurement of the outcomes difficult (Huber & Craig, 2007). However, research has documented positive outcomes for clients when nurse case managers were used (Cronin & Maklebust, 1989; Ethridge & Lamb, 1989). Heart failure patients participating in a home-based, advanced practice nurse–directed program reported positive outcomes and improved patient satisfaction (Anderson, 2007). In an effort to improve outcomes for patients with type 2 diabetes, nurse practitioners (NPs) focused on behavior changes for patients via coaching. This was done during office visits, and although outcomes were not formally researched, the anecdotal reports appeared to be positive for patients (Hayes, McCahon, Panaki, Hamre, & Pohlman, 2008).

DIFFERENTIATING THE LEVELS OF NURSE CASE MANAGEMENT PRACTICE

Recently, discussion has been centered on the use of nurse case managers prepared at the baccalaureate versus the advanced practice graduate level (Bower, 1992; Cesta & Tahan, 2003; Connors, 1993; Mahn & Spross, 1996). The American Nurses Association (ANA; 1992) asserts that minimum preparation for a nurse case manager is a bachelor's degree with 3 years of relevant experience. However, in practice, nurses functioning in case management positions have differing clinical and educational backgrounds, including in some settings, registered nurses (RNs) without a master's degree or even a bachelor of science in nursing (BSN). Their roles and responsibilities are also quite varied and defined in different ways, depending on the clinical site. The Tahan and Huber study (2006) provides an analysis of changes that occurred in the practice of case management over the 5-year period between the mid-1990s and early 2000s and highlights the activities, relationships, knowledge, and skills most required in the more recent years.

Connors (1993) suggested that because case managers serve clients with varying levels of care across the continuum, not every client who is case managed is complex or catastrophic. He pointed out that even though the nurses with master's degrees may be best suited to fill case management positions, this may not be possible given the practice demands. One approach would be to have baccalaureate degree–prepared nurses manage most clients and have APNs manage those cases with more complex needs. In other words, the nurse's expertise "should be matched with the complexity of the situation and amount of autonomy required to fulfill the role" (Connors, 1993, p. 196).

Support for the APN case management role, particularly with high-risk or high-cost client populations has been made in the literature (Connors 1993; Cronin & Maklebust, 1989; Hamric, 1992; Krichbaum, 1999). The APN has expert knowledge regarding the clinical population for which standards and pathways are written, and sees the whole client and understands his or her needs on a continuum-of-care basis. Moreover, the APN has the additional benefit of outcome accountability (Krichbaum, 1999).

An expanding use of APNs is noticed in the case management of patients with chronic diseases. As a result of their education and clinical skills, APNs are able to focus on the multidimensional nature of chronic illness. A group of hospital-based clinics called on APNs to join a team effort that successfully improved clinical outcomes for patients with diabetes (Boville, Saran, Salem, & Clough, 2007).

Similarly, Mahn and Zazworsky (2000) pointed out that APNs are well suited to perform case management for complex client populations because of their advanced education, autonomy, ability to conduct extensive assessments, and initiate and modify treatment regimens. These authors cited the work of Connors (1993), Hamric (1992), and Mahn and Spross (1996) to describe how the competencies of the APN role mirror those of the nurse case manager. Umbrell (2006) and Curtis, Lien, Chan, Grove, and Morris (2002) demonstrated the effectiveness of the APN in trauma management. The APN possesses specialized knowledge in providing "direct care, consultation, research utilization/continuous quality improvement, collaboration, data analysis and information management, change agency, ethical decision making and expert guidance and coaching" for a specific client population (Mahn & Zazworsky, 2000, p. 568). Such competencies are all congruent to those of nurse case managers. A research study to evaluate the impact of a nurse-directed educational activity that focused on lifestyle modification, such as diet and medication compliance, showed improved quality of life and functional capacity in people with heart disease (Kutzleb & Reiner, 2006).

To a lesser extent, arguments have also been presented for separate graduate programs in case management versus increasing case management content in existing advanced practice specialist master's programs (Falter, Cesta, Concert & Mason, 1999; Sowell & Young, 1997). One argument is that nurse practitioners (NPs) and clinical nurse specialists (CNSs) who are prepared at the master's level have the advanced clinical knowledge needed to care for clients with complex health-care needs and that these nurses can be effectively used to work with high-risk clinical populations. On the other hand, graduates who are master's prepared in case management have in-depth knowledge and skill in case management models, systems, and tools, health-care financing, reimbursement, and community resource use. These nurses can provide case management services and provide the leadership to design systems of care coordination and quality management in health-care organizations. Graduates from both types of master's programs can make a significant contribution to case management practice, administration, education, and research. More research demonstrating the effectiveness of nurses who have baccalaureate and master degrees needs to be conducted. Moreover, it is important that a distinction be made among nurses prepared at the baccalaureate, master's—advanced practice (NP or CNS), and master's—case management levels. See **Box 16-1** for a description of the levels of nurse care management practice.

BOX 16-1

Differentiating Between Advanced Practice Nurse Case Manager with a Baccalaureate or Master's Degree and a Nurse with a Master's Degree Prepared Specifically for Case Management

LEVELS OF CASE MANAGEMENT:

Baccalaureate Registered Nurse (RN) Case Managers have foundational theoretical and clinical knowledge in nursing. These nurses are able to manage the care of patients who are less complex and more predictable, often with the assistance of critical paths. These nurses may work in collaboration with an advanced practice nurse (APN) case manager prepared at the master's level or a nurse case manager prepared at the master's level.

Master's-APN Case Managers have clinical expertise and advanced knowledge in health and wellness promotion and illness intervention models for specific patient populations. These nurses can manage patients with complex health needs such as those in high-risk, vulnerable populations, and those who require high resource consumption. Additionally, these nurses are expected to conduct research related to case management practice, disease management, and clinical outcomes.

Nurses with Master's Level Preparation Specifically for the Functional Role of Case Manager possess expert knowledge and skill in case management models, processes and tools, health-care financing, reimbursement, outcome monitoring, and measurement. These nurses are able to design and monitor systems of care coordination and deliver case management services, and are expected to conduct research related to case management practice and clinical outcomes.

NURSE CASE MANAGEMENT MODELS

A review of the literature provides many types of case management models and differentiates the contributions each makes within a designated field. The common aspects of these models are advocacy, services brokering, risk management, care coordination, and a process designed to accomplish these objectives (Huber, 2000). Knollmueller (1989) identified seven models of case management: (a) social, (b) primary care, (c) medical/social, (d) HMO, (e) independent, (f) insurance, and (g) in-house. Stempel, Doerge, Van Mie, and Combs (1997) describe four types of nurse case management: (a) clinical case management, (b) payer-based case management, (c) program case management, and (d) community case management. Another breakdown of models of nurse case management is offered by Lamb (1992): (a) hospital based, (b) hospital-to-community based, and (c) community-based **(Table 16-1).**

The literature on nurse case manager practice within the different models reflects some dilemmas regarding the purpose, scope, and functions of the nurse case manager role. Although there is a large body of anecdotal stories, research in the field is still working to control the effect of extraneous variables in studies and developing nursing-sensitive outcomes. Qualitative descriptions of nurse case management practice have pointed to some common themes across all nurse case management practice. They include (a) working with individuals, families, and populations at risk; (b) applying the nursing process to enhance quality and cost outcomes; (c) accessing individuals and families in more than one setting; and (d) coordinating and advocacy integration (Lamb, 1995). With regard to the advocacy role, Hellwig, Yam, and DiGiulio (2003) proposed an advocacy model for nurse case management practice. In the authors' qualitative study, hospital-based nurse case managers described that their advocacy was based on the needs of the patient and their family, payer issues, and obstacles and opportunities for advocacy. Participants indicated the obstacles included time constraints and examples of opportunities were physician support, rapport with insurance companies, and use of a team approach (Hellwig et al., 2003).

The nurse case management models used in practice today are as rich and diverse as the individuals, families, and populations they serve. Current practice within hospital-based models in many organizations has moved from a primarily clinical case manager role to one of an intense use/discharge planning model. Conversely, the hospital-to-community-based and community-based

TABLE 16-1

Nurse Case Management Models

Model	Role Description	Example
Hospital-based; "within the walls"	Individual nurses as case managers coordinate services, unit based or disease based. Usually follow patients inside hospital.	New England Medical Center (Zander, 1996)
Hospital-to-community based	Case managers work with high-risk populations in acute-care and community settings.	See Naylor et al. (1999)
Community-based; "beyond the walls"	Case managers work with individuals in their homes and other community settings.	Carondelet St. Mary's (Forbes, 1999)

models have experienced an increasing need for a high level of clinical expertise in their case managers, as well as the traditional knowledge of community resources. Historically, nursing case management moved into the foreground with public health nursing at the beginning of the 20th century. As models continue to evolve in response to practice needs and environmental changes, the models for the 21st century must continue to include and enhance the role APNs can and do play in community-based practice models.

CASE MANAGER RESPONSIBILITIES AND SKILLS

Quality of care and efficient use of limited resources have been a hallmark of case management since the 1860s, with the intervening influence of early settlement houses, public health nursing, federal government legislation, and managed care. Regardless of who drives the process (e.g., insurance company, employer, federal government, or private entrepreneur), the outcome expectations are similar. The definitions of quality and efficiency may differ by source, but all models require a skill and knowledge set of their case managers. The setting in which the case manager practices, the model design, and patient population dictate the overall knowledge base and clinical expertise required. The national quality agenda will be supported by the involvement of nurse case managers. Case managers in all settings are alert to the importance of evaluation of quality and the appropriateness of care delivered to patients (White, 2004).

Successful nurse case management mandates a wide variety of both management and clinical skills. Some of the most typical management skills include delegation, conflict resolution, collaboration, crisis intervention, coordination, direction, consultation, and fiscal accountability. Clinical skill requirements vary from model to model and may include nurses educated from the diploma/associate degree to master's level. The suggested practice areas for differing levels of education (baccalaureate to master) are also discussed in this chapter. Nurses educated at the diploma/associate degree level frequently find themselves in positions in nurse case management similar to the baccalaureate RN case manager described in Box 16-1. A summary of the most common skills and competencies of nurse case managers is found in **Table 16-2.** This table is not meant to be an exhaustive listing of skills and competencies, but rather a snapshot view of what is needed by nurse case managers in varying situations.

Nurse case management continues to be a hybrid within nursing and has led many to examine the issue of "clinical expertise" as listed in the job descriptions of case managers. Calkin (1984), in attempt to differentiate between the expertise of a nurse case manager and APN case manager, defined the former as experts by experience and the latter as prepared by a combination of clinical experience and education. The advanced practice case managers retain their use of experience-based intuition, but use their additional academic and clinical preparation to manage more highly complex and unpredictable individuals and populations. Although the focus of advanced practice case managers is still on providing direct patient care, they also make significant contributions toward coordination of multidisciplinary care. This advanced practitioner in a case manager role can continue to monitor, advocate, and coordinate care for patients across the continuum and can develop programs and systems to support both community-based and private-practice-based care (Erickson, 1997).

Not all case managers practice the duties and responsibilities of managing patient care at the same advanced level. As nurse case managers become involved in more complex cases the need for advanced education becomes apparent. This growth in complexity has resulted in the need for APNs to join the ranks of case managers (Stanton, Swanson, Sherrod & Packa, 2005).

TABLE 16-2

Skills and Competencies of Nurse Case Manager

Skill/Competency	Goal
Patient advocacy	Assist patient in achieving autonomy and self-determination
Guardian of confidentiality	Preserve dignity and privacy
Case selection expert	Identify recipients of case management
Care coordinator	Procure and broker services; seamless continuum
Assessment and reassessment	Problem identification/resolution; monitor outcomes
Discharge planner	Facilitate movement in care continuum
Follow-through	Optimum care within resources available
Use management	Appropriateness of resources used
Knowledge of insurance structures/benefits	Interpret resources available to patient
Cost-benefit analysis (fiscal advocacy)	Demonstrate case management affect on care, usually monetary
Negotiation	Procure what patient requires for health purposes
Clinical expertise*	Appropriate care interventions, improvement in outcomes
Critical thinker	Think out of box to find creative solutions and increase case manager autonomy
Competent professional (includes accountability, knowledge of standards of practice, legal issues, and research ability)	Do the right thing at the right time for the right reason
Outcomes management	Evaluating and managing outcomes
Interpersonal (communication, assertiveness, collaboration, and tact/diplomacy)	Gather information and channel to appropriate sources
Organizational (time management, marketing/networking, prioritization, and report writer)	Use time and people resources wisely

*Depends on case management model and setting.

Adapted from Powell, S. K. (2000). *Case management a practice guide to success in managed care*. Philadelphia: Lippincott Williams & Wilkins; and More, P. K., & Mandell, S. (1997). *Nursing case management: an evolving practice*. New York, NY: McGraw-Hill.

TOOLS AND STRATEGIES

Through the development of clinical expertise, knowledge of research processes, communication skills, critical thinking, decision making, and leadership skills the APN is uniquely qualified to influence case management and disease management practice in a variety of health-care environments. The strategic use of APNs in the case management role to improve communication and collaboration with treating physicians is an effective tool, given the importance of physician involvement in the success of case and disease management interventions. Evidence-based interventions and standardized outcome measures are important strategies used in disease management programs to improve the quality of health-care services. These same principles and strategies are beginning to be applied to case management practice. In an effort to assist case managers and program designers to identify effective tools and evidence-based guidelines for case management, and to standardize the evaluation of the outcomes of case management interventions, the CMSA created the Council for Case Management Accountability (CCMA) in 1996 (CMSA, 2002). Through the use of expert case management researchers and practitioners, the CCMA has identified five care domains and outcomes in which case management has been shown or believed to have an affect:

- *Patient knowledge:* Case management patients need adequate knowledge on a number of fronts, including knowledge about health benefits and services, knowledge about their health conditions, and knowledge about their treatment plans. Successful case management results in improved patient knowledge.
- *Patient involvement in care:* Health care is a cooperative endeavor; patients play a key role in quality, cost-effective care. Successful case management involves clients in the decisions and actions of self-care.
- *Patient empowerment:* Case management should help patients build a sense of self-efficacy regarding their ability to manage their own health, as well as an ability to negotiate the care system successfully.
- *Patient adherence:* Cost-effective health care is predicated on patients' consistent adherence to their treatment programs. Successful case management results in higher rates of patient adherence.
- *Coordination of care:* Case managers provide consistency of care across the continuum while eliminating redundancy and waste (CMSA, 2002).

The CCMA's goal is to publish state of the science "white papers" in each of these domains, with the goal of providing case managers with the latest evidence-based intervention strategies and tools along with standardized outcome measures. Through the use of these tools, case managers increase the likelihood of successful case management interventions and form a basis for consistent research and comparison of case management results. The work of the CCMA also helps to focus program development in the domains in which case management is thought to have an effect—it is through the principles "manage what you measure" and "measure what you manage" that case management programs may demonstrate their value. As stated previously, the standardization of outcome measures allows for the comparison of the effectiveness of specific case management interventions applied in a variety of settings with a range of populations.

Little is known to date regarding the amount or type of nursing (or "dose of nursing") needed to affect patient outcomes. This knowledge is necessary in applying case and disease management interventions (Brooten & Naylor, 1995). For example, there have been a number of published studies highlighting the effectiveness of APNs as case managers for Medicare-aged members with heart failure. The question becomes is it necessary for the APN to have direct patient interaction or contact at the physician's office or clinic or in the home, or is it just as effective to use telephonic outreach with this population? Should the use of the APN be relegated to high-risk case management only, or should APNs be included in health education and promotion? What interventions seem to provide the most excellent outcomes cost effectively? The work of the CCMA will help to answer these important research questions. To date, two white papers have been published regarding patient adherence since the inception of the program.

Similar to the work of the CMSA-CCMA project, the University of Iowa College of Nursing has been involved since 1995 in research supported by the National Institute of Nursing, titled "The Iowa Nursing Intervention and Outcomes Projects—NIC [Nursing Interventions Classifications] & NOC [Nursing Outcomes Classification]." The NIC is a comprehensive standardized language used to describe evidence-based nursing interventions and provide the documented literature and research on which each is based. Each intervention reflects current clinical practice and research. All interventions are accompanied by a list of background readings that support the development of the intervention; all interventions have been reviewed by experts in clinical practice and by relevant clinical practice specialty organizations; a feedback process to receive suggested changes has been developed (Iowa Interventions and Outcomes Project, 2002).

The NOC is standardized language that describes patient outcomes sensitive to the nursing interventions noted in NIC. When tied to the work of the CCMA (focusing on those interventions and outcomes linked to the five core domains of case management), NIC and NOC can assist case managers in using evidence-based nursing interventions for care planning and the identification of appropriate outcome measures. This work is comprehensive, readily available, and updated on a regular basis. In addition, NIC and NOC are available on CD-ROM, which allows for easy access by case managers. Unfortunately, few case managers and administrators are aware of the work of the CCMA or of NIC and NOC.

Another strategy used to ensure high-quality, effective case management processes and outcomes is the development of case management database systems using national case management standards and guidelines such as the Utilization Review Accreditation Commission/American Accreditation Health Care Commission case management standards. In the absence of existing outcomes data, those who routinely evaluate the quality of programs consider the following equation as an indicator of the potential for good outcomes: GOOD STRUCTURE + GOOD PROCESSES = GOOD OUTCOMES.

Good structure in case management is achieved, primarily, through the use of highly skilled and educated case managers. Researchers have proven many benefits of using APNs in the case management role (Brooten & Naylor, 1995; Lamb & Stempel, 1994). Case management administrators need to ensure that good orientation and continuing education experiences are available for case managers and further that they are tailored to the specific setting and populations served to ensure competent case management practice and promote exemplary care management techniques. Encouraging the attainment of certification and recognizing and rewarding the various levels of case management practice is another strategy designed to develop high-performing case management teams.

Good processes can be realized through the development and use of case management systems that follow national case management standards and guidelines and provide links to important resources and information, such as NIC and NOC and case management industry Web sites. Skiba and Cohen (2000) highlight the critical importance of technology in case management practice, stating, "data-based decision making in case management is crucial for ensuring quality of care and the appropriate management of patient outcomes, and it underpins the viability of this delivery model of care" (p. 132). Although there are few examples of systems that incorporate all the business requirements of case management practice, many are being developed with the goal of integration between patients, providers, and payors of health-care services. Through the use of standardized outcome measures linked to the use of evidence-based case management interventions, case managers can be assured that what is measured is being managed and what is managed is being measured—all in a reportable fashion necessary to demonstrate the value of case management services to our customers and to answer the questions regarding cause and effect with a highly divergent population.

Finally, and most importantly, tools used to identify those individuals who can most benefit from exceptional case management services and interventions that focus on communication and relationship building are critical. Predictive models, algorithms that produce registries of the highest-risk patients, and specific, at-risk diseases have become important tools in identifying the 5% of the population that can account for 50% of the medical costs—these are the individuals who can most benefit from case management services (Forman & Kelliher, 1999). Additional training and development in techniques such as motivational interviewing and intrinsic coaching increases the case manager's ability to improve a person's ability to make choices and to seek relevance and value in making health changes that directly relate to his or her life goals (Miller & Rollnick, 2002).

DISEASE MANAGEMENT AND THE ROLE OF THE ADVANCED PRACTICE NURSE

Case management versus disease management—what is the defining difference? Many establish a difference in scope: Disease management is a population-focused approach to case management. Frequently, disease management uses a systematic approach designed to assist individuals with a specific condition or combination of related conditions. Interventions are designed using established national care standards and guidelines. In comparison, case management uses available evidence-based interventions and tailors them to meet the individual needs of persons who are identified as at high risk for health-care service use or are highly complex; frequently, this may include those individuals whose health status does not improve with participation in a disease management program (an outlier).

APNs have had an active role in both case and disease management, particularly as a case manager within the acute and community care settings. Research has found many benefits of using APNs in the case management role, in particular, qualities such as clinical expertise and improved access and communication with treating physicians in the community. This improved access and communication, along with the expert clinical knowledge regarding a particular disease state, can result in observed improved outcomes for individual patients receiving interventions with these targeted conditions within disease management programs.

Program managers, however, struggle regarding the employment of the APN in population-focused disease management programs. As noted previously, there have been numerous published studies that have demonstrated the positive effects of using the APN in the case manager role. To reiterate, although patient outcomes are generally positive, the amount and type of nursing ("nurse dose") needed to affect patient outcomes is not known and continues to confound the employer (Brooten & Naylor, 1995). Research regarding the effectiveness of disease management interventions has focused on "total program" effectiveness (Outcomes Guidelines Report, Volume II, DMAA, Washington, DC, 2007).

It is difficult to discern the value of the use of APNs in disease management programs that have demonstrated success with employment of a number of interventions such as telephonic outreach to members with chronic conditions, by experienced or specially educated RNs, mailing of health-related brochures and educational materials, and use of technology such as e-mail reminders and interactive voice response systems.

Additionally, although these programs have demonstrated success, published research has focused on two distinct populations: individuals in the Medicare age range and individuals who receive care within a staff model HMO environment. Commercial disease management came into being as a market driven request by health insurance plans to control the cost of caring for the chronically ill (Howe, 2006). Therefore, little is known regarding the effectiveness of interventions which focus on the use of the APN among commercial network model health plan populations. This is critical because the primary purchasers of disease management services are currently commercial managed care organizations and employer groups. Nursing interaction and calls are considered by most to be the most effective intervention in disease management programs (Freudenheim, 2002).

However, commercial populations are frequently not available for telephonic interventions and consider these types of strategies to be intrusive in their very busy lifestyles. Therefore, interventional strategies may change. APNs may be useful for those individuals with the highest risk or need; frequently these are individuals who do not respond to the usual pathway that has been developed for telephonic education, continued monitoring, and support. In these instances, assessing the individual's relationship with his or her treating physician, and collaboration with the physician is essential to ensure that care is being delivered according to evidence-based guidelines, and that the patient understands and adheres to prescribed regimens.

The APN, with excellent clinical knowledge and communication skills, may be effective in this strategy especially as care models evolve to support the use of the advanced medical home, which emphasizes the need for the chronically ill to have a personal health-care provider. Some research has been conducted on the cost-effectiveness of APN management of patients with chronic illness. Paez and Allen (2006) evaluated the cost-effectiveness of APN case management to lower blood lipids in patients with coronary heart disease. Their findings "suggest that case management by a APN is a cost-efficient and therapeutically effective strategy in managed care, to improve the of patients with cardiovascular disease." Using what the authors call a chronic care model, a group of hospital-based clinics incorporated APNs into the multidisciplinary team to treat patients with chronic diseases. The pilot sample improved clinical outcomes and economic performance as well (Boville et al., 2007).

THE ADVANCED PRACTICE NURSE: DISEASE MANAGEMENT EXAMPLES

Example 1: The Advanced Practice Nurse in the Disease Manager Role in a Managed Care Setting

K is a typical APN disease case manager within the managed care setting. She has a strong clinical background in oncology. As part of her role in the medical management department, K was recently asked to participate in the strategic planning for the development of a new disease management program.

Expert clinical knowledge and an ability to apply this knowledge is critical in the development of successful disease management intervention for managed care. Knowledge of a particular disease process is essential to identify the applicability of disease management interventions. For example, many conditions are considered to be potential targets for disease management primarily because of a high prevalence or high costs associated with the particular disease. However, not all diseases can effectively be managed using disease management program principles. The hallmark of these programs is coordination of health-care services and improving self-care measures. The APNs' expert clinical knowledge of a particular disease state and their knowledge of the care provided within the health-care system can identify critical junctures at which disease management interventions can be the most effective.

K used both of these skills in her evaluation of cancer as a potential target for disease management. Although cancer is prevalent among commercial populations and is also a high-cost disease state, it is considered to be a difficult disease to manage. K noted that many individuals with cancer are admitted to the hospital as a result of the side effects of chemotherapeutic agents. With education and improved self-care measures, could these admissions be avoided? Could this be the critical juncture in managing avoidable costs? She then proceeded to recommend the design of an education packet and telephonic outreach protocol focusing on prehydration for members undergoing chemotherapy to prevent dehydration admissions, and dietary considerations in the prevention of anemia. She designed an educational packet to include reputable Web sites for lay review of the national cancer treatment protocols and a number of community resources and support groups. Through her knowledge of the disease process and an opportunity for improved care, K identified a key juncture for focused disease management intervention. The rate of admissions for the complications of chemotherapy—specifically dehydration and anemia—are the clinical outcome measures that will determine the success of this program.

Additionally, collaboration with the treating oncologist to support the physician's treatment plan and encourage patient participation in the program is critical. The APN, working with the health plan's medical director can assist in meeting this goal.

Example 2: The Advanced Practice Nurse's Role in Continuous Quality Improvement

M is an APN with an extensive experience in hospice care. Many cancer patients are successfully treated; however, many other cancers result in terminal conditions. Few terminal cases receive the benefits of hospice care. M, as a case manager in the managed care setting, has noted this trend and has suggested that there be an evaluation of end-of-life care for disease management. Improvements in the quality of care provided in these circumstances may result in the reduction of acute service admissions and improved quality of life, particularly through pain management and support of individuals and families through death and dying. This example demonstrates the need to have APNs in the managed care setting consistently in search of areas for improvement and disease management intervention. With frequent review of the literature and observations of trends, the APN frequently identifies, plans, and implements disease management solutions. Rather than reacting to market forces and trends, the APN as a member of the managed care team, consistently seeks areas for continued improvement and service to clients. The health plan that uses this intellectual capital is provided with managed care solutions that not only provide value to its customers facing escalating health-care costs and the challenges of variability in the quality of care received, but also can differentiate itself from reactionary competitors.

REIMBURSEMENT AND MARKETING OF CASE MANAGEMENT PRACTICE

Physicians' current procedural terminology (CPT) codes are available for the reimbursement of case management services in a fee-for-service environment. Therefore, clinicians who normally bill for services using the CPT coding system, such as physicians and APNs, can bill for time used for the delivery of case management services in the outpatient setting. Marketing of case management services is also becoming more prominent, particularly among competing managed care organizations. It is not unusual for these organizations to run print or radio advertisements denoting the individual benefits of case management, capitalizing on the humanistic qualities of this important service. Additionally, with the advent of predictive modeling and promotion of case management as the solution to managing the health risk of the small percentage of individuals who drive the large percentage of health-care expenditures, case management companies and services are actively marketing the benefits of their services. In this competitive environment, it is not uncommon for case management to be a value-added program to plan subscribers. In December of 2007 the CMSA sent an e-mail message to all members to write to Congress in support of a measure to make care coordination services payable by Medicare. CMSA requested that several CPT codes be changed from non-payable to Medicare payable codes. See Chapter 6 for more on the history of reimbursement.

EDUCATION FOR NURSE CARE MANAGEMENT PRACTICE

Outside academic settings, education on case management can occur via continuing education courses, institutes, and on-the-job training. Within academic settings, case management concepts may be integrated into baccalaureate- and master-level curricula or taught in required or elective courses. Also, at the graduate level there are master's programs in case management. Another model is to offer case management as a concentration in which students take a required number of courses in addition to training in a clinical specialty.

On-the-job training or short training courses are not likely to be adequate because offering content solely as an elective course cannot expose all nurses to essential knowledge bases necessary to assume case management functions. To best prepare nurses for case management practice within a managed care environment, it is recommended that educators adopt a systematic approach to the integration of case management in nursing curricula. Approaches to incorporating such content are described elsewhere (Mundt, 1996; Sinnen & Schifalaqua, 1996; Sowell & Young, 1997).

Overall, at the baccalaureate level, case management should be considered a core curriculum concept and threaded throughout the undergraduate program. At the graduate level, in addition to core graduate and specialty content, advanced practice curricula should contain theory and clinical experiences related to case management, care coordination across the continuum, community resource use, and managed care concepts including reimbursement and health-care financing. Because nurse case managers look to the skills of other health-care professionals in their care planning, an interdisciplinary course would also prove invaluable.

The curriculum sponsored by the CMSA notes that there are essential elements of study. These include managed care, use management, and legal and ethical issues, among others. It is also noted that change is constant and case managers must keep up with the changes in the health care system (Powell & Ignatavicius, 2001).

Finally, there is a need for graduate programs to prepare nurse case management specialists. In 1993, Villanova University College of Nursing in Pennsylvania offered the first designated graduate track in case management in the country. Master's programs in case management should include core graduate content, as well as, specialized content related to case management models, strategies, tools, quality management, health-care financing and reimbursement systems, managed care, health-care outcomes, client education, community resources, clinical practice in case management, and role development. Course work and clinical experiences with specific aggregate populations is highly recommended. Moreover, such curricula need to prepare graduates who can practice case management in hospitals and outpatient settings, including insurance companies. Offering master's programs in case management and integrating case management content at the master's level for APNs will produce practitioners who can deliver nursing case management services, create systems of care coordination, and institute policy that will reflect quality outcomes. An example of a graduate program in case management is outlined in **Box 16-2.**

CERTIFICATION AND ASSOCIATIONS FOR CASE MANAGEMENT

There are numerous certification bodies available for case management and for related areas such as quality management. Some of these certifying organizations are interdisciplinary and others are specific to nursing case management. Many do not require advanced degrees and each has different eli-

BOX 16-2
Saint Peter's College's Master of Science Program in Case Management

At institutions such as Saint Peter's College, innovative curricula have been designed to prepare nurse case managers at the master's level. The Department of Nursing offers a 37-credit masters' program in case management with a functional concentration in nursing administration. Curriculum core and specialty content areas are listed in the following.

OBJECTIVES OF THE MASTER OF SCIENCE IN NURSING PROGRAM:
Students will be able to do the following

■ Analyze case management models from a broad systems perspective and project changes for future models.

■ Implement the role of nurse case manager, employing case management strategies and therapeutic nursing interventions to ensure that quality care is provided.

■ Incorporate the nursing and case management process and advanced learning to coordinate care and services for individuals, families, and client aggregates across the health-care continuum.

■ Synthesize knowledge of organizational theory and financial concepts to design, direct, and evaluate the delivery of care.

■ Incorporate research in nursing case management and administrative practice.

KEY CONTENT AREAS
■ Nursing theory and research
■ Health care/human diversity issues and policy
■ Ethical frameworks
■ Clinical standards/legal issues
■ Communication theory and skills
■ Technological applications
■ Educational theory and skills
■ Clinical concepts (e.g., health promotion/disease prevention, advocacy, aggregate care, culturally relevant interventions and continuum-based care)
■ Leadership and organizational theories
■ Health-care financing and managed care
■ Outcomes: monitoring and measurement
■ Case management: models, processes, tools, and strategies
■ Case management role development

gibility requirements in terms of practice, testing, educational preparation, and recertification. Currently, there is not a specific certification for advanced practice case management. Employers may or may not require certification for case management practice. According to Tahan, "certification is an important way for case management professionals to distinguish themselves as having the educational background, experience, skills, knowledge, and competencies to perform the multifaceted and complex job of a case manager today" (2005, p.19).

It is recommended that APNs maintain their clinical specialty certification and adhere to the licensure laws of the state in which they practice. APNs who are recruited to be program managers or clinical leaders in the field of case management, given their advanced education and skill sets, should consider obtaining case management administrator certification. This certification is offered through the Center for Case Management and is intended to validate the knowledge and experience necessary for case management administration. APNs who function in case management roles may also want to consider joining professional associations related to case management and managed care. See the list of Web sites linked to this chapter for some examples. Such associations provide information related to continuing education, relevant publications, conferences, as well as, the opportunity to network with colleagues.

CONCLUSION

This chapter has explored the historical roots of the case manager role, case manager role competitors, levels of practice for nurse case managers, various case management models, case management roles and skills, tools and strategies, including disease management for APNs, and issues such as reimbursement and marketing, education for practice, as well as, certification programs and associations. This is an exciting and challenging time to be an APN within a case management practice environment. Those who successfully grasp the role and function will be the pacesetters for tomorrow's health-care challenges. This will also ensure a place at the table for nursing as it grows and develops and provides the nation with innovative care models.

References

Anderson, J. H. (2007). Nursing presence in a community heart failure program. *Nurse Practitioner, 32(10)*, 14–18.

American Nurses Association. (1992). *Case management by nurses.* Kansas City, MO: American Nurses Association.

American Nurses Credentialing Center. (1998). *Nursing case management catalog.* Washington, DC: Author.

Boville, D., Saran, M., Salem, J. K., & Clough, L. (2007). An innovative role for nurse practitioners in managing chronic disease. *Nursing Economic$, 25*(6), 359–364.

Bower, K. S. (1992). *Case management by nurses* (2nd ed., pp. 13–15). Kansas City, MO: American Nurses Association.

Brault, G. L., & Kissinger, L. D. (1991). Case management: Ambiguous at best. *Journal of Pediatric Health Care, 5*(4), 179–183.

Brooten, D., & Naylor, M. D. (1995). Nurses' effect on changing patient outcomes. *Image, 27*(2), 95–99.

Buhler-Wilkerson, K. (1993). Public health then and now: Bringing care to the people. *American Journal of Public Health, 83*(12), 1778–1786.

Calkin, J. (1984). A model for advanced nursing practice. *Journal of Nursing Administration, 14*(1), 24–30.

Case Management Society of America. (1995). *Standards of practice for case management.* Little Rock, AR: Case Management Society of America.

Case Management Society of America. (2002). Center for Case Management Accountability. Retrieved September 9, 2002 from the Case Management Society of America Web site: www.CMSA.org/ccma-main.

Cesta, T. G., & Tahan, H. A. (2003). *The case manager's survival guide.* St. Louis: Mosby.

Cohen, E. L., & Cesta, T. G. (1993). *Nursing care management: From concept to evaluation.* St. Louis: Mosby.

Connors, H. R. (1993). Impact of care management modalities on curricula. In K. Kelly & M. Maas (Eds.), *Managing nursing care* (pp. 190–207). St. Louis: Mosby.

Cronin, C. J., & Maklebust, J. (1989). Case-managed care: Capitalizing on the CNS. *Nursing Management, 20*(3), 38–47.

Curtis, K., Lien, D., Chan, A., Grove, P., & Morris, R., (2002). The impact of trauma case management on patient outcomes. *Journal of Trauma: Injury, Infection and Critical Care, 53(3)*, 477–482.

Daniels, S., & Ramey, M. (2005). *The leaders guide to hospital case management.* Sudbury, MA: Jones and Bartlett Publishers.

Dock, L. (1937). Whence the term "public health nursing"? *Public Health Nursing, 29*(12), 712–714.

Erickson, S. M. (1997). Managing case management across the continuum: An organized response to managed care. *Seminars for Nurse Managers, 5*(3), 124–128.

Ethridge, P., & Lamb, G. (1989). Professional nursing case management improves quality, access and costs. *Nursing Management, 20*(3), 30–35.

Falter, E. J., Cesta, T. G., Concert, C., & Mason, D. J. (1999). Development of a graduate program in case management. *Journal of Care Management, 5*(3), 50–56, 72, 74, 76–78.

Forbes, M. A. (1999). The practice of professional case management. *Nursing Case Management, 4*(1), 28–33.

Forman, S., & Kelliher, M. (1999). *StatusOne: Breakthroughs in high risk population health management.* San Francisco: Jossey-Bass.

Frachel, R. R. (1988). A new profession: The evolution of public health nursing. *Public Health Nursing, 5*(2), 86–90.

Freudenheim, M. (2002, February 17). Bedside visits, on the telephone. *New York Times,* p. C2.

Hamric, A. B. (1992). Creating our future: Challenges and opportunities for the clinical nurse specialist. *Oncology Nursing Forum, 19*(1 Suppl), 11–15.

Hayes, E., McCahon, C., Panaki, M. R., Hamre, T., & Pohlman, K. (2008). Alliance not compliance: Coaching strategies to improve type 2 diabetes outcomes. *Journal of the American Academy of Nurse Practitioners. 20*(3), 155–162.

Hellwig, S. D., Yam, M., & DiGiulio, M. (2003). Nurse case managers' perceptions of advocacy. *Lippincott's Case Management, 8*(2), 53–63.

Howe, R. (2006). Population care management. *Lippincott's Case Management, 11*(6) 331–337.

Huber, D. L. (2000). The diversity of case management models. *Case Management, 5*(6), 248–255.

Huber, D. L., & Craig, K. (2007). Acuity and case management. *Professional Case Management, 12*(3), 132–146.

Intagliata, J. (1982). Improving the quality of community care for the chronically mentally disabled: The role of case management. *Schizophrenia Bulletin, 8*(4), 655–674.

Iowa Interventions and Outcomes Projects. (2002). *Nursing interventions classification.* Retrieved August 10, 2002, from the University of Iowa, College of Nursing Web site: www.nursing.uiowa.edu/centers/cncce/nic/nicquestions.htm.

Kersbergen, A. L. (1996). Case management: A rich history of coordinating care to control costs. *Nursing Outlook, 44*(4), 169–172.

Knollmueller, R. N. (1989). Case management: What's in a name? *Nursing Management, 20*(10), 38–42.

Krichbaum, K. (1999). Advanced practice nurse case managers and care pathways. In M. Snyder, & M. P. Mirr (Eds.), *Advanced practice nursing: A guide to professional development* (2nd ed., pp. 99–116). New York: Springer.

Kutzleb, J., & Reiner, D. (2006). The impact of nurse directed patient education on quality of life and functional capacity in people with heart failure. *Journal of the American Academy of Nurse Practitioners, 18*(3), 116–124.

Lamb, G. S. (1992). Conceptual and methodological issues: Nursing case management research. *Advances in Nursing Science, 15*(2), 16–24.

Lamb, G. S. (1995). Case management. *Annual Review of Nursing Research, 13,* 117–136.

Lamb, G. S., & Stempel, J. E. (1994). Nurse case management from the client's view: Growing as insider-expert. *Nursing Outlook, 42*(7), 7–13.

Mahn, V. A., & Spross, J. A. (1996). Nurse case management as an advanced practice role. In A. B. Hamric, J. A. Spross, & C. M. Hanson (Eds.), *Advanced nursing practice: An integrative approach* (pp. 445–465). Philadelphia: WB Saunders.

Mahn, V. A., & Zazworsky, D. (2000). Nurse case management as an advanced practice role. In A. B. Hamric, J. A. Spross, & C. M. Hanson (Eds.), *The advanced practice nurse case manager: An integrative approach* (2nd ed., pp. 549–606). Philadelphia: WB Saunders.

Miller, W. R., & Rollnick, S. (2002). *Motivational interviewing—Preparing people for change* (2nd ed.). New York: The Guilford Press. Retrieved April 1, 2008 from the Totally Coached Web site: www.totallycoached.com/en/about_us/intrinsic_coaching/.

More, P. K., & Mandell, S. (1997). *Nursing case management: An evolving practice.* New York: McGraw-Hill.

Mundinger, M. (1984). Community-based care: Who will be the case managers? *Nursing Outlook, 323*(6), 294–295.

Mundt, M. H. (1996). Key elements of nurse case management in curricula. In E. L. Cohen (Ed.), *Nurse case management in the 21st century* (pp. 48–54). St. Louis: Mosby.

Naylor, M., Brooten, D., Campbell, R., Jacobsen, B. S., Mezey, M. D., Pauly, M., et al. (1999). Comprehensive discharge planning and home follow-up of hospitalized elders. *Journal of American Medical Association, 28*(7), 613–620.

Outcomes Guidelines Report, Volume II. (2007). Washington, DC: DMAA.

Paez, K. A., & Allen, J. K. (2006). Cost effectiveness of nurse practitioner management of hypercholesterolemia following coronary revascularization. *Journal of the American Academy of Nurse Practitioners, 18*(9), 436–445.

Palmer, R. E. (1969). *Hermeneutics.* Evanston, IL: Northwestern University.

Powell, S. K. (2000). *Case management: A practice guide to success in managed care.* Philadelphia: Lippincott Williams & Wilkins.

Powell, S. K., & Ignatavicius, D. (2001). *Core curriculum for case management.* Philadelphia: Lippincott Williams & Wilkins.

Profession of promoting health. (1919). *Public Health Nurse, 11*(1), 10–12.

Reverby, S. M. (1987). *Ordered to care: The dilemma of American nursing, 1850–1945.* New York: Cambridge University.

Reynolds, C. G., & Smeltzer, C. H. (1997). Case management: Past, present, future—The drivers for change. *Journal of Nursing Care Quality, 12*(1), 9–19.

Shonick, W. (1988). Public health services: Background and present status. In S. J. Williams, & P. R. Torrens (Eds.), *Introduction to health services.* (3rd ed., pp. 85–123). New York: Delmar.

Sinnen, M., & Schifalaqua, M. (1996). The education of nurses: Nurse case managers' view. In E. L. Cohen (Ed.), *Nurse case management in the 21st century* (pp. 55–62). St. Louis: Mosby.

Skiba, D. J., & Cohen, E. (2000). Case management and technology: A necessary fit for the future. *Nursing Administration Quarterly, 25*(1), 132–141.

Sowell, R. L., & Young, S. W. (1997). Case management in nursing curriculum. *Nursing Care Management, 2*(4), 173–176.

Stanton, M. P., Swanson, M., Sherrod, R. A., & Packa, D. R. (2005). Case management evolution: From basic to advanced practice role. *Lippincott's Case Management, 10*(6), 274–284.

Stempel, J., Doerge, J., Van Mie, K., & Combs, J. (1997). Nurse case management. In B. Case (Ed.), *Career planning for nurses* (pp. 133–160). Albany: Delmar.

Tahan, H. A. (1998). Case management: A heritage more than a century old. *Nursing Case Management, 3*(2), 55–60.

Tahan, H. A. (2005). Clarifying certification and its value for case managers. *Lippincott's Case Management, 10*(1), 14–21.

Tahan, H. A., & Huber, D. L. (2006). The CCMC's national study of case manager job descriptions. *Lippincott's Case Management, 11*(3), 127–144.

Umbrell, C. E., (2006). Trauma case management: A role for the advanced practice nurse. *Journal of Trauma Nursing, 13*(2), 70–73.

Wald, L. D. (1915). *The house on Henry Street.* New York: Henry Hold & Co.

Weil, M., & Karls, J. (1985). Historical origins and recent developments in case management. In Weil, M. (Ed.), *Case Management in Human Service Practice.* San Francisco: Jossey-Bass.

White, A. B. (2004). Case management and the national quality agenda: Partnering to improve the quality of care. *Lippincott's Case Management, 9*(3), 132–140.

Zander, K. (1990). Case management: A golden opportunity for whom? In J. C. McCloskey & H. K. Grace (Eds.), *Current issues in nursing* (3rd ed., p. 201). St. Louis: Mosby.

Zander, K. (1996). The early years: The evolution of nursing case management. In D. L. Flarey, & S. S. Blancott (Eds.), *Handbook of nursing case management* (pp. 23–45). Gaithersburg, MD: Aspen.

Zerwekh, J. V. (1992). Public health nursing legacy: Historical practical wisdom. *Nursing and Health Care, 13*(2), 84–91.

17

The Advanced Practice Nurse and Research

Pamela F. Cipriano

Suzanne M. Burns

RESEARCH AS A ROLE COMPONENT

The advanced practice nurse (APN) role has always included a component of research as a standard expectation. This expectation has evolved characteristically over the years from one of simple participation in the support of research to one of participating in the generation of research questions, facilitating research studies, implementing findings, establishing evidence-based best practices, and conducting research.

As a trusted knowledge source, the APN is positioned to apply innovations from nursing research into practice. The APN infuses experience and intuition, as well as, valid clinical research findings, together with the patient's input to influence the most effective care. Promoting evidence-based practice (EBP) is the key to bridging the theory-research-practice gap (Profetto-McGrath, Smith, Hugo, Taylor, & El-Hajj, 2007).

The clinical nurse specialist (CNS) was one of the first APN roles identified to include research as an essential component for the clinical expert prepared at the master's level. The American Nurses Association (ANA) identified the five dimensions of the CNS role as specialist in clinical practice, educator, consultant, researcher, and administrator. CNSs contribute to their areas of specialization by generating and refining research questions, promoting scientific inquiry to improve practice, interpreting and applying research findings in clinical practice, disseminating findings to other nurses, and collaborating in designing as well as conducting research including sharing findings through publication (ANA, 1986; Hamric, 2000; McGuire & Harwood, 2000).

Today, given the increase in nurses who are doctorally prepared, and the maturation of the discipline, many programs prepare APNs primarily to participate in phases of the research process, act as consumers of research, and apply knowledge of research methods to processes requiring scholarly inquiry. In 2004, the American Association of Colleges of Nursing (AACN) called for a transformation in the education of professional nurses practicing at the highest level, to doctoral education (AACN, 2006). The doctorate of nursing practice degree (DNP), a new alternative to the research-focused doctor of philosophy (PhD) program, retains the expectations of scholarly practice, practice improvement, and the innovation and testing of care delivery models. The DNP addresses the educational move from master's to the doctorate level, by focusing on clinical scholarship and analytic methods for EBP (Sperhac & Clinton, 2008). The DNP also provides an opportunity for collaboration between the academician researcher and the clinician, blending the art and science of nursing (Burman, Hart, & McCabe, 2005).

The ANA's *Scope and Standards of Practice* (2004) includes a standard of professional performance addressing the integration of research findings into practice. The standard for competent behavior for the role requires that "the APN: contributes to nursing knowledge by conducting or synthesizing research that discovers, examines, and evaluates knowledge, theories, criteria, and creative approaches to improve healthcare practice," (p. 40). The APN can provide evidence of meeting this standard through a variety of activities. These include critically evaluating existing practice using relevant research findings, identifying clinical research questions, and disseminating relevant research findings in practice consultation or in education of nurses and others.

APNs, especially beginning APNs, are often concerned about their ability to effectively develop a research-based practice. Further, they wish to instill the importance of research in others, yet struggle with how to accomplish the goal. This chapter describes essential APN attributes and behaviors consistent with successful integration of research into practice. Ways to develop research skills, solutions to common barriers, and examples of clinical research-based projects are also discussed.

Attributes

To be successful, the APN first assesses how others perceive the strengths and contributions one brings to the practice environment. A sense of self-awareness is important to measure capacity for success in any part of the APN role. The APN's credibility is essential to earn the trust and respect of other caregivers in nursing and in other disciplines. In turn, the APN demonstrates trust and respect for others and values their contributions to care.

Achieving effective working relationships with other caregivers is a primary factor in successful role development. Personal confidence is important, as are traits of adaptability, flexibility, motivation, and creativity to develop the role. Negotiation skills to resolve conflicts and manage change are personal characteristics that enable the APN to build support and overcome barriers to effective role implementation. Ensuring there is clarity in role definition and expectations also helps others understand the relationship of the APN to their work (Jones, 2004).

Knowledge is used to inform and influence APN practice. To be effective in a team environment, the ability to be flexible and demonstrate tolerance for differences in others' styles, personalities, and opinions is important. Likewise, the ability to compromise as a team member is essential.

Self-direction in most aspects of the role, and in particular in pursuing knowledge and skills within the specialized area of clinical practice, is an important attribute of the APN. Learning beyond the master's degree is a requirement if the APN is to develop as an expert, and research skills are often acquired through venues other than formal learning. Participating in research projects, presenting findings, joining in performance improvement or product evaluation activities, and serving on a research committee are all effective ways to acquire research skills. Working as a research assistant also provides invaluable experiential learning.

The successful researcher has in-depth knowledge and mastery of basic research methods relevant to the area of clinical investigation. For example, the APN who works with critically ill neonates and their families needs to understand methods for analyzing developmentally appropriate interventions and patient reactions. The APN working with chronically ill adults is able to administer tools to assess functional ability and changes in clinical status.

All nurses engaged in any form of research are required to understand the values, expectations, and sanctions of research (Mateo & Kirchoff, 1999). Awareness of the changing regulatory requirements related to the protection of human subjects, privacy of information, and ethical standards of data integrity is the responsibility of all those involved in research-related projects regardless of the level of participation. The APN demonstrates an understanding and awareness of the need to maintain high standards, protect the public, and maintain the integrity of the work.

The maintenance of scholarly habits related to research activities is central to the APN's success. A commitment to the work, scheduling time to devote to projects, and the ability to work on multiple initiatives at one time are necessary to succeed and complete research activities. The APN is also expected to help develop a research attitude in others, particularly registered nurses (RNs), to publish and to promote research and the implementation of relevant research findings. In addition to these more work-related attributes, the APN must be highly motivated and creative, and must have well-developed interpersonal skills.

Research Skill Development

APN practice is founded on research findings that define practice. The need for the nurse to question and find answers to validate practice techniques and care processes drives the APN to place greater emphasis on application of research findings in clinical practice. This may, in turn, require the APN to pursue continuing self-education to be able to competently implement this part of the role, as well as assume a leadership position when facilitating research.

New skills in using and conducting research can be acquired through a variety of activities such as solving clinical problems, presenting research findings, participating in performance improvement and patient classification systems analyses, conducting product evaluation, and evaluating practice protocols for evidence of needed change. The APN usually progresses from being a facilitator of research to later assuming a leadership role. Facilitation usually involves serving as a collaborator or assisting others to assess the literature for relevant clinical information. Leadership involves conducting research and integrating findings into clinical practice (Brown, 2000). To this end, the Association of Clinical Nurse Specialists identified over 68 CNS research studies and reported on outcomes of CNS practice published in the nursing literature over the last decade. (Fulton & Baldwin, 2004). The relatively small number may be because care is often provided in teams making the identification of CNS specific outcomes difficult.

Facilitative Role and Collaboration

APNs have frequent opportunities to assist other staff through the use of relevant research literature. The APN should not only respond to inquiries by staff, but also lead them to understand and change their practice based on findings from research. The APN can help frame and examine problems identified in a defined patient population and can provide consultation in routine forums such as grand rounds and patient conferences when challenging issues are raised. The APN also has the responsibility to do the same with his or her own practice by evaluating practice protocols, patient outcomes, new findings from the literature, or phenomena specific to a patient population. Other industries are finding the expertise of APNs invaluable in product evaluation, conduct of clinical trials, justification of patient care, and evaluation of outcomes.

The APN can also act as collaborator by assuming a role as a coinvestigator or consultant on a research team. Early research experience as a team member helps build skills in tool development, protocol testing, and publication of results. As the clinical expert, the APN contributes knowledge for protocol or tool development. In turn, the APN receives valuable advice and experience from experienced researchers. Teams can also provide ongoing positive reinforcement, as well as support for completion of the work and translation of results into publications.

A number of models for collaboration among APNs and researchers have been proposed. Benefits of collaboration include shared expertise of a number of individuals and disciplines, enhanced resources, access to clinical populations, synergy between APN and nurse researchers to gain increased power and influence, and improved relevance of the research (Goldberg & Moch, 1998). At the institutional level, a number of academic medical centers affiliated with schools of nursing have developed collaborative models that support APNs, doctoral students, and faculty, resulting in a road range of activities that support research use and the conduct of research. Benefits of academic collaboration models include more rapid integration of new knowledge focused at the unit level, tangible support for research, development opportunities for APNs to hold joint appointments and teach clinical application of research findings to staff, and the creation of an environment that promotes the application of scientific knowledge in patient care (Berger et al., 1999; Mercer, 2008).

The first practice-based research network for advanced practice registered nurses (APRNs) was recently established under the leadership of Dr. Margaret Grey at the Yale University School of Nursing. Six founding university schools of nursing helped establish the APRN network, APRNet, with the purpose of facilitating and conducting research to study APRN primary care practices, developing EBP models for APRNs, and translating research findings into primary care practice (Deshefy-Longhi, Swartz, & Grey, 2002). This network will greatly facilitate the study of primary care nursing practice and will link with other primary care providers to accomplish collaborative studies.

Leadership

The APN may conduct research as an individual or as a member of a team. Conducting research begins with clinical problem identification, with careful attention paid to limiting the focus as much as possible to ensure answerable questions. Research provides the systematic process for finding the answers to questions that challenge the methods of care nurses provide. APNs are strategically positioned to pilot different interventions and strategies of care on a daily basis (Nugent & Lambert, 1996). Conducting one phase or a complete study can make significant contributions.

Integrating research, or using research findings to change practice, requires a number of steps. Once a practice problem is identified, the pertinent patient outcomes must be documented so that future measurement of change will indicate whether or not improvement was achieved. Review of literature and synthesis of current research findings about a specific practice then guides thinking about possible interventions to change and improve practice. The next step is to plan for and implement changes in practice, taking into account readiness for change, resource requirements, education, lead time, institutional approvals, if required, and design of measurement and evaluation techniques. Finally, measuring the effectiveness of the change on specific outcomes and resource use, with final decision making about sustaining the change, completes the process (Mateo & Kirchoff, 1999).

ADVANCED PRACTICE NURSE BEHAVIORS AND THE DEVELOPMENT OF A PHILOSOPHY OF "RESEARCH IS PART OF WHAT WE DO"

Although the APN's academic preparation includes how to evaluate and conduct research, few practicing APNs feel adequately prepared to lead a research program in their practice arena without "practical experience." Clinicians trying to apply research concepts find that many of the principles learned in school fall short when applied to clinical practice. This is complicated by the insidious and widely held belief that real research can only be conducted by those with a doctorate (Burns, 2002; Burns & Keeling, 1999; Campbell & Chulay, 1990; Granger & Chulay, 1999).

For the research gap to narrow so that research is part of what clinicians do, the APN's ability to develop a milieu that promotes the philosophy is essential (Burns, 2002; Titler et al., 1994). To successfully engineer a scientific milieu in a clinical setting, selected APN behaviors such as problem solving, change agency, mentoring, leadership, and ability to work with a multidisciplinary team are required.

Problem Solving and Evidence-Based Practice

The APN is often called on to develop solutions to problems in the clinical setting. The imperative for implementing evidence is improving outcomes. Oddly enough, even when strong evidence exists, practice changes may occur slowly or not at all. An example is the ubiquitous practice of instilling normal saline into endotracheal tubes before suctioning. Though evidence continues to strongly suggest that the practice is both ineffective and potentially harmful, it continues to be a common practice in critical care units (Hanberg & Brown, 2006)

Thus, the ability to use a logical yet creative approach to applying the evidence or conducting clinical research serves to support the philosophy that research is an integral and important part of everyday practice.

The APN begins by helping clinicians (referring throughout to any nurses involved in research) understand the meaning of EBP. The term means that the clinician is aware of the evidence that exists for a practice and the strength of the evidence. Professional and regulatory agencies often perform systematic reviews to determine the existing evidence for selected practices, especially high-risk procedures or practices. Practice guidelines are developed from these reviews and generally identify the level of scientific evidence for each recommendation from the lowest (e.g., consensus statements by professional organizations) to the highest (e.g., meta-analyses of randomized controlled studies). The decision to implement the guidelines is made by considering the relevancy of the practice change to the specific population of interest and by considering the potential for "unintended consequences" that may ensue. EBP changes may also be required by regulatory agencies in which case the hospital must comply. APNs are often the individuals charged with implementation. An example is the use of restraints. Health-care agencies must ensure that they are appropriately applied and that use is rigorously monitored. Another example is the implementation of a technique that could potentially affect the rate of line infections. Because of the high potential risk associated with such a change, rigorous follow-up evaluation or outcomes tracking following implementation is required. In contrast, implementation of a low-risk intervention such as the use of "bagged baths" in the place of traditional options may require only periodic audits of clinicians using the products and oversight by institutional wound, ostomy, and continence nurses.

When authoritative guidelines do not exist to help with EBP changes, consensus statements by professional organizations may be available and are quite helpful. These statements are based on systematic reviews of the available evidence. Similar to guidelines, the statements help the user understand the level of evidence so that careful application may occur. Other similar resources that may also be referenced are practice alerts. These tend to be published by professional organizations and are generally narrowly focused on a specific practice such as the use of blue food coloring in tube feedings. Finally, a literature review on the topic of interest will help the APN guide the clinicians in determining the need for a practice change or for a clinical study to answer the question.

Although some EBP changes may be initiated using existing research, the vast majority of practice traditions that exist have little science to validate their efficacy. For example, while the Centers for Disease Control (CDC) and the Infusion Nursing Society both recommend specific timing related to the use of selected site dressings used to cover and secure central venous (CV) catheter lines, they do not help the clinician decide among many commercially available products. Related questions such as how long the methods adhere, which are best for the skin, and which method types work best with specific catheters, remain unanswered. In these cases the design and conduct of a clinical study to determine the answer is a reasonable and expected part of the APN's role.

APNs integrate evidence from many realms and also blend experiential knowledge of the culture and support systems to shape recommendations for clinical practice changes (Profetto-McGrath et al., 2007). If the APN determines that a clinical study is necessary to answer a practice question, it is essential to determine the project feasibility. A well thought-out, narrowly focused, well-designed study is essential for clinician buy-in. In fact, selection of projects, especially first-time projects, should be carefully done to ensure a "quick win." More difficult projects can follow as the clinicians and APN become more sophisticated in the conduct of clinical studies. The following questions are helpful to determine the potential feasibility and subsequent success of conducting a clinical study.

1. *Is proposed study a topic of interest to the clinicians?* Without clinician interest in the topic, the study is unlikely to move forward. In fact, it may be seen as the "APN's project" versus one owned by the unit or clinicians.

2. *Can it be done in a reasonable amount of time?* This is especially important for first-time projects. The project should be able to be completed in a couple of months or interest and enthusiasm will diminish. In a recent study by Winfield, Davis, Schwaner, Conaway, and Burns (2007), clinicians in a postanesthesia care unit questioned the best method for securing peripheral intravenous (PIV) lines. Because they were able to estimate the number of PIVs placed in a month, they were able to complete their study in approximately 3 months. Interest in the study stayed high throughout the study period.

3. *Can the data be collected in the course of a clinical day?* Although qualitative studies are important to practice and are quite attractive to nurses, they are time consuming and difficult to accomplish in a clinical setting. Quantitative studies, on the other hand, are easier to accomplish. Nurses are used to collecting data. If the study is focused on a clinical problem, such as the PIV study noted previously, much of the data collection can be accomplished in the course of providing patient care. In addition, data that are routinely collected may also contribute to evaluating nursing interventions, and when aggregated and analyzed, can help establish best practices (Resnick, 2006).

4. *Will the study require informed consent?* Studies that measure the effect of an intervention or practice or that challenge a "policy" or established practice standard require informed consent. From a practical perspective, it is desirable, especially for beginning clinical researchers, to design studies that do not require consent. The time that practicing clinicians must spend to obtain consent is often beyond that reasonably taken from normal care responsibilities and may be especially complicated if the patient is unable to give consent, and the family must be approached.

    Studies that do not require informed consent are relatively common and are better choices for beginning researchers. For example, in the PIV study noted previously, four different PIV securing methods were compared. Consent was waived because no standard of care was breached (there was no existing standard securing method).

5. *Will the study require funding?* Many clinical projects such as the PIV example do not require a funding source. Supplies are often those used in the course of patient care and complex analyses are rarely necessary. However, some may require financial support and this should be

considered before beginning. If an institutional budget is not available for such support, other avenues may be explored.

Small amounts of money are fairly easy to obtain, but they do require time and energy to acquire. Examples include funding sources such as institutional quality assurance grants or small project monies ($100 to $500) provided by professional organizations. Another source may be unit funds; the manager or administrator should be consulted ahead of time to determine if this is a viable solution. Another option is to collaborate with an academic colleague or a statistician from the beginning so they are part of the project team. Regardless, to be feasible, funding sources for selected elements of the project should be considered early in the development and design of the project. It is desirable to have an infrastructure in place that ensures support for statistical analyses, so that each project does not require a unique solution.

6. *Are there barriers to evidence use?* Some cultures resist the APN's efforts to implement practice changes. It may be useful to develop a strategy for delivering the findings in a less formal manner. Staff often prefer one-on-one coaching, inservices, staff meetings, and learning methods that are not intimidating. Involving others from the start helps reinforce the premise that the work does not belong solely to the APN. Regardless, everyone is not successful implementing research findings. The process requires strong critical thinking and facilitation skills. APNs can enhance the growth of clinicians in these areas by meeting their learning needs early on, exchanging expertise, and stimulating participation throughout the study (Ferguson, Milner, & Snelgrove-Clarke, 2004). These and other successful strategies are discussed later in this chapter.

Mentoring and Leadership

To encourage clinicians to accept that research is a necessary part of what they do every day, the APN's ability to mentor them in the process goes a long way to encouraging the acceptance of such a philosophy. Although this statement seems somewhat obvious, it is far from being so. Many individuals are good at envisioning projects, and some may even inspire others to participate in the projects. Unfortunately, a less appreciated behavior linked with success is the APN's ability to ensure that all steps of the project are completed. This is hard work and often requires dogged determination to support, lead, and mentor others throughout the course of the project. Past performance speaks to this ability, and it is essential that the APN be able to realistically assess his or her previous experience in completing projects and mentoring others. An APN who is working with clinicians on a clinical or service line quality improvement project for example, should not assume that participating individuals can independently accomplish the assigned tasks. Clinicians working on the project may have selected a project to learn how to do clinical research; experience in some of the steps of the process, however, such as how to accomplish a literature review, may be lacking. The APN needs to anticipate this and help the individual accomplish the review. This one-on-one teaching is important to demystify the process, eliminate barriers, move the process along, and to ensure success. The support and teaching provided by the APN also helps with the APNs credibility and ensures the development of others.

The APN's enthusiastic leadership goes a long way to making others excited about the process. This leadership extends to all aspects of the clinical project, from project identification to application. Most importantly, the projects should be fun! As noted previously, many bedside clinicians feel that research is for others, and they are fearful of embarking on any project that remotely looks like a study. A sense of humor, as in all aspects of nursing practice, goes a long way toward eliminating the fear of doing research and making it fun to do.

Change Agency and a Systems Approach

Perhaps one of the most important behaviors of the APN is the ability to navigate the environment in which she or he practices. This understanding of the system is essential if appropriate changes are to be implemented. The APN must be able to identify the need to change an existing practice and the effect of this practice change. The APN's clinical knowledge and understanding of how to get something done in a clinical environment helps ensure that quality is maintained. To that end, the APN has a responsibility to the institution to evaluate clinical and system-focused initiatives. In fact, these initiatives may be another way of demonstrating that "research is part of what we do" and is essential to a widespread scientific approach to practice. An example is an initiative that is instituted to decrease the cost of care by employing a greater number of unlicensed personnel. The APN's role is to help determine whether studies on staffing patterns using a higher ratio of unlicensed personnel to RNs exist so that a rational and logical discussion on the topic might follow. This kind of scientific approach to the problem helps administrators and clinicians proactively avoid outcomes that will adversely affect clinical and financial results.

In some cases, data do not exist to guide the system changes. The role of the APN is to help evaluate the outcomes associated with the system change so that the initiatives can be adapted as needed or to maintain and sustain positive outcomes. These kinds of projects often fall under the title of quality improvement (QI). Although slightly different from research studies in that they are rarely as rigorous in design or conduct, they can be popular projects for clinician participation. An example includes a project in a medical intensive care unit (MICU) designed to determine the effect of an outcomes management approach to the care of long-term mechanically ventilated patients using an APN to manage and monitor the patients, a clinical multidisciplinary pathway, and weaning and sedation guidelines (Burns et al., 1998; Burns & Earven, 2002). The project was a popular one for the clinicians involved in the project, and the institution was especially interested because both clinical and financial outcomes for this patient population needed improvement. The favorable results of the project (shorter weaning times and length of stay) coupled with improved financial outcomes were the stimulus for the initiation of a hospital-wide initiative to replicate the model successfully in all adult intensive care units in the system (Burns et al., 2003).

The behaviors discussed previously, in addition to the attributes of the APN, determine the effectiveness of the APN in making research come to life in a clinical setting. However, barriers to success do exist (Carroll et al., 1997; Lekandder, Tracy, & Lindquist, 1994). The most commonly cited barriers to the development of a research milieu include clinical access to patient populations, buy-in from clinicians, administrative support, attaining resources (i.e., time and money), and completing and publishing the results. Barriers and potential solutions are addressed in the following section.

REMOVING BARRIERS TO ADVANCED PRACTICE NURSE RESEARCH

Although the application of evidence to practice has been an expectation of the APN role in the past, the actual conduct of clinical research has not been strongly emphasized. This is changing as regulatory agencies, such as the Joint Commission, and professional groups that reward hospitals for demonstrating an evidence-based nursing practice, such as the American Nurses Credentialing Center (ANCC) and the AACN, include the conducting of research as part of their expectation for recognition. These organizations have identified that clinical outcomes improve when nursing care is evidence-based (AACN, 2008a; ANCC, 2008). In addition, the presence of an active formal nursing research program demonstrates the hospital's commitment and support.

Clinical research and APN involvement is critical to the profession. To that end a variety of methods are necessary to remove barriers and facilitate the role of the APN in conducting clinically relevant research activities.

Clinical Access and Clinician Buy-In

Selecting a patient population to study is not generally difficult; the choice is driven by the question and the practice or service setting in which the APN works. It is important to remember that for clinical research to become a useful and real part of everyday practice, the research must be relevant. Greater buy-in is achieved when there is harmony or mutual interest of the involved participants. APNs can foster a spirit of inquiry and reinforce the idea that research is a journey. The culture of inquiry can evolve one question at a time (Rivers, Cohen, & Counsell, 2006; Pepler et al., 2006). The APN acts as a clinical intermediary to influence practice changes by sharing evidence through clinical rounds, in staff education, and by demonstrating practice changes. In this way APNs can bridge the gap between theory and clinical practice (Ferguson et al., 2004).

Clinical access may be denied (or even covertly discouraged) if the research is seen as not important to the clinical practice. When clinicians are involved, and buy-in is high, access to patients is rarely an issue. Unfortunately, APNs who seek to only pursue their own research interests will quickly find that clinicians may not be supportive.

Strategies that have been suggested to encourage a research philosophy and buy-in include traditional solutions such as the development of journal clubs. In reality, journal clubs tend to last only for a few meetings, may be poorly attended because they are often held away from the clinical setting, and are often less than inspiring. Although they may be one way of infusing a research focus into practice, they are rarely the complete answer. Instead, the evaluation of scientific articles may be more acceptable and interesting if used in conjunction with a clinical question that emerges from a practice committee meeting or clinical dilemma.

As previously noted, clinicians are interested in research that has direct application to their practice. In a series of taped interviews with MICU nurses who had been engaged in unit-based research, participants stated that the choice of project was important to the clinicians' belief that research is a necessary part of practice (Burns, 2002). In these unit-based studies, data collection was integrated, whenever possible, into the regular patient care day. Additionally, the clinicians all noted the importance of how the research was used to change practice routines. And finally, clinicians also noted the importance of having a research mentor to guide them through each step of the process.

Administrative Support

Administrative support for clinical projects (especially those requiring clinician time or money) heavily hinges on the APN's previous accomplishments. Generally, many of the same attributes (e.g., perseverance, follow-through, and attention to detail) are required for any project to be successful. In addition, communication is essential for a true partnership built on trust and mutual respect between the administrator and the APN. Updates on the project progress, barriers to the process, and plans for dissemination of the results help ensure administrative understanding and future support.

It is helpful for the APN and administrator to have a discussion about goals for developing a research-based practice early in the partnership. That way a logical and sequential set of steps can be designed to ensure the APN's success. It is important as well that the APN and administrator agree on the program philosophy and define the boundaries for the program (e.g., support of various aspects such as meeting times, statistical analyses, and financial or educational support for clinicians who present study results outside of the institution).

Fueled in part by the growth in the Magnet Recognition Program, more organizations are implementing dedicated clinical nursing research roles. A more formal framework for research enhances the APN's opportunity to lead or participate in some aspect of clinical research.

Time and Money

In today's practice environment, it is sometimes difficult to believe that there is also time to do research or even to evaluate existing research in an effort to determine whether practice changes should be implemented. The refrains, "we're too busy" or "we will do it when we have more time" are common.

The APN's ability to demonstrate how research activities can be accomplished as part of a normal clinical day is essential to ensuring success. In fact, as discussed previously, when considering the feasibility of a research project or EBP change, a realistic assessment of the clinical environment should be accomplished first. Feasibility includes the cost of the project and potential financial outcomes associated with it. Both feasibility and financial solutions were addressed previously in this chapter.

COMPLETING THE RESEARCH ("CLOSING-THE-LOOP"): ADVANCED PRACTICE NURSE SCHOLARSHIP

A mark of true scholarship is to "close-the-loop" by presenting the outcomes of the research project to key stakeholders. In some cases this means providing an update in the form of a study summary at the unit level, or if generalizable, to other patient care areas. The outcomes may also be presented at local or national meetings and may be published as well. Unfortunately, many APNs accomplish wonderful research-based practice changes or research studies, but they do not disseminate the results.

Learning how to present the material is an important skill and improves with practice. Initially, the APN should seek a mentor who is experienced in presenting and publishing. Although writing and presenting skills may be difficult for the beginning APN, the importance of working to improve the skills cannot be understated.

AN APPROACH TO CLINICAL RESEARCH: THE EXPERIENCE OF ONE INSTITUTION

As discussed throughout this chapter, the APN's level of development largely determines the scope of the clinical research that is attempted. It is essential to start slow and small; the unit level is appropriate at the early stages. Subsequent projects may be attempted at a service line level or with more than one unit. Finally, institutional research projects can be initiated. Regardless of the level, the support of the institution is essential and good communication and a team approach are required. One institution's experience is described to illustrate key components of a successful clinical research program.

A Professional Nursing Staff Organization Research Program

Our Professional Nursing Staff Organization (PNSO) set a goal of establishing a program of clinical nursing research that is productive, widely disseminated within the hospital and sustainable. To accomplish this goal the PNSO sought the help of one of the hospital's APNs who had a background in clinical unit-based research.

The philosophy of the program is that clinical research is a necessary part of nursing practice and that clinicians at all levels should be included. To that end the infusion of a research milieu is essential. A formal institutional research program designed for professional nurses is a key component.

To ensure that the PNSO research program is successful and sustainable, the focus of the program is the development of bedside clinician researchers. The program director's role is to teach research, one step at a time, to selected clinicians. This oversight is quite time intensive because the director provides formal classes to teach aspects of research and subsequently helps the clinicians as needed to develop studies with their teams.

The clinician researchers are carefully selected and are called *research mentors* (RM). The term is one coined by Granger and Chulay (1999) and is used for two reasons. First, the clinicians are taught by the director how to guide their teams in conducting a project. The mentoring skills that the RMs learn are transferable to other aspects of leadership and are at the core of the APN role. Second, one of the major objectives of the program is to develop a *sustainable* program. Following the completion of the RMs first study, the expectation is that they develop second-generation projects with *less* need for intensive oversight and guidance from the director. The research mentor program is one of the best ways to build research capacity and create a sustainable structure for the organization and conduction of research.

This successful model is popular, and over 400 bedside clinicians are currently involved in research projects of some type. The study topics vary widely, but all are fairly narrowly focused to ensure completion. Three examples are described in the following sections to illustrate this concept.

Temperature Changes with Oral Fluid Intake

Clinicians on a surgical acute care unit questioned the timing related to oral temperature measurement following hot or cold liquid ingestion. Although most nursing textbooks note that between 15 and 30 minutes should elapse following oral intake, a literature review demonstrated that previous studies had been done with mercury thermometers and mostly in men. The clinician researchers felt a study testing the practice with digital thermometers (now the dominant technology) would be valuable. To that end they designed their study (Quatrara, et al., 2007).

The study was done testing the effect of cold and hot beverages on health-care volunteers' temperatures over time. All liquid temperatures were strictly controlled, as was the room temperature and the length of time the liquids were in the mouth. The researchers learned that waiting 30 minutes before temperature measurement yielded more accurate readings. The study resulted in a change in practice within the hospital and was published so that others might also make appropriate practice changes.

Blood Pressure Measurement in an Ambulatory Cardiology Clinic

Clinicians in an ambulatory cardiology clinic had noted that the method used to measure blood pressure (BP) in their clinic varied greatly among clinicians. They were concerned because they were aware that the American Heart Association (AHA) had published guidelines stating that the patient should be in a chair with feet on the ground and with the arms supported. In addition, the guidelines recommended that the heath-care provider wait for a few minutes before measurement.

Despite the existence of the guidelines, the clinicians noted that buy-in to changing the practice did not exist and that variation in BP measurement technique was the norm throughout the ambulatory clinics at the institution. They believed that a study to test the effect of using the AHA guidelines on their clinic patients' would be a useful method to teach the value of research, confirm the AHA recommendations, and help convince others that EBP changes were essential to quality care.

They designed a study that randomly assigned the patients to different positions and wait times. Their findings supported the AHA recommendations, and in addition demonstrated that an average of 14 points may be noted with improper technique (Turner et al., 2008). As a result of their study, BP measurement technique was changed in their clinic and others throughout the institution. They presented the content at a number of national meetings, and a manuscript on the study is in press.

Peripheral Intravenous and Central Venous Line Securement Methods

Two different unit teams lead by RMs in the postanesthesia care unit (PACU) and acute care medicine units questioned the efficacy of the current methods used to dress and secure PIV and CV lines. Both designed studies comparing methods approved by the CDC to their existing methods (Trotter, Brock, Schwaner, Conaway, & Burns, 2008; Winfield et al., 2007). The two groups found that the methods commonly used in their practice were inferior to other tested methods. The results were used to change and standardize PIV and CV catheter dressing and securement practices throughout the institution. In addition to the positive effect on practice that resulted from the work, the changes also resulted in an institutional cost savings. Both projects were presented at a variety of professional forums and were published in clinical journals.

Summary

The three examples of clinical projects demonstrate a number of important outcomes of clinical research. Projects that emerge from a specific service line or unit are especially popular to clinicians because the results of the projects are directly applicable to unit practice. In addition, the conduction of the research makes the importance of research come alive for the clinicians. As in the BP study, buy-in for change was ensured with the involvement of clinicians in the study, the short time frame, and the "doable nature" of each study. They saw firsthand the effect of positioning and timing on BP. It also demonstrated the validity of the AHA evidence-based guidelines, and by extension, others as well. Finally, the clinicians grew professionally and felt empowered that their research was making a real difference in the field, as they shared their results with others locally, and even beyond their own hospital.

CONCLUSIONS

Excellence in advanced practice depends on "acquiring, analyzing, synthesizing and applying evidence to inform the practice process" (Dickenson-Hazard, 2002). For the APN to guide and shape practice, research must be integrated. Whether we serve as consumers of research by reading and applying results of scientific reports or actually conduct studies to determine the answer to a clinical question, research must be evident as an important element of everyday practice. The role of the APN as a research mentor is essential to ensure that EBP is integrated and widespread. Only then will research truly be "part of what we do!"

References

American Association of Colleges of Nursing. (2006). The essentials of doctoral education for advanced nursing practice. Retrieved April 18, 2008, from the American Association of Colleges of Nursing Web site: www.aacn.nche.edu/DNP/pdf/Essentials.pdf.

American Association of Colleges of Nursing. (2008a). Beacon award. Retrieved April 17, 2008, from the American Association of Colleges of Nursing Web site: www.aacn.org/AACN/ICURecog.nsf/vwdoc/toc.

American Association of Colleges of Nursing. (2008b). Clinical inquiry grants. Retrieved April 17, 2008, from the American Association of Colleges of Nursing Web site: www.aacn.org/AACN/aacnnews.nsf/GetArticle/ArticleTwo1710#grants.

American Nurses Credentialing Center. (2008). Magnet designation. Retrieved April 17, 2008, from the American Nurses Credential Center Web site: www.nursecredentialing.org/magnet/.

American Nurses Association. (1986). *The role of the clinical nurse specialist.* Kansas City, MO: Author.

American Nurses Association. (2004). *Nursing: Scope and standards of practice.* Washington, DC: nursebooks.org.

Atherton, S., Church, V., Locke, C., & Tjoelker, R. (2007). Clinical nurse specialists: Bridging the gap between evidence and practice using evidence-based fact sheets. *2007 NACNS National Conference Abstracts: February 28-March 3, Phoenix, Arizona. Clinical Nurse Specialist, 21,* 102.

Berger, A. M., Eilers, J. G., Heermann, J. A., Warren, J. J., Franco, T., & Triolo, P. K. (1999). State-of-the-art patient care: The impact of doctorally prepared clinical nurses. *Clinical Nurse Specialist, 13*(5), 259–266.

Brown, S. J. (2000). Direct clinical practice. In A. B. Hamric, J. A. Spross, & C. M. Hanson (Eds.), *Advanced nursing practice: An integrative approach* (2nd ed., pp. 137–173). Philadelphia: WB Saunders.

Burman, M. E., Hart, A. M., & McCabe, S. M. (2005). Doctorate of nursing practice: Opportunity amidst chaos. *American Journal of Critical Care, 14*(6) 463–464.

Burns, S. M. (2002). Clinical research is part of what we do! The experience of one medical intensive care unit. *Critical Care Nurse, 22*(2), 100–113.

Burns, S. M., & Earven, S. (2002). Improving outcomes for mechanically ventilated medical intensive care patients using advanced practice nurses: A six-year experience. *Critical Care Nursing Clinics of North America, 14*(3), 231–243.

Burns, S. M., & Keeling, A. W. (1999). The ACNP as researcher: Strategies for practice. In P. Logan (Ed.), *Principles and practice of the acute care nurse practitioner* (pp. 91–97). Stamford, CT: Appleton and Lange.

Burns, S. M., Marshall, M., Burns, J. E., Ryan, B., Wilmoth, D., Carpenter, R., et al. (1998). Design, testing and outcomes of an outcomes managed approach to patients requiring prolonged ventilation. *American Journal of Critical Care, 7*(1), 45–57.

Burns, S. M., Earven, D., Fisher, C., Lewis, R., Merrel, P., Schubart, J., et al. (2003) Implementation of an institutional program to improve clinical and financial outcomes of patients requiring mechanical ventilation: One year outcomes and lessons learned. *Critical Care Medicine, 31*(12), 2752–2763.

Campbell, G., & Chulay, M. (1990). Establishing a clinical nursing research program. In J. Spicer & M. A. Robinson (Eds.), *Environmental management in critical care nursing.* Baltimore: Williams & Wilkins.

Carroll, D. L., Greenwood, R., Lynch K. E., Sullivan, J. K., Ready, C. H., & Fitzmaurice, J. B. (1997). Barriers and facilitators to the utilization of nursing research. *Clinical Nurse Specialist, 11*(5), 207–212.

Deshefy-Longhi, T., Swartz, M. K., & Grey, M. (2002). Establishing a practice-based research network of advanced practice registered nurses in Southern New England. *Nursing Outlook, 50*(3), 127–132.

Dickenson-Hazard, N. (2002). Evidence-based practice: the "right approach." *Leadership,* second quarter, 6.

Ferguson, L., Milner, M., & Snelgrove-Clarke, E. (2004). The role of intermediaries, getting evidence into practice. *Journal of Wound Ostomy and Continence Nursing, 31*(6), 325–327.

Fulton, J. S., & Baldwin, K. (2004). An annotated bibliography reflecting CNS practice and outcomes. *Clinical Nurse Specialist 18*(1), 21–39.

Goldberg, N. J., & Moch, S. D. (1998). An advanced practice nurse–nurse researcher collaborative model. *Clinical Nurse Specialist, 12*(6), 251–255.

Granger B., & Chulay, M. (1999). *Research strategies for clinicians.* Stamford, CT: Appleton and Lange.

Hamric, A. B. (2000). A definition of advanced nursing practice. In A. B. Hamric, J. A. Spross, & C. M. Hanson (Eds.), *Advanced nursing practice: An integrative approach* (2nd ed., pp. 53–73). Philadelphia: WB Saunders.

Hanberg, A., & Brown, S. C. (2006). Bridging the theory-practice gap with evidence-based practice. *The Journal of Continuing Education in Nursing, 37*(6), 248–249.

Jones, M. L. (2004). Role development and effective practice in specialist and advanced practice roles in acute hospital settings: Systematic review and meta-synthesis. *Journal of Advanced Nursing, 49*(2), 191–209.

Lekandder, B. J., Tracy M. F., & Lindquist, R. (1994). Overcoming the obstacles to research based clinical practice. *AACN Clinical Issues, 5*(2), 115–123.

Mateo, M. A., & Kirchhoff, K. T. (1999). *Using and conducting nursing research in the clinical setting* (2nd ed.). Philadelphia: WB Saunders.

McGuire, D. B., & Harwood, K. Y. (2000). Research. In A. B. Hamric, J. A. Spross, & C. M. Hanson (Eds.), *Advanced nursing practice: An integrative approach* (2nd. ed., pp. 245–278). Philadelphia: WB Saunders.

Mercer, T. A. (2008). Research settings, regional consortium provides much-needed resource, networking opportunity for nurse researchers. *Advance for Nurses, 10*(4), 23.

Nugent, K. E., & Lambert, V. A. (1996). Advanced-practice nurses: Approaches to collaborative research. *Nursing Connections, 9*(2), 5–16.

Pepler, C. J., Frisch, S., Rennick, J., Swidzinski, M., White, C., Brown, T., et al. (2006). Strategies to increase research-based practice. *Clinical Nurse Specialist, 20*(1), 23–31.

Profetto-McGrath, J., Smith, K. B., Hugo, K., Taylor, M., & El-Hajj, H. (2007). Clinical nurse specialist use of evidence in practice: A pilot study. *Worldviews on Evidence-Based Nursing, 4*(2). 86–96.

Quatrara, B., Coffman, J., Jenkins, T., Mann, K., McGough, K., Conaway, M., et al. (2007) The effect of respiratory rate and ingestion of hot and cold beverages on the accuracy of oral temperatures measured by electronic thermometers. *Medsurg Nursing, 16*(2), 105–108.

Resnick, B. (2006). Outcomes research: You do have the time! *Journal of the American Academy of Nurse Practitioners, 18*(11), 505–509.

Rivers, R., Cohen, L., & Counsell, C. (2006). Science critical to patient care. *Nurse Leader, 4*(3), 40–44.

Sperhac, A. M., & Clinton, P. (2008). Doctorate of nursing practice: Blueprint for excellence. *Journal of Pediatric Health Care, 22*(3), 146–151.

Titler, M., Kleiber, C., Steelman, V., Goode, C., Rakel, B., Barry-Walker, J., et al. (1994). Infusing research into practice to promote quality care. *Nursing Research, 43*(5), 307–314.

Trotter, B., Brock, J., Schwaner, S., Conaway, M. R., & Burns, S. M. (2008). Central venous catheter dressings put to the test. *American Nurse Today, 3*, 43–44.

Turner, M., Chaney, C., Dame, M., Parks, C., Staggers, S., Stell, M., et al. (2008). Measuring blood pressure accurately in an ambulatory cardiology clinic setting—Does patient position and timing really matter? *Journal of Medical Surgical Nursing, 17*(2), 93–98.

Winfield, C., Davis, S., Schwaner, S., Conaway, M., & Burns, S. M. (2007) Evidence: The first word in safe I.V. practice. *American Nurse Today, 2*, 31–33.

Winters, C. (2007). CNS education: Using a faculty-supervised research practicum to build context for CNS competencies and quality outcomes. *2007 NACNS National Conference Abstracts: February 28-March 3,* Phoenix, Arizona. *Clinical Nurse Specialist,* 21, 119.

The Advanced Practice Nurse and Complementary Therapies

Rothlyn P. Zahourek

18

INTRODUCTION

Interest in "natural remedies" and Eastern and indigenous healing has grown in the last 30 years as consumers become more knowledgeable in accessing health and illness information from the Internet. The field of what used to be called *alternative medicine* has evolved and is now called *complementary-alternative medicine (CAM)* or *integrative* care. That term may again change to *complementary-integrative* (CI) or simply to *holistic care*. Each term has a slightly different meaning **(Table 18-1).** For advanced nursing, CI or holistic are preferable because both imply a philosophical framework that is greater than the modality. Much of the data presented in this chapter will use the term *CAM* because the practice and research literature still use that term. CAM, however, implies an emphasis on modality, rather than on a philosophical approach. In this chapter the terms *CAM, CI,* and holism will reflect "the integrative nature of nursing practice rather than . . . an alternative method of health care" (Sparber, 2001, p.2).

Historically, nurses have been at the forefront of developing holistic care and CI modalities. Florence Nightingale's (1859/1969) early statistical and clinical work taught the health-care community about the importance of environment and spirituality on health and healing. Nightingale believed that nurses put the patients in the best condition for nature to act upon them, and that all disease is essentially a reparative process. She argued for cleanliness, fresh air, color, fresh food, and the presence of pets to aid healing to heal the sick and injured.

The holistic bio-psycho-social-spiritual-cultural model is introduced in fundamental nursing texts. Nurses value the role of the interpersonal relationship in their healing work, and they incorporate the role of environmental health and culture. Nursing has pioneered in the integration of comfort enhancing mind-body therapies such as prepared childbirth education, preparation for surgery programs, and the use of gentle massage. Relaxation, imagery, fostering a therapeutic relationship and communication, and the development of therapeutic touch (TT) and healing touch (HT) have been part of our nursing lexicon for decades. However, this holistic nursing foundation has waxed and waned throughout our development as a profession. As the nurse practitioner (NP) movement developed in the late 1960s, nurses became more "medicalized" and specialized in both focus and practice. Consequently, many nurses may be marginally or unprepared to meet their patients' holistic needs. Advanced practice nurses (APNs) need to be aware that they may be focusing more on the medical side of their practice, and they need to rediscover the richness of nursing theory created since Nightingale.

According to Helen Erickson (2007), as nurses developed group-specific knowledge and skills (i.e., children, women, and mental health clients), we recognized the *parts* of the person or group

TABLE 18-1

Terms Associated with Complementary Integrative Therapies and Holistic Nursing

Term	Definition	Source
Holism	(a) Identifying the interrelationships of the bio-psycho-social-spiritual dimensions of the person, that is, recognizing that the whole is greater than the sum of its parts; and (b) understanding the individual as a unitary whole in mutual process with the environment.	American Holistic Nurses Association
Complementary and alternative medicine	Practices that include various medical and health-care systems and practices and products that are not presently considered to be part of conventional medicine.	National Center for Contemporary and Alternative Medicine at the National Institutes of Health
Conventional allopathic medical and nursing practice	Practices that have been well accepted, have some research support, and are taught in standard educational programs, and for which some degree of understanding exists for the mechanism of action. This mechanism of action is in question for many of our treatments particularly in psychiatry.	
Alternative therapies	Used in place of conventional medicine. An example of an alternative therapy is Bach flower remedies for diabetes.	
Complementary therapies	A diverse group of health-care systems and not necessarily proven therapies that are used in conjunction with conventional medicine/nursing. An example is encouraging exercise, meditation, and massage to manage hypertension.	National Center for Contemporary and Alternative Medicine
Integrative medicine (nursing)	"[H]ealing-oriented medicine that takes account of the whole person (body, mind, and spirit) including all aspects of lifestyle. It emphasizes the therapeutic relationship and makes use of all appropriate therapies, both conventional and alternative."	Rakel, 2007, p. 7

but not the integral whole. In response, Kubsch et al. (2007) advocate for a paradigm shift from reductionism (i.e., characteristic of our current allopathic health-care system and some NP programs) to a holistic philosophy that includes complementary approaches and suggest that health is synonymous with well-being. Tension exists as this paradigm shift is occurring between physicians, nurses, and consumers.

According to the American Holistic Nurses Association (AHNA), holistic nurses recognize two views of holism: (a) identifying the interrelationships of the bio-psycho-social-spiritual dimensions of the person, that is, recognizing that the whole is greater than the sum of its parts; and (b) understanding the individual as a unitary whole in mutual process with the environment. Both views are valued, and the goals of nursing can be achieved within either framework (AHNA, 2004). A holistic philosophy is congruent with the theoretical base for advanced nursing practice of CAM modalities and holistic integral nursing practice. This holistic emphasis is the framework for this chapter. A modality (complementary or conventional), therefore, is less important than the holistic intent of the practitioner. A danger for APNs lies in placing too great an emphasis on the modality rather than the theoretical ad philosophical foundations for practice.

Healing is basic to nursing practice. It is a term often used in conjunction with holistic nursing and CI modalities. It is a process rather than an endpoint. It may include cure, but it implies recovery from a state of feeling shattered or fragmented into one of new or restored wholeness. The person becomes aware of a shift in their perception of a life experience, finds new meaning, and often develops new behaviors (Zahourek, 2004).

At the First American Samueli Symposium, a panel that included six nurse leaders grappled with issues of definition and research in healing. Quinn, Smith, Ritenbaugh, Swanson, and Watson's paper (2003) discusses the process and potential outcomes of a "healing relationship" as the basis for both research and practice. This relationship is the "quality and characteristics of interactions between healer and healee that facilitate healing" and includes "empathy, caring, love, warmth, trust, confidence, credibility, honesty, expectation, courtesy, respect, and communication" (Dossey, 2003, p. A11).

Holistic Nursing

Donnelly (2006) explains that "[h]olistic nursing interventions have always originated from the perspective of the person, community or family" (p. 215) and suggests that holistic nursing can help transform today's health-care system. Holistic nursing is "all nursing practice that has healing the whole person as its goal" (AHNA, 1998). Holistic nurses become "therapeutic partners" to strengthen human responses by facilitating the healing process and promoting wholeness (Mariano, 2007, p. 166).

In 2006, the American Nurses Association (ANA) in collaboration with the AHNA updated the holistic nursing scope and standards for practice and a section on advanced practice was added (Mariano, 2007). As a specialty, holistic nursing is based on "a philosophy, a body of knowledge, and an advanced set of nursing skills applied to practice that recognize the totality of the human being, the interconnectedness of body, mind, spirit, energy, social/cultural relationship context, and environment. Philosophically it is a world view, and not just a modality" (Mariano, 2007, p. 166). Practice is drawn from various healing systems, incorporates CAM modalities, and through "unconditional presence and intention" creates healing environments; self-care and self-responsibility are essential components.

For decades, nurses have used holistic interventions that are defined by National Center for Complementary and Alternative Medicine (NCCAM) as CAM. These include relaxation, art, guided imagery, massage, meditation, music, sound therapy, and prayer (Dossey, Frisch, Forker, & Lavin, 1998). Nurses incorporate energy therapies such as TT, HT, aromatherapy, and Reiki in their work in various clinical settings.

MILESTONES IN THE DEVELOPMENT OF COMPLEMENTARY-INTEGRATIVE HOLISTIC PRACTICE

The research base for CAM continues to grow. NCCAM was founded at the National Institutes for Health (NIH) in 1999 as an outgrowth of the Office of Alternative Medicine. It now funds research in more than 260 institutions and supplies information for practitioners, researchers, and consumers including Internet accessible information sheets, up-to-date research compilations on modalities and supplements.

NCCAM has categorized CAM modalities into four "domains" that include: *biologically based practices, energy medicine, manipulative and body-based practices, mind-body medicine* **(Box 18-1).** Some CAM practices involve personal or self-care activities (e.g., exercise, meditation, and prayer), products (e.g., over the counter nonregulated dietary supplements, herbs, and megavitamins), or treatments given by specialized practitioners (e.g., acupuncturists, chiropractors, and doctors of oriental medicine). Some practices are grounded in culture and tradition (Auyurveda) and others are original nursing interventions (TT and HT). Modalities considered to be CAM continue to change as practice becomes more standardized because the research supports its mechanism, efficacy, or safety. Acupuncture, acupressure, aromatherapy, biofeedback, chiropractic care, diet, exercise, guided imagery, some herbal medicine, some homeopathy, humor, hypnosis, magnets, massage, meditation, music, prayer, and relaxation techniques all currently enjoy a substantial research base; reports of these modalities can be found on the NCCAM Web site. A fifth category, "whole medical systems" is not included as a domain but is researched at NCCAM. These systems, built on whole theoretical and practice approaches, evolved apart from our conventional system (i.e., traditional Chinese medicine, homeopathy, and Ayurvedic medicine).

White House Commission on Contemporary and Alternative Medicine Policy

In March 2000, President Bill Clinton appointed the White House Commission on Contemporary and Alternative Medicine Policy (WHCCAMP; 2002) to explore society's need for safe and effective CAM practices. Two of the commissioners were nurses; other members included conventional practitioners, consumers, alternative practitioners, and business people (goals listed in **Box 18-2).**

BOX 18-1

National Center for Contemporary and Alternative Medicine's Classification System: Contemporary and Alternative Medicine Domains with Examples

- Biologically based practices: substances found in nature; herbs, special diets, amino acids, probiotics, and vitamins in doses in excess of standard practice
- Energy medicine: use of energy fields: (a) magnetic energy, which can be measured (i.e., magnets for pain) and (b) biofields, which are not currently measurable, and believed to surround and penetrate the body like auras (i.e., Reiki, therapeutic touch, and healing touch)
- Manipulative and body-based practices: manipulation of body parts (i.e., massage, reflexology, or chiropractic)
- Mind-body medicine: uses techniques to enhance the mind's ability to affect bodily functions (i.e., relaxation, imagery, hypnosis, biofeedback, and spiritual practices such as prayer)
- Alternative medical systems is not a domain but includes whole philosophical schools of thought and practice including: traditional Chinese medicine, Ayurveda, and homeopathy

Adapted from National Center for Contemporary and Alternative Medicine Web site, Retrieved March 20, 2008.

BOX 18-2
White House Commission on Complementary
and Alternative Medicine Policy 2000 Goals

- Coordinating research to increase knowledge about contemporary and alternative medicine (CAM) practices and products.
- CAM therapies should be researched aggressively.
- Conventional practitioners should be educated in CAM.
- Dietary supplements should receive increased research and safety checks guiding appropriate access to, and delivery of, CAM.
- A national coding system available to complementary practitioners.
- Providing health-care professionals with reliable useful information about CAM that is accessible and understandable to the general public.
- Individual styles of CAM practice should be maintained rather than subsumed into a standard medical model.

The complete report is available at www.whccamp.hhs.gov.
(Muscat, 2000; report in *Integrative Nursing,* Sept/Oct. 2002).

A particular emphasis of the report is the caveat that safe and effective practices established for one condition may introduce new safety concerns when used with conventional medications. Individuals with chronic conditions may be particularly vulnerable.

A Nursing Summit on Integrative Care

In 2002, a select group of nurse leaders met at the Minnesota Center for Spirituality and Healing and formalized a plan for nurses in integrative care (Eliopoulos, 2002). They emphasized that nurses' practice of CAM should be grounded on a holistic model such as that developed by AHNA. They developed recommendations for clinical practice, education, research, and "positioning" for faculty and students to become educated in integrative care and for certification and credentialing to support reimbursement. State boards of nursing (BON) needed to become better informed about CAM. Nurses should participate in developing research agendas and be included on panels and multidisciplinary projects. Positioning implied that nurses should clarify and articulate their values about healing and avoid the disease-based medical model when describing and implementing CI therapies.

RESEARCH ON CONTEMPORARY AND ALTERNATIVE MEDICINE USE

A consistent pattern of increased CAM use has been demonstrated through numerous national surveys over the last 20 years. The most recent survey by NCCAM, released in December 2008, shows that about 38% of U.S. adults aged 18 years and above and 12% of children use some form of CAM (NCCAM, 2008). The first landmark utilization survey (Eisenberg et al., 1993) found that approximately 33% of individuals in the United States had used one or more unconventional therapy during the preceding year. In a follow-up study, Eisenberg et al. (1998) found an increased use—42.1% of Americans had used one or more CAM therapies. The NCAAM report released in May 2004 was conducted with the National Center for Health Statistics (NCHS) in the Centers for Disease

Control and Prevention (CDC). The study surveyed 31,044 adults and found that 55% believed CAM was beneficial particularly when combined with conventional approaches; 36% used some form of CAM, and when prayer was included as a modality, up to 62% used CAM. When prayer was included, the mind-body domain was most commonly used; when prayer was excluded, biologically based therapies (22%) were most common (mind-body therapies: 17%). Prayer continued to be the most commonly used modality for specific health reasons. According to all the epidemiological studies, in addition to prayer, the most commonly used modalities include: mind-body interventions, herbs, supplements, and homeopathy, acupuncture, massage, chiropractic, stress management procedures, and energy work such as Reiki and TT. As previously noted, prayer and seeking spiritual guidance are prevalent, which has implications for the APN (NCCAM, 2008).

In this most recent survey (2008), CAM users are women in greater numbers than men; people with higher education; people who have been hospitalized in the last year; and former smokers. Participants used CAM for a wide variety of problems: painful conditions such as back, neck, and joint pain; colds; anxiety and depression; sleep problems; and gastrointestinal problems. People used CAM most often (55%) to improve their health and in combination with conventional medicine. Another 50% were simply interested in trying CAM; others believed conventional medicine would not help. For others, their conventional provider suggested CAM or the person felt conventional treatments were too expensive. This 2004 survey did not query the amount of money people spent on CAM. The previous report (Eisenberg et al., 1998) estimated that the U.S. public spent $36 to $46 billion on CAM; between $12 and $20 billion was spent out of pocket, $5 billion of which was spent on herbal products. The common emphasis on "natural" products and remedies in everything from shampoo to hormone replacement therapy reflect this trend. Continued research may show that the reasons and purposes for CAM use are as diverse as the consumers who use them.

Consumers incorporate complementary therapies in designing their own integrative health plans. Success of these plans is demonstrated by the findings that 79% of respondents using both CAM therapies and traditional medicine "perceived the combination to be superior to either one alone" (Eisenberg et al., 2001, p. 1). Jonas (1997) concluded that consumers' complementary therapy use does not always mean dissatisfaction with conventional medicine, but rather it is part of their social network, or they are not satisfied with the process or results of their conventional care (p. 34). One might speculate, however, from simply listening to the evening news, that in the 11 years since his article, dissatisfaction with health-care accessibility, expense, and quality has grown significantly.

An important finding from all the surveys is that more than half of the respondents do *not* share their use of CAM practices with their health-care provider. Reasons for nondisclosure included feeling that it was not important for the provider to know; the provider did not ask; the patient felt it was none of the provider's business; or that the provider would not understand. It is important to note that primary care providers were mandated in 1998 to question patients about the use of complementary practices and record the information in their permanent records (United States Department of Health & Human Services [USDHHS], 1998).

National Center for Contemporary and Alternative Medicine as a Resource

NCCAM is a vitally important link for health-care professionals and consumers (**Box 18-3**). Information about the research status of CAM therapies is also available for consumers and health-care providers through links to other NIH centers and programs. A regular free newsletter

---

BOX 18-3
National Center for Contemporary and Alternative Medicine

The NCCAM Web site includes new and updated fact sheets; these are in the public domain and duplication is encouraged:

- 10 things to know about evaluating medical resources on the Web.
- What is complementary and alternative medicine (CAM)?
- CAM use and children.
- Who uses CAM: Statistics.
- Domains.
- About clinical trials and CAM.
- Most frequent health topics: acupuncture, arthritis, black cohosh, cancer, chelations, chiropractic, dietary supplements, depression, echinacea, ephedra, gingko, ginseng, glucosamine, homeopathy, herbs at a glance, meditation, menopause, and St. John's wort.
- Links to valuable reports by the National Center for Contemporary and Alternative Medicine (NCCAM) can be found on DavisPlus.

For information about NCCAM or any aspect of CAM contact the Clearinghouse at 1-888-644-6226, fax at 1-866-464-3616, or e-mail info@nccam.nih.gov. Send written requests to NCCAM Clearinghouse, P.O. Box 7923, Gaithersburg, MD, 20898-7923

NCCAM PUBLICATIONS:

- *Complementary and Alternative Medicine at NIH* is a quarterly publication by NCCAM highlighting current research, research funding opportunities, calendars of activities, and clearinghouse information. Available by mail, on NCCAM's Web site, or via e-mail by contacting the NCCAM Clearinghouse. The publication is not copyrighted.
- Treatment information: by treatment or therapy and disease or condition available at http://nccam.nih.gov/health/bytreatment.htm.
- National Institutes of Health consensus development program Available at http://consensus.nih.gov.
- Live help, video lectures, CAM on PubMed, and research results.

National Center for Contemporary and Alternative Medicine Web site: http://nccam.nih.gov.

---

is available that contains listings and abstracts of recent research results, as well as, more substantial articles on such topics as placebo response or prayer and spirituality.

Consumers are engaging in CI health-care practices whether the health-care professional guides them or not. Health-care providers must be knowledgeable about the safety and efficacy of complementary therapies to help clients choose safe and potentially effective modalities. (See DavisPlus for additional Web sites.)

COMPLEMENTARY-INTEGRATIVE MODALITIES AND ADVANCED HOLISTIC NURSING PRACTICE

The role of the APN is to support patients in their choice of holistic-integrative practices, make recommendations, and deliver safe and effective complementary therapies when appropriate.

Examples of Complementary-Integrative Holistic Practice Modalities

Several years before the landmark Eisenberg et al. study (1993), nurses were publishing about CAM modalities. Snyder (1985) completed a book titled *Independent nursing interventions* that included CAM approaches (e.g., relaxation, imagery, massage). Clark published *Wellness nursing* (1986), and *Holistic nursing: a handbook for practice* was first published in 1988. Clements and Martin published *Nursing and holistic wellness* (1990), Zahourek published early papers on the use of hypnosis with pain (1982a, 1982b), *Clinical hypnosis and therapeutic suggestion in nursing* (1985) and *Relaxation and imagery* or nurses (1988). Delmar has published *The nurse as healer,* a series of small books edited by Lynn Keegan on such topics as *Creative imagery in nursing* (Shames 1996) and *Awareness in healing* (Rew, 1996). It is also paradoxical that McCloskey and Bulechek (1992) classified several of these same therapies as nursing interventions in the year before Eisenberg's report (1993). Their 7-year research project funded by the National Institute of Nursing culminated in the publication of the *Nursing Interventions Classification* (NIC). This comprehensive standardized classification of research-based nursing interventions (McCloskey & Bulechek, 2000) included "simple guided imagery" (p. 595), "simple massage" (p. 596), and "simple relaxation therapy" (p. 598).

Mind-Body Therapies and Advanced Nursing Practice

Relaxation, imagery, and therapeutic suggestion (hypnosis) have become standard practice to help relieve pain. Kwekkeboom and Gretarsdottir (2006) reviewed randomized trials of relaxation interventions for the treatment of pain in adults from 1996 to 2005. Although many of the studies had weak methodology, 8 of the 15 studies showed support of relaxation techniques (e.g., jaw relaxation and systematic relaxation) for arthritis and postoperative pain. Kitko (2007) describes rhythmic breathing as an easy way to learn intervention for reducing pain. The nurse helps the patient focus on an activity (e.g., purposeful breath), enhancing the relaxation response.

NCCAM reviewed studies on mind-body interventions with cancer patients and found that evidence exists that these interventions aid in improving mood, coping, and quality of life, as well as, ameliorate chemotherapy-induced nausea and vomiting and pain. According to this report, strong evidence exists that these techniques also are effective in the treatment of coronary artery disease and enhance cardiac rehabilitation.

A major report on the mechanism and value of the placebo as a mind-body response can be found in the *CAM at the NIH* newsletter (2007). In this newsletter, the placebo effect is treated as a potentially positive therapeutic tool rather than a research problem. The use of positive suggestions, no matter what the modality, has greater chance of success than if communication is negative or fosters a poor response to an intervention. Saying "this will hurt" (negative), or "this may cause some brief discomfort but is so powerful we know it can make you better" (positive), may both set off a "placebo" response but in opposite directions.

Guided Images

Human imagery is a holistic phenomenon described as a "multidimensional mental representation of reality and fantasy that includes not only visual pictures but also remembrance of situations and experiences such as sound, smell, touch, movement and taste" (Bright, 2002, p. 113). There are many different forms of imagery, including imagery for behavioral rehearsal, impromptu imagery, and biologically based imagery, and symbolic and metaphoric imagery (Schaub & Dossey, 2005). Ashen (1977) developed an old, but still relevant, theory of imagery: images are stored in the mind as an experiential unit that includes the image, somatic response, and its meaning. In this context, imagery is used as a therapeutic tool for aiding anxiety and pain and behavioral rehearsal for change.

Imagery is used in healing trauma and posttraumatic stress disorder, often combined with cognitive behavioral therapy. It is used to treat numerous acute problems such as preparation for childbirth and for surgery and augmenting and minimizing side effects from medications and treatments. Grief resolution is, in part, an imagery process because people imagine their loss and themselves as strong and coping and subsequently find meaning in their experience. Reed (2007) describes several uses of imagery in clinical practice in which the study groups who received the imagery intervention had significantly more pain relief and required less pain medication.

Eslinger (2000a, 2000b) encourages nurse anesthetists to incorporate some of the techniques to "greatly enhance patient comfort and satisfaction" (2000a, p. 159). The use of hypnosis in childbirth is explained by Oster (2000), and Breurer (2000) discusses hypnosis in primary care settings, including quick induction for children and managing painful procedures. Eslinger (2000b) also presents case studies of hypnosis combined with guided imagery to help patients with hemophilia and migraine headaches.

Energy Therapies and Holistic Complementary-Integrative Nursing Practice

A "disruption in the flow of energy surrounding a person's being that results in disharmony of body, mind and/or spirit" is a nursing diagnosis (North American Nursing Diagnosis Association [NANDA], 2005). Energy therapies are listed as NCCAM modalities and currently are taught in continuing education, as well as, in holistic nursing programs and courses. Energy therapies are both intentional nontouching and hands-on therapies that work in the person's biofield of energy that, so far, cannot be measured. Energy therapies most often used by nurses include TT, HT, and Reiki. These therapies are purported to facilitate a person's bodily, as well as energetic, balance. Research on energetic modalities has been difficult in both nursing and in CAM. Engebretson and Wardell (2007) discuss in detail the methodological issues and problems for this modality that apply to research on many of these therapies. In general, these energetic approaches produce comfort and relaxation and do not cause harm unless an important conventional treatment is avoided and the person becomes more ill.

Therapeutic Touch, Healing Touch, and Reiki

In the early 1970s, nurse Doloris Krieger and healer Dora Kunz developed TT to help people with comfort and healing. Many nurses have been taught this technique. According to meta-analyses of studies on the effects of TT (including quantitative, qualitative, and mixed methods research), TT is useful in decreasing anxiety and promoting comfort (Peters, 1999; Winstead-Fry & Wijeck, 1999). Some studies have also been conducted on its affect on wound healing, but these effects are not sufficiently consistent.

HT, also considered a biofield energy modality by NCCAM, evolved from TT in the early 1980s and was more extensively developed as a training program by Janet Mentgen in 2002. Similar to TT, HT incorporates other theories and practices and is based on the idea that the body is a complex energy system that can be influenced by another's intention for healing and well-being. In a review of over 30 studies on HT, Wardel and Weymouth (2004) found that although the studies reported positive results in reducing stress, anxiety, and pain and enhancing healing time and quality of life, the quality of the research was such that generalizable results could not be determined. Wardell of Healing Touch International (HTI) has compiled an annotated bibliography that is available on the HTI Web site (http://healingtouch.net).

Originally practiced outside of conventional health care, the Japanese spiritual practice of Reiki has become an increasingly popular modality. Reiki is an energy-based therapy in which the practitioner's vibrational energy is connected to a universal source (e.g., chi, qi, prana) and is transferred to a recipient for healing (Miles & True, 2003). Additional nursing reports are beginning to appear on such topics as reducing anxiety and pain after abdominal hysterectomy (Vitale & O'Conner, 2006), self-care for nurses (Brathovde, 2006), and orthopedic pain (DiNucci, 2005). According to the NCCAM report, some areas of controversy include:

1. Little scientific evidence about Reiki, so accepting teaching about ki is a matter of faith.
2. Speculation that the effects of treatment are placebo.
3. Some feel Reiki is incompatible with their religious beliefs.
4. Governmental regulation and licensing is controversial.

Reiki is similar to HT and TT, but these modalities have substantially more research and are grounded in nursing theory and practice.

Biological Remedies

Biologically based practices according to NCCAM include, but they are not limited to, botanicals, animal-derived extracts, vitamins, minerals, fatty acids, amino acids, proteins, pre- and probiotics, whole diets, and functional foods. Although these products have not been regulated, the FDA is currently developing good manufacturing practices (GMPs) for dietary supplements. Newly marketed products are not subject to premarket approval or surveillance. Americans use supplements and herbs to promote overall health, to improve performance and energy, to treat depression, and to treat and prevent such illnesses as colds and flu. People with multiple illnesses, those who have a specific illness, consume large amounts of alcohol, or are obese tend to be frequent users (NCCAM, 2008).

Sutherland (2001) describes the use of four commonly used herbs for mild or moderate hypertension (*Rauwolfia serpentina, Staphania tendra, Panax notogensing,* and *Crataegus hawthorn* extract) and discusses recommendations for nursing assessment, intervention, and client education. The *American Nurse Today* (Fitzgerald, 2007) did a continuing education article on the use of herbs that included descriptions of six herbs (feverfew, gingko biloba, red yeast rice, saw palmetto, St. John's wort, and valerian) and their potential drug-herb interaction. Rosenfeld (2008), in a popular magazine, *Parade,* reviews the safety and effectiveness of ginseng, garlic, echinacea, chamomile, St. John's wort, ginkgo biloba, valerian, ginger, saw palmetto, hawthorn, black cohosh, and feverfew. His information coincides with the office of dietary supplements fact sheets, which review the research, uses, and side effects of these and other herbs and supplements. Currently more studies are being conducted on black cohosh for menopausal symptoms and vitamin D for bone health. Health effects of omega-3 fatty acids for people with depressions and B vitamins and berries in age-related neurodegenerative diseases are also being reported on the Web site.

Because many patients may use supplements without knowledge of their dosages, effects, or potential side effects, APNs need to know how to access accurate information. Patients' use of herbal remedies is important, particularly to APN's with prescriptive authority. Used for centuries and in many cultures, herbs can be as effective as our manufactured medications; therefore, some of the same cautions and precautions exist. NCCAM has several Web pages devoted to herbs and supplements.

The page "Herbs at a Glance" lists 42 herbs that can be accessed including black cohosh, cranberry, ephedra, ginger, gingko biloba, kava, milk thistle, green tea, etc. Consult the NCCAM Web site for the most current information on the effectiveness, as well as, drug-herb-supplement interactions. Numerous cautions for herbs and supplements listed by NCCAM include being aware:

- If a person has substituted an herb or supplement for a conventional medication
- What impact the supplement might have on the client's overall condition
- What interactions might occur between the supplement or herb and other medications
- Particular risks for people with diabetes, hypertension, or mental health problems such as depression and for people facing invasive procedures
- If a woman is pregnant or if treating children

It is important to ask the patient what he or she is taking, even if it is over the counter, "natural," or seems benign. A practitioner well educated in supplements and herbs can be a useful resource.

Aromatherapy

Aromatherapy is another popular nursing intervention (Smith & Kyle, 2008). Nurse Jane Buckle (2005) pioneered its development in nursing. Aromatherapy uses essential oils that are derived from plants (common herbs). The oils are either placed on cotton and near a person or in a steam distiller. Aromatherapy is often used in conjunction with conventional therapies for pain, anxiety, spasms, insomnia, and infection. Scientific evidence is growing about its efficacy. Many anecdotal reports describe positive effects in nursing homes, hospitals, and emergency rooms (Buckle, 2005; Garner, 2007). As with herbs and supplements, the practitioner needs to be aware of potential side effects and interactions. These oils should never be used internally because they are many times stronger than the herb itself.

Spirituality

One of the most frequently reported uses of CAM is prayer and spirituality. The impact of prayer in healing has been controversial for the last 15 years. Because the studies on prayer are contradictory, the controversy most likely will continue. However, dealing with patients' spiritual needs, and our own, is important. For many, coping with this rapidly changing, and increasingly technological world is causing existential crises of disconnectedness and a sense of alienation. Threats of devastation from global warming, wars, and conflict dominate the news compounding the anxiety with futility. When illness or injury occurs, or when a loved one dies, the need for solace and sense of connection, purpose, and meaning become even greater.

The North American Nursing Diagnosis Association (NANDA) recognizes spiritual distress as a diagnosis, and the ANA's Code of Ethics states nurses must consider a person's value system and religious beliefs. Burkhardt and Nagai-Jacobsen (2002) did early work on spirituality in nursing. They believe spirituality is different from religion. Spirituality is the "essence of our being . . . it permeates our living in relationships and infuses our unfolding awareness of who and what we are, our purpose in being, and our inner resources" (Burkhardt & Nagai-Jacobsen, 2005, p. 137). In practice, spirituality is related to active intentional listening and presence. It often employs the use of story and metaphor. Elders, for example, derive a sense of meaning from reminiscing and telling their life story to someone who is genuinely interested. Spiritual practices, such as mindfulness meditation, centering, and developing the capacity to be present, are useful for nurses themselves to prevent burnout and create a sense of purpose and meaning in busy and demanding practices. Praying with patients has been discussed at the annual Harvard Spirituality Conference and prayer groups for people who are ill are now common.

Baldacchino and Draper (2001) reviewed the literature from 1975 related to spiritual coping (187 articles) and concluded that illness often rendered feelings of a loss of control. Support of spiritual coping strategies in holistic care seemed to enhance self-empowerment, leading to a sense of purpose and meaning. Eldridge (2007) emphasizes that nurses need to know how to address patients' spiritual needs as they arise. She lists nine spiritual interventions: be there; listen actively; use touch; reflect and remember; laugh; share the experience; pray or encourage the patient to pray; use inspirational words or music; and evaluate spiritual needs. In addition, nurses need to remember the difference between spirituality and religion and respect the religious beliefs and practices, or lack of, in those they care for. Nurses do not force their own beliefs on others.

Burkhardt and Nagai-Jacobsen (2005) emphasize that "care of the spirit is a professional nursing responsibility and an intrinsic part of holistic nursing" (p. 149). Nurses must nurture their own spirits by pausing and reflecting about what is going on around them. This seems a challenge in our demanding health-care environment, which is often not healing in how it values and treats its caregivers.

Creating a Healing Environment

Modern health-care facilities are more aware of the need to create healing environments. Newer hospitals have largely private rooms that are bright with pleasant views. More space is provided in patient rooms to allow for families. The impact of noise and aromas are considered. The old locker room for the staff is being replaced in some forward-thinking institutions with stress reducing, peaceful spaces with recliners, soft lighting, and music where staff can rest.

Healing gardens, meditation spaces, animals and fish tanks, and attention to color and use of space to create calm and rest is becoming the norm. McCaffery (2007) compared the effect on mildly depressed older adults of participation in different environmental strategies: walking in a beautiful Japanese garden, a walk with guided imagery, and art therapy. Using focus groups she determined that all three groups' symptoms improved. Cole and Gawlinski (2000) reported a pilot study that explored the effects of animal-assisted therapy using an aquarium with fish on the stress levels of patients awaiting orthotopic heart transplantation in a cardiac care unit. Both patients and nurses were satisfied with the program.

PRACTICE ISSUES FOR THE ADVANCED PRACTICE NURSE AND COMPLEMENTARY-INTEGRATIVE THERAPIES

The APN's responsibility to society's changing health-care needs can be interpreted through the ANA's *Social Policy Statement* (2003). In this document, *expansion* "refers to the acquisition of new practice knowledge and skills and legitimizing role autonomy within areas of practice that overlap traditional boundaries of medical practice." Advancement includes "both specialization and expansion and is characterized by the integration of theoretical, research-based, and practical knowledge (as part of graduate education)" (p. 4). New practice knowledge and skills related to complementary therapies for APNs may include CAM science, nursing science, research-based nursing interventions, and guidelines for integrative or holistic practice.

Activities for the registered nurse and for APNs are outlined in the *Holistic Nursing Scope and Standards of Practice* (ANA/AHNA, 2007). Specific APN roles include consultation and prescriptive authority. Within that standard, the APN "uses advanced knowledge of pharmacology, psychoneuroimmunology, nutritional supplements, herbal and homeopathic remedies" and is cognizant of and evaluates potential effects, side effects, and interactions (Mariano, 2007, p. 183).

Educational Considerations for Complementary-Integrative and Holistic Nursing

Preparing APNs with the education and experiences to support patients in their integrative plans, to recommend therapies, and to deliver safe and effective CI nursing interventions is a challenge for nurse educators, continuing education providers, administrators, and accrediting agencies. CAM has been included in medical education and is now more often discussed in nursing undergraduate and graduate programs. The inclusion of complementary and alternative therapies in graduate nursing curricula is vital for the current graduate student population (Gaydos, 2001). According to Burman (2003), most NP programs include some CAM education. Sok, Erlen, and Kim (2004) evaluated the integration of CAM material into nursing education and advanced practice programs and suggest that graduate programs develop a recognized course of CAM study. They propose a 2-year program for NPs that includes content on the basics of CAM the first year followed by a second of intensive specialization. Fenton and Morris (2003) completed an electronic Web survey of deans of schools of nursing to determine the degree of integration of CAM into their curricula. They concluded from a sample of 125 schools that 60% used the definition of holistic nursing practice in their curricula and 84.8% included complementary modalities.

For more than two decades members of AHNA have been committed to developing resources for nurses seeking to expand their practice. The AHNA has an active and well-developed education committee that addresses both curriculum development in formal education, as well as, monitors and endorses continuing education programs **(Box 18-4).** As AHNA develops its Web site, more educational opportunities and online modules will be available, as well as, resources for accessing the scope of knowledge and research in holistic nursing **(Box 18-5).** Guidelines for curriculum development, advanced practice, and certification are available in the form of *Standards of Advanced Holistic Nursing Practice for Graduate-Prepared Nurses* (AHNA, 2002b; ANA/ANHA, 2007). The American Holistic Nursing Credentialing Center (AHNCC) now certifies holistic nurses at basic (HNC) and advanced level (AHN-BC). They endorse several basic and graduate programs **(Table 18-2).** Most graduate and many certificate programs are now taught online, which is the wave of the future.

Complementary-Integrative Therapies in Regulated Nursing Practice

Requirements for education and training, licensure, and reimbursement for CAM practitioners and advanced nursing practice are regulated by states. Understanding the qualifications and practice domains of nurses and other practitioners is the foundation for integrative practice.

BOX 18-4

Certificate Programs from American Holistic Nurses Association

- Certificate program in integrative aromatherapy
- Healing touch certification program
- Integrative reflexology
- Certificate program in integrative imagery
- Whole health education certificate
- Holistic stress management instructor certification workshop
- Integrative healing arts
- Great River Craniosacral Therapy Institute training program
- Aromatherapy for health professionals

BOX 18-5

Examples of Resources from American Holistic Nurses Association

- *AHNA Standards of Holistic Nursing Practice: Guidelines for Caring and Healing* (Frisch, Dossey, Guzzetta, & Quinn, 2000)
- *Holistic nursing: Scope and standards of practice* (American Nurses Association & American Holistic Nurses Association, 2007)
- *Holistic nursing: A handbook for practice* (Dossey, Keegan, & Guzzetta, 2005)
- *Core curriculum for holistic nursing* (Dossey, 1997)
- *Journal of Holistic Nursing,* the official Journal of American Holistic Nurses Association (AHNA) published by Sage publications
- *Beginnings* the newsletter published by AHNA
- AHNA Web site www.ahna.org
- Certificate continuing education programs endorsed by the AHNA

Sparber (2001) surveyed state BON to identify policies regarding registered nurses' (RNs) use of complementary therapies. At that time "Forty-seven percent of the BONs had taken positions that permitted nurses to practice a range of complementary therapies; thirteen percent were in the process of discussing this matter; and forty percent, although they had not formally addressed the topic, did not necessarily discourage these practices" (p. 1). In 1991, the Arizona BON was one of the first to issue a formal advisory on CAM. Kentucky, Massachusetts, and Pennsylvania followed by recognizing energy therapies of TT, HT, and massage therapies (now recognized in 25 states and an additional 7 are considering). Sparber's 2001 report has not been updated, but more recently, Denner (2007) and Radzyminski (2007) reviewed the legal status of nurses and CI modalities **(Box 18-6).**

TABLE 18-2

Programs Endorsed by the American Holistic Nurses' Certification Corporation

Department	Location	Program(s)
Xavier University Department of Nursing	Cincinnati, OH	BSN
Metropolitan State University School of Nursing	St. Paul, MN	BSN
Humboldt State University, School of Nursing	Arcata, CA	BSN
Western Michigan University, Bronson School of Nursing	Kalamazoo, MI	BSN
University of Colorado at Colorado Springs	Colorado Springs, CO	BSN and MSN
New York University, Department of Nursing	New York, NY	APN
Indiana University School of Nursing, South Bend	South Bend, IN	BSN
West Virginia University School of Nursing	Morgantown, WV	BSN
University of Texas Medical Branch at Galveston, School of Nursing	Galveston, TX	BSN, generic and flexible option tracks
Dominican University of California, School of Arts and Science	San Rafael, CA	BSN and MSN
University of Colorado—Denver	Denver, CO	BSN and MSN
University of Texas at Brownsville and Texas Southmost College	Brownsville, TX	BSN
Tennessee State University	Nashville, TN	BSN and MSN

APN, advanced nurse practitioner program; BSN, baccalaureate program; MSN, master's program.

These are the endorsed programs as of April 4, 2008. American Holistic Nurses' Certification Corporation endorsement indicates that the school of nursing provides a program of study based on the standards of practice for holistic nursing.

BOX 18-6
Legal Cautions

1. Is the modality within the scope of practicing nursing, or is it practicing medicine without a license? This is a particular problem as APN practice begins to look more like medical practice with overlapping roles and functions. Here a firm grounding in nursing theory and diagnosis will add clarity.

2. Standards of care for contemporary and alternative medicine (CAM) may be less clear than for conventional practice. Consider risk management guidelines of the institution and state nurse practice acts.

3. Is the practice in concert with the guidelines of the nurse practice act in the state in which the nurse practices?

4. Has the practice or modality been limited to another discipline? Some disciplines have their own licensure (i.e., chiropractic might limit the nurse's practice of craniosacral therapy).

5. Nurses traditionally counsel clients regarding nutrition and supplements. Does the state in which the nurse practices limit that counseling or prohibit prescribing over-the-counter herbs and supplements? Most often APNs with prescriptive authority are the only nurses qualified to prescribe such substances.

The Advanced Practice Nurse and Holistic Nursing Research and Complementary Therapies

The holistic and CI nursing research base has grown substantially in recent years. Graduate nursing programs have supported research focused on both theory development and the evaluation of modalities. Enzham-Hagedorn and Zahourek (2007) provide both a theoretical model and an extensive chart of studies on all aspects of holistic nursing. It is imperative that APNs become aware of the evidence and precautions derived from various research approaches to make informed choices about using any modality or encouraging their clients to do the same. (For specific case studies, please refer to the bibliography located on DavisPlus.)

Role Development and Avenues and Models for Advanced Practice Nurses as Complementary-Integrative Practitioners

Nontraditional, holistic interventions are common APN practices. Sohn and Loveland Cook (2002) surveyed NP's degree and source of CAM knowledge and their referral practices and found that APNs from both liberal and conservative communities were making efforts to meet the demands for CAM.

More nurses are becoming independent CI or holistic practitioners. Health coaching has become a role. A 2006 issue of *Beginnings* is devoted to holistic nurses developing private practices. Nurses describe practices that include HT, massage, counseling, a radio show, work in cardiology, aromatherapy, and developing an online journal, *The Alternative Journal of Nursing*). APNs interested in developing complementary therapy practices or delivering holistic nursing interventions must take responsibility for obtaining the necessary education, experience, and when appropriate, certification.

APNs may be involved in an integrative practice in which patients have a choice between a conventional and an alternative practitioner. Broad and Allison (2002) describe a Hawaiian healing community-based clinic where both NPs and *kahunas* (Hawaiian health practitioners) were available to provide services to "uninsured and underinsured people in an atmosphere that assures respect for the culture and the health needs" (p. 50). They learned in their pilot study examining the preferences and choices of practitioners, that NP services were sought for predominantly acute conditions and kahunas provided treatment for chronic conditions. Of the respondents, 67% reported satisfaction with the combination of both practices.

The Shuler Nurse Practitioner Model is a guiding framework for providing holistic health care to the elderly (Shuler, Huebscher, & Hallock, 2001). This model includes a comprehensive assessment and suggested therapies for general well-being and stress management. The tool is grounded in holistic philosophy and the treatment plan considers four components: problem/diagnosis judgments, self-care activities, disease-prevention activities, and health-promotion activities. Patient outcomes are based on improved health status and wellness.

APNs recommend complementary therapies, which require being informed about which therapies are safe and effective for integrating into the patient's plan of care, being cognizant about the patient's condition. Rauckhorst (2001) suggests that recommending CI therapies to Alzheimer disease patients and their caregivers can be quite empowering in a situation characterized by helplessness and frustration (p. 53). Similarly, after reviewing the scientific base for CIs, Huebscher (2000) suggests that health-care providers consider preventing further damage and providing symptomatic comfort measures by encouraging patients to make informed choices about CI interventions.

For nurses in acute and critical care settings, Kreitzer and Jensen (2000) recommend giving patients "control of their lives by making complementary therapies available" (p. 11). They identify criteria for determining whether a complementary therapy is appropriate. **Box 18-7** contains questions that APNs can use as a guide to recommending CI therapies.

The NCCAM home page offers guidance for recommending therapies on the section "Be an informed consumer." This includes such issues as selecting a CAM practitioner, paying for CAM, and 10 things to know about evaluating medical resources on the Web. In bold letters is the statement "Tell your doctor about your CAM use." NCCAM and the Office of Dietary Supplements continue to be valuable resources for updated reviews and meta-analyses of research. Sufficient understanding of both the patient's disease process and the specific therapy are mandatory requirements before referral is made. Communication and collaboration with the CI practitioner is useful in providing comprehensive care.

Ethical Considerations

The APN has the obligation to foster patients' choices about the care they receive and must function within the *ANA Code of Ethics for Nurses with Interpretative Statement* (2001). According to Mariano (2007), the ethical stance of the holistic nurse is as an "option giver," a partner, and a "co-prescriber." "The relationship is a copiloting of the individual's health experience whereby one respects the person's decision about his or her own health. It is a process of engagement rather than compliance" (p. 169).

The ethical principles of autonomy, nonmalfeasance, beneficence, and justice must be considered when advising or referring patients who use or consider using complementary therapies that are beyond advanced nursing practice. Patients have the right to choose treatments consistent with their

---

BOX 18-7

Question Guide for Advanced Practice Nurses Recommending Complementary-Integrative Therapies

- Has the therapy been used to manage the symptom or initial treatment?
- Is there research evidence that the therapy is safe and effective?
- Is the therapy appropriate for the patient?
- Does the patient want or expect the therapy to work?
- Are there providers who are skilled in providing the therapy (Kreitzer & Jensen, 2000, pp. 11–12)?
- Has the patient had prior or current experience with complementary therapies?
- What modality does the patient's cultural group tend to use most frequently?
- When you refer a patient to a complementary-integrative health-care provider do you know the provider's credentials and licensing requirements, the qualifications of the practitioner, and some evidence of competence (Corless, Abrams, Nicholas, & McGibbon, 2000; Manzella, 2000)?
- Counseling patients in their decision to use complementary therapies also includes consideration for the cost of the treatments (Corless et al., 2000). Although insurance companies cover some complementary modalities (e.g., chiropractic, hypnosis, and massage), most modalities are paid for out of pocket and are often quite expensive.
- Counsel patients about access to herbs and supplements on the Internet. Which are legitimate and is the cost reasonable?

own values and culture. The APN's ethical obligation "involves not only respecting patient decisions but also fully informing the patient about the potential risks and benefits of CAM therapies" (Kaler & Ravella, 2002). The constructs of nonmalfeasance, beneficence, and autonomy in three holistic organizations were studied by Wardell and Engebretson (2001). They concluded that:

> *By appreciating the value of diverse healing modalities and sharing the decision making with clients, clinicians preserve patient autonomy and honor the principle of beneficence. Providers risk malfeasance if they ridicule, trivialize, or discourage patients' access to therapies from which they could benefit (p. 333).*

Ensuring that all patients have equal access to complementary therapies requires monitoring changes in insurance coverage and community resources. Kaler and Ravella (2002) state, "Keeping abreast of the research and making care decisions with ethical principles in mind will help optimize patient benefits and minimize risks from these modalities" (p. 42).

CONCLUSION

It is a holistic philosophy and evidence-based nursing science that facilitates the development of an integrative practice rather than a fragmented approach of adding optional therapies. As role models for other nurses and health-care professionals, APNs have the potential to affect the entire health-care system. Because of our holistic philosophic legacy, APN's have much to offer in the field of CAM, CI, and holistic nursing. Although modalities are important, they are more powerful for patients' and our own well-being if that practice is grounded in a strong commitment to holistic care, no matter what the modality. With this commitment to practice we can participate in creating a future that enriches ourselves, our patients, and society at large **(Box 18-8).**

BOX 18-8
Expanding and Advancing Contemporary and Alternative Medicine

To integrate contemporary and alternative medicine (CAM) into conventional health care and enable clients to benefit from the best of all treatments available, the advanced practice nurse (APN) will need to:

- Acquire and maintain current knowledge and competency in holistic nursing practice, including CAM therapies and practices integrated within that practice.
- Provide care and guidance to persons through nursing interventions and therapies consistent with research findings and other sound evidence.
- Adhere to a professional code of ethics and healing that seeks to preserve wholeness and dignity of self and others.
- Recognize each person as a whole: body-mind-spirit.
- Assess patients holistically, using appropriate traditional and holistic methods.
- Create a plan of care in collaboration with the patients and their significant others, if they wish, consistent with cultural background, health beliefs, sexual orientation, values, and preferences that focuses on health promotion, recovery or restoration, or peaceful dying so that the person is as independent as possible (p. 1).

Based on American Holistic Nurses Association. (2002a). *AHNA: position on the role of nurses in the practice of complementary and alternative therapies.* Retrieved July 15, 2002, from American Holistic Nurses Association Web site: www.ahna.org/limited/cam.rtf.

References

American Holistic Nurses Association. (1998). *Description of holistic nursing.* Flagstaff, AZ: Author.

American Holistic Nurses Association. (2002a). *AHNA: Position on the role of nurses in the practice of complementary and alternative therapies.* Retrieved July 15, 2002, from the American Holistic Nurses Association Web site: www.ahna.org/limited/cam.rtf.

American Holistic Nurses' Association. (2002b). *AHNA standards of advanced holistic nursing practice for graduate-prepared nurses.* Flagstaff, AZ: Author.

American Holistic Nurses Association. (2004). What is holistic nursing? Available from American Holistic Nurses Association Web site: www.ahna.org.

American Nurses Association. (2001). *Code of ethics for nursing with interpretative statements.* Washington, DC: Author.

American Nurses Association. (2003). *Nursing's social policy statement* (2nd ed.). Washington, DC: Author.

American Nurses Association, American Holistic Nurses Association. (2007). *Holistic nursing: Scope and standards of practice.* Washington, DC: Author.

Ashen, A. (Spring 1977). Eidetics: An overview. *Journal of Mental Imagery 1,* 5–38.

Baldacchino, D., & Draper, P. (2001). Spiritual coping strategies: A review of the nursing research literature. *Journal of Advanced Nursing, 34*(6), 833–841.

Brathovde, A. (2006). A pilot study: Reiki for self-care of nurses and healthcare providers. *Holistic Nursing Practice, 20*(2), 95–101.

Breuer, W. C. (2000). The use of hypnosis in a primary care setting. *CRNA: The Clinical Forum for Nurse Anesthetists, 11*(4), 186–189.

Bright, M.A. (2002). *Holistic health and healing.* Philadelphia: F.A. Davis Co.

Broad, L. M., & Allison, D. M. (2002). Nurse practitioners and traditional healers: An alliance of mutual respect in the art and science of health practices. *Holistic Nursing Practice, 16*(2), 50–57.

Buckle, J. (2005). Aromatherapy. In B. Dossey, L. Keegan, & K. Guzetta (Eds.), *Holistic nursing: A handbook for* practice (4th ed., pp. 829–848). Sudbury, MA: Jones and Bartlett.

Burkhardt, M. A., & Nagai-Jacobsen, M. G. (2002). *Spirituality: Living our connectedness.* Albany, NY: Delmar Thompson Learning.

Burkhardt, M. A., & Nagai-Jacobsen, M. G. (2005). Spirituality and health. In B. Dossey, L. Keegan, C. Guzetta (Eds.), *Holistic nursing: A handbook for practice* (4th ed., pp. 137–168). Sudbury, MA: Jones & Bartlett.

Burman, M. E. (2003). Complementary and alternative medicine: Core competencies for family nurse practitioners. *Journal of Nursing Education, 42*(1), 28–34.

CAM at the NIH Newsletter. (2007). *The placebo effect as a therapeutic tool.* Retrieved December 15, 2008, from the NCCAM Web site: http://nccam.nih.gov/news/newsletter/.

Clark, C. C. (1986). *Wellness nursing: Concepts, theory, research and practice.* New York: Springer.

Clements, I., & Martin, E. J. (1990). *Nursing and holistic wellness: A new beginning.* Dubuque, IA: Kendall/Hunt Publishing.

Cole, K. M., & Gawlinski, A. (2000). Animal-assisted therapy: The human-animal bond. *AACN Clinical Issues, 11*(1), 139–149.

Corless, I. B., Abrams, D., Nicholas, P. K., & McGibbon, C. A. (2000). The use of complementary and alternative therapies. *AACN Clinical Issues, 11*(1), 4–6.

Denner, S. S. (2007). The advanced practice nurse and integration of complementary and alternative medicine. *Holistic Nursing Practice, 21*(3), 152–159.

DiNucci, E. M. (2005). Energy healing: A complementary treatment for orthopaedic and other conditions. *Orthopaedic Nursing, 24*(4), 259–269.

Donnelly, G. F. (2006). From the editor: The transformation of healthcare: A wicked problem. *Holistic Nursing Practice, 20*(5), 215–216.

Dossey, B. M. (1997). *Core curriculum for holistic nursing.* Boston: Jones & Bartlett.

Dossey, B. M., Frisch, N. C., Forker, J., & Lavin, J. (1998). Evolving a blueprint for certification: Inventory of professional activities and knowledge of a holistic nurse. *Journal of Holistic Nursing, 16*(1), 33–56.

Dossey, B. M., Keegan, L., & Guzzetta, C. E. (2005). *Holistic nursing: A handbook for practice* (4th ed.). Gaithersburg, MD: Aspen.

Dossey, L. (2003). Samueli conference on definitions and standards in healing research: Working definitions and terms. Definitions and standards in healing research: The first American Samueli symposium (Ed.), W. Jonas & R. A. Chez. A supplement to *Alternative Therapies in Health and Medicine, 9*(3), A10–A12.

Eisenberg, D. M., Davis, R., Ettner, S. L., Appel, S., Wilkey, S., VonRompay, M., et al. (1998). Trends in alternative medicine use in the United States, 1990–1997. *Journal of the American Medical Association, 280*(18), 1569–1575.

Eisenberg, D. M., Kessler, R. C., Foster, C., Norlock, F. E., Calkins, D. R., & Delbanco, T. L. (1993). Unconventional medicine in the United States: Prevalence, costs, and patterns of use. *The New England Journal of Medicine, 328*(4), 246–252.

Eisenberg, D. M., Kessler, R. C., Van Rompay, M. I., Kaptchuk, T. J., Wilkey, S. A., Appel, C., et al. (2001). Perceptions about complementary therapies relative to conventional therapies among adults who use both: Results from a national survey. *Annuals of Internal Medicine, 135*(5), 344–351.

Eldridge, C. R. (2007). Meeting your patients' spiritual needs. *American Nurse Today, 2*(10), 51–52.

Eliopoulos, C. (2002). Leading the way to integration. *Integrative Nursing, 1*(1), 1.

Engebretson, J., & Wardell, D. W. (2007). Energy-based modalities. *Nursing Clinics of North America, 41*(2), 243–260.

Enzham-Hagedorn, M., & Zahourek, R. P. (2007). Research paradigms and models for investigating holistic nursing concerns. *Nursing Clinics of North America 41*(2), 335–353

Erickson, H. L. (2007). Philosophy and theory of holism. *Nursing Clinics of North America, 41*(2), 139–163.

Eslinger, M. R. (Ed.). (2000a). Complementary therapies in anesthesia [Special Issue]. *CRNA: The Clinical Forum for Nurse Anesthetists, 11*(4), 190–196.

Eslinger, M. R. (2000b). Foreword. *CRNA: The Clinical Forum for Nurse Anesthetists, 11*(4), 159.

Fenton, M. V., & Morris, D. L. (2003). The integration of holistic nursing practices and complementary and alternative modalities into curricula of schools of nursing. *Alternative Therapies in Health and Medicine, 9*(4), 62–67.

Fitzgerald, M. A. (December 2007). Herbal facts, herbal fallacies. *American Nurse Today, 2.*

Frisch, N. C., Dossey, B. M., Guzzetta, C. E., & Quinn, J. A. (2000). *AHNA standards of holistic nursing practice: Guidelines for caring and healing.* Gaithersburg, MD: Aspen.

Garner, B. (2007). Aromatherapy for you and your patient. *American Nurse Today, (2)*9, 53–54.

Gaydos, H. L. (2001). Complementary and alternative therapies in nursing education: Trends and issues. *Online Journal of Issues in Nursing, 6*(12). Retrieved October 13, 2002, from the American Nurses Association Nursing World Web site: www.nursingworld.org/ojin.

Huebscher, R. (2000). Peripheral neuropathy: Alternative and complementary options. *Nurse Practitioner Forum, 11*(2), 73–77.

Jonas, W. B. (1997). Alternative medicine: Editorial. *Journal of Family Practice, 45*(1), 34.

Kaler, M. M., & Ravella, P. C. (2002). Staying on the ethical high ground with complementary and alternative medicine. *The Nurse Practitioner, 27*(7), 38–42.

Kitko, J. (2007) Rhythmic breathing as a nursing intervention. *Holistic Nursing Practice 21*(2), 85–88.

Kreitzer, M. J., & Jensen, D. (2000). Healing practices: Trends, challenges, and opportunities for nurses in acute and critical care. *AACN Clinical Issues, 11*(1), 7–16.

Kubsch, S., O'Shaughnessy, J., Carrick, J., Willihnganz, T., Henricks-Soderberg, L., & Sloan, S. A. (2007). Acceptance of change in the healthcare paradigm from reductionism to holism. *Holistic Nursing Practice, 21*(3), 140–151.

Kwekkeboom, K. L., & Gretarsdottir, E. (2006). Systematic review of relaxation interventions for pain. *Journal of Nursing Scholarship, 38*(3), 269–277.

Manzella, S. M. (2000). Complementary healthcare practices and the implications for nurse practitioners. *Clinical Excellence for Nurse Practitioners, 4*(4), 205–211.

Mariano, C. (2007). Holistic nursing as a specialty: Holistic nursing-scope and standards of practice. *Nursing clinics of North America, 41*(2), 165–188.

McCaffery R. (2007). The effect of healing gardens and art therapy on older adults with mild to moderate depression. *Holistic nursing practice, 21*(2), 79–84.

McCloskey, J. C., & Bulechek, G. M. (1992). *Nursing interventions classification.* St. Louis: Mosby.

McCloskey, J. C., & Bulechek, G. M. (2000). *Nursing interventions classification* (3rd ed.). St. Louis: Mosby.

Miles, P., & True, G. (2003). Reiki—A review of biofield therapy history, theory, practice and research, *Alternative Therapies, 3*(9), 62–71.

Muscat, M. (2000). James Gordon selected to chair White House CAM Policy Commission. *Complementary and Alternative Medicine at NIH, VII*(2), 1, 4–5.

National Center for Complementary and Alternative Medicine (NCCAM). (2008). *2007 statistics on CAM use in the United States.* Retrieved December 15, 2008, from the NCCAM Web site: http://nccam.nih.gov/news/camstats.htm.

North American Nursing Diagnosis Association. (2005) *NANDA: Nursing diagnoses: Definitions and classification, 2005–2006.* Philadelphia: Author.

Nightingale, F. (1859/1969). *Notes on nursing.* New York: Dover Publishing.

Oster, M. I. (2000). Contemporary methods in hypnotic preparation for childbirth. *CRNA: The Clinical Forum for Nurse Anesthetists, 11*(4), 160–166.

Peters, R. M. (1999).The effectiveness of therapeutic touch: A meta-analytic review. *Nursing Science Quarterly, 12*(1), 52–61.

Quinn, J. F., Smith, M., Ritenbaugh, C., Swanson, K., & Watson, M. J. (2003). Research guidelines for assessing the impact of the healing relationship in clinical nursing. Definitions and standards in healing research: The first American Samueli symposium, Ed. Jonas, W., & Chez, R. A. A supplement to *Alternative Therapies in Health and Medicine, 9*(3), A65–A79.

Radzyminski, S. (2007). Legal parameters of alternative-complementary modalities in nursing practice. *Nursing Clinics of North America, 41*(2), 189–212.

Rakel, D. (2007). *Integrative medicine* (2nd ed.). Philadelphia: WB Saunders.

Rauckhorst, L. (2001). Integration of complementary and conventional health care in Alzheimer's disease and other dementias. *Nurse Practitioner Forum, 12*(1), 44–55.

Reed, T. (2007). Imagery in the clinical setting. *Nursing Clinics of North America 41*(2), 279–294.

Rew, L. (1996). *Awareness in healing.* Albany, NY: Delmar Thompson Publishers.

Rosenfeld, I. (2008, March 16). Do herbal remedies work? *Parade Magazine.* Available from the Parade Web site: www.parade.com.

Schaub, B. G., & Dossey, B. M. (2005). Imagery: Awakening the inner healer. In B. M. Dossey, L. Keegan, & C. E. Guzzetta (Eds.), *Holistic nursing: A handbook for practice* (pp. 567–610). Sudbury, MA: Jones & Bartlett Publishers.

Shames, K. H. (1996) *Creativity in nursing.* Albany, NY: Delmar.

Shuler, P. A., Huebscher, R., & Hallock, J. (2001). Providing wholistic health care for the elderly: Utilization of the Shuler nurse practitioner practice model. *Journal of the American Academy of Nurse Practitioners, 13*(7), 297–303.

Smith, M. C., & Kyle, L. (2008). Holistic foundations of aromatherapy for nursing. *Holistic Nursing Practice, 22*(1), 3–9.

Snyder, M. (1985). *Independent nursing interventions.* New York: John Wiley & Sons.

Sohn, P. M., & Loveland Cook, C. A. (2002). Nurse practitioner knowledge of complementary alternative health care: Foundation for practice. *Journal Advanced Nursing, 39*(1), 9–16.

Sok, S. R., Erlen, J. A., & Kim, K. B. (2004). Complementary and alternative therapies in nursing curricula: A new direction for nurse educators. *Journal of Nursing Education 43*(9), 401–405.

Sparber, A. (2001). State boards of nursing and scope of practice of registered nurses performing complementary therapies. *Online Journal of Issues in Nursing, 6*(3), 1–10. Retrieved October 3, 2002, from the American Nurses Association Nursing World Web site: www.nursingworld.org/ojin.

Sutherland, J. A. (2001). Selected complementary methods and nursing care of the hypertensive client. *Holistic Nursing Practice, 15*(4), 4–11.

United States Department of Health and Human Services. (1998). *Healthy people 2010 objectives: Draft for public comment.* Washington, DC: Government Printing Office.

Vitale, A., & O'Connor, P. C. (2006). The effect of Reiki on pain and anxiety in women with abdominal hysterectomies. *Holistic Nursing Practice, 20*(6), 263–272.

Wardell, D. W., & Engebretson, J. (2001). Ethical principles applied to complementary healing. *Journal of Holistic Nursing, 19*(4), 318–334.

Wardell, D. W., & Weymouth, K. (2004). Review of studies of healing touch. *Journal of nursing scholarship, 36*(2), 147–154.

White House Commission on Complementary and Alternative Medicine Policy. (2002). *White House Commission on Complementary and Alternative Medicine Policy: Final report.* Retrieved July 19, 2002, from the White House Commission on Complementary and Alternative Medicine Policy Web site: http://whccamp.hhs.gov/finalreport.html.

Winstead-Fry, P., & Wijeck, J. (1999). An interpretative review and meta-analysis of therapeutic touch research. *Alternative Therapies in Health and Medicine, 5*(6), 58–67.

Zahourek, R. P. (1982a). Hypnosis in nursing practice—Emphasis on the problem patient who has pain, [Part 1]. *Journal of Psychosocial Nursing and Mental Health Services, 20*(3), 13–17.

Zahourek, R. P. (1982b). Hypnosis in nursing practice—Emphasis on the problem patient who has pain. [Part 2]. *Journal of Psychosocial Nursing and Mental Health Services, 20*(4), 21–24.

Zahourek, R. P. (1985) *Clinical hypnosis and therapeutic suggestion in nursing.* Orlando: Grune and Stratton, Inc.

Zahourek, R. P. (1988). *Relaxation and imagery: Tools for therapeutic communication and intervention.* Philadelphia: WB Saunders.

Zahourek, R. P. (2004). Intentionality forms the matrix of healing: A theory. *Alternative Therapies in Health and Medicine, 10*(6), 40–49.

19

Basic Skills for Teaching and the Advanced Practice Nurse

Marilyn H. Oermann

In today's health-care environment, the advanced practice nurse (APN) serves a critical role in educating patients, students, staff, and other learners. The extensive knowledge base, clinical competencies, and communication skills of the APN prepare the nurse for carrying out this role across practice settings. Patient education is an important part of managing the patient's care to achieve optimal outcomes. Through this education, patients gain an understanding of their health problems and treatments, how to care for themselves at home, and health-promoting behaviors. By learning about their conditions and treatment options, patients can participate more fully in health-care decisions.

Teaching patients and their families, however, is only one role of the APN. For some APNs the educator role extends to nursing students, with the APN serving as a preceptor to nursing students and guiding their learning in the practice setting. In many settings the APN also teaches staff, assisting them in developing the knowledge and skills essential for providing care, keeping them up to date with advances in clinical practice, and mentoring nurses in the practice setting, ultimately improving the quality of patient care.

The purposes of this chapter are to describe the qualities of an effective teacher in nursing, the educational process from assessment through evaluation, strategies for teaching, and the role of the APN as educator. The chapter provides an overview of these topics as a way of preparing the APN for teaching patients, students, staff, and others.

FRAMEWORK FOR TEACHING

Every APN needs an understanding of the concepts of learning and teaching. These concepts provide a framework for the APN to use when making educational decisions.

Learning

Learning is a process of gaining new knowledge and skills as a result of experiences in which the learner engages. These experiences may be planned activities intended to guide the learner in acquiring this knowledge and these skills, or they may be unplanned experiences that lead to a new understanding. Learning may result in an overt and measurable change in behavior, such as a higher test score or ability to perform a procedure, or the outcomes of learning may not be readily apparent, such as gaining a new perspective on a chronic illness or insight about a patient's condition. Although learning has occurred, it may be more difficult to assess those outcomes.

Teaching

Teaching is a series of planned actions by the APN to facilitate learning. Teaching is not merely giving information, although that might be included in the process. Instead, teaching is identifying individual needs, setting goals in collaboration with the learner, planning experiences that guide the learner toward meeting those goals, and monitoring the learner's progression and determining where further learning is indicated (Gaberson & Oermann, 2007). Teaching is facilitating learning through experiences that actively involve the learner. Rather than telling a staff nurse what care to provide, the APN asks the nurse questions about that patient to guide the nurse in deciding on interventions.

Supportive Environment for Learning

The relationship between teacher and learner is critical to the educational process. Learning is facilitated in a supportive environment in which there is mutual trust and respect (Gaberson & Oermann, 2007). Establishing this environment is particularly important when working with students and staff in the clinical setting. Clinical practice is stressful for students (Oermann & Lukomski, 2001; Shipton, 2002) and new graduates (Beecroft, Santner, Lacy, Kunzman, & Dorey, 2006; Oermann & Garvin, 2002).

Although education is a shared experience between the APN and learners, the APN has the ultimate responsibility for establishing a supportive learning environment. When working with students and new graduates, the APN should remember that they are beginning practitioners and have varying clinical knowledge and competencies. The expectations set by the APN for these learners should be realistic considering their background and prior experiences.

Qualities of Effective Teachers in Nursing

Research conducted over the years has established the qualities of an effective teacher in nursing, particularly for teaching in the clinical setting. The findings of this research are significant because they guide the APN in developing skills that promote learning and avoiding behaviors that might impede learning. There are five predominant qualities of effective teaching: (a) expert knowledge, (b) clinical competence, (c) teaching skills, (d) positive relationships, and (e) personal characteristics. **Table 19-1** goes into more detail about these qualities.

ASSESSMENT OF LEARNER

The teaching process begins with an assessment of learning needs and other determinants of learning and progresses through planning, implementation, and evaluation. The process, however, is not linear; teaching does not necessarily start with assessment and end with evaluation. For example, the APN may plan a program for staff development following a needs assessment, but he or she may realize at the start of the program that most of the nurses lack the knowledge base for understanding the new content. This in turn suggests that different content should be presented to assist staff in gaining the prerequisite knowledge.

Assessment of Learning Needs

Assessment is the first step in the teaching process because it determines the learner's present knowledge and skills and examines other characteristics, such as readiness to learn and health status, which may influence achieving the objectives. The goal of assessment is to identify the

TABLE 19-1

The Five Predominant Qualities of Effective Teaching

Quality	Details	Research
Expert knowledge	■ Have expertise in content area to be taught ■ Stay up to date with interventions and new developments in that area ■ Be both aware of and able to translate current research findings and evidence into clinical practice	Beitz & Wieland, 2005; Gaberson & Oermann, 2007; Gignac-Caille & Oermann, 2001; Niederhauser & Kohr, 2005; Oermann, Blair, Kowalewski, Wilmes, & Nordstrom, 2007
Clinical competence	■ Know how to care for patients ■ Arrive at sound clinical judgments ■ Have advanced clinical skills in their area of practice and can guide learners in developing these skills	Gaberson & Oermann, 2007; Gignac-Caille & Oermann, 2001; Tang, Chou, & Chiang, 2005
Teaching skills	■ Know how to teach and have the ability to use those principles in teaching ■ Assess learning needs and plan instruction that meets those needs ■ Explain ideas clearly at a level each learner can understand ■ Ask thought-provoking questions that promote critical thinking and clinical judgment ■ Effectively demonstrate procedures and technical skills ■ Evaluate learners fairly, correct mistakes without embarrassing them and decreasing their self-confidence, and give immediate feedback	Gaberson & Oermann, 2007; Gignac-Caille & Oermann, 2001
Positive relationships	■ Bring strong interpersonal skills and an understanding of the importance of communication to the student-teacher relationship ■ Provide caring support for students ■ Communicate clearly	
Personal characteristics	■ Include: enthusiasm for teaching, patience, a sense of humor, friendliness, and willingness to admit mistakes	Berg and Lindseth (2004)

knowledge and skills the learner has already acquired and the needs for learning. Assessment reveals gaps in learning to be met through education. Questions that guide assessment of learning needs are highlighted in **Box 19-1.**

Learners frequently have more needs than the time and resources available for teaching. As a result, the APN prioritizes the learning needs focusing the instruction on the essential knowledge

---

BOX 19-1
Questions That Guide Assessment of Learning Needs:

What does the learner know already about the content?
What competencies does the learner already have?
Is this knowledge and are those competencies sufficient to learn the new content?
Based on this information and the goals or objectives to be achieved, what should be taught?

---

and skills for meeting immediate needs and for situations in which safety is a concern (Bastable, 2003). For example, the mother of a toddler recently diagnosed with asthma needs to know warning signs of an asthma episode and how to manage it, her child's asthma medications, the correct use of inhalers, asthma triggers for her child and how to prevent them, and when to seek treatment. These are immediate learning needs and should be the priorities for teaching by the APN. Although the mother may ask about the relationship of asthma and participating in organized sports, this information is not essential and is a low priority for teaching.

There also is limited time for educating staff, and the APN needs to focus the instruction on knowledge and skills essential for safe and competent practice. What are the most common practice problems new graduates and nursing staff are likely to encounter? What content must be learned to understand those problems and provide effective nursing care? What knowledge and competencies are required for safe care of patients? Once these essential learning needs are met, then the APN can extend the instruction to other areas of learning.

Assessment of Readiness to Learn

A second area to assess is the learner's readiness to learn. Readiness is the point in time when the learner demonstrates an interest in learning and is able to participate in the teaching process (Bastable, 2003). The learner must be ready physically, psychologically, and cognitively to engage in learning, otherwise, learning will not occur regardless of the importance of the content and skills.

In assessing *physical readiness,* the APN focuses on whether the learner has the physical ability to learn the skill. For example, a patient must have a certain degree of strength to learn to transfer from bed to wheelchair. Health status also affects physical readiness because it often influences the energy the learner has to engage in learning and degree of comfort. A patient experiencing acute pain following a surgical procedure or who is fatigued because of a treatment may not have the energy to learn and may be too uncomfortable to participate. Teaching the family or planning instruction for the follow-up visit may be more appropriate.

Psychological readiness includes the degree of anxiety and stress experienced by the learner, motivation to learn, and developmental stage. The learner needs to be able to focus on learning and be actively involved in it. The stress associated with the diagnosis of a serious health problem, fear of losing one's job because of illness, and concern about not being successful in an educational program, to name a few, may influence readiness to learn. In assessing psychological readiness, it is important for the APN to get a sense of the learner's state of mind and determine whether the learner is emotionally ready to engage in learning.

Motivation is the desire of an individual to learn—the drive to gain new knowledge and skills or to change a behavior. Differences among students and staff in their motivation to learn are often apparent in the effort they give to learning, their desire to achieve at a high level of performance rather than meet minimal expectations, and their willingness to engage in remedial learning and practice. Motivation may change over time and with different learning situations. Strategies for motivating learners as part of the teaching process are presented in **Box 19-2.**

Readiness to learn also is determined by the learner's developmental stage. Pediatric nurses are well aware of differences in how children learn based on their ages and development. Knowledge of growth and development guides the APN in determining the complexity and outcomes of learning and the types of teaching strategies that are appropriate.

Cognitive readiness relates to the knowledge base of the learner—whether or not the learner has the prerequisite knowledge and skills for beginning the instruction. This is a critical area of assessment, particularly for content and skills that build on one another. When lacking the prerequisites, it is up to the APN to fill in these gaps and guide learners to resources and experiences they can complete on their own. Assessment of cognitive readiness also allows the APN to determine whether or not the learner has already mastered the objectives and is ready to progress to a new area of learning.

Other Assessment Areas

Other areas to assess depend on the educational situation and type of learner. In teaching patients and families, the APN should be aware of their culture and how that might influence their education and methods selected for teaching. Chang and Kelly (2007) described the importance of including cultural values, health practices, and literacy as part of assessing learning needs and readiness. Cultural differences also may exist when teaching students and staff and should be assessed by the APN. The educational level of learners is often an important area for assessment, although the highest grade achieved in school does not necessarily indicate the learner's knowledge of a health problem or how that person will respond to the instruction.

BOX 19-2
Strategies for Motivating Learners as Part of Teaching

Teach *for* the learner, based on the learner's needs not the educator's needs.

Teach when ready to learn or develop alternate strategies, such as teaching family members and planning instruction for follow-up visits.

Set small and attainable goals so learners can meet them.

Focus the learner's attention on what needs to be learned.

Explain why this content and these skills are important.

Divide information to be learned in small segments, organize them logically, and teach only the amount learners can retain at a time.

Provide frequent and positive reinforcement (e.g., praise, for correct answers and accurate performance of skills).

Give immediate feedback at the time of learning, clarifying incorrect responses and errors in performance and reteaching as needed.

Allow for practice of skills so the learner develops confidence in abilities.

Review essential content and skills over a period of time to improve retention.

Strategies for Assessment

Questioning Learners

One of the most effective strategies for assessment is questioning learners about their understanding of the content and what they believe are their educational needs. These questions can be planned in advance and asked in a structured interview, or they can be integrated in the interactions between the APN and learner, a more informal means of assessing needs. For patient education, it is valuable to develop a list of questions about the conditions and treatments commonly found in the APN's practice; a standardized list of questions facilitates assessment and enables the APN to document the learning needs, instruction provided to patients and family, and outcomes.

Questions for assessment need to be open ended and probing to be effective. Asking patients, "Do you have any questions about your asthma?" is of limited value in assessing their understanding of asthma and self-care. A more effective line of questioning is, "Tell me about the medications you are taking for your asthma and whether they are helping. What problems are you still having, and what are you doing about them?" Using open-ended and higher level questions is particularly important when assessing the learning needs of students and staff. Learners may be able to answer questions that ask for recall of facts and specific information but be unable to answer those that require application to new situations, analytical thinking, drawing relationships among data, and evaluation. By asking different levels of questions, the APN can identify more clearly the actual learning needs.

Questionnaires

A second strategy for assessment is to develop a questionnaire that lists content areas and asks learners to identify where they need further instruction. One problem with questionnaires, however, is that learners rate their own instructional needs, which may not reflect an accurate assessment. A second problem when used for staff development is the length of time between conducting the assessment and planning and implementing the educational program. In that period, the learning needs of staff may change significantly.

Pretests

Written tests given before the instruction provide a reliable and valid means of assessing learning needs. By using pretest results, the APN can determine the content already mastered and identify gaps in learning that become the focus of the instruction. An advantage of using written tests is the opportunity to administer both a pretest and posttest as a means of evaluating the effectiveness of the instruction and educational programs offered throughout a facility. Although students and staff are conditioned to testing as a way of measuring learning, patients may be uncomfortable with written tests, and care must be used to write questions at a level patients can understand.

Observations

There is no better means of assessing psychomotor and technical skills than by observation of the learner performing them. Ideally, the APN should observe performance more than once.

Development of Objectives

Assessment reveals the knowledge and skills that the learner needs to acquire to meet the educational goals and the characteristics that might influence the learning process. From these needs the APN specifies the objectives to be met by the learner. These objectives reflect the outcomes of learning—the knowledge, psychomotor and technological skills, and values to be attained by the learner. The objectives also guide the selection of content and teaching strategies; evaluation determines the extent to which learners have achieved the objectives and where further learning is indicated (Oermann & Gaberson, 2006). The planning phase of the teaching process includes the development of objectives and the selection of content, teaching methods, and learning experiences.

Some educators prepare detailed objectives such as, "After reading an article on nursing management of patients in heart failure, the staff nurse identifies two nursing interventions with supporting evidence." Other educators prepare more general objectives that specify at minimum who the learners are and what they will know or be able to do at the end of the instruction. Using the previous example, a general objective would be: "The staff nurse identifies two nursing interventions with supporting evidence for care of patients in heart failure." In most teaching situations, a general objective is sufficient.

Objectives should be clear, measurable, and attainable considering the level of the learner and time frame allotted for the instruction. Behaviors such as list, identify, apply, and compare are measurable in contrast to terms such as know and understand. The time frame for teaching also dictates the number of objectives and their complexity.

Taxonomies of Objectives

There are three domains or areas of learning: cognitive, psychomotor, and affective. Objectives may be written in each of these domains and leveled using the taxonomies, which are classification systems for objectives.

Cognitive Domain

Learning in the cognitive domain relates to the acquisition of knowledge and development of intellectual skills such as problem solving. In many teaching situations, the outcome of learning is memorizing facts and specific information; however, at other times, the goals are learning to apply concepts to new situations, analyze complex data about patients, arrive at decisions about patient problems and alternative possibilities that exist, and make decisions about the most appropriate course of action.

The taxonomy of the cognitive domain enables the teacher to organize the learning outcomes in a logical way from memorization to increasingly more complex cognitive skills. There are six levels in the cognitive taxonomy, beginning with recall of specific facts and information, the lowest, and progressing through comprehension, application, analysis, synthesis, and evaluation (Bloom, Englehart, Furst, Hill, & Krathwohl, 1956). A definition and sample objective for each of the six levels of the cognitive taxonomy are found in **Table 19-2.**

Anderson and Krathwohl (2001) updated the taxonomy, rewording the categories as verbs (e.g., remembering instead of knowledge) and reordering synthesis and evaluation. The highest level of learning in the adapted taxonomy is creating—synthesizing elements to form a new or different product.

Psychomotor Domain

Psychomotor learning results in the development of technological skills, ability to perform technical procedures, and other competencies that involve physical coordination. There are two aspects of psychomotor learning. One aspect relates to the knowledge base of the skill, which are the scientific principles and rationale underlying the performance, and the second is the actual technique of carrying out the skill. These two aspects of skill learning should be kept separate in the teaching process, beginning with a discussion of the principles on which the skill is based and then progressing to demonstration and practice of the motor components. It inhibits skill learning when the teacher asks

TABLE 19-2	
Cognitive Taxonomy and Sample Objectives	
Levels of Cognitive Taxonomy	**Sample Objective**
Knowledge: Ability to recall facts and specific information	The patient identifies side effects of medications.
Comprehension: Ability to understand and explain information	The nurse explains the underlying pathophysiology of the patient's condition.
Application: Ability to use knowledge in a new situation and apply concepts and theories to practice	The student plans interventions for critically ill patients that are based on current evidence.
Analysis: Ability to identify relevant parts and their relationships	The manager analyzes the outcomes of the new staffing pattern on patients and nursing staff.
Synthesis: Ability to develop a new product	The nurse designs a protocol for pain management.
Evaluation: Ability to arrive at judgments based on internal and external criteria	The student evaluates research studies on relaxation for use in clinical practice.

a cognitive question related to the principles of the skill, while the learner is trying to develop and refine performance of the procedure itself. When learning to drive a car, the teacher does not ask how the engine works. Similarly, as the patient is learning to draw up the insulin, or student is setting up an intravenous pump, the focus of the teacher should be on guiding those movements, not on the underlying principles of the skills.

Different taxonomies have been developed for the psychomotor domain. One taxonomy useful in nursing education specifies five levels in the development of psychomotor skills. The lowest level is imitation learning, in which the learner observes a demonstration of the skill and imitates that performance. In the second level, the learner is able to perform the skill following written guidelines. By practicing skills the learner refines the ability to perform them without errors (precision) and in a reasonable time frame (articulation) until they become a natural part of care (naturalization; Oermann & Gaberson, 2006). Although objectives can be written using the psychomotor taxonomy, similar to the cognitive domain, in most situations skills are taught using a checklist of the steps of the procedure.

Affective Domain

In some educational situations, the APN assists learners in developing values important in professional practice. Value development in this context builds on an understanding of the values and beliefs that are essential to practice as a professional, such as confidentiality and privacy. From this knowledge base, learners need to then accept these values and beliefs as their own and internalize them as a basis for their own professional practice (Oermann & Gaberson, 2006). In most teaching situations, the APN would not specify values to be taught to patients and other learners in the form of objectives but would be aware of these outcomes when planning the instruction.

DEVELOPMENT OF A TEACHING PLAN

The objectives represent the outcomes of learning based on the APN's assessment and form the basis for the teaching plan. The aim of the teaching plan is to guide learners in achieving the objectives considering other characteristics of the learner also examined during the assessment. The APN plans and organizes content related to the objectives, selects teaching methods, and plans learning activities, all with the intent of assisting the learner in meeting the objectives or outcomes of learning.

In developing the teaching plan, the APN should consider the level of learning to be achieved as a result of the instruction. If the outcome of learning is to recall facts, then the teaching methods could be lecture, discussion, and readings. When the objective is to *use* the knowledge gained from the teaching to decide on the most effective nursing management for a patient (application) or to determine the priority problem (analysis), then the teaching strategies need to extend beyond lecture and discussion. For example, with those outcomes of learning, the APN might develop a short case in which the learner applies the concepts to a hypothetical patient scenario or have a discussion with staff about how to best manage a patient's care considering the current priorities.

Although teaching often occurs without a written plan or by adapting standardized plans, written teaching plans serve five purposes. They: (a) communicate to the learner and others in the agency the intended outcomes of learning, strategies for achieving them, and allotted time; (b) provide an opportunity for learners to review and modify the plan so it is mutually acceptable; (c) guide the teacher in organizing the instruction; (d) serve as written documentation of the educational goals and plan, which is essential when more than one person is participating in the instruction; and (e) document that a teaching plan was developed and implemented (Bastable, 2003).

There are many formats for developing teaching plans, but generally they include at least six components that relate to each another: (a) purpose or goal of the education, (b) objectives or outcomes to be met, (c) outline of the content, (d) teaching methods for presenting the content and guiding learners to meet each objective, (e) time frame for the instruction, and (f) evaluation methods. **Figure 19-1** provides a sample teaching plan developed for a continuing education program; this can be used as a template for the development of teaching plans by the APN.

The content is organized logically from simple to complex, with prerequisite content presented first. The extent of content to include depends on the objectives and the amount of time allotted for the instruction. If there is only a limited time available, the goal is to present the content that is critical to foster achievement of the outcomes. The content is usually listed on the teaching plan in outline format with sufficient detail for other educators to know what to teach and in what order. If only a brief outline is required in the setting, the APN can develop a more detailed one for personal use in delivering the instruction.

The next component of the plan is a list of the teaching methods, the strategies the APN will use to help learners achieve the outcomes and gain the knowledge and skills they need. Methods should be appropriate for the content to be presented and achieving the objectives. The type of learner, patients, students, new graduates, and experienced staff; size of the group; and time frame also influence the selection of teaching methods.

With patient education, discussion, handouts, visuals, and demonstration are effective because they lend themselves to individualized instruction and allow the APN to gear the teaching to the particular needs of the patient. With students and staff, there are many teaching methods from which to choose, but some, such as written assignments, are more appropriate for students rather than staff.

The group size is significant in that some methods are best used for individual instruction and with small groups such as discussion, case studies for analysis, and demonstration, whereas others are useful for larger groups such as lecture and PowerPoint presentations. Along the same line, some strategies are more time consuming to implement. For example, games and simulations provide for experiential learning, foster critical thinking, and actively involve learners, but they often are time consuming to set up and implement (Gaberson & Oermann, 2007). Discussion and small group

Continuing Education Offering: Documentation Form
Title of Offering: Teaching Critical Thinking in the Practice Setting
Purpose: Prepare preceptors and educators to promote critical
thinking abilities of nursing staff

Objectives	Content	Teaching Methods	Time Frame	Evaluation Methods
1. Describe characteristics of critical thinking.	I. What is critical thinking? A. Characteristics of critical thinking B. Need for clinical knowledge base	Lecture PowerPoint Handout	10 min	Questioning group
2. Identify strategies for teaching and assessing critical thinking in the clinical setting.	II. Teaching and assessing critical thinking in the clinical setting A. Strategies 　1. Observation of nurse combined with questions 　2. Discussion (one-to-one, small group); discussion about patients that leads to improved thinking 　3. Conferences	Lecture/ Discussion PowerPoint Handouts	50 min	Questioning group
	4. Critical thinking/problem-solving strategies (case method) for orientation, in-service programs	Small group activity: Develop strategies for teaching critical thinking to nursing staff	30 min	Review of strategies
3. Examine the use of questions for promoting critical thinking in clinical practice.	B. Use of questions for critical thinking 　1. Levels of questions, why important 　2. Sequencing questions to lead to critical thinking	Examples of sequencing questions		
	3. Making your interaction count C. Summary and evaluation	Role-play of interaction between preceptor and new graduate	10 min	Self-evaluation of learning

FIGURE 19-1 Sample teaching plan.

activities add time to the instruction compared with presenting the content in a lecture format, but activities such as these might be critical considering the outcomes to be met and learner needs.

The next component of the teaching plan specifies the time frame for the instruction. As indicated previously, the time allotted for teaching determines the depth and complexity of the content and also influences the selection of teaching strategies. The APN should carefully plan the content to avoid running out of time and not including essential information that the learner needs. It is less of a problem when the instruction is completed early because the APN can review the content, ask questions to ensure learner understanding, use small group activities for critical thinking, and provide additional practice for skills.

The last component of the teaching plan is the evaluation methods used to measure achievement of the objectives. Evaluation may be formative, providing feedback to learners on their progress in meeting the objectives, or summative, measuring achievement of the outcomes of learning. Evaluation methods are described in a later section of this chapter.

Teaching Methods

There are many teaching methods available for use by the APN in educating patients, students, and staff. This section of the chapter presents a number of these strategies. The goal is to choose methods that facilitate achievement of the objectives and are appropriate for the learner.

Lecture

Lecture is a structured means of presenting information to a group. In recent years with the focus on critical thinking, there has been a shift from lecturing, in which students are usually passive participants, to more active learning methods. However, a lecture that synthesizes from multiple sources, is well organized, is delivered with skill, and allows for questions and open discussion is a highly effective method for presenting a large body of content in a short period (Oermann, 2007). Lectures can be efficient in that the teacher can emphasize key points to learn and can draw on different sources of information not available to the learners. For critical thinking and higher level objectives, the teacher can include examples that apply concepts and theories from the lecture to clinical situations and can ask questions about alternative perspectives and different possibilities (Oermann, 2007). By adapting the traditional lecture with minimal learner involvement to an interactive format with questions and discussion, lecture can be used for higher level learning.

A lecture begins with an introduction that presents the objectives to be met, an overview of the content, and why this information is important. The content presented during the lecture should reflect a synthesis from multiple sources of information rather than repeating what could be read in an article or a textbook. The intent of the lecture is to draw from resources not available to learners. Content should be clear and organized logically, beginning with simple concepts and progressing to more complex ones, consistent with the outline in the teaching plan. Questions and examples integrated throughout allow for higher level learning and actively involve the participants. Small group activities within the lecture or at the end serve a similar purpose, as well as encourage collaborative learning. The lecture ends with a summary that reviews the main points, and for students and staff, their relevance to clinical practice.

The use of multimedia in the lecture provides for visualization of the content, allows the teacher to highlight key points as the lecture progresses, and adds variety to the presentation. Some important principles for developing media for presentations are shown in **Box 19-3**. In addition, there are many online tutorials that prepare teachers for developing quality media for their lectures and other

BOX 19-3
Guidelines for Presentations (Lectures, Speeches, and Other Types)

IDENTIFY LEARNERS AND OBJECTIVES

Know your learners and their background.

If presenting to learners about whom you have limited information, review materials that describe the educational program and ask program planners about learners.

Review objectives for presentation.

PLAN PRESENTATION

Plan content to meet objectives considering learners and time allotted.

Do not develop content from one article or textbook; synthesize literature and resources not available to learners.

Develop list of topics and subtopics to be presented or use outline format.

Prepare introduction that includes objectives to be met, an overview of content, and why the information is important.

Do not write out presentations in sentence form to avoid reading to group; use short phrases.

Next to list of topics or outline, include sample questions to ask learners.

Develop clinical scenarios and examples of how content applies to practice; integrate these throughout presentation, use for small group work, or save for end of presentation if presentation is finished early.

Underline or highlight with color key points to make during presentation so they are easy to see in notes.

List key points to include in summary.

DEVELOP MEDIA

Develop media, such as a PowerPoint presentation, that emphasize major points.

Check that each slide presents one idea and begins with clear title.

Use key words and short phrases rather than sentences and keep to a minimum so slide is not too "busy."

Make sure font is large enough, at least 24-point or larger, for everyone to read.

Choose contrasting colors for text and background so text is easy to read.

Avoid changing format, such as adding underlining, **bold**, *italics*; changing font size; or using different fonts on same slide.

Combine uppercase and lowercase letters instead of all uppercase.

Avoid varying transitions between slides so to avoid distracting learner from content.

Mark on list of topics or outline when to change slides or introduce new media.

DELIVER PRESENTATION

Practice in front of mirror or be videotaped to assess style and gauge time.

Open with interesting anecdote, question, photo, humor, or another statement to get learner's attention.

During presentation, repeat and emphasize important points.

Include transitions between different content areas.

Continued

> **BOX 19-3**
> **Guidelines for Presentations (Lectures, Speeches, and Other Types)—cont'd**
>
> Be enthusiastic.
> Speak clearly, loud enough for everyone to hear, and at appropriate speed.
> Scan learners as you speak to gauge their attentiveness.
> Never tell learners you "ran out of time"; if you finish early, move to your clinical
>   scenarios and extra learning activities, then summarize the content.

types of presentations. Other guidelines for presenting an effective lecture or speech are also found in Box 19-3. Inexperienced teachers should practice their lectures in front of a mirror or have them videotaped for self-assessment or critique by a colleague.

Discussion

Discussion is an exchange of ideas between teacher and learner to meet an educational goal (Gaberson & Oermann, 2007). Although the teacher often plans the topic, the intent of the discussion is for learners to express their views, not to provide a forum for teachers to express their own views. Both teacher and learner should actively participate.

Discussions are particularly valuable for affective objectives because they allow students and staff to express their feelings and beliefs about a situation, examine values that influence patient care and their interactions with others, and explore ethical issues. Discussions also are effective for critical thinking because the teacher can ask the "right" questions—open-ended questions that ask learners to think beyond the obvious, consider alternative perspectives, and examine different decisions possible in a situation (Alfaro-LeFevre, 2004; Oermann & Gaberson, 2006; Oermann, Truesdell, & Ziolkowski, 2000). The cognitive taxonomy described previously in the chapter is a valuable tool to guide the level of questions asked in a discussion. The APN can begin with recall questions that assess the knowledge of facts and can then progress toward higher level questions. **Table 19-3** illustrates questions at each level of the taxonomy.

A discussion can occur on a one-to-one basis with a learner or in a small group. Gaberson and Oermann (2007) recommended limiting small group discussions to 10 people to provide an opportunity for everyone to talk. Learners need to know that their views and opinions in a discussion are accepted even if different from the teacher's. Some guidelines for conducting an effective discussion follow.

- Focus the discussion on the objectives to be met.
- Encourage the participation of each learner but do not force a learner to participate.
- Actively participate as a means of guiding the discussion toward the outcomes but do not dominate the discussion.
- Ask open-ended questions that cannot be answered with a "yes-no" response.
- Sequence questions from low to high level; the taxonomy is useful for this purpose.
- Do not accept the first answer to a question, even if correct; explore other possibilities and ask for a rationale.
- Prevent side-tracking of ideas and help learners return to the topic.
- Summarize what was learned and how it relates to the objectives set for the discussion (Gaberson & Oermann, 2007).

TABLE 19-3	
Levels of Questions for Discussion	
Level	**Sample Questions**
Knowledge: Questions that ask for recall of facts and specific information	What is this type of breath sound called? Define peak expiratory flow rate.
Comprehension: Questions that explore understanding of content	What is the difference between emphysema and chronic bronchitis? Give an example of a short acting bronchodilator.
Application: Questions that examine ability of learners to relate content to new or different situation	How do your patient's symptoms compare with what you read about chronic obstructive pulmonary disease or chronic obstructive pulmonary disease? Why is it important to monitor these symptoms?
Analysis: Questions about analyzing data and relationships	What data support your diagnosis, and why are these data relevant? What are alternative interventions that might work in this situation and why?
Synthesis: Questions that ask for development of new ideas and plans	How would you modify this teaching plan to better meet your patient's needs? Tell me about two new interventions that would be effective in your patient's care, their evidence base, and how you would decide whether to use them.
Evaluation: Higher level questions that ask for judgments, critical thinking	Are your interventions effective, and how can you determine that? Your patient is still coughing. What changes can be made in the plan of care, and why would these be appropriate?

Clinical Conference

Clinical conferences are specific types of discussions held with students and staff in the clinical setting. They can precede the clinical experience to ensure that learners have the prerequisite knowledge and skills to provide patient care and engage in other learning activities planned by the teacher. Often the APN can use these conferences to explain patient problems, interventions, and underlying rationales to learners if they lack the knowledge base to care for those particular patients.

Conferences held after the clinical experiences provide an opportunity to review patient care; discuss patient problems, interventions, and other possible approaches; apply theory to clinical practice; and explore issues in clinical practice. Conferences also provide a forum for learners to express feelings about patients and experiences in clinical practice and to develop support systems (Stokes & Kost, 2005). In clinical conferences, similar to other types of discussions with staff and students, the APN should ask open-ended and probing questions that encourage learners to think about alternative ways of addressing clinical problems. The need for these questions and examples of them were described previously. The APN should be creative in planning conferences to provide variety and maintain learner interest, particularly at the end of a tiring clinical day.

Depending on the objectives, clinical conferences also may involve other disciplines. In these conferences learners participate with other health-care providers in analyzing patient needs, planning care, and developing protocols and proposals that extend beyond a single profession. Interdisciplinary conferences are good learning experiences for nursing students and beginning staff because they demonstrate how different health professionals work together to solve patient and system problems. This is critical in today's health-care system with the emphasis on teamwork for patient safety (Baker, Gustafson, Beaubien, Salas, & Barach, 2005).

Clinical Case

Clinical cases are actual or simulated scenarios for analysis. This method is effective for learning how to apply theory to practice and gaining skill in analyzing data, identifying problems, and deciding on possible solutions (Gaberson & Oermann, 2007). The value of cases for analysis is that they provide experience for learners in thinking through clinical decisions before they are faced with those decisions in actual practice.

With this strategy, the APN develops a case followed by questions about it. The cases should be short, a few sentences to a paragraph, and present only essential information. Questions can be directed toward assessment, focusing on missing data in the case, and what additional information is needed for decision making. They also can be geared to identifying problems in the case, interventions for immediate action and for planning care, alternative decisions and consequences, and how concepts and theories can be used as a framework for understanding the case and answering the questions.

The questions focus on the objectives to be met by analyzing the case. For example, if the outcome is to select appropriate nursing management for a patient with diabetes, the questions would ask learners about possible interventions and how they would manage the patient's care. In analyzing a case, learners should describe the thought process they used and the rationale for their answers (Gaberson & Oermann, 2007). Because these cases are short, they can be integrated easily within a lecture, can be used at the end of the class as small group work, and can be used in clinical conferences. Examples are provided in **Box 19-4.**

Case Study

A case study provides an in-depth description of a patient, family, or community, including background information. Case studies can be developed around actual or simulated clinical situations, similar to shorter cases. With case studies learners can identify significant data, from nonsignificant information in the case, and can explore the effect of the patient's background on current problems and situation. A sample case study is presented in Box 19-4.

Unfolding Cases

Cases can be developed to represent a simulated clinical situation that changes over time, similar to patients whose conditions change. These are often called unfolding cases (Ulrich & Glendon, 2002). A simulated or hypothetical case is presented first, followed by questions for learners. After they analyze the case, the teacher presents more information that modifies the clinical scenario, for example, by adding data or changing the patient's health status. Learners critique the new scenario and again answer questions about it. The teacher can continue to add data to the case to demonstrate changes in the patient's condition and related nursing care.

Grand Rounds

One other teaching method that also revolves around analysis of a case is grand rounds. In grand rounds the teacher presents an update on a clinical topic or care of a patient with a particular diagnosis or treatment. Observation and assessment of the patient, typical patient problems encountered, interventions, and evaluation of outcomes are often described. In some settings the grand rounds presentations are videotaped and available on the Web for nurses to view at a time and place convenient

BOX 19-4
Examples of Clinical Case and Case Study

CLINICAL CASE

Mrs. B, 46-year-old, is brought to the clinic by her husband with complaints of weakness of the left arm and difficulty "getting her thoughts." The husband tells you that his wife was treated a few months ago for a cerebral aneurysm but has been fine since then. Mrs. B's blood pressure is 210/90. She slowly answers your questions with long pauses in between sentences.

1. What information would you collect from the husband as a priority? Provide a rationale why this information is critical to deciding on the diagnosis and actions to take.

2. What are possible problems that Mrs. B might be encountering? Describe why each of these is a possibility.

You are working in home health care and have a new patient with edema of both legs and extreme fatigue. The patient has no family in the area.

1. What additional data would you collect in your first home visit?

2. Summarize the information you might obtain in the home visit and identify a priority problem. What resources are needed for this patient's care?

You believe your patient may be experiencing side effects from her medication, but your preceptor does not agree and tells you to give the medication to the patient.

1. What are two possible approaches you could take in this situation?

2. What are the advantages and disadvantages of those options?

3. What would you do? Why?

Your patient, who is increasingly restless, pulls out her endotracheal tube. What should you do first?

You are working in the emergency department when a young man is admitted following a motor vehicle accident. His larynx appears to be fractured, and there are many facial cuts and bruises. You suction him only to find large amounts of blood; you determine that the only way to keep the airway clear is by suctioning.

1. What are your options for managing his airway?

2. What observations would you make, and what other data would you collect that might affect your decision about how to manage his airway?

3. How would you manage this patient's airway? Provide a rationale.

CASE STUDY

Sally is a 6-year-old who has been complaining of pain in her abdomen off and on for the last week. Two weeks ago, she was seen by the pediatrician for a respiratory flu. Sally's current symptoms are two episodes of vomiting this morning, abdominal cramps, no appetite, and a rash on her back. Vital signs, blood pressure, height, and weight are normal. Sally is holding her abdomen and tells you it hurts. When you palpate her abdomen, you find diffuse tenderness without any rebound. There are no masses that you can detect. Sally's past medical history is unremarkable. She has never had any serious illnesses and has never been hospitalized. Her mother tells you that there are no changes in the family or home situation; they recently returned from a camping trip that Sally enjoyed.

1. What laboratory tests would you expect to be ordered? Explain each test and its relationship to this case.

2. What is the significance of "diffuse tenderness without any rebound"?

3. Name all possible problems Sally might have and why.

4. If Sally asks you what's wrong, how would you respond? Provide a rationale based on her age and development.

for them. For example, at Cincinnati Children's Hospital Medical Center (2008), nursing grand rounds are available on the Web via streaming media. Some of the programs are offered for continuing education contact hours. Nursing grand rounds also can be conducted in the clinical setting with observation of the patient and discussion about care.

Multimedia

Multimedia provide for multisensory learning. Depending on the type of media, they teach by using different sensory modes. In many teaching situations, it is easier to learn when more senses are involved in communicating the message. Learners can see a patient in a video clip or watch a DVD rather than imagining what the patient looks like or how the intervention should be implemented from the verbal description by the teacher or from their readings. Multimedia are useful for demonstrating procedures and technological skills, from gathering the equipment through each step to follow. As learners practice their skills, they can replay the media when questions arise or they are unsure about their performance.

Multimedia also are valuable for affective objectives. A short segment from a DVD or a CD-ROM, for example, can be used to present clinical situations for learners to examine their values and beliefs and consider how they would respond in those situations. Scenarios can be used to present ethical dilemmas for individuals and groups of students and staff to analyze; small group activities accompanying the media can teach valuable lessons in analyzing and resolving ethical issues.

The growth of the Internet and related technological innovations has resulted in new strategies for educating patients, students, and staff. It is beyond the scope of this chapter to examine the multiple types of technology available for teaching in nursing, but the APN should keep current with the development of these technologies and their use in nursing education.

Selecting Media for Teaching

Considering the variety of multimedia available for teaching, the APN first needs to evaluate the quality of any multimedia program or Web-based method under consideration. Not every teaching situation needs the addition of multimedia. The goal is to use media when they clarify the content better than an explanation alone such as by depicting a patient with the condition being discussed or demonstrating a procedure. Multimedia should not be used only for the sake of incorporating technology into teaching; instead they should be selected based on the outcomes to be achieved and individual learner needs. In addition to evaluating the quality of the multimedia as a basis for their selection, the second area of concern is their appropriateness for the intended learners.

Questions the APN can use to guide this evaluation are the following:

1. Is the content presented in the multimedia accurate?
2. Is the content up to date?
3. Is the content organized effectively and presented clearly?
4. Are procedures and techniques illustrated consistent with current practice in the setting, or can they be adapted easily?
5. Are the multimedia of high technical quality (e.g., graphics, sound, interaction with learner, feedback mechanism, and so on)?
6. Are the multimedia appropriate for the outcomes to be met, and will they meet the learner's needs?
7. Are the multimedia appropriate for the learning situation (e.g., patient versus student education, setting for the education, time frame, etc.)?

Readability

One additional consideration in evaluating print materials and Web sites for use in patient education is their readability. The reading level of patient education materials should be *less than the sixth grade level* (Badarudeen & Sabharwal, 2008); however, most educational materials for patients are written above this level. This discrepancy inhibits many patients from understanding the information in written materials, including important documents such as consent forms, medication package inserts, educational pamphlets, handouts, and discharge instructions, among others.

Early research on readability focused on print materials, but patients accessing health information on the Internet also need to understand what they are reading on the Web. Studies have examined the readability of Web sites for patients, revealing that much of the health information on the Web is at too high a reading level for many consumers (Badarudeen & Sabharwal, 2008; Dornan & Oermann, 2006; Eysenbach, Powell, Kuss, & Sa, 2002; Oermann, Gerich, Ostosh, & Zaleski, 2003; Oermann, Lowrey, & Thornley, 2003; Oermann, & McInerney, 2007).

There are different readability formulas for assessing patient education materials. These include the Flesch formula for use with materials between the fifth grade and college level, the Fog Index that is easy to use and can be applied to a short sample of words from fourth grade through college level materials, the Fry formula for use with a wide range of materials from the first grade through college, and the SMOG formula (Bastable, 2003). One easy way of estimating readability is by using the spelling and grammar function in Microsoft Word.

The APN has an important role in assessing the readability of patient education materials, discharge instructions, and documents given to patients. Before recommending health Web sites to patients, the quality of those sites including readability should be first evaluated. When teaching patients and families who lack the ability to read and understand the information, the APN should focus on key concepts to be learned, use easy-to-understand words, and use varied teaching strategies that rely on visuals. Murphy-Knoll (2007) recommended always speaking in "simple and non medical terms" and asking patients and families to repeat back the information in their own words (p. 207).

Self-Directed Instructional Methods

Self-directed instructional methods are completed by learners on their own to meet remedial needs, acquire prerequisite knowledge and skills, and fulfill personal interests. These methods include modules, independent study, and multimedia programs that learners complete independently; many of these are now available online. Self-directed methods are well suited for learners who are motivated, committed, and independent because they can be completed at a time and in a setting of the learner's choice. A major advantage from an educational point of view is the ability of learners to progress through the instruction at their own rates of learning. This affords learners the opportunity to repeat the instruction when unsure or until competent and to omit content areas already mastered.

Although self-directed methods may be planned for all students, the advantages they offer in terms of individualizing the instruction make them a better resource for meeting remedial needs and gaining prerequisite knowledge and skills. That way, learners who have already met the objectives and can demonstrate the competencies can progress to new areas of learning. Self-directed learning places the responsibility for achieving the competencies on the learner rather than the teacher. The teacher, however, might establish time frames for completion for certain activities and monitor learner progress by asking for a self-assessment or by periodic quizzing.

Demonstration

Demonstration is the presentation of how to perform a procedure or skill with the intent for learners to model that performance and implement the skill on their own. Before demonstrating the procedure, the APN should explain its purpose, equipment to gather, and steps to follow. Any explanation of the principles underlying the skill and discussion about its use in clinical practice should occur at this point in the instruction. As learners practice, explanations by the APN should focus on the performance itself, not on the cognitive base of the skill. Because psychomotor learning is egocentric, learners need to focus on manipulating the equipment and refining their performance (Gaberson & Oermann, 2007).

All learners must be able to see each step to be performed and hear any explanations. By observing the demonstration, learners develop an image of what the skill looks like and how to perform it, which then guides their practice of the skill. The return demonstration is when the learner performs the skill with cues from the APN as needed (Bastable, 2003). Cues are prompts given by the teacher to guide performance but without telling the learner the exact steps to follow. Once competent, learners can practice skills on their own; practice helps refine performance so the procedure can be implemented in a reasonable time frame. With human patient simulators, students and nurses can practice and develop competency in the skill before performing it in the clinical setting.

Simulations

Simulations provide experiences with patient care and in making decisions outside of the actual clinical setting. Learners have an opportunity to practice and develop their skills in a safe environment. Human patient simulators offer a high degree of realism for learners; with simulators learners can practice their technological skills, make decisions and view the outcomes of those decisions, and develop their critical thinking abilities before caring for a real patient. With procedures that require costly equipment and supplies, learners need an opportunity to practice those procedures in a controlled environment before trying them with patients in the clinical setting. Jeffries (2006) indicated that simulations are useful as a competency check for new graduates and individuals being oriented to the clinical setting.

With simulations, learners should have an opportunity to review and reflect on their experiences and decisions; this occurs in the debriefing session after the simulation. In the debriefing, the discussion also may include how their personal values influenced their decisions. In developing values, learners need to experience situations to determine how they will respond to them; simulations provide this type of experience and help learners develop a sensitivity to how others may feel in a situation.

Evaluation of Learning

Evaluation is an integral part of any teaching situation and serves different roles. In working with patients, students, and staff, individually and in small groups, the APN continually assesses how well learners are acquiring an understanding of the content and developing ability to perform skills. Using this information, the APN modifies the teaching, perhaps explaining the content again and in a different way, adding media, suggesting remedial instruction, and allowing the individual more practice time for skills. This type of evaluation is diagnostic; it represents feedback to the learner about progress in meeting the objectives and provides the basis for developing a plan for improvement (Oermann & Gaberson, 2006). This is referred to as formative evaluation.

A second type of evaluation is summative. As the name suggests, this type of evaluation summarizes what has been learned rather than providing feedback to learners. Examples of summative evaluation are final examinations in a course and annual performance evaluations.

With both formative and summative evaluation, the objectives to be met serve as the framework for evaluation. The evaluation determines the progress of learners in meeting those objectives or for summative evaluation if they have achieved them. For many diagnoses and procedures, standard teaching plans are available for patient education that specify the objectives of the instruction; evaluation then measures the extent to which these were met.

There are many methods for evaluating learning. The APN selects methods that provide information on the outcomes to be assessed and are appropriate for the learner. Evaluation methods include the following:

- Questioning: Questions are asked to assess the extent of learning.
- Observation of performance: Learners are observed while performing procedures, providing care, and carrying out interventions in clinical practice. Often a summary of the observations is recorded in a narrative note or on a checklist of performance.
- Rating scale: Performance of competencies is rated on a scale.
- Checklist: Steps in a procedure or skill are checked off as the learner performs them.
- Test: The learner is asked to answer a set of written questions about the content.
- Written assignment: Students complete papers of varying length.

ROLE OF ADVANCED PRACTICE NURSE AS EDUCATOR

Providing education to patients, students, and staff is an integral part of the APN role. The APN has a critical role in teaching patients about their illness and preventing further complications, treatments and medications, how to provide self-care, and the importance of follow-up care. In many settings it is up to the APN to prepare the patient for discharge and managing own care at home.

Teaching about the illness and self-care is only one of the areas of education provided by the APN. The APN also teaches patients and families about preventing illness and staying healthy. Without education by the APN, few patients would be informed about their health and how to maintain it. APNs are well suited to provide health-related patient education because they understand interventions for both health and illness.

In some settings, the APN also may be involved in teaching graduate and undergraduate nursing students. The APN may serve as a preceptor for students or guide student learning for individual clinical experiences. Because of their extensive clinical knowledge and skills, APNs may participate in classroom teaching and give lectures and speeches in their area of expertise.

Another component of the APN role is to educate nursing staff and health providers. This education may be informal, teaching in the clinical setting as the need arises, and through formal continuing education programs. As APNs become known for their particular areas of expertise, they are often asked to organize and present continuing education programs.

CONCLUSION

The APN has an important role in educating patients, students, and staff. The teaching process described in this chapter, assessing learner needs, planning instruction, selecting varied teaching methods, and evaluating learning, provides a framework for teaching any of these groups of learners. Nurses in advanced practice are well prepared for their role as educator with their extensive knowledge base, expert clinical skills, and strong communication skills. The knowledge and expertise of the APN combined with an understanding of the educational process prepare the APN to meet the learning needs of patients, families, students, and staff regardless of the setting in which the APN chooses to practice.

References

Alfaro-LeFevre, R. (2004). *Critical thinking and clinical judgment* (3rd ed.). St. Louis: Saunders.

Anderson, L. W., & Krathwohl, D. R. (Eds.). (2001). *A taxonomy for learning, teaching, and assessing: A revision of Boom's taxonomy of educational objectives.* New York: Longman.

Badarudeen, S., & Sabharwal, S. (2008). Readability of patient education materials from the American Academy of Orthopaedic Surgeons and Pediatric Orthopaedic Society of North America web sites. *The Journal of Bone and Joint Surgery. American Volume, 90*(1), 199–204.

Baker, D. P., Gustafson, S., Beaubien, J., Salas, E., & Barach, P. (2005). *Medical Teamwork and Patient Safety: The Evidence-based Relation* [Literature Review] (AHRQ Publication No. 05-0053, April 2005). Rockville, MD: Agency for Healthcare Research and Quality.

Bastable, S. B. (2003). *Nurse as educator: Principles of teaching and learning for nursing practice* (2nd ed.). Sudbury, MA: Jones and Bartlett.

Beecroft, P. C., Santner, S., Lacy, M. L., Kunzman, L., & Dorey, F. (2006). New graduate nurses' perceptions of mentoring: Six-year programme evaluation. *Journal of Advanced Nursing, 55*(6), 736–747.

Beitz, J. M., & Wieland, D. (2005). Analyzing the teaching effectiveness of clinical nursing faculty of full- and part-time generic BSN, LPN-BSN, and RN-BSN nursing students. *Journal of Professional Nursing, 21*(1), 32–45.

Berg, C. L., & Lindseth, G. (2004). Students' perspectives of effective and ineffective nursing instructors. *Journal of Nursing Education, 43*(12), 565–568.

Bloom, B. S., Englehart, M. D., Furst, E. J., Hill, W. H., & Krathwohl, D. R. (1956). *Taxonomy of educational objectives: The classification of educational goals. Handbook I: Cognitive domain.* White Plains, NY: Longman.

Chang, M., & Kelly, A. E. (2007). Patient education: Addressing cultural diversity and health literacy issues. *Urologic Nursing, 27*(5), 411–417.

Cincinnati Children's Hospital Medical Center. (2008). *Nursing grand rounds.* Retrieved February 14, 2008, from the Cincinnati Children's Hospital Medical Center Web site: www.cincinnatichildrens.org/ed/cme/streaming-media/library/nursing/.

Dornan, B. A., & Oermann, M. H. (2006). Evaluation of breastfeeding Web sites for patient education. *MCN: Maternal and Child Nursing, 31*(1), 18–23.

Eysenbach, G., Powell, J., Kuss, O., & Sa, E. (2002). Empirical studies assessing the quality of health information for consumers on the World Wide Web: A systematic review. *Journal of American Medical Association, 287*(20), 2691–2700.

Gaberson, K., & Oermann, M. H. (2007). *Clinical teaching strategies in nursing* (2nd ed.). New York: Springer.

Gignac-Caille, A. M., & Oermann, M. H. (2001). Student and faculty perceptions of effective clinical instructors in ADN programs. *Journal of Nursing Education, 40*(8), 347–353.

Jeffries, P. R. (2006). Designing simulations for nursing education. In M. H. Oermann & K. T. Heinrich (Eds.), *Annual review of nursing education* (Vol. 4, pp. 161–177). New York: Springer.

Murphy-Knoll, L. (2007). Low health literacy puts patients at risk. *Journal of Nursing Care Quality, 22*(3), 205–209.

Niederhauser, V. P., & Kohr, L. (2005). Research endeavors among pediatric nurse practitioners (REAP) study. *Journal of Pediatric Health Care, 19*(2), 80–89.

Oermann, M. H. (2007). Lectures for active learning in nursing education. In L. E. Young & B. Paterson (Eds.), *Teaching nursing: Developing a student centered environment* (pp. 279–294). Philadelphia: Lippincott Williams & Wilkins.

Oermann, M. H., Blair, D., Kowalewski, K., Wilmes, N., & Nordstrom, C. (2007). Citation analysis of the maternal/child nursing literature. *Pediatric Nursing, 33*(5), 387–391.

Oermann, M. H., & Gaberson, K. (2006). *Evaluation and testing in nursing education* (2nd ed.). New York: Springer Publishing

Oermann, M. H., & Garvin, M. F. (2002). Stresses and challenges of new graduates in hospitals. *Nurse Education Today, 22*(3), 1–6.

Oermann, M. H., Gerich, J., Ostosh, L., & Zaleski, S. (2003). Evaluation of asthma websites for patient and parent education. *Journal of Pediatric Nursing, 18*(6), 389–396.

Oermann, M. H., Lowrey, N. F., & Thornley, J. (2003). Evaluation of Web sites on management of pain in children. *Pain Management Nursing, 4*(3), 99–105.

Oermann, M. H., & Lukomski, A. P. (2001). Experiences of students in pediatric nursing clinical courses. *Journal of the Society of Pediatric Nurses, 6*(2), 65–72.

Oermann, M. H., & McInerney, S. M. (2007). An evaluation of sepsis Web sites for patient and family education. *Plastic Surgical Nursing, 27*(4), 192–196.

Oermann, M. H., Truesdell, S., & Ziolkowski, L. (2000). Strategy to assess, develop, and evaluate critical thinking. *Journal of Continuing Education in Nursing, 31*(4), 155–160.

Shipton, S. P. (2002). The process of seeking stress-care: Coping as experienced by senior baccalaureate nursing students in response to appraised clinical stress. *Journal of Nursing Education, 41*(6), 243–256.

Stokes, L., & Kost, G. (2005). Teaching in the clinical setting. In D. M. Billings, & J. A. Halstead (Eds.), *Teaching in nursing: A guide for faculty* (2nd ed., pp. 325–346). St. Louis: Saunders.

Tang, F., Chou, S., & Chiang, H. (2005). Students' perceptions of effective and ineffective clinical instructors. *Journal of Nursing Education, 44*(4), 187–192.

Ulrich, D., & Glendon, K. (2002). Managers forum: Unfolding case study instruction. *Journal of Emergency Nursing, 28*(2), 246–247.

20 Culture as a Variable in Practice

Mary Masterson Germain

This chapter is an invitation to step into other worlds—worlds where experiences may be quite different from your own. You will be asked to reflect on the beliefs and values that make you who you are and to examine how they affect you as a healer and caregiver. Through your direct and indirect roles as an advanced practice nurse (APN), you play a pivotal role in shaping the quality of care that patients receive. In the service of others, you are privileged to share in some of your patient's most profound and intimate experiences. To fully enter into the patient's experience and to provide comprehensive care that is respectful of the patient's cultural beliefs and practices, nurses need to find ways to bridge the linguistic and cultural challenges that are inherent in caring for increasingly diverse populations. It is uncomfortable to stretch our ethnocentric boundaries; it is much easier to care for replicas of ourselves. However, if you are open to learning from your patients, the transient discomfort that you experience from having your time-honored interventions and teaching strategies tested and found wanting by patients with different cultural perspectives, will be rewarded by gaining rich insights into cultural beliefs and practices that will inform your practice for years to come. With that said, let us begin the journey.

SCOPE OF THE NEED

The challenge for APNs is to operationalize care in populations and practice settings that are increasingly diverse. **Table 20-1** shows comparative U.S. resident population data by racial and ethnic grouping for 2000 and 2006.

In 2000, the U.S. Department of Health and Human Services (USDHHS) published Healthy People 2010. The document established two overarching goals for improving the health of U.S. residents and communities in the first decade of the 21st century:

Goal 1: Increase quality and years of healthy life
Goal 2: Eliminate health disparities

These two goals, representing 28 focus areas and 467 measurable objectives, have a single, overarching purpose of promoting health and preventing illness, disability, and premature death, and a unifying vision: healthy people living in healthy communities. (USDHHS, 2000a). Note that goal 2 does not say *reduce*. It says *eliminate*; a lofty goal. It is also critical to note that ethnicity and the social determinants of health care are inextricably linked in the discussion of the disparities in health status and access and use of health-care services presented in Healthy People 2010. This chapter will approach cultural competence in advanced practice nursing from a similar frame of reference.

The Agency for Healthcare Research and Quality (AHRQ), in collaboration with the USDHHS Interagency Work Group, produces an annual National HealthCare Disparities Report (NHDR) on

TABLE 20-1

Comparative U.S. Resident Population Data by Racial and Ethnic Grouping, 2000 and 2006

Race	Number in 2000[a]	Percent of Total Population (%)	Estimated Number in 2006[b]	Estimated Percent of Total Population (%)
Total population	281,421,906	—	299,398,485	—
Number of race responses	274,595,678	—	—	—
White	211,460,626	75.1	221,331,507	73.9
Black or African American	34,658,190	12.3	37,051,483	12.4
American Indian and Alaska Native	2,475,956	0.9	2,369,431	0.8
Asian	10,242,998	3.6	13,100,095	4.4
Native Hawaiian and other Pacific Islander	398,835	0.1	426,194	0.1
Some other race alone	15,359,073	5.5	19,007,129	6.3

[a]U.S. Census Bureau. (2000). Census. PHC-T-1: Table 3. *Population by race alone, race in combination only, race alone or in combination, and Hispanic or Latino origin, for the United States: 2000*. Retrieved March 10, 2008, from U.S. Census Bureau Web site: www.census2000/phc-t1/tab04.pdf.

[b]U.S. Census Bureau. (2006a). *American Community Survey. B02001: Race—universe: total population*. Data Set: 2006 American Community Survey. Retrieved March 10, 2008, from U.S. Census Bureau Web site: www.factfinder.census.gov.

behalf of the USDHHS. The 2007 NHDR is the fifth report issued by the agency. It indicates that the number of persons living in the United States who are foreign born rose from 20 million in 1990 to 33.3 million in 2003. Approximately 70% of persons of Asian descent and 40% of persons of Hispanic descent are foreign born, in contrast to only 6% of whites and blacks (AHRQ, 2007b, p.174).

Because these data represent nationwide statistics, they do not capture the complexity of delivering culturally competent care, especially in urban settings that traditionally house large immigrant populations. The data on racial origin reported by the Bureau of the Census are associated with significant differences in health status and disease, condition-specific morbidity and mortality, and socioeconomic status:

■ The infant mortality rate (2004) for non-Hispanic black women in 2004 was 13.60 per 1000 live births, which is more than two times greater than that of white, non-Hispanic women, which was 5.66 per 1000 live births (Mathews & MacDorman, 2007, p. 5). In addition, analysis of causal factors related to infant deaths between 1999 and 2004 revealed that 41% of deaths of infants to Puerto Rican mothers and 46% of deaths to infants of non-Hispanic, black women were associated with preterm causes (Mathews & MacDorman, 2007, p.11; MacDorman, Callaghan, Mathews, Hoyert, & Kochanek, 2007).

■ The death rate for blacks from diabetes per 100,000 in 2005 was more than twice that for whites: 47 compared to 22.5 (Henry J. Kaiser Family Foundation, 2005). In addition, analysis of data from the SEARCH for Diabetes in Youth study revealed the prevalence of at least two cardiovascular risk factors in 21% of the study population. The racial/ethnic disparities in prevalence were pronounced: 16% in non-Hispanic whites, 35% in Hispanics, 32% in African Americans, 37% in Asian-Pacific Islanders, and 68% in American Indians (Rodriguez et al., 2006).

Clearly racial origin alone does not account for these disparities in health outcomes. Health status is influenced by a multiplicity of factors, as reflected in **Figure 20-1.**

Key determinants associated with poor health status and outcomes also tend to reflect racial origin, ethnicity, and household composition. In 2005, 25% of blacks, 22% of Hispanics, 11% of Asians, and 8% of whites were poor (AHRQ, 2007b, p. 181). Regarding household composition, 9.8% of families with children under 18 years reported living below the poverty level. Of this group, 4.7% of married-couple households reported living below the poverty level, which is in stark contrast to the 28.6% of poor households headed by women with no husband present. Poverty in female-headed households with children ranged from a low of 21.8% for White households to 38.6% for Hispanic or Latino origin, 36.1% black or African American, and 41.8% for American Indian and Alaska Native (U.S. Census Bureau, 2006e)

There is also a direct relationship between education and income. Data from the 2006 American Community Survey (U.S. Census Bureau, 2006d) demonstrates the dramatic association between educational attainment and economic well-being:

- In the population 25 years and older, 6.3% have less than a ninth grade education and another 9.1% have some high school, but have not earned a high school diploma. 30.3% are high school graduates, and the remainder of the respondents have at least some college level study (U.S. Census Bureau, 2006d).

- Only 3.1% of respondents age 25 or older reporting graduate or professional degrees were living in poverty, compared to 23.7% of those surveyed who reported less than a high school education (U.S. Census Bureau, 2006d). *Note:* in 2005, the federal poverty threshold for a family of two adults and two children was $19,806 (AHRQ, 2007b, p. 181).

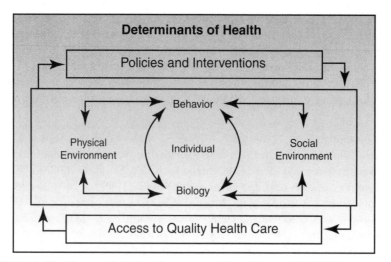

FIGURE 20-1 Healthy people in healthy communities. *(Source: USDHHS, 2000a, p. 18.)*

Education may also play a part in the survival of children. The health status and survival of children of undereducated women differs significantly from that of their better-educated peers. In 2004, 92.7% of whites, 90.2% of Asian-Pacific Islanders, and 93.5% of non-Hispanic whites who were college-educated accessed prenatal care during the first trimester (AHRQ, 2007b, p. 191). In comparison, only 73.% of women with less than a high school education and 82.4% of high school graduates met this goal in 2004 (AHRQ, 2007b, p. 190). One goal set by Healthy People 2010 was to have a minimum of 90% of pregnant women accessing prenatal care during the first trimester.

Another goal set by Healthy People 2010 was for 100% of Americans to have health insurance. In 2005, the proportion of persons with insurance was almost one-third lower for people with less than a high school education than for people with some college: 59.9% versus 89.3% (AHRQ, 2007b, p. 115). Hispanics of every income, and education level were significantly less likely to have health insurance than were their non-Hispanic peers (AHRQ, 2007b, p. 117). Based on these findings, education equals more income, which relates to health-care access.

The 2007 NHDR measures the progress being made in reducing disparities in access to, and quality of, health care for priority populations in the United States. The priority populations include ethnic and racial minorities, women, children, the elderly, low-income groups, persons with disabilities or special needs, and persons living in rural areas. The report addresses four components related to health care: quality, stages of care, and barriers and facilitators to access, and effective use of care. The three key themes identified by the 2007 NHDR (p. 1) are:

- Overall, disparities in health-care quality and access are not getting smaller.
- Progress is being made, but many of the biggest gaps in quality and access have not been reduced.
- The problem of persistent uninsurance is a major barrier to reducing disparities.

Some of the data that led to the NHDR's conclusions are given in **Box 20-1.** It is clear that there is no simplistic solution to the issue of disparities in health care. The causal factors are multiple and interactive. What is clear is that issues of access and quality will become even more pronounced as the health-care needs of an ever growing elderly population compete for already limited resources. Designing and funding a system of care that will ensure equitable access to high-quality health-care services for all is a challenge that APNs must play a pivotal role in solving.

As is evident from the 2007 NHDR, the goals and objectives espoused in Healthy People 2010 continue to present APNs with an unparalleled opportunity to lead, to practice, to develop high-quality, cost-effective health-care delivery systems that empower patients and promote self-care, and to conduct seminal research documenting the positive health outcomes associated with advanced practice nursing interventions. This demands a passionate commitment to professional activism, basic human rights, and a vision of quality health care for all peoples in the United States. The visionaries among you who accept the leadership challenge will be revered by those vulnerable populations for whom you advocate and reviled by those whose actions are determined by political expediency, maintenance of professional turf, and monetary gain. Never before has the choice been so clear. We can lead, follow, or get out of the way. Which path will you choose? As Robert Frost, the renowned Pulitzer Prize winning poet, wrote, "I took the road less traveled by, and that has made all the difference" (Frost, 1961, p. 84).

APNs frequently face a dual challenge: to provide high-quality, evidence-based care to culturally diverse populations and to do so in communities that are often socially and economically disadvantaged. Our profession's response to this challenge is found in the American Nurses Association's (ANA) *Code of Ethics for Nurses*, particularly Provision 1:

BOX 20-1
2007 National Health Disparities Report Data

■ Poverty is related to race and ethnicity. In 2005, 25% of blacks, 22% of Hispanics, 11% of Asians, and 8% of whites were poor. In functional terms, two of the results of these economic differences are that a significantly greater percentage of poor persons have no health insurance compared to high-income persons (69.4% versus 93.7%), and they are 50% less likely to have a consistent, primary care provider and (AHRQ, 2007b, pp. 115, 182).

■ Educational level is a major determinant of insurance status. In 2005, the percentage of persons with some college education and persons with less than a high school education reporting insurance coverage were 89.3% and 59.9%, respectively (AHRQ, 2007b, p. 115).

■ In 2005, children totaled 73.5 million people, 24.8% of the population. Almost 40% of these children came from racial and ethnic minority groups, and 17.6% lived in families whose incomes were below the federal poverty level (AHRQ, 2007b, p. 196).

■ Poverty had major implications for communication and for access to care. Parents of poor children reported experiencing difficulty communicating with their childrens' providers at a rate three times that of high-income parents. Poor adults were twice as likely to experience delays in being able to access care for an illness or injury, than did high-income persons (AHRQ, 2007b, p. 8).

■ Uninsured individuals do worse than privately insured individuals on almost 90% of the 42 quality measures and on *all* of the eight measures of access (AHRQ, 2007b, pp. 1, 9).

■ Hispanics of every income and education level were significantly less likely than their non-Hispanic peers to have health insurance (AHRQ, 2007b, p. 117).

■ No group has yet achieved the Healthy People 2010 target of 100% of Americans with health insurance (AHRQ, 2007b, p. 117).

■ Insurance status was a primary determinant of mammogram usage. In 2005, 58.6% of black women age 40 and over covered by public insurance reported having had a mammogram within the past 2 years, compared to 76.3% of privately insured black women. Uninsured black women fared even worse, with only 44.2% reporting having had a mammogram within the previous 2 years (AHRQ, 2007b, p. 154).

The nurse, in all professional relationships, practices with compassion and respect for the inherent dignity, worth and uniqueness of every individual, unrestricted by considerations of social or economic status, personal attributes, or the nature of health problems (ANA, 2001, p. 7).

Central to the concept of ethical practice is the principle of justice: fair and equitable access to quality health-care services. That this access is not available for many Americans is indisputable, and it has served as the focal point for the debate over whether health care is a right or a privilege. In a quote attributed to the late Dr. Martin Luther King Jr., he addressed the inherent injustice in disparities in health care by saying, "Of all the forms of inequality, injustice in health is the most shocking and inhumane." The racial, ethnic, and social factors creating existing disparities in health and access to health-care services create a moral imperative for APNs to integrate cultural competence into all their direct and indirect care roles. Cultural competence demands not only incorporation of our patient's cultural beliefs and practices into our caregiving, but also broader application of the principles of cultural competence in the management of clinical services and professional activities such as the formulation of health policy. It is inadequate for APNs to simply do no harm. APNs represent the majority of our profession's most highly educated nurses. It is their responsibility to do more than just render high-quality care on a one-to-one basis with their patients. They are also accountable for continually improving the systems within which that care occurs.

WALK A MILE IN SOMEONE ELSE'S SHOES

Imagine that you are an elderly U.S. tourist participating in an Elder Hostel tour abroad. This is the first time that you have ever been out of the United States. You have a history of hypertension and coronary artery disease, as well as myopia and moderate, bilateral hearing loss. While abroad, you experience recurrent chest pain. The tour guide tries unsuccessfully to locate an English-speaking physician, so you are brought to the local hospital where you are admitted for observation. Your glasses and clothing have been removed, and you are on bedrest and are receiving nitroglycerin intravenously and oxygen by nasal cannula. You are unable to reach the bedside table and you cannot see the other patients or the staff in the ward clearly. You are unable to speak or understand the language, so you have no idea of the severity of your condition or its treatment. The tour guide, who initially served as your translator, has had to return to the group that is departing for the next tour destination in the morning.

If this were you, how would you feel? Vulnerable? Frightened? At the mercy of a health-care system and care providers whose language, and perhaps beliefs and practices, are totally foreign to you? Now imagine that you and your family recently immigrated to the United States. You may or may not speak and read English. The health-care beliefs and practices of your culture may differ significantly from those of Western medicine. You may be an undocumented alien, fearful of detection, and reticent to seek care. Superimposed on your ethnic and racial statuses may be the social implications of coming from the culture of poverty, or the drug culture.

In short, you would be a prototype for many of the patients cared for by APNs. How would you want to be treated if the roles were reversed and you were the patient?

THEORETICAL BASIS FOR CULTURAL COMPETENCE IN ADVANCED NURSING PRACTICE

Leininger's (2001) pioneering work in transcultural nursing and the development of her culture care theory provides a framework for the practice of APNs who care for culturally diverse populations. Care and caring, distinguishing characteristics of professional practice to which APNs lay particular claim, are central to her theory: "Care is the essence of nursing and the central, dominant and unifying focus of nursing" (p. 35). Leininger holds that for too long, caring has been the "covert, unknown, and almost invisible aspect of nursing and health services" (p. 32).

Leininger's commitment to the development of a theoretical framework that would assist nurses and other health-care providers to deliver culturally congruent care to patients from diverse populations evolved from a commitment to improve the health of clients, families, and cultural groups; to better help patients from diverse cultural groups to maintain or regain their health; or to experience death in a manner compatible with their cultural beliefs and practices. Leininger's theory of culture care acknowledges both universal and culture-specific care patterns. For instance, although beliefs and expressions associated with caring may vary widely from one cultural group to another, human care practices have been documented from the beginning of recorded history.

Formulated from an anthropological perspective, the theory questions nursing's traditional reliance on the concepts of person, health, and the environment. Leininger (2001) notes that, in many non-Western cultures, family and social institutions are primary and that the language may not even have a word for person. She also notes that although nurses and nursing exert significant influence over individual and societal health and the environment, these concepts are hardly unique to our profession or its practice. In place of these generic concepts, Leininger proposes that care and caring are the central core of nursing, stating, "Care is the nurse's way of being with and helping people" (p. 40).

Leininger's theory and the Sunrise Model **(Figure 20-2),** which depicts both the universality and diversity of cultural care, provide a framework for the APN to examine the dynamic interplay of the many forces that influence the delivery of care.

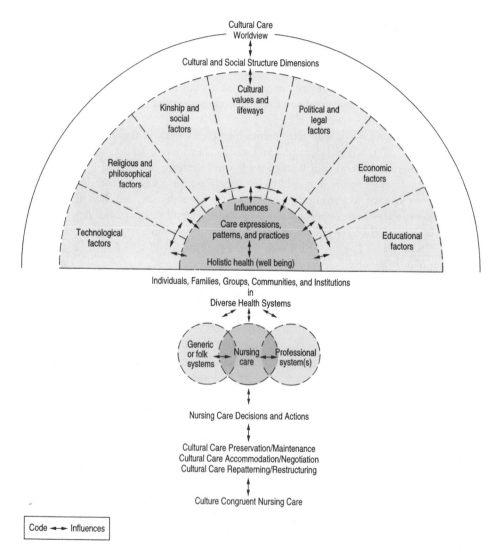

FIGURE 20-2 Leininger's sunrise model to depict theory of cultural care diversity and universality. (*Source: Leininger, 1991, p. 43, with permission of the National League for Nursing.*)

The culture care theory incorporates three major approaches to the delivery of culturally congruent nursing assessment, decision making, and interventions. Leininger defines these modalities as the following:

1. **Cultural care preservation and maintenance.** "Professional actions and decisions that help people of a particular culture to retain and/or preserve relevant care values so that they can maintain their well being, recover from illness, or face handicaps and/or death" (p. 48).
2. **Cultural care accommodation and negotiation.** "Creative professional actions and decisions that help people of a designated culture to adapt to, or to negotiate with others for a beneficial or satisfying health outcome with professional care providers" (p. 48).
3. **Cultural care repatterning or restructuring.** "Professional actions and decisions that help a client(s) reorder, change, or greatly modify their lifeways for new, different, and beneficial health care patterns while respecting the client(s) cultural values and beliefs and still providing a beneficial or healthier lifeway than before the changes were coestablished with the client(s)" (p. 49).

Inherent in each of these modalities are three of the core values that underlie all of advanced practice nursing: respect, advocacy, and partnership. The culturally competent APN is knowledgeable and respectful of diverse cultural beliefs and practices, partners with the patient to develop a care regimen that produces the desired health outcomes within the context of the patient's cultural values, and advocates for the development of culturally appropriate patient care services.

APNs who apply these modalities in their care of patients provide what Leininger (2001) terms *cultural congruent (nursing) care.* Leininger states that this term:

> . . .*refers to those cognitively based assistive, supportive, facilitative, or enabling acts or decisions that are tailor made to fit with individual, group or institutional cultural values, beliefs, and lifeways in order to provide or support meaningful, beneficial, and satisfying health care, or well-being services (p. 49).*

MOVING FROM THEORY INTO PRACTICE

There are multiple definitions of cultural competence. The definition used in this chapter was developed by the Maternal and Child Health Bureau (MCHB) of the Health Resources and Services Administration (HRSA) of the USDHHS. It speaks to the requirements for achieving organizational, as well as individual, competence. In an environment in which health-care delivery systems are increasingly held accountable for continuous quality improvement and cost containment, APNs often straddle dual roles as clinicians and managers of clinical services. Thus, the APN must not only be skilled in the direct delivery of culturally congruent care, but also in the implementation of policies and procedures that ensure cultural competence at the organizational level. Cultural competence is defined as a set of values, behaviors, attitudes, and practices within a system, organization, program, or among individuals that enables APNs to work effectively cross-culturally. Further, it refers to the ability to honor and respect the beliefs, language, interpersonal styles, and behaviors of individuals and families receiving services, as well as staff who are providing such services. Striving to achieve cultural competence is a dynamic, ongoing, developmental process that requires a long-term commitment. Cultural competence mandates that organizations, programs, and individuals must have the ability to do the following (USDHHS, MCHB, 1999):

- Value diversity and similarities among all people.
- Understand and effectively respond to cultural differences.

- Engage in cultural self-assessment at the individual and organizational levels.
- Make adaptations to the delivery of services and enabling supports.
- Institutionalize cultural knowledge.

The elements in the MCHB's definition complement the definition currently employed by the Office of Minority Health (OMH) and used by HRSA in 2001 when they sponsored a major project to develop a framework and evaluation measures for assessing cultural competence in health-care settings. The HRSA study used the definition of cultural competence developed by Cross, Bazron, Dennis, Isaac, and Campinha-Bacote (1989): Cultural competence is a set of congruent behaviors, attitudes, and policies that come together in a system, in an agency, or among professionals and enable that system, agency, or those professionals to work effectively in cross-cultural situations.

The American Hospital Association's (AHA) Patient's Bill of Rights, first adopted in 1973 and revised in 1992, contained a statement in its introduction that read:

> *Hospitals must ensure a health care ethic that respects the role of patients in decision making about treatment choices and other aspects of their care. Hospitals must be sensitive to cultural, racial, linguistic, religious, age, gender, and other differences as well as the needs of persons with disabilities (AHA, 1992).*

The Patients' Bill of Rights has been replaced with a document titled *The Patient Care Partnership*. It is in the form of an easy-to-read brochure and describes what patients should expect during their hospitalization with respect to their rights and responsibilities. It is available in eight languages: English, Arabic, traditional and simplified Chinese, Spanish, Russian, Vietnamese, and Tagalog. A brief excerpt from the brochure appears in **Box 20-2**. It conveys a desire on the part of the hospital to integrate the patient's values and beliefs into their care. The AHA has also produced two products for staff use to enhance culturally competent care within U.S. hospitals: a toolkit for collecting race, ethnicity, and primary language information from patients (Hasnain-Wynia et al., 2007) and the diversity assessment tool.

Health Literacy

Cultural competence must be operationalized in the context of health literacy. The definition of health literacy that was used in Healthy People 2010 (USDHHS, 2000a) was presented by the National Library of Medicine (Selden, Zorn, Ratzan, & Parker, 2000):

> *the degree to which a person can obtain, process and understand basic health information and services needed to make appropriate health decisions (Ratzan & Parker, 2000).*

Several tools are available to clinicians to assess the literacy of their patients. These include the rapid estimate of adult literacy in medicine (REALM), which is available in both the original and shortened version; the rapid assessment of adolescent literacy in medicine (REALM-Teen); and the test

---

BOX 20-2
Excerpt from the Patient Care Partnership

"You may have health care goals and values or spiritual beliefs that are important to your well-being. They will be taken into account as much as possible throughout your hospital stay. Make sure your doctor, your family and your care team know your wishes" (AHA, 2003).

of functional health literacy in adults (TOFHLA), available in both the original and shortened versions, and in Spanish **(Table 20-2).** Although these assessment tools are often described as assessing health literacy, this description may be somewhat misleading. As examination of Table 20-2 reveals, these tools assess the literacy component of health literacy. Although reading comprehension and an understanding of commonly used medical terms are essential components of health literacy, such understanding does not necessarily translate into the ability to navigate the system to obtain the health-care services that promote improved health outcomes.

Citing data from the National Assessment of Adult Literacy (Kutner, Greenberg, & Baer, 2003), the AHRQ reports that 9 out of 10 adults in the United States are not health literacy proficient, and as a result, may lack the skills to engage in successful health promotion, disease prevention, and management of acute and chronic diseases for themselves and their families (AHRQ, 2007a, p. 1). Health literacy is directly linked to English language proficiency. The American Community Survey (U.S. Census Bureau, 2006c) reported that 37,547,789 foreign-born persons resided in the United States, and almost 21,780,058 were not U.S. citizens. Most were of Hispanic (47.2%) or Asian (23.4%) descent and lived within married-couple households. Of those 25 years and older, 32% had not completed high school. The poverty rate for families of foreign-born persons ranged from a low

TABLE 20-2

Literacy Assessment Tools

Name of Tool	Format of the Tool	Test Administration	Approximate Completion Times
Rapid estimate of adult literacy in medicine (REALM)	66-item word recognition test of commonly used medical terms.	The individual is asked to pronounce words in ascending order of difficulty.	2–6 minutes (Wallace, 2006)
Rapid estimate of adult literacy in medicine-revised (REALM-R)	8-item, rapid screening, word recognition test.	The individual is asked to pronounce words in ascending order of difficulty.	Under 2 minutes (Bass, Wilson, & Griffith, 2003)
Rapid estimate of adolescent literacy in medicine: REALM-Teen (Davis et al., 2006)	66-item word recognition test. Appropriate for adolescents in grades 6–12. Available only in English.	The individual is asked to pronounce words in ascending order of difficulty.	Under 3 minutes
Test of functional health literacy in adults: original and short versions (Wallace, 2006)	Timed, reading comprehension test in which every fifth to seventh word in a written passage is omitted. Available in both English and Spanish.	The individual replaces the missing words from four multiple-choice options for each missing word.	22 minutes (TOFHLA); 7 minutes (S-TOFHLA)

of 11.1% for married-couple families to 43.3% for families with children under 5 years of age and 40.2% for families with children under 18 years of age. Most (46%) lived in rental housing units (U.S. Census Bureau, 2006c).

Of those, 52.4% reported that they spoke English less than "very well," and 90.3% of native-born Americans reported that English was the only language spoken at home. This finding is in stark contrast to foreign-born respondents, only 15.6% of whom reported English as the only language spoken in the home. Spanish or Spanish-Creole (12.2%) was the major language other than English that was spoken in the home, followed by Indo-European languages (3.7%) and Asian-Pacific Islander languages, reported by 3% of the respondents. Of the households of foreign-born persons, 31.4% were described as being "linguistically isolated" (U.S. Census Bureau, 2006c). These data paint a picture of millions of potential patients, many of whom are children, who are at high risk for limited access, inadequate care, and inability to acquire the self-care management knowledge and skills essential to maintain health and optimum function. Cultural beliefs and practices, limited education and English proficiency, and poverty are all barriers to accessing and effectively using health-care resources. When they converge, the negative effects of each individual barrier are magnified.

In 2000, the Institute of Medicine (IOM) issued a report titled *America's Health Care Safety Net: Intact but Endangered* (Lewin & Altman, 2000). As if anticipating the demographic data previously cited and the AHRQ's definition of health literacy, the report states: "Compared with privately insured persons, Medicaid beneficiaries tend to be far more vulnerable, their needs more diverse, and their experience with and capacity for exercising choice more limited. . . . In addition, non-medical services of special importance to vulnerable populations (e.g., enabling services such as translation services, transportation to clinic visits, and the provision of child care services, and outreach) may not be part of a managed care contract or amenable to managed care infrastructure" (Lewin & Altman, 2000, p. 7).

In 2004, the IOM conducted a comprehensive study of health literacy and its impact on health outcomes. Key findings can be found in **Box 20-3.** The report brings the impact of deficient health literacy dramatically to light in a case example:

> *A two-year-old is diagnosed with an inner ear infection and prescribed an antibiotic. Her mother understands that her child has an ear infection and knows she should take the prescribed medication twice a day. After looking at the label on the bottle and deciding that it does not tell how to take the medicine, she fills a teaspoon and pours the antibiotic into her daughter's ear" (Parker, Ratzan, & Lurie, 2003, p. 150).*

For many of us, our practice environments have seen an exponential growth in patients from a wide variety of cultures; our knowledge of these cultures may be limited at best. For example, the University of Washington's Medical Center in Seattle reported 20,000 patient encounters requiring the use of interpreters in 1999 (Abbott et al., 2002). The five major non-English languages spoken by these patients were Russian, Spanish, Korean, Vietnamese, and Chinese. In contrast, the caregivers at the medical center are white (64%), African American (7%), Native American (1%), Hispanic (3%), and Asian (25%). The influx of culturally diverse patients, many with multiple health and social needs, may tax an organization's ability to provide translators. Similarly, patient education materials, essential to patient welfare and to meeting institutional accreditation standards set by The Joint Commission (TJC) are often not available in languages other than English and Spanish. These are but two of the challenges that confront the practitioner in a multicultural care environment.

BOX 20-3
Institute of Medicine Key Findings

■ Finding 3-1: "The majority of these adults are native-born English speakers. Literacy levels are lower among the elderly, those who have lower educational levels, those who are poor, minority populations, and groups with limited English proficiency such as recent immigrants" (Nielsen-Bohlman, Panzer, & Kindig 2004, p. 8).

■ Finding 3-2: "On the basis of limited studies, public testimony, and committee members' experience, the committee concludes that the shame and stigma associated with limited literacy skills are major barriers to improving health literacy" (Nielsen-Bohlman et al., 2004, p. 8).

■ Finding 3-3: "Adults with limited health literacy, as measured by reading and numeracy skills, have less knowledge of disease management and of health-promoting behaviors, report poorer health status, and are less likely to use preventive services" (Nielsen-Bohlman et al., 2004, p. 8).

■ Finding 3-4: "Two recent studies demonstrate a higher rate of hospitalization and use of emergency services among patients with limited literacy. This higher utilization has been associated with higher health-care costs" (Nielsen-Bohlman et al., 2004, p. 9).

■ Finding 4-1: "Culture gives meaning to health communication. Health literacy must be understood and addressed in the context of culture and language" (Nielsen-Bohlman et al., 2004 p. 10).

■ Finding 5-5: "Health professionals and staff have limited education, training, continuing education, and practice opportunities to develop skills for improving health literacy" (Nielsen-Bohlman et al., 2004, p. 11).

■ Finding 6-2: "Health literacy is fundamental to quality care, and relates to three of the six aims of quality improvement described in the IOM Quality Chasm Report: safety, patient-centered care, and equitable treatment. Self-management and health literacy have been identified by IOM as cross-cutting priorities for health-care quality and disease prevention" (Nielsen-Bohlman et al., 2004, p. 12).

Health literacy is not simply about English proficiency. Even if one is proficient in speaking, reading, and writing English, all of us process communication with our health providers in terms of interpersonal dynamics and the lens of cultural beliefs and practices. Literal translation of patient education materials, discharge instructions, consent forms, and other written and multimedia patient materials often do not achieve their intended purpose because the content is not presented in a culturally congruent manner. We need to move from translation to transcreation, which is development of all forms of information within a cultural context. A recent study (Guerra, Krumholz, & Shea, 2005) of 145 Latino women receiving care in community health clinics in Philadelphia, revealed that 70% had marginal or inadequate health literacy. The study examined the relationship between health literacy, as assessed by the short test of functional health literacy in adults (S-TOFHLA) and the short acculturation scale for Hispanics, and knowledge, beliefs, attitudes about and use of breast self-examination and screening mammography. The findings revealed no relationship between health literacy and beliefs and attitudes, and only a weak relationship to knowledge. However, there was a significant association with ever having had a mammogram; Latinas with poor functional health literacy were significantly less likely to undergo screening mammographies.

Another study (Aguirre, Ebrahim, & Shea, 2005) compared the performance of three groups of Medicaid and Medicare patients on the English and Spanish versions of the TOFHLA. The 2,370 participants in the study attended eight clinics in Philadelphia, which serve predominantly African American and Hispanic populations. The English S-TOFHLA was completed by 1,034 participants (936 self-identified as non-Hispanic, 91% of whom were African American, and 368 as Hispanic) and 1,066 completed the Spanish version of the S-TOFHLA (self-identified as Hispanics, 93% of whom reported being Puerto Rican). Analysis of the findings revealed that 33% of the Hispanic, Spanish-version participants received scores indicating inadequate health literacy, compared to 19% of the non-Hispanic, English version subjects and 8% of the Hispanic, English-version participants (p. 334). Hispanic participants who chose to complete the English version of the S-TOFHLA achieved the highest scores of all subgroups of participants. Hispanics who indicated a preference for speaking Spanish and who chose to complete the Spanish S-TOFHLA, had the lowest scores (p. 338). Of particular interest in this study was the finding of significant differences in health literacy between men and women, a finding not seen in previous studies. Women performed better than men in this study on both the English and Spanish versions of the S-TOFHLA (p. 337).

Asian Americans are one of the fastest growing population groups in the United States, increasing at a rate faster than the general population between 1990 and 2000 (Barnes & Bennett, 2002, p. 3). The trend continues, with persons of Asian descent estimated at 113,100,095 (4.4% of the total population) in 2006, up from 3.6 % in 2000 (U.S. Census Bureau, 2006b). This population is more at risk for developing type 2 diabetes than non-Hispanic whites, even though their body weight is lower. Chinese Americans, 50% of whom self-report being "linguistically isolated," constitute the greatest percentage of Asian Americans. The Joslin Clinic, a teaching affiliate of the Harvard Medical School, took the lead in developing culturally appropriate care sites and educational materials for Asian Americans with, or at risk for, diabetes. All of the educational materials, including the Joslin Clinic's clinical guidelines for the prevention, detection, and treatment of diabetes, are available in English, traditional Chinese, and simplified Chinese.

A driving force for the development of the transcreated educational materials and interactive Web site were findings from a pilot study of Chinese Americans between the ages of 18 and 70 who were diagnosed with diabetes for at least 1 year and who were taking either oral agents or insulin. The study, conducted by Hsu et al. (2006), consisted of 52 subjects, 91% of whom had type 2 diabetes. Twenty-two of the subjects indicated a preference for English, and 30 indicated Chinese as their preferred language. The Chinese American subjects, who indicated a preference for Chinese as their preferred language, demonstrated less knowledge about their disease process and had higher hemoglobin A1C levels than did the subjects for whom English was the preferred language. These differences occurred even though the care to all subjects in the study was delivered in culturally competent sites with ready access to translation services. Another interesting finding of the study was that a significantly greater proportion of the English-language preference Chinese immigrant subjects (36.4%) reported diabetes educators as a source of information, compared to Chinese-language preference Chinese immigrant subjects (3.3%).

An increasing number of other health-care organizations are developing educational materials and programs that reflect transcreation; that are both linguistically and culturally appropriate for the target populations that they serve. Two more notable examples are New York University, School of Medicine's Center for Immigrant Health, and the National Cancer Institute's (NCI) Office of Education and Special Initiatives. The NCI transcreated an English-language booklet titled *Facing Forward: Life After Cancer Treatment (Siga adelante: la vida después del tratemiento del cancér)*, designed for cancer survivors. NYU's Center for Immigrant Health, in collaboration with the NYU Cancer Institute, established a Cancer Awareness Network for Immigrant Minority Populations (CANIMP), which seeks to address disparities in cancer prevention, detection, and treatment in minority populations through transcreated materials and outreach. In 2002, the CANIMP produced "Survivor", an educational video designed for the English-speaking Caribbean community, emphasizing the importance of prostate screening for men at high risk, age 40 and older. A companion video—"*Rete Vivan*"—was developed in 2004 specifically for members of the Creole-speaking Haitian community. The video begins in the heart of the community, in a Haitian owned barbershop in Brooklyn and features a Haitian prostate cancer survivor. The borough of Brooklyn is home to approximately 60,000 Haitian immigrants (CANIMP, 2004, p. 1).

Patient Navigator Programs

In addition to empowering patients through the development of transcreated educational materials, vulnerable populations are known to experience significant difficulty in "navigating" the health-care system. The interplay of barriers—poverty, limited English proficiency, dependence on over burdened, publicly funded health facilities that often lack evening and weekend services for nonurgent care—leave many patients feeling overwhelmed by the complexity of the system. Patients' failures to follow through on diagnostic tests and referrals, to obtain and take their medications as prescribed, and the like are usually ascribed to being "noncompliant." If you dig deeper, often noncompliance represents an inability to access the services necessary to facilitate adherence to their prescribed health-care regimen. In *Crossing the quality chasm*, The IOM, quoting the Picker Institute and the AHA, put it bluntly:

> It is not surprising, then, that studies of patient experience document that the health system for some is a "nightmare to navigate" (IOM, 2001, p. 4).

Two recent studies attest to the importance of patient navigators in minority populations.

Researchers at the City University of New York and Mount Sinai School of Medicine in New York City conducted a cohort study of patients referred for screening colonoscopies from their primary care clinics between November 2003 and May 2006. Of the 688 patients who were eligible to participate in the study, 532 had a female, bilingual, Hispanic patient navigator assigned to assist them with successfully completing the procedure. Of the navigated patients, 66% completed their screening colonoscopies. The vast majority—95%—had adequate bowel preparation; 16% were found to have adenomas. The "no-show" rate for urban minority patients dropped from a high of 40% before implementation of the navigator program, to a low of 9.8%. Most (98%) of the patients reported being satisfied with the navigator program, and 66% indicated that they probably, or definitely, would *not* have completed the procedure if the patient navigator program had not been in effect. (Chen et al., 2008).

A randomized control trial was conducted by members of the Departments of Medicine and Oncological Sciences at Mount Sinai School of Medicine in New York City (Christie et al., 2008). Citing data from New York State for 2004 that reported that only 43% of residents of East Harlem reported having a colonoscopy in the last 10 years, compared to 54% of residents of Manhattan, the researchers investigated the effect of using a patient navigator on compliance with referrals for screening colonoscopies from primary care physicians in a local community health center. The subjects were randomized into two groups—navigator ($n = 13$) and no navigator ($n = 8$). The average age of the subjects was 58; 75% were female and 71% were Hispanic. Most of the subjects were low income, had less than a high school education, and were uninsured or covered by public insurance. The patient navigator assisted patients with completion of forms, scheduling, organized and coordinated transportation, and explained the procedure in English or Spanish, using the colonoscopy preparation protocol. A significantly greater percentage of the navigated patients completed their screening colonoscopies than did the nonnavigated patients: 53.8% versus 13%. Only one of the nonnavigated patients completed the screening colonoscopy. In addition, 86% of the navigated patients who had colonoscopies were rated as having good or excellent colon preps.

The potential for wide-scale implementation of patient navigator programs to reduce disparities in health and access to high quality health-care services garnered support in Congress. On April 25, 2005, Representative Robert Menendez (D-N.J.) introduced H.R. 1812: The Patient Navigator, Outreach and Chronic Disease Prevention Act of 2005 to amend the Public Health Service Act. The amendment authorized the secretary of Health and Human Services (HHS), acting through the administrator of the HRSA, to award grants for up to 3 years, with provision for a 1 year extension, to health-care facilities to develop and implement patient navigator services to reduce barriers to care and to improve health outcomes. Facilities receiving the grants would be required to establish benchmarks and identify outcome criteria to measure the effectiveness of the program. Its companion bill in the Senate was S. 898, introduced by Senator Kay Bailey Hutchison (R-TX). The proposed legislation had broad, bipartisan support and passed both houses of Congress. On June 29, 2005, President George W. Bush signed the Patient Navigator, Outreach and Chronic Disease Prevention Act (P.L. 109-18, Section 340A) into law (GovTrack, 2005). In fiscal year 2008, $2,948,000 was appropriated for competitive grants, of which five were awarded.

HRSA's fiscal year 2009 Justification of Estimates for Appropriations Committees of the United States Congress, is presented in the context of its mission and the agency's seven strategic goals **(Box 20-4).**

Despite multiple research studies that demonstrate the effectiveness of patient navigator programs, especially in minority communities, and a mission statement and goals that speak to improving the health care of vulnerable populations, HRSA is not requesting funding for the Patient Navigator program for fiscal year 2009: "Funding for this program has been eliminated in FY 2009"

BOX 20-4
Health Resources and Services Administration's Mission Statement

Health Resources and Services Administration's (HRSA) mission, as articulated in its Strategic Plan for 2005–2010, is to provide the national leadership, program resources, and services to improve access to culturally competent, quality health care for uninsured, underserved, and special needs populations.

The agency's seven strategic goals are to:

- Improve access to health care
- Improve health outcomes
- Improve the quality of health care
- Eliminate health disparities
- Improve the public health and health-care systems
- Enhance the ability of the health-care system to respond to public health emergencies
- Achieve excellence in management

(USDHHS, 2008, p. 6). The agency has also eliminated all program funding for public health improvement ($304,500,000) in fiscal year 2009 (USDHHS, 2008, p. 6). The cuts reflect the fiscal year 2009 president's budget request for HRSA, which is $5,864,511,000, a decrease of $991,681,000 below the amount enacted for fiscal year 2008 (USDHHS, 2008, p. 3). This is a good object lesson about competing demands in an environment of increasingly scarce resources. It is incumbent on APNs to translate their patient advocacy role into political and legislative activism. Public laws that are unfunded, such as the Patient Navigator, Outreach and Chronic Disease Prevention Act (P.L. 109-18, Section 340A), cannot deliver on the legislative intent for which they were enacted.

Even in the best of worlds, with full funding of P.L. 109-18, Section 340 A, successful patient navigator programs present a real conflict to their parent health-care institutions. Implementation of a successful program requires a substantial investment in personnel and training. A successful program will produce measureable improvements in patient outcomes, such as fewer patient visits to emergency departments for routine care, decreased incidence and severity of complications in patients with chronic disease processes, fewer hospital admissions, etc. Although all these are highly desirable outcomes for patients, these outcomes translate into significantly less reimbursement to health-care facilities and providers. From a business perspective, it makes no sense to implement a program that will generate less revenue. A similar situation is seen in managed care programs weighing the pros and cons of implementing or expanding health promotional programs. If a few managed care plans take the lead in offering such expanded programs, they run the real risk that the long-term benefits that would accrue to the programs through a reduction in the care costs of their enrollees, will not be realized to their corporations if the enrollees subsequently switch to another managed care plan. The managed care plans who exhibited a commitment to health promotion could end up bearing all the costs for implementing these programs and realize none of the benefits. Indeed, the benefits could flow to other managed care plans who had not made such an investment in the health of their enrollees. Reimbursement needs to be redesigned to incentivize and reward delivery systems that produce positive health outcomes and lower overall health-care costs. APNs need to be actively engaged in the development of health policy at all levels, and they need to bring an understanding of the economics of health care, as well as their expertise in patient care to those decision-making tables. Their advocacy role must extend beyond institutional boundaries into the political and legislative arenas.

Assessment

The first step in meeting these challenges is assessment—of ourselves, of our patients needs, and of our existing organizational resources. Each of us brings the influence of our own cultural heritage, experiences, biases, beliefs, and expectations about patient-provider relationships to the care that we give. Evaluation of the effect of these influences on our caregiving practices is the first step to achieving cultural competence as a practitioner. The National Center for Cultural Competence (NCCC) at the Georgetown University Center for Child and Human Development offers an exceptional array of assessment tools for assessing cultural competence in individuals and organizations, as well as a wealth of instructional materials. Two of the self-assessment tools deserve particular mention. The Cultural Competence Health Practitioner Assessment (CCHPA) tool may be completed online in about 20 minutes. The tool contains six subscales: Values and Belief Systems; Cultural Aspects of Epidemiology; Clinical Decision-Making; Life Cycle Events; Cross-Cultural Communication, and Empowerment/Health Management. On completion of the tool, the practitioner receives immediate assessment of their performance on each of the subscales, as well as a list of recommended resources for addressing any identified deficiencies. Another excellent self-assessment tool is a 37-item checklist titled Promoting Cultural and Linguistic Competency for Personnel Providing Primary Health Care Services. Its content is applicable to all four advanced practice nursing specialties. The individual responds to specific examples about values, attitudes, communication styles, the practice environment, and patient materials and resources. For example, item 7 asks the practitioner to indicate the frequency with which he or she would do the following:

> *For individuals and families who speak languages or dialects other than English, I attempt to learn and use key words so that I am better able to communicate with them during assessment, treatment or other interventions.*

The individual would respond that this is something that they do frequently, occasionally, or rarely, if ever. The tool may be downloaded by visiting the NCCC Web site at http://gucchd.georgetown.edu and clicking on Products and Tools.

Language gives voice to cultural expression. Many cultures have rich oral traditions that transmit the stories, traditions, and beliefs that define their cultural heritage from generation to generation. Language serves as the primary vehicle for most of our interpersonal communication, from patients' descriptions of their health-care needs to interprofessional collaboration. Linguistic competence is essential to the delivery of culturally competent health care. A fundamental tenet of advanced practice nursing is patient empowerment: patients as informed, full partners in decision making about their health care. Operationalizing this core belief clearly requires effective provider-patient communication, a condition that does not exist when linguistic barriers are present. At the very least, lack of linguistic competence makes patient assessment and intervention difficult. At worst, patient safety may be fundamentally compromised (**Box 20-5**).

BOX 20-5
Buenos Días, Señora

Mrs. W, a 43-year-old married Hispanic woman with three children, came to the neighborhood health center complaining of tightness in her chest and difficulty in coughing up her secretions. Her usual bilingual care provider was unavailable, so she was seen by another practitioner who was not proficient in Spanish. Her records revealed that she had been diagnosed with mild intermittent asthma, for which she had been prescribed albuterol to be used as necessary. Mrs. W reported that she had not filled her last prescription because of the cost.

Mrs. W's physical examination was unremarkable except for a slight increase in respiratory rate and scattered expiratory wheezes. To save her the cost of prescription medication, the provider recommended that she purchase the over-the-counter product Robitussin and take it four times per day. She was advised to return to the clinic if her symptoms did not improve. No written follow-up instructions were available in Spanish.

Four days later, Mrs. W came to the clinic in acute distress. Because of her limited understanding of English, she had purchased Honey Cough by Robitussin. The provider had not thought to explain, or to give her written instructions, about the difference between guaifenesin (the active ingredient in plain Robitussin, which acts to liquefy pulmonary secretions and promote expectoration) and Honey Cough, which contains only dextromethorphan, a potent cough suppressant. Instead of relieving Mrs. W's symptoms, the provider's lack of linguistically appropriate intervention significantly worsened her condition by depressing the very mechanism that would have allowed her to loosen and expel her secretions.

The process of self-assessment must be approached with a willingness to confront and modify or discard those inaccurate and uninformed preconceived cultural beliefs and attitudes that detract from the care we provide. Many of our attitudes and beliefs are so ingrained that we may never scrutinize them in the course of our daily practice until, and if, we become aware of their negative effect on our care. Even then, long-held biases may limit our introspection. Ethnocentrism, or the belief in the relative superiority of one's own cultural group, is a common phenomenon. Often operating at an unconscious level, ethnocentrism can exert a powerful influence on our patient interactions and care practices.

The NCCC has also produced another excellent tool that details the process for conducting an organizational self-assessment (Goode, Jones, & Mason, 2002). The process, which stresses community involvement and a nonpunitive approach with an emphasis on self-knowledge and growth, is also available at the NCCC Web site listed previously. Knowledge of our individual and institutional strengths and weaknesses in the area of cultural competence is a prerequisite to corrective action.

Culturally competent patient assessment is indispensable to appropriate diagnosis and treatment and promotes patient participation in decision making about health and treatment regimens. Although an understanding of the beliefs and practices of a patient's cultural group facilitates such assessment, respectful questioning wherein the patient becomes the teacher about his or her culture produces data to support your clinical judgments and helps build trust between patient and provider. A particularly valuable resource for drawing out a patient's beliefs about health and illness is *Understanding, eliciting and negotiating multicultural health beliefs* (Jackson, 1993). The reader is referred to **Box 20-6.**

Note that all of the questions are framed from the perspective of the patient. They acknowledge the patient's ownership of his or her unique illness experience. Framing the questions in this way allows the APN to enter into the patient's lived experience. By exploring the patient's perceptions and expectations, the provider is better able to propose a treatment plan that is compatible with the patient's cultural beliefs and practices.

BOX 20-6

Questions to Elicit Beliefs and Treatment Expectations from Patients Seeking Illness Care

- What do you think caused your problem?
- Why do you think it started when it did?
- What do you think your sickness does to you?
- How does it work?
- How severe is your sickness?
- Will it have a short or long course?
- What kind of treatment should you receive?
- What are the results you hope to receive from this treatment?
- What are the problems your sickness has caused you?
- What do you fear most about your sickness?

Adapted from Jackson, 1993, p. 30.

Culturally competent assessment also requires that the clinician apply ethnically appropriate parameters when interpreting physical findings. Body mass index (BMI) is widely used as a tool to assess patients' risk for diabetes and cardiovascular disease. There is a growing body of evidence to suggest that the current, European derived, "one size fits all" BMI classifications for overweight (25.0 kg/m² or greater, but less than 30.0 kg/m²) and obese (equal to or greater than 30 kg/m²), may not be appropriate across all ethnic groups. A recent study (Razak et al., 2007) reported in *Circulation* sought to determine if the current cut point for determining obesity that is used in clinical practice is appropriate for use in non-European populations. A random sample of 1,078 subjects were recruited from participants in the Study of Health Assessment and Risk in Ethnic Groups (SHARE) and Risk Evaluation in Aboriginal Peoples (SHARE-AP). The subjects, from four ethnic groups—South Asians (n = 289), Chinese (n = 281), Aboriginals (n = 207), and Europeans (n = 301)—were evaluated for 14 variables: 2 clinical (systolic and diastolic blood pressure) and 12 biochemical (fasting and 2-hour glucose; fasting and 2-hour insulin; HbA1C, Homeostasis Model Assessment-insulin resistance (HOMA-IR); high density and low density lipids and triglycerides; fasting and 2-hour free fatty acids) cardiometabolic markers. Factor analysis revealed three latent factors that accounted for 56% of the variation in the subjects' cardiometabolic markers and blood pressure. The main effect of ethnicity was highly significant for each factor (P < 0.001). Compared to European subjects for a given BMI, South Asian, Chinese, and Aboriginal subjects had elevated glucose and lipid metabolism-related factors. The South Asian subjects had the worst glucose and lipid profiles—the highest 2-hour oral glucose tolerance tests levels, the highest LDL levels, and the lowest HDL levels (Razak et al. 2007, p. 2113). Elevated blood-pressure-related factor was found in Chinese subjects; at a BMI of 25.3 kg/m² compared to a BMI of 30.0 kg/m² in Europeans (p. 2114). In discussing their findings, the authors conclude:

> *Use of BMI cut points derived among Europeans understates the cardiometabolic risk associated with weight gain in other ethnic groups. The pathway linking obesity to clinical events is mediated partially through its strong association with the development of diabetes, hypertension, and dyslipidemia. . . . This suggests that to minimize the development of cardiometabolic risk factors, lower BMI targets should be used by healthcare professionals in some non-European populations (Razak et al., 2007, p. 2114).*

Major sources of best practices, such as the Joslin Clinic, have already incorporated ethnospecific BMI recommendations in their clinical guidelines. The Joslin Diabetes Center and Joslin Clinic clinical nutrition guideline for overweight and obese adults with type 2 diabetes, those with prediabetes, or those at high risk for developing type 2 diabetes defines as high risk Asian populations (South Asian Indians, East Indians and Malays) with a BMI > 23 kg/m² and a waistline > 35"/90 cm in men or > 31"/80 cm in women. This is in contrast to the guideline's generic criteria of BMI > 25 kg/m² and/or a waistline > 40"/102 cm (men) and 35"/88 cm (women).

Treatment regimens should always strive to incorporate the cultural practices and preferences that are most valued by the patient. For example, Muslim patients observe strict dietary laws that include a prohibition against eating any pork products. Practicing Muslims also pray five times a day and may be reluctant to eat or to take medications during daylight hours at certain periods of the year—for example, tradition dictates that Muslims fast while the sun is up during the observance of Ramadan. Treatment plans that are congruent with patients' valued cultural beliefs and practices are more likely to generate positive outcomes. Outcomes data are key determinants of reimbursement, provider recognition by third-party payors, and institutional accreditation. Culturally and linguistically competent patient assessment is the foundation of successful outcomes.

Knowledge

As an APN, you are well aware of the value of knowledge. Evidence- and research-based practice is the standard to which you are held. Many of the new national guidelines for clinical assessment of major health conditions affecting large segments of the U.S. population reflect a cultural congruence not seen in previous guidelines, as in the Centers for Disease Control and Prevention (CDC) growth charts released in 2000. Before the release of the new guidelines, clinicians had to rely on growth charts developed in 1977 by the National Center for Health Statistics, which were derived from data drawn primarily from 10,000 White, middle class infants and children living in Ohio between 1929 and 1975. In contrast, the CDC guidelines are based on survey data for different ethnic and racial groups and incorporate data on breastfed children in proportion to the rate of breastfeeding in the general population. Fourteen percent of the data from which the new guidelines were developed represent information collected in surveys of African American children. This figure reflects the proportion of African American children living in the United States from 1971 to 1994 ("New Growth Charts a Welcome Improvement," 2002).

Just as you are expected to incorporate the latest clinical guidelines for the management of conditions such as diabetes and lipid disorders into your practice, so, too, must you inform yourself about the beliefs and practices of the cultural groups in your patient population. This can seem like a daunting task, especially if your patient population is quite diverse. The task becomes even more complex if you have a rapid influx of immigrants from a cultural group new to the setting. Many sources of help are available to assist the individual practitioner and organization to care effectively for diverse populations. Every cultural group has its community leaders. Often they are religious leaders and professionals who are more than willing to assist local health and social agencies in meeting the needs of their community. Many culturally affiliated church and social organizations have developed literature and other materials to help noncommunity members better understand their cultural beliefs and practices.

All APNs are partners with their patients in providing culturally competent care. Recognizing that individual patients may or may not adhere to cultural norms, key questions to explore about any cultural group for whom you care are in **Box 20-7.** Here is a phrase that may help you to remember these key questions and be a better partner:

Partners in delivering culturally competent research-based care for diverse populations.

The Internet is an extremely valuable resource for gathering information on various cultural groups. The culture-specific materials developed by the University of Washington Medical Center are invaluable to APNs practicing in culturally diverse settings. A 1996 survey of the staff conducted by the Center's Patient and Family Education Committee identified a need for support in giving culturally and linguistically appropriate care (Abbott et al., 2002). The resultant culture clues, are brief, provider-friendly overviews of the dominant beliefs and practices of the major cultural groups cared for by the medical center staff. Examples of the types of information included in the clues are essential information about the cultural group's perception of illness, how medical decisions are made, how prognostic information should be handled, and cultural norms about touch and modesty, among others. Culture clues have been developed for the care of African American, Albanian, American Indian/Alaska Native, Chinese, Korean, Latino, Russian, Somali, and Vietnamese patients, as well as deaf and hard-of-hearing patients. They are available on the Internet at www.depts.washington.edu/pfes/cultureclues.html. An additional case presentation is included in **Box 20-8.**

BOX 20-7
Key Questions Used to Explore Cultural Groups: PIDCCRCFDP

Partners in delivering culturally competent research-based care for diverse populations

- **P**erceptions: How are health and illness defined?
- **I**nterpersonal behavior: Does the cultural group have particular norms for interpersonal behavior regarding beliefs about touch, eye contact, personal space, modesty, sexuality, or others?
- **D**ecision-making: Who makes health-care decisions?
- **C**ommunication needs: Be particularly sensitive to how the patients wish to be addressed and to how and by whom health-care information is communicated (see Box 20–6).
- **C**omplementary medicine: What are the group's folk medicine beliefs and practices to maintain wellness and to treat illness or injury? Explore their use of complementary and alternative medicine.
- **R**eligion/spirituality: To what extent does spirituality or religious belief affect health-care beliefs and practices (e.g., specific dietary practices, prayer rituals, and such)?
- **C**are: What are the patient's expectations for the outcomes of health and illness care? What cultural preferences and practices does the patient wish to have incorporated into his or her plan of care (e.g., the diet of some Chinese patients may include the use of selected foods or herbs to maintain a balance between complementary forces [yin and yang] of hot and cold, light and dark)? Is this the patient's first formal experience with receiving care in a structured health-care setting? The first experience of being cared for by an APN?
- **F**amily: What is the primary social unit—the individual, the family, or the community? What are the family and kinship structures and roles in health care?
- **D**eath and dying: Explore the meaning of and rituals associated with death and dying.
- **P**sychiatric/mental health: How are mental health issues perceived by the group?

Each of the culture clues provides the reader with additional resources about the cultural group and health care. The University of Washington also maintains a Web site called EthnoMed at www.ethnomed.org that is a treasure trove of information on different cultural groups, including the Soviet Jewish and Arab communities. The culture-specific materials include comprehensive discussion of the barriers to health care. You may also download the site's extensive EthnoMed cross cultural bibliography (Abbott et al., 2002). Diversity Rx (www.diversityrx.org) and the National Multicultural Institute (www.nmci.org) are additional useful sites.

The AHA is a rich source of cultural information that improves patient care. Two products designed to improve cultural competence in individual caregivers and health-care facilities are a toolkit for collecting race, ethnicity, and primary language information from patients and the diversity assessment tool, both retrievable from www.aha.org.

The AHA was also instrumental in the development of an Institute for Diversity in Health Management, founded in 1994, which is a nonprofit organization that works with educational institutions and health-care organizations to expand leadership opportunities for ethnic minorities in management of health care. Its Web site is: www.DiversityConnection.org. The AHA also has a particular focus on end-of-life care. A national center to improve the palliative care of patients has been established at the Mount Sinai School of Medicine in Manhattan. Known as the

> **BOX 20-8**
> ## My Name is Mr. Roberts
>
> Mr. John Roberts, a widower, was a 68-year-old black man of African American descent. Retired for 10 years, he lived independently in his private home. His civilian and military pensions allowed him to live comfortably and to meet his health-care costs. He was active in several church and community groups and expressed a high degree of satisfaction with his life. A heavy smoker for many years, he had recently agreed to enroll in a smoking cessation program in an effort to better control his hypertension. A chest x-ray examination performed during a comprehensive physical examination revealed a large, previously undetected mass in his right lung. Further testing determined that the mass was malignant and that metastases had occurred. Mr. Roberts declined any treatment, saying that he wanted to live out his remaining life as fully as possible.
>
> When his condition deteriorated to the point at which his comfort and safety were at risk, he agreed to enter a hospice home-care program. The APN coordinating Mr. Robert's care collaborated with him and his son in ensuring that all aspects of his physical and psychosocial needs were respected and met. Late in the terminal phase of his illness, Mr. Roberts fell and fractured his right hip, necessitating hospitalization. In the hospital, he was frequently addressed by his first name, especially by younger staff members. Despite his repeated admonishment that his name was Mr. Roberts, many of the staff persisted in calling him John.
>
> Mr. Roberts died while hospitalized. He had been brought up in a traditional home in which older persons were addressed by their last name by all except family members and close friends. Younger individuals never presumed to call an older person by their first name. To do so would have been considered disrespectful and rude.
>
> An accident denied the fulfillment of Mr. Robert's wish to die at home. However, the indignities that he experienced while hospitalized were totally preventable, had his caregivers been more respectful of his communication needs.

Center to Advance Palliative Care (CAPC), it receives funding from multiple sources, including major funding from the Robert Wood Johnson Foundation. The CAPC (www.capc.org) has a broad mission ranging from developing and achieving consensus on best practices in palliative care to increasing the number of hospitals capable of providing high-quality palliative care. A stated goal of the center is to make such care standard practice in the delivery of comprehensive, hospital-based patient care.

For assistance in meeting the psychologic needs of your patients, the American Psychological Association (APA) has an extensive collection of resources, among them guidelines for psychologic counseling of multicultural populations (APA, 2002). It is available at www.apa.org. Although some of APA's materials are restricted to use by their members, the APA offers a wide variety of materials to help health-care professionals better meet the needs of their patients, ranging from resources on elder abuse and the psychologic issues faced by gays, lesbians, and bisexuals to information on the recognition and care of patients with trauma-related stress.

Finally, honesty is the best policy. If you are unsure whether your approach to a patient is culturally appropriate, acknowledge your unfamiliarity with the patient's cultural norms and ask for guidance in how to best deliver care. Most patients perceive this as being a thoughtful response to their right to respect and will be happy to help inform you. They may become your best teacher. It will enhance their trust in you and allow you to provide care until you research additional information on the patient's cultural group.

Communication

Communication is a critical element in the self- and institutional-assessment process. It encompasses provider-patient communication in all its forms, from assessment to patient education, counseling, and documentation. How do you assess a patient or community whose primary language is other than English? What tools or personnel are at your disposal to facilitate assessment, intervention, and teaching? What is your own level of proficiency in languages other than English? Linguistic competence is essential to quality patient care. With our multicultural patient populations, most of us are, or soon will be, linguistically challenged. This becomes a practice issue only if we ignore the need and make no attempt to modify our practice environment to meet the comprehensive needs of our patient base. Multiple texts and computer-based programs exist to develop basic foreign language skills.

Patient teaching raises major ethical issues regarding equality of treatment. Whether the patient is an individual, family, or community, the vast majority of patient education materials are available primarily in English. A substantial number have also been translated into Spanish. For most other languages, the practitioner depends on translators or English-speaking family members to assist in the education process. The availability of these supports may be limited, and as we know, patients need supplemental materials to reinforce direct teaching, especially if the patient is anxious or the encounter is hurried. Cost-containment efforts focus on increased staff productivity, which translates into more patients in less time. This, coupled with a linguistic barrier to teaching, is a recipe for a poor outcome. Collaborative decision making with your patients, a defining characteristic of advanced nursing practice, mandates the ability to communicate effectively. Advocacy begins in your own practice environment, with your own patients. You have an ethical and legal obligation to work toward ensuring equality in the treatment of all patients. The National Institute of Diabetes and Digestive and Kidney Diseases Web site, at: www.niddk.nih.gov/health/spanish.htm, is an example of a site that can provide a fairly extensive listing of patient education materials that are available in Spanish, as well as English in urologic health, kidney disease, diabetes, and digestive diseases. Many of the materials are in portable document format (pdf) and may be downloaded and reproduced. Another helpful resource is the Babel Fish Translation Service (www.babelfish.altavista.com). The latter resource allows you to input up to 150 words per entry, which can then be translated into multiple languages ranging from Spanish to Japanese and Korean. A word of caution, however: The "*translation*" may only be a rough approximation of the English content that you entered. It is helpful if you want to translate basic patient instructions such as—"Do not eat for 8 hours before your blood tests," but in most cases a translator who is proficient in the language should review the material obtained from this source before you give it to patients. As the provider, you are ultimately responsible for the accuracy of the patient education materials that you use.

Many additional organizations and concerned individuals are actively engaged in addressing health literacy. Two of the most innovative resources now available to APNs are The Asian American Diabetes Initiative (AADI) www.aadi.joslin.harvard.edu) offered by the Joslin Diabetes Center and "The Debilitator." The ADDI has developed a wide range of teaching-learning tools, ranging from video clips to its interactive Asian Wok, which teaches the viewers how to calculate the caloric value, fat, and sodium content of Asian recipes and commonly used foods. Materials developed by the AADI may be found on the Internet at: www.aadi.joslin.harvard.edu. "The Debilitator," developed by African American independent filmmaker Maurice Madden, is a 30-minute DVD designed to increase awareness of the devastating effects of diabetes in the black community. "The Debilitator" won a 2006 "Life Making a Difference in Diabetes Award" and is available through the National Diabetes Education Program (NDEP) available at: www.ndep.nih.gov (Chwedyk, 2007).

Another thought for consideration is your indirect role as a nurse researcher. Do you, or the institutions with which you are affiliated, conduct evaluation research to determine whether you are accomplishing desired patient outcomes in your area of specialty practice? Would it be interesting to collect and analyze outcomes data and not only compare the relative efficacy of the different types of practitioners, but also to examine outcomes as a function of patient cultural groupings, primary languages spoken and read, and other factors? Outcomes data from evaluation research are often the catalyst for bringing about organizational change.

Professional Accreditation and Legal Considerations

Commitment to the provision of culturally competent care is an integral component of advanced practice nursing, as reflected in *Nursing: scope and standards of practice* (ANA, 2004). The document reemphasizes the client's right to self-determination, privacy, confidentiality, full and truthful disclosure, and care that is respectful and inclusive of their cultural beliefs and practices. The client advocacy role of the nurse is stressed, as is the importance of empowering the patient for effective clinical decision making and self-care.

In addition to the professional imperative, three other major external forces mandate that APNs be culturally competent. Of most immediate importance are the legal implications of failing to practice in a culturally appropriate manner. The care that is documented in a patient's clinical record is a direct reflection of your practice. If cultural and linguistic barriers exist between you and your patients and you have not taken action to address these in your history taking, clinical decision making, and patient education, treatment failure and adverse outcomes may well occur. From a legal perspective, what is not documented has not been done. In our increasingly litigious society, failure to document culturally appropriate care may well serve as an ethical and legal indictment of your practice with very real professional repercussions.

Individual and organizational and system vulnerability to legal action may also result from failure to comply with the provisions of Section 601 of Title VI of the Civil Rights Act of 1964, as amended, 42 U.S.C. §2000d et seq. which provides that:

> *No person in the United States shall, on the ground of race, color, or national origin, be excluded from participation, be denied the benefits of, or be subjected to discrimination under any program or activity receiving Federal financial assistance [emphasis by this author] (U.S. Department of Justice [USDOJ], Civil Rights Division, 1998).*

Previous court decisions involving Title VI have employed the Fourteenth Amendment's standard of proof of intentional discrimination, as well as Title VI's requirement for demonstration of "disparate impact." Health-care institutions receiving federal assistance whose programs or policies discriminate against particular cultural groups are liable to be held accountable under the provisions of Title VI. For example, the Supreme Court has held that undocumented aliens fulfill the definition of "persons" in the context of the Fifth and Fourteenth Amendments to the Constitution of the United States. As such, they are by extension, included under the protections afforded by Title VI. Keep in mind that federal assistance has been broadly defined as encompassing not only direct financial assistance, but also forms of indirect aid such as subsidies, loans of federal personnel, and federal training (USDOJ, Civil Rights Division, 1998).

On August 11, 2000, Executive Order 13166 was issued: "Improving Access to Services for Persons with Limited English Proficiency." The Executive Order required any federal agency that funded any nonfederal program(s), publish guidance to recipients of such funding as to how they could comply with the provisions Title VI which forbid "restrict[ing] an individual in any way in the enjoyment of any advantage or privilege enjoyed by others receiving any service, financial aid, or other benefit under the program" or from "utiliz[ing] criteria or methods of administration which have the effect of subjecting individuals to discrimination because of their race, color, or national origin, or have the effect of defeating or substantially impairing accomplishment of the objectives of the program as respects individuals of a particular race, color, or national origin" (USDHHS, 2004, p. 2).

In response to the Executive Order, the USDHHS issued a guidance document for its own recipients of funding on August 30, 2000. During the time period that various federal agencies were developing such guidance and seeking public comment and input, the United States Department of Justice (USDOJ) was developing criteria by which both recipients and federal agencies funding external programs could assess their compliance with the provisions of the Executive Order. To minimize confusion and maximize compliance across all federal agencies, adoption of the uniform criteria established by the USDOJ was encouraged. The current regulatory guidelines of the USDHHS went into effect in October of 2004. Limited English proficiency (LEP) persons are defined as:

Individuals who do not speak English as their primary language and who have a limited ability to read, write, speak, or understand English may be limited English proficient, or "LEP," and may be eligible to receive language assistance with respect to a particular type of service, benefit, or encounter (p. 27).

The guidelines identify the types of USDHHS recipients who must comply with the provisions of Title VI, as well as identifying four criteria that programs and institutions can use to determine the level of resources that must be invested to ensure compliance. Examples of recipients range from hospitals and nursing homes to state Medicaid programs, Head Start Programs, managed care programs, state, county, and local health agencies, and providers who receive financial assistance from the USDHHS. The four criteria are: (a) The number or proportion of LEP persons eligible to be served or likely to be encountered by the program or grantee; (b) the frequency with which LEP individuals come in contact with the program; (c) the nature and importance of the program, activity, or service provided by the program to people's lives; and (d) the resources available to the grantee/recipient and costs (USDHHS, 2004).

TJC is increasingly incorporating culturally and linguistically appropriate care as a key element in the accreditation standards that are used in their institutional evaluation process. The overview to TJC 2007 requirements related to ethics, rights and responsibilities states: "Patients/residents/clients deserve care, treatment, and services that safeguard their personal dignity and respect their cultural, psychosocial, and spiritual values. These values often influence the patient/resident/client's perceptions and needs. By understanding and respecting these values, providers can meet care, treatment, and service needs and preferences."

In support of health-care institutions accredited by, or seeking TJC accreditation, the organization has developed materials to assist institutions in implementing culturally congruent care, especially as it relates to spirituality and pain management. TJC recommends that the minimum data set for assessment of a patient's spirituality include their denomination (if any), beliefs, and important spiritual practices. The standards require that the organization define the elements and breadth of its spiritual assessment of patients, as well as the qualifications of the practitioners conducting the assessment. In an effort to assess the potential impact of patients' spiritual beliefs on care requirements and service delivery, TJC has made available examples of questions that may improve the spiritual assessment process. Although the following elements are not formally required in the standards, they serve as a useful tool for institutions seeking to be more responsive to their patients' spiritual needs (TJC, 2004). The reader is referred to **Box 20-9.**

> **BOX 20-9**
> **Sample Questions for Spiritual Assessment**
>
> - Who or what provides the patient with strength and hope?
> - Does the patient use prayer in his or her life?
> - How does the patient express his or her spirituality?
> - How would the patient describe his or her philosophy of life?
> - What type of spiritual or religious support does the patient desire?
> - What is the name of the patient's clergy, ministers, chaplains, pastor, or rabbi?
> - What does suffering mean to the patient?
> - What does dying mean to the patient?
> - What are the patient's spiritual goals?
> - Is there a role of church or synagogue in the patient's life?
> - How does faith help the patient cope with illness?
> - How does the patient keep going day after day?
> - What helps the patient get through this health-care experience?
> - How has illness affected the patient and his or her family?
>
> Adapted from TJC, 2004.

Although one may quibble with the noninclusive and abstract language of some of these questions (e.g., for many patients, their place of worship is neither a church nor a synagogue), the intent to promote more comprehensive spiritual assessment of patients is clear and is to be commended. The questions are equally applicable to inpatient and ambulatory settings, although some of the questions may need to be rephrased to increase their clarity. If we have this level of information about the role of spirituality in our patients' lives and their perception of health and illness, our ability to individualize their care is taken to new heights.

NEXT STEPS

A landmark study, published in the *Journal of the American Medical Association* (Mundinger et al., 2000) reported the results of a randomized trial conducted between August 1995 and October 1997 in which medical outcomes, patient satisfaction, laboratory test results, and service use of 1,316 urban patients who had no regular source of care were reviewed to compare nurse practitioner ($n = 806$) and physician ($n = 510$) outcomes. Patient outcomes were comparable. In fact, for patients with hypertension, diastolic values were significantly lower for the group of patients managed by the nurse practitioner than for the physicians' patients.

Studies, such as the one cited previously, are leading even major financial publications to tout the advantages of using APNs. Kiplinger's Retirement Report carried an article, "Nurse Practitioners for Routine Health Care," encouraging readers to seriously consider using a nurse practitioner for their routine health care. In addition to citing the demonstrated comparability of physician and nurse practitioner care, the article speaks to the quality of nurse practitioner-patient relationships, stating, "Another plus of using nurse practitioners is that they typically spend more time with patients than doctors and often develop closer relationships" (Nurse Practitioners for Routine Health Care, 2002, p. 18).

I submit that the defining characteristic that has led to widespread use of APNs across multiple care settings and earned them unparalleled patient acceptance is their ability to truly partner with their patients to provide care that the patient perceives as being respectful and inclusive of his or her uniqueness as a human being. That patients value this level of caring is incontrovertible, as evidenced by the success of nurse-midwives. They not only provide outstanding gynecological and obstetrical care to some of our nation's most vulnerable populations, but are often selected as the preferred care provider by women who can afford any provider.

Dr. Nancy Dickenson-Hazard, who recently stepped down as the CEO of Sigma Theta Tau International, after 14 years of exemplary leadership, wrote of the excellence with which her care provider, a nurse practitioner, employed evidence-based practice in a truly collaborative partnership with her patients. Writing of her care experience, she says:

> As a consumer, I felt so informed, so empowered to make decisions and so cared for as a whole person that it reignited and renewed my commitment to evidence-based practice as the standard of care. . . . The nurse who invests his or her intellect, expertise and emotion in the patient creates a therapeutic, welcoming environment. Blending these traits with active engagement of the patient and family in decisions while addressing their uniqueness through creativity and innovation fosters trust, respect and caring (Dickenson-Hazard, 2002).

The demand for our services accelerates. The delivery of culturally congruent care is mandated by the ethical standards of our profession, as well as by legal and accreditation requirements. What remains is for us as individual APNs and collectively as practitioners within a variety of health-care institutions, to consistently practice in a manner that differentiates us from other health-care providers. In 2001, the IOM's report outlined 10 basic rules for improving health care and minimizing medical errors. Five of the IOM's recommendations are particularly relevant to advanced nursing practice and encompass the care characteristics that we claim to demonstrate in our practices. They are the following:

- Care is based on continuous healing relationships.
- Care is customized according to patient needs and values.
- The patient is the source of control.
- Decision making is evidenced based.
- Needs are anticipated.

The IOM's recommendations are a prescription for success. Our patients deserve nothing less. The rest is up to you.

References

Abbott, P. D., Short, E., Dodson, S., Garcia, C., Perkins, J., & Wyant, S. (2002). Improving your cultural awareness with culture clues. *Nurse Practitioner, 27*(2), 44–47, 51.

Agency for Healthcare Research and Quality. (2007a). *Health literacy program brief.* Rockville, MD: U.S. Department of Health and Human Services, Agency for Healthcare Research and Quality. Retrieved November 19, 2007, from the Agency for Healthcare Research and Quality Web site: www.ahrq.gov.

Agency for Healthcare Research and Quality. (2007b). *2007 National healthcare disparities report* (AHRQ Pub. No. 08-0041). Rockville, MD: U.S. Department of Health and Human Services, Agency for Healthcare Research and Quality.

Aguirre, A. C., Ebrahim, N., & Shea, J. A. (2005). Performance of the English and Spanish S-TOFHLA among publicly insured Medicaid and Medicare patients. *Patient Education and Counseling, 56*(3), 332–339.

American Hospital Association. (1992). *A patient's bill of rights.* Retrieved July 6, 2002, from American Hospital Association Web site: www.hospitalconnect.com/aha/about/pbillofrights.com.

American Hospital Association. (2003). *The patient care partnership.* Retrieved March 10, 2008, from the American Hospital Association Web site: www.aha.org/aha/content/2003/pdf/pcp english_030730.pdf.

American Nurses Association. (2001). *Code of ethics for nurses with interpretive statements* (Publication No. CEN21). Silver Spring, MD: American Nurses Publishing.

American Nurses Association. (2004). *Nursing: Scope and standards of practice* (Pub No. 03SSNP). Silver Spring, MD: American Nurses Publishing.

American Psychological Association. (2002). *Guidelines on multicultural education, training, research, practice and organizational change for psychologists.* Washington, DC: Author.

Barnes, J. S., & Bennett, C. E. (2002). *Census 2000 brief: The Asian population 2000.* Washington, DC: U.S. Census Bureau.

Bass, P. F., Wilson, J. F., & Griffith, C. H. (2003). A shortened instrument for literacy screening. *Journal of General Internal Medicine, 18*(12), 1036–1038.

Cancer Awareness Network for Immigrant Minority Populations. (2004, Winter/Spring). *Newsletter.* New York: New York University Center for Immigrant Health.

Chen, L. A., Santos, S., Jandorf, L., Christie, J., Castillo, A., Winkel, G., et al. (2008). A program to enhance completion of screening colonoscopy among urban minorities. *Clinical Gastroenterology and Hepatology, 6*(4), 443–450.

Christie, J., Itzkowitz, S., Lihau-Nkanza, I., Castillo, A., Redd, W., & Jandorf, L. (2008). A randomized controlled trial using patient navigation to increase colonoscopy screening among low-income minorities. *Journal of the National Medical Association, 100*(3), 278–284.

Chwedyk, P. (2007). Targeted tools: Resources for creating culturally competent diabetes interventions. *Minority Nurse, 16*(1), 34.

Cross, T. L. Bazron, B. J., Dennis, K. W., Isaac, M. R., and Campinha-Bacote, J. (1989). *Towards a cultural competent system of care: A monograph on effective services to minority children who are severely emotionally disturbed.* Washington, DC: Georgetown University Child Development Center, CASSP Technical Assistance Center.

Davis, T. C., Wolf, M. S., Arnold, C. L., Byrd, R. S., Long, S. W., Springer, T., et al. (2006). Development and validation of the rapid estimate of adolescent literacy in medicine (REALM-Teen): A tool to screen adolescents for below-grade reading in health care settings. *Pediatrics, 118*(6), 1707–1714.

Dickenson-Hazard, N. (2002). Evidence-based practice 'the right approach'. *Reflections on Nursing Leadership, 28,* 5.

Frost, R. (1961). *You come too.* New York: Holt, Rinehart and Winston.

Goode, T., Jones, W., & Mason, J. (2002). *A guide to planning and implementing cultural competence organization self-assessment.* Washington, DC: National Center for Cultural Competence, Georgetown University Child Development Center.

GovTrack. (2005). U.S. H.R. 1812-109th Congress. *Patient Navigator Outreach and Chronic Disease Prevention Act of 2005.* Retrieved March 10, 2008, from the Gov Track Web site: www.govtrack.us.

Guerra, C. E., Krumholz, M., & Shea, J. A. (2005). Literacy and knowledge, attitudes and behavior about mammography in Latinas. *Journal of Health Care for the Poor and Underserved, 16*(2), 152–156.

Hasnain-Wynia, R., Pierce, D., Haque, A., Hedges-Greising, C., Prince, V., & Reiter, J. (2007). *Health research and educational trust disparities toolkit.* Retrieved March 8, 2008, from the Health Research and Education Trust Disparities Web site: www.hretdisparities.org.

Henry J. Kaiser Foundation. (2005). *Number of diabetes deaths per 100,000 population by race/ethnicity.* Retrieved April 9, 2008, from the State Health Facts Web site: www.statehealthfacts.org.

Hsu, W. C., Cheung, S., Ong, E., Wong, K., Lin, S., Leon, K., et al. (2006). Identification of linguistic barriers to diabetes knowledge and glycemic control in Chinese Americans with diabetes. *Diabetes Care, 29*(2), 415–416.

Institute of Medicine. (2001). *Crossing the quality chasm: A new health system for the 21st century.* Retrieved February 20, 2008, from National Academies Press Web site: www.nap.edu/catalog/10027.html.

Jackson, L. E. (1993). Understanding, eliciting and negotiating clients' multicultural health beliefs. *Nurse Practitioner, 18*(4), 30–32, 37–38, 41–43.

Kutner, M., Greenberg, E., & Baer, J. (2003). *2003 National assessment of adult literacy.* Washington, DC: U.S. Department of Education, Institute of Education Sciences, National Center for Education Statistics.

Leininger, M. M. (1991). *Ethnonursing: A research method with enablers to study the theory of culture care.* New York: National League for Nursing.

Leininger, M. M. (2001). *Culture care diversity and universality—A theory of nursing.* Boston: Jones and Bartlett.

Lewin, M. E., Altman, S. (Eds.). (2000). *America's health care safety net: Intact but endangered.* Washington, DC: Institute of Medicine of the National Academies.

MacDorman, M. F., Callaghan, W. M., Mathews, T. J., Hoyert, D. L., & Kochanek, K. D. (2007). *Trends in preterm-related infant mortality by race and ethnicity: United States, 1999–2004.* Hyattsville, MD: US Department of Health and Human Services, CDC, National Center for Health Statistics.

Mathews, T. J., & MacDorman, M. F. (2007). Infant mortality statistics from the 2004 period linked birth/infant death data set. *National Vital Statistics Reports, 55*(15). Hyattsville, MD: National Center for Health Statistics.

Mundinger, M. O., Kane, R. L., Lenz, E. R., Totten, A. M., Twai, W. Y., Cleary, P. D., et al. (2000). Primary care outcomes in patients treated by nurse practitioners or physicians: a randomized trial. *Journal of the American Medical Association, 283*(1), 59–68.

New growth charts a welcome improvement. (2002). *Clinician Reviews, 12,* 75.

Nielsen-Bohlman, L., Panzer, A. M., & Kindig, D. A. (Eds.). (2004). *Health literacy: A prescription to end confusion.* Washington, DC: Institute of Medicine of the National Academies.

Nurse practitioners for routine health care. (2002). *Kiplinger's Retirement Report, 9,* 13.

Parker, R. M., Ratzan, S. C., & Lurie, N. (2003). Health literacy: A policy challenge for advancing high-quality health care. *Health Affairs, 22*(4), 147–153.

Ratzan, S. C., Parker, R. M. (2000). Introduction. In C. R. Selden, M. Zorn, S. C. Ratzan, and R. M. Parker (Eds.), *National Library of Medicine current bibliographies in medicine: Health literacy* (NLM Pub. No. CBM 2000-1). Bethesda, MD: National Institutes of Health, U.S. Department of Health and Human Services, p. 5.

Razak, F., Anand, S. S., Shannon, H., Vuksan, V., Davis, B., Jacobs, R., et al. (2007). Defining obesity cut points in a multiethnic population. *Circulation: Journal of the American Heart Association, 115,* 2111–2118.

Rodriguez, B. L., Fujimoto, W. Y., Mayer-Davis, E. J., Imperatore, G., Williams, D. E., Bell R. A., et al. (2006). Prevalence of cardiovascular disease risk factors in U.S. children and adolescents with diabetes. *Diabetes Care, 29*(8),1891–1896.

Selden, C. R., Zorn, M., Ratzan, S. C., & Parker, R. M. (2000). *National Library of Medicine current bibliographies in medicine: health literacy* (NLM Pub. No. CBM 2000-1). Bethesda, MD: National Institutes of Health, U.S. Department of Health and Human Services.

The Joint Commission. (2004). *Spiritual assessment (Revised 01-01-04).* Retrieved March 30, 2008, from The Joint Commission Web site: www.jointcommission.org/AccreditationPrograms/Hospitals/Standards.

The Joint Commission. (2007). *The Joint Commission 2007 requirements related to the provision of culturally and linguistically appropriate health care: Version 2007-1, May 2007.* Division of Standards and Survey Methods, The Joint Commission. Retrieved March 30, 2008, from The Joint Commission Web site: www.jointcommission.org.

U.S. Census Bureau. (2000). Census, PHC-T-1: Table 3: Population by race alone, race in combination only, race alone or in combination, and Hispanic or Latino origin, for the United States: 2000. Retrieved March 10, 2008, from the U.S. Census Bureau Web site: www.census2000/phc-t1/tab04.pdf.

U.S. Census Bureau. (2006a). American Community Survey. B02001: Race—Universe: Total population. *Data set: 2006 American Community Survey.* Retrieved March 10, 2008, from U.S. Census Bureau Web site: www.factfinder.census.gov.

U.S. Census Bureau. (2006b). R0204: Percent of the total population who are Asian alone. *Data set: 2006 American Community Survey.* Retrieved March 10, 2008, from U.S. Census Bureau Web site: www.factfinder.census.gov.

U.S. Census Bureau. (2006c). S0501: Selected characteristics of the native and foreign-born populations. *Data set: 2006 American Community Survey.* Retrieved March 10, 2008, from the U.S. Census Bureau Web site: www.factfinder.census.gov.

U.S. Census Bureau. (2006d). S1501: Educational attainment. *Data set: 2006 American Community Survey.* Retrieved March 10, 2008, from the U.S. Census Bureau Web site: www.factfinder.census.gov.

U.S. Census Bureau. (2006e). S1702: Poverty status in the past 12 months of families. *Data set: 2006 American Community Survey.* Retrieved March 10, 2008, from the U.S. Census Bureau Web site: www.factfinder.census.gov.

U.S. Department of Health and Human Services, Maternal and Child Health Bureau. (1999). *Guidance for SPRANS grant.* Washington, DC: Health Resources and Services Administration, U.S. Department of Health and Human Services.

U.S. Department of Health and Human Services. (2000a). *Healthy People 2010: Understanding and improving health* (Volume I, Conference edition). Washington, DC: Author.

U.S. Department of Health and Human Services. (2004) *Guidance to federal financial assistance recipients regarding Title VI prohibition against national origin discrimination affecting limited English proficient persons* (Revised). Washington, DC: Author.

U.S. Department of Health and Human Services. (2008). *Health resources and services administration justification of estimates for appropriations committees for fiscal year 2009.* Washington. DC: Health Resources and Services Administration, U.S. Department of Health and Human Services. Retrieved March 21, 2008, from the Health Resources and Services Administration Web site: www.hrsa.gov/about/budgetjustification09.

U.S. Department of Justice, Civil Rights Division. (1998). *Title VI legal manual.* Retrieved March 21, 2008, from the U.S. Department of Justice Web site: www.usdoj.gov/crt/grants_statutes/legalman.html.

Wallace, L. 2006. Patients' health literacy skills: The missing demographic variable in primary care research. *Annals of Family Medicine, 4*(1), 85–86.

Conflict Resolution: An Essential Competency in Advanced Practice

Phyllis Beck Kritek

Lucille A. Joel

Conflict happens. Few nurses find this startling news, and most nurses can, with little effort, describe in detail several conflicts currently swirling about them in their daily practice. As scope of practice expands, so do the conflicts nurses face. This chapter explores that reality, and its implications for the nurse facing the challenges of advanced practice. It also posits that expanding conflict resolution competency is an opportunity to improve our work environments, and a choice worth making.

Conflict resolution, also called alternative dispute resolution (ADR), is a relatively young but burgeoning academic discipline developing a sophisticated body of literature, including formal research, best practices commentary, compelling case histories, and evocative emerging theories. As such, it provides a rich array of insights for persons confronted with conflict in their work situations. Interestingly, the discipline has only minimally explored the use of ADR in health care. Were it to do so, it would find a gold mine.

Because the ADR community has had limited involvement within health-care environments, most health-care professionals also have limited information about ADR. In addition, early efforts to address health-care conflicts tended to focus on malpractice, union disputes, and other structural conflicts that may have seemed remote to the practicing nurse. Yet even a casual assessment of health-care environments reveals the central role conflict plays in the daily life of the practicing nurse. Recent studies about the dissatisfactions of nurses clearly support the centrality of such conflict. Some examples may help.

The June 2002 issue of the *American Journal of Nursing* reported on a survey about nurse-physician relationships in Voluntary Hospitals of America (VHA) on the West Coast, part of a national network of community-owned hospitals and health-care systems (Rosenstein, 2002). Reporting on the analysis of the first 1,200 responses to the survey, Rosenstein, himself a physician, reports that "although all respondents saw a direct link between disruptive physician behavior and nurse satisfaction and retention," the three respondent groups of administrators, physicians, and nurses differed in their beliefs about the outcomes of these conflictual situations (p. 26). Nurses scored the administrative support they received in nurses' conflicts with physicians significantly lower than either administrators or physicians. Their lowest rating in the study, also statistically significant, was their reported perception of physician support in nurse-physician conflict. Nurses do not feel supported in such conflicts, either by their bosses or by physicians. They also fear retribution and do not believe that physician counseling processes are adequate. Research has shown that patient outcomes are adversely affected by team conflict. Coworker interactions are among the most essential to quality of care. Effective teamwork becomes even more critical as care becomes more complex (Baker Gustafson, Beaubien, Salas, & Barach, 2005).

These findings substantiate some significant job dissatisfiers for nurses, that is, reasons they may leave practice and never return. They are more compelling when juxtaposed with the growing body of literature focusing on the importance of registered nurses to quality patient care and their impact on outcomes. By way of example, concurrent with Rosenstein's study, *The New England Journal of Medicine* published two related articles. Needleman, Buerhaus, Mattke, Stewart, and Zelevinsky (2002) reported on a nurse-staffing levels and quality-of-care study that concluded that "a higher proportion of hours of nursing care provided by registered nurses and a greater number of hours of care provided by registered nurses per day are associated with better care for hospitalized patients" (p. 1716). Steinbrook (2002), a physician, provided his analysis of the current nursing shortage. He noted that many of the tensions currently shaping the health-care environment "will be difficult, if not impossible, to resolve" (p. 64). He then offered an example of a path to better care as one linked to nurses with advanced education. Steinbrook stated, "Such a workforce, however, would expect more responsibility and greater independence and would be more expensive to hire and retain" (p. 64). This statement sets the stage for advanced practice nurses (APNs) and development of skills in conflict resolution as part of the required course of studies.

Knickle and McNaughton (2008) find nurses are statistically more active and effective in resolving conflict with clients and students than we are with peers. These researchers have incorporated simulations and components of role-playing and role reversal in learning conflict resolution skills, allowing the participants to move from adversarialism to an effective dialogue with their simulated colleague. The results have been positive, but require more investigation of the retention of these skills and long-term application in the real world. This represents one piece of research that is contributing to a body of knowledge comparing classroom-based techniques with simulations in teaching conflict resolution strategies.

These examples point toward some of the inherent glitches in health-care environments today and strategies that offer hope. Conflict is a reality, and it is guaranteed to be an escalating and intensifying phenomena. Avoiding conflict is simply not an option, so we had best learn how to understand and deal with it.

CONFLICT MANAGEMENT STRATEGIES OF NURSES

The issue of conflict avoidance is critical. Valentine (2001) reported a synthesis of research findings about nurses' conflict management strategies as identified by use of the Thomas-Kilmann Index (TKI). The TKI is a conflict mode index that identifies preferred conflict management strategies from a set of five options: avoiding, compromising, collaborating, competing, and accommodating. Eight studies were analyzed.

Two conflict strategies were used predominantly by all categories of nurses: avoiding and compromising. The third strongest preference was for accommodation. These findings are sobering because avoiding and accommodating lead to outcomes in which one disadvantages oneself. Compromising runs a weak second because in this strategy all parties are equally disadvantaged. The remaining two strategies least often used by nurses, collaborating and competing, are the only strategies that ensure some type of gains for oneself. Richard Shell (1999), the director of the Wharton Executive Negotiation Workshop, observes, "Among the professional groups I have taught, hospital nurses are characteristically accommodating. Sometimes this works well for them. But they can also get squeezed between the demands of angry patients and impatient, authoritative physicians" (p. 12). A similar observation is made by Kelly (2006), who sees conflict within the nursing profession as traditionally generating negative feelings.

Taback and Orit (2007) studied the effect that different ways of resolving conflicts have on those involved. They examined the tactics nurses adopt to resolve conflicts with doctors and how these tactics affect their level of stress and job satisfaction. What they have called the integrating (collaborating) and dominance (competing) approaches to conflict resolution are associated with low occupational stress levels, whereas the obliging (compromising and accommodating) and avoidance approaches are linked to higher stress. In this study, there was evidence that the seniority and status of nurses drive both their choice of tactics and the associated stress and satisfaction levels. Similar outcomes were found in a study that focused on the occurrence of conflict in an assisted living facility and nursing home and how staff as compared to residents of each handled the situation. Results indicate that staff in each care context showed a preference for a solution-oriented approach, whereas residents reported an equal use of nonconfrontational and solution-oriented approaches. The authors propose that the conflict resolution style may vary most as a function of the role of the communicator (Small & Montoro-Rodriguez, 2006). Do not residents often see themselves as being at the mercy of staff, powerless and unsupported in their interpersonal disputes?

In a recent study by Siu, Spence Laschinger, and Finnegan (2008), investigators identified a link between the nurses' perception of the quality of their practice environment and their self-evaluation to success in conflict resolution. A positive professional practice environment and a high self-evaluation explained over 46% of the variability in nurses' constructive conflict management and effectiveness of the solutions. Put simply, if you see yourself as a skilled participant in a quality work environment, you have a good chance of resolving disputes in an effective manner.

Hence, we find that although the levels of conflict in health-care environments, and quite specifically those faced by nurses, are indeed escalating, the strategies nurses are using are often those most likely to ensure an undesirable outcome. As the shortages deepen and as nurses seek advanced practice responsibilities, this troublesome state of affairs will quite readily worsen. Increasing one's scope of competence, expertise, and authority is actually a sufficient catalyst to increasing one's exposure to conflicts.

It would seem nursing is at something of a crossroads in relationship to conflict and the possibilities of ADR. Reframing our options and learning new strategies appears to be in our best interest, and probably, therefore, also in the best interest of those for whom we care. Becoming a skillful manager of conflict is a goal that would wisely replace our naïve embrace of conflict avoidance and delimiting compromise.

A simple literature review indicates that there is a growing consciousness about this concern. Five years ago, the *Cumulative Index to Nursing and Allied Health Literature* identified few sources connected with the terms *conflict* and *conflict resolution*. Today, the listings number more than 3000. Most of these manuscripts advocate for ADR and encourage nurses to master this area. However, we do not yet have comprehensive research in this area, and the options for learning about ADR are too often incongruous with nursing's realities. There is work to be done here.

CHANGING PARADIGMS OF ALTERNATIVE DISPUTE RESOLUTION

Initial development in ADR was heavily influenced by the work done by a network of innovators at Harvard University, perhaps best exemplified by the best-selling primer on ADR, *Getting to Yes: Negotiating Agreement Without Giving In* by Roger Fisher and Bill Ury (1991). This classic in ADR sets forth the basic tenets of interest-based negotiation, an approach that encourages disputing parties to find common interests that could serve as the basis for a settlement of the conflict. Because both Fisher and Ury were part of my earliest training in ADR, it is a perspective that shaped my original understanding of the field and also evoked some degree of resistance. I have since learned that this is a resistance shared by many nurses.

Happily, the field of ADR is expanding its horizons, and supplementing this initial theoretical posture with several that probably will be experienced as more congruent with professional nursing's values and traditions. Nurses often find themselves negotiating on behalf of patients and their families. Hence, although they may be able to identify the interests of a given disputant with whom they are in conflict, trying to present their interests as "representing the patient's interests" can be viewed as offensive and presumptuous and can simply escalate the conflict. Alternatives are needed.

Bush and Folger (1994) broke new ground by positing an approach to ADR they called *transformative practice,* in which the goal shifted from interest-based settlement to empowerment and recognition of the disputing parties, a model more deliberately focused on the relational and social interaction dimensions of conflict. Others have followed. Mayer (2000), with more than 25 years of ADR experience, looks back reflectively on what he has learned and posits that communication and attitudes toward conflict are more compelling than settlement. He views ADR as a process that can help people solve their problems in ways that are not only collaborative but also just and powerful.

Winslade and Monk (2000) have recast the initial model of ADR to one congruent with postmodernity, creating a process they call *narrative mediation,* building relationships that start with story. They, too, focus on collaboration as a central dimension of hearing and understanding the stories of disputants. Cloke and Goldsmith (2000) also use stories as a central component of their approach to ADR. They posit a model of mediation that focuses on transformation and forgiveness, once more focusing on relationship.

Shell (1999), referenced previously, makes a case for switching from interest-based to information-based negotiation. He places emphasis on the uniqueness of each conflict, and actively discourages the illusion of thinking a single approach or set of guidelines can ensure mastery of ADR. He also posits that the essential attributes of an effective negotiator are "a willingness to prepare, high expectations, the patience to listen, and a commitment to personal integrity" (p. 15). His description stands in sharp contrast to many interest-based descriptions of ADR in which manipulation and cunning are covertly posited as indicators of skill.

Each of these ADR experts is providing leadership in moving away from perceiving conflicts as situations in which the personal interests of two or more parties are dissonant and require intervention and settlement. They are ushering in an alternative viewpoint, one with an emphasis on relationship building, collaboration, authenticity, and self-management. These models bode well for nurses interested in ADR.

THE WORD FROM THE TRENCHES

My personal interest in ADR emerged from a growing frustration with the negative effect of conflict in our practice settings and a personal hunger for "something better." This led me to 3 years of intensive ADR training during a Kellogg Leadership Fellowship (1986–1989). Since then, I've been involved in a variety of negotiation and mediation program initiatives, the writing of a book on the subject (Kritek, 2002), and an ever-expanding investment in training nurses in ADR. If we are going to have to manage a good deal of conflict anyway, I believed that it made sense to learn how to do it well. Hence, the lion's share of my energy in ADR has focused on training nurses throughout the United States to become more knowledgeable and competent in their management of conflict.

The training work with nurses has taught me a good deal about conflict in our times. I have done workshops all over the United States (and abroad), and I have developed some insights, and some convictions, along the way. Sharing some of each makes up the central message in this chapter. All emerge from repetitious experiences during training sessions with nurses, and hence lack formal empirical grounding. Nonetheless, their repetitiousness is instructive. Although this results in something of a "grocery list" of the following observations, it is hoped that these ideas can be catalytic in propelling APNs toward exploration and mastery of ADR and its potential for good.

- *Many nurses are extremely conflict avoidant.* Some, trying to overcome this tendency, become attacking and aggressive. Neither posture appears to meet the ADR needs of nurses and those with whom they work.
- *Many nurses want an "easy" answer to learning ADR.* They want a set of rules or guidelines that can be applied much like one applies the step-by-step process of learning how to use a new piece of equipment. Conflict is about relationship. The values that have made nursing a powerful health-care force—the respect for humans, the compassion, and the commitment— are the factors that also shape the ADR enterprise. There are no shortcuts.
- *Many nurses make snap judgments about a conflict rather than conducting a conflict analysis.* They create a quick story in their minds that explains the conflict, preferably one that casts "the other" as at fault or "in the wrong." This pattern of snap judgments short-circuits the process of ADR before it can get started. All conflicts are complex, and it takes time to really understand them.
- *Many nurses believe they should prevail in conflicts because they know that they have good motives and feel comfortable questioning the motives of others.* Others sometimes contribute to this tendency by indeed having questionable motives. Resolving conflict, however, is *not* about differentiating the good guys from the bad guys. Judgment and blaming rarely further the effort or assist in meeting the goal. The search is for common ground, points of agreement and collaboration, not the creation of moral hierarchies.
- *Many nurses hope to resolve conflicts they confront, although remaining personally unchanged by the process.* All effective conflict resolution changes the parties involved, for good or ill. It is the intent of ADR to make the outcome for the "good." Conflict unveils the dark and edgy side of all of us, and running from it can seem quite reasonable. Working hard to avoid authenticity and self-insight keeps conflicts going. Wanting to resolve them does require change, even transformation, of both oneself and one's relationships.
- *Many nurses make declarative sentences to insist on their viewpoint during a conflict.* They might more constructively ask questions that evoke from the other disputants needed information and understanding of the issues. Declarative sentences tend to lock positions; questions open avenues of thought.
- *Many nurses confuse accommodation and collaboration.* They smooth over a conflict without resolving it, only to find it will return the next day or the next week . . . with a vengeance. Part of conflict resolution is truth telling, and this means neither verbal assault nor coy innuendo, but simple candor without judgment and blaming. One has to slog through the messy part of conflict to get to a real resolution.
- *Many nurses deny or avoid recognition of the overt structured inequity designed into health-care systems in the United States.* They ignore this when it involves patients, and they deny it when it involves nurses. Many believe that to honestly face these facts will be disempowering, an admission of disadvantage. However, although persons can treat me as a victim,

it does not mean I must become one or act as one. To deny the efforts of others to diminish or victimize me usually leads to my collusion in this process. This may be difficult to accept.

■ ***Many nurses rush to settlement too quickly, eager to end the discomfort of conflict.*** Hence, they fail to look at the range of choices they have available to resolve the conflict and the consequences of each. Rather than seeing ADR as a creative process, they are eager to make it a quick process. This diminishes the outcomes and their potential for good.

■ ***Many nurses give away their personal power as a solution to keeping conflict at bay.*** They keep silent, or go along, or compromise their integrity. Somewhere, their authentic selves know that they have done this. This can enrage or depress them and make them cling even more tenaciously to their conflicts. This is a sad thing, and not seeing it in oneself is often tragic.

This list is not exhaustive, but it does capture the challenges before nurses, and the options they have to change their current conflict styles. In addition, it highlights some of the serious losses nurses are taking by their unwillingness to become conflict experts. Few disciplines are as well equipped as nursing to actually become ADR-proficient. The time has come to lay claim to this unique possibility.

RESPONDING TO THE CHALLENGE: EXERCISES IN ALTERNATIVE DISPUTE RESOLUTION

Nurses who take on expanded practice roles often experience a sense of personal satisfaction about this achievement. They tend to have worked hard to get where they are and know the path before them will evoke new professional experiences that will enhance their sense of personal satisfaction. Conflict can sometimes seem like the "spoiler," the irritating situation that distracts from the task at hand.

One thing is obvious: we as nurses can decide to become more proficient at conflict management. Having previously provided a list that essentially serves as a self-assessment inventory, the following second list of opportunities that address the inventory outcomes may prove useful. These exercises are available for APNs to improve their participation in ADR activities. This list is not exhaustive, but it does provide a "reality map" of options for the path unfolding before us.

■ Read about ADR. The reference list at the end of this chapter can be a starting point. The books that have been identified as more recent may offer paradigms of conflict management more attractive to nurses.

■ Participate in an ADR training program. There are a variety of options out there. Watch for opportunities, and sign on. Make it part of your planned continuing education.

■ Look in your phone book for available mediation programs and services available in your area. Call to find out what opportunities might be available for you.

■ Go to the Internet and search for options that might fit your needs, including additional books, programs, training options, and online courses.

■ Find an ADR mentor. Any of the resources listed previously might reveal one and give you a chance to start working with an expert.

■ Start deliberately practicing what you are learning. Take a small, easy conflict and try your new skills.

■ Systematically study your own conflict behaviors. Find out what ways you tend to engage in conflict. Keep a journal of this, if possible, to increase your self-honesty and your awareness. Determine whether your current practices are enough, and what added skills you would like to acquire.

■ Ask peers or colleagues to critique your conflict behaviors. Ask them to tell you how they see you responding to conflict. After you ask, listen carefully. Many people do not like to answer this question for fear of starting a conflict, so assure your informant of your openness before you ask.

■ Do environmental scans of your workplace. Train yourself to conduct comprehensive and objective conflict analyses, and observe the ways that your understanding of conflict shifts as you expand your understanding of a given conflict. Systematically teach yourself new modes of thought about conflict and reinforce them through practice.

■ Form a coalition with other colleagues interested in improving their conflict management skills; share learning experiences, assessments, and analyses of conflict situations. Learn from one another and *normalize* dealing with conflict as a group expectation.

This is a starter set of ideas. Any or all of them can be helpful in moving toward enhancing your conflict management skills and in accessing the many skills you currently have that can be helpful in conflict situations. You elected to prepare yourself for an APN role because you wanted to give care, not slog through conflicts. The efficient and skillful management of conflict as it emerges can ensure that you spend as much time as possible focused on your primary goal of patient care and as little time as possible on the sometimes onerous, yet often transformative task of resolving conflict.

Surprisingly, your patients are watching. They may find your new skills and competencies worthy modeling, and assuredly worthy of their trust. It is nice to know that the person taking care of you knows what to do with conflict. It increases one's sense of safety, a belief that the care provider is an advocate with the necessary ability to advocate well, even in the face of conflict.

CONCLUSION

Nurses who elect to expand their practice roles will find that along with the increased ability to deliver care, they will also confront a larger and more complex array of conflicts in their work settings. To date, nurses have not invested in increasing their ability to improve their conflict management skills. This has a deleterious effect not only on nurses, but also on other providers, and more poignantly, on patients and their families. Hence, improved mastery of ADR abilities is an idea whose time has come.

The field of ADR has minimally invested in health-care environments to date. More recent theoretical developments in the field have yielded models of ADR that show high congruence with the values and traditions of nursing. Nurses who wish to enhance their ADR competencies would be wise to first conduct an honest self-assessment of current skill levels, both acknowledging existing strengths and also identifying learning needs. Having done this, they have a wide range of options available that can be accessed as resources for further building conflict management skills. The decision to do such building benefits not only the nurse, but also all persons who come in contact with the nurse, particularly patients and their families. ADR is indeed an idea whose time has come for the nursing profession.

References

Baker, D. P., Gustafson, S., Beaubien, J. M., Salas, E., & Barach, P. (2005). Medical team training programs in health care. In *Advances in patient safety: From research to implementation. Volume 4: Programs, tools and products* (AHRQ Publication No. 05-0021-4). Rockville, MD: Agency for Healthcare Research and Quality and the Department of Defense-Health Affairs.

Bush, B. R. A., & Folger, J. P. (1994). *The promise of mediation: Responding to conflict through empowerment and recognition.* San Francisco: Jossey-Bass.

Cloke, K., & Goldsmith, J. (2000). *Resolving personal and organizational conflict.* San Francisco: Jossey-Bass.

Fisher, R., & Ury, W. (1981). *Getting to yes: Negotiating agreement without giving in*. Boston: Houghton Mifflin and Company.

Kelly, J. (2006). An overview of conflict. *Dimensions of Critical Care Nursing, 25*(1), 22–28.

Knickle, K., & McNaughton, N. (2008). Collegial conflict: Experiencing attribution theory through simulation. *Medical Education, 42*(5), 541–542.

Kritek, P. B. (2002). *Negotiating at an uneven table: Developing moral courage in resolving our conflicts* (2nd ed.). San Francisco: Jossey-Bass.

Mayer, B. (2000). *The dynamics of conflict resolution: A practitioner's guide*. San Francisco: Jossey-Bass.

Needleman, J., Buerhaus, P., Mattke, S., Stewart, M., & Zelevinsky, K. (2002). Nurse-staffing levels and the quality of care in hospitals. *New England Journal of Medicine, 346*(22), 1715–1722.

Rosenstein, A. H. (2002). Nurse-physician relationships: Impact on nurse satisfaction and retention. *American Journal of Nursing, 102*(6), 26–34.

Shell, G. R. (1999). *Bargaining for advantage: Negotiation strategies for reasonable people*. New York: Penguin Books.

Siu, H., Spence Laschinger, H. K., & Finegan, J. (2008). Nursing professional practice environments: Setting the stage for constructive conflict resolution and work effectiveness. *Journal of Nursing Administration, 38*(5), 250–257.

Small, J. A., & Montoro-Rodriguez, J. (2006). Conflict resolution styles: A comparison of assisted living and nursing home facilities. *Journal of Gerontological Nursing, 32*(6), 39–45.

Steinbrook, R. (2002). Nursing in the crossfire. *New England Journal of Medicine, 346*(22), 1757–1766.

Tabak, N., & Orit K. (2007). Relationship between how nurses resolve their conflicts with doctors, their stress and job satisfaction. *Journal of Nursing Management, 15*(3), 321–331.

Valentine, P. E. B. (2001). A gender perspective on conflict management strategies of nurses. *Journal of Nursing Scholarship, 33*(1), 69–74.

Winslade, J., & Monk, G. (2000). *Narrative mediation: A new approach to conflict resolution*. San Francisco: Jossey-Bass.

UNIT 4

Ethical, Legal, and Business Acumen

Evaluation of the Advanced Practice Nurse: Cost Efficiency, Accomplishments, Trends, and Future Development

Jane M. Flanagan

Dorothy A. Jones

INTRODUCTION

Historically, the clinical nurse specialist (CNS) and the nurse practitioner (NP) were major roles within the framework of the advanced practice nurse (APN). Nursing knowledge, knowledge from other disciplines along with specialty knowledge, including information about populations and settings further defined each APN role. With academic advancement and the requirement of the master's degree, role implementation of the APN expanded rapidly to every venue within the health-care delivery system, including large medical centers, physicians' offices, community health centers, ambulatory care clinics, and emergency rooms, as well as the traditional community and rural hospitals and clinics.

Today, APNs work with increasingly diverse populations, often in large cities and towns and remain educated at the master's level and in some cases with doctoral preparation. Historically, the advanced practice roles developed out of an identified need for continuity of care and better access to health care. In the current health-care environment, many APNs work with a variety of people, including the insured, as well as uninsured clients, in a variety of settings where access to health care is limited or is available from multiple providers, including physicians and physician assistants.

According to the International Council of Nurses (ICN; 2002) key components of the role of the APN include the integration of research, education, practice, and management; autonomy; having a direct case load; possession of advanced health assessment and decision-making and diagnostic reasoning skills; having the skill to independently consult and the aptitude to plan, implement, and evaluate programs; and having an ability to be a first point of contact for patient care. The ICN also recognizes that individual countries and states within countries have regulations limiting implementation of the full potential for APNs, including the right to diagnose, prescribe, consult, and admit in the course of patient care. Today there is increasing attention to the APN role within the United States, with some states further restricting APN practice, regulating the title of who can be considered to be an APN.

Over the years, the role of the APN has enjoyed much success. Patients, administrators, family, and physicians have all acknowledged the contributions made by nurses working as NPs, CNSs, certified nurse-midwives (CNMs), and nurse anesthetists (Horrocks, Anderson, & Salisbury, 2002; Ingersoll, McIntosh, & Williams 2000; McGee & Kaplan, 2007). Satisfaction with the communication and information sharing has been recognized as an important component of the role. The value and contributions of APNs have expanded well beyond the United States, and the APN is now a role gaining increased attention worldwide. In areas of the world where there is pandemic disease and concerns about childbirth, the demand for nurses, and especially nurse-midwives and NPs, is even more pronounced (Schober, 2006; World Health Organization, 2006).

This chapter will explore the impact of the APN on health care over the years. In addition, trends including the demands of a changing health-care environment, outcome-driven reimbursement and the demands of insurers, along with a decreased number of primary care physicians, and the impact of shifts from primary care to the role of acute care NPs managing patients in hospitals in place of physician residents and the changing work rules will be explored. A discussion of the APN role within the context of nursing science and its link to changes in advancing the clinical practice environment will be addressed.

PRACTICE SETTINGS OF THE ADVANCED PRACTICE NURSE

APNs work within a wide range of health-care settings. Whereas the CNS continues to practice primarily within the hospital, the NP role initially focused on primary care for underserved populations within the inner city, rural health care, and other nonhospital settings. The NP still provides care to patients in settings in which traditional physician providers are unavailable but has increasingly expanded in the hospital setting, often as a physician extender in disease-based specialty care (Steven, 2004). CNMs, as well as pediatric NPs, originally provided care in nontraditional settings such as the home, transition care units, and schools (American Nurses Association [ANA], 1997; American College of Nurse-Midwives, 2002), but over the last several years especially in the United States, they, too, practice in the hospital setting.

The certified nurse anesthetist role (CRNA) was developed by surgeons who desired to reduce the high mortality rates associated with anesthesia (Dexter, Macario, & Traub, 2000; Gunn, 2000). Because of their knowledge and many competencies, including biophysical and psychosocial knowledge and advanced assessment skills, surgeons recognized that these nurses were the providers who could holistically attend to the patient's needs during surgery (American Association of Nurse Anesthetists [AANA], 2002). Although there has been a rise in the number of anesthesiologists over the past 15 years, the only providers of anesthesia in many rural hospitals continue to be the CRNAs (Gunn, 2000).

The role of the CNS developed in an effort to reduce fragmentation and improve continuity of care (Reiter, 1966). The development of this role was advanced by the 1965 Nurse Training Act. With increased educational preparation, many nurses focused on advanced practice with specialized populations and worked to develop staff in the delivery of safe, cost-effective, quality care, usually within the acute care environment. The early introduction of the role in the 1960s focused on promoting continuity and quality care. Over the years, however, the impact of cost containment measures in many hospital settings has threatened the CNS role. Administrators have challenged the CNS to provide evidence that linked their care contributions to improved patient outcomes, enhanced quality of care, and cost effectiveness (Fulton, 2002).

The growth of the NP role and the challenges around merging the CNS and NP roles (Elsom & Happel, 2006) continue to challenge the CNS role. The National Association of Clinical Nurse Specialists (NACNS) was established to support and renew the growing need for expert clinicians and evidence-based practice, particularly in the acute care settings. To this end, NACNS has generated new interest in the CNS role with an increase in the number of CNSs from 69,071 in 2000 to 75, 521 in 2004 (Health Resources and Services Administration [HRSA], 2007). Many hospitals have begun hiring CNSs to develop staff; mentor a growing number of inexperienced nurses, especially during their first year in practice; increase educational opportunities for staff, patients, and families; and promote the development and use of research to inform knowledge-based patient outcomes.

CHANGES AND CHALLENGES IN HEALTH CARE

The past decade has presented many challenges to health-care organizations and the delivery of safe, quality, timely, cost-effective patient care (Institute of Medicine [IOM], 1999, 2001). Proposed plans to reform the system will have a significant impact on the APN role. Currently, the suggested reforms include an overhaul of the current health-care system with increased emphasis on (a) the need for continued cost reduction, (b) the identification of potential risks to existing and new services, and (c) vigilance and monitoring over "never events." In 2006, the National Quality Forum released a list of 28 events that they termed "serious reportable events," which are extremely rare medical errors that should never happen to a patient. Often termed *never events,* these include errors such as surgery performed on the wrong body part or on the wrong patient, leaving a foreign object inside a patient after surgery, or discharging an infant to the wrong person. See www. qualityforum.org for more information.

These suggested reforms may effect reimbursement for clinicians, as well as impact patient length of hospitalization and recovery. Since 1980, there has been emphasis placed on preparation of primary care physicians. Despite this emphasis, 75% of physicians choose specialty practice over primary care and in the years between 1999 and 2006, the trend toward specialization continued despite federal government cuts in funding for residency programs in areas of specialization (Steven, 2004).

New federal regulations, which limit the resident work week to 80 hours, have added a new burden to health-care delivery, creating a void in medical management within the acute care setting. Within this environment, NPs have recently become more visible, especially in areas of specialized care. This trend is creating added burden for the NP, often requiring them to gain additional education and competency acquisition beyond the traditional curriculum to prepare for advanced practice. Often, these new skills focus more on medical specialty knowledge, such as interpreting echocardiograms, than on advanced nursing knowledge, such as being with, listening to, and coming to know the patient as a whole and complex person and assisting them and their families in a process of informed decision making. Within the context of these challenges many nurses are learning new skills on the job to respond to the demands of the patient population they are serving. This change is shifting the focus of NP education and clinical practice away from the core of advanced nursing knowledge to skill acquisition within a medical realm, and it has caused some to question whether APNs are practicing in a way that reflects the goals of the discipline (Bryant-Lukosius, Dicenso, Browne, & Pinelli, 2004; Flanagan, 2008; Grace, 2008; Newman, Smith, Pharris, & Jones, 2008).

As the number of nurses in advanced practice continue to increase, competition for reimbursement and questions about quality of care and evidenced-based patient/family practice continue to present challenges. In addition, limited time with patients during the patient visit and reduced opportunities for follow-up due to cost constraints potentially compromise the full impact nurses can have on patient care.

THE IMPACT OF ADVANCE PRACTICE NURSES

Findings from many individual, as well as systematic, reviews of research comparing the effectiveness of APN practice as compared to the physician suggest that APNs provide care that is comparable to care provided by medical doctors. Several authors suggest that APNs can complete much of primary and preventive care more cost effectively, than care traditionally handled by physicians (Hoffman, Tasota, Zullo, Scharfenberg, & Donaue, 2005; Horrocks et al., 2002; Steven, 2004). These cost factors are associated with the sophistication they require in the places where they give care and the cost of their liability insurance and education. Many nursing studies have examined the relation of the APN to preventive care provided, actual costs incurred, patient satisfaction, hospital recidivism rates, and the actual quality and safety of care delivered. The results indicate high satisfaction for both the patient and nurse. Key components of the APN role across specialties include: direct and comprehensive patient care, support and advocacy within the health-care system, monitoring and ensuring quality of service, education, research, publication, and professional leadership (Cumbie, Conley, & Burman, 2004; Mick & Ackerman, 2000). A recent review of research suggests that research supporting APN practice is lacking.

In 2000, the American Nurses Association (ANA) identified nurse-sensitive indicators for APNs in both the acute care and community-based settings. These indicators include care related to activities around pain management, patient satisfaction, cardiovascular disease prevention, pressure ulcer prevention and treatment, identification and prevention of risk for patient falls, nosocomial infection rate, and nurse satisfaction. The concept of nurse-sensitive outcomes was further explored by Ingersoll et al. (2000), who found that the nine highest ranked indicators were satisfaction with care delivery; symptom resolution or reduction; perception of being well cared for; complication or adherence with treatment plan; knowledge of patients and families; trust in care provider; collaboration among care providers; frequency and type of procedures ordered; and quality of life. In addition, Kring (2008) suggested five domains to promote CNS practice, and they include "discovery, summary, translation, integration and evaluation" (p. 179). The author linked these competencies with CNS practice in the areas of expert practice, research, consultation, education, and leadership. Such indicators can offer the APN a focus, as well as an opportunity to research and disseminate findings about practice outcomes amenable to the efforts of the APN.

OUTCOMES OF CARE AND THE ADVANCED PRACTICE NURSE

Professional nursing associations have identified research-based outcomes that can be used by the APN to evaluate practice and identify complementary policy changes that may be in order. Much of the research addressing the impact of NPs, CRNAs, and CNMs has focused on comparing the care delivered by APNs to that of their physician counterparts (Mundinger, et al. 2000; Paine, et al., 2000). As APNs continue to grow in number, and their impact on health care is more widely acknowledged, there have been new challenges about their efficacy. The movement toward the preparation of the "doctor nurse" and arguments that suggest care by the APN is as "good as the physicians" may require a careful analysis of the role and its future within the domain of nursing. Some have argued that this expansion is a "natural evolution" of the APN role, whereas others have argued that the recent changes foster professional abandonment and that this blurring and lack of a nursing theoretically driven model of care results in a diminished voice for nursing, decreased collaboration, a loss of professional autonomy, and reduced public legitimacy (Bryant-Lukosius et al., 2004; Fawcett, Newman, & McAllister, 2004; Flanagan, 2008; Grace, 2008; Jones, 2006; Newman et al., 2008).

Certified Nurse-Midwives

The Health Resources and Services Administration (HRSA; 2007) reports that there are 13,684 CNMs with an average of 1 and a half years of specialized education beyond nursing school and with increasing numbers prepared at the master's level. In general, CNMs provide gynecological care to healthy women and low-risk obstetrical care.

A meta-analysis by the ANA reported that CNMs performed fewer forceps deliveries and administered less intravenous medication during birth and had higher rates of mothers who chose to breastfeed their newborns (ANA, 1997). These findings are consistent with other studies that have demonstrated that CNMs were able to provide prenatal, labor, and delivery care in patient's homes, which resulted in more an accessible, low-cost delivery model for obstetric care. Home births offer a safe, inexpensive modality of care with lower rates of neonatal mortality and cesarean births.

In hospital settings, the CNM is becoming increasingly visible. Studies have demonstrated that CNMs have improved reports of patient satisfaction with care, lower incidences of cesarean births, decreased use of forceps delivery, less medication use, decreased length of hospital, and overall, fewer complications with the delivery (Davidson, 2002; Declercq, 2002; De Koninck, Blais, Joubert, & Gagnon, 2001). Other studies have demonstrated that mothers cared for by CNMs have a greater tendency to breastfeed their babies, which improves infant's immunity and reduces infant mortality (De Koninck et al., 2001; Raisler, 2000; U.S. Department of Health and Human Services, 2002). Hellings and Howe (2000) suggest that not only did NPs and CNMs have a better understanding of problems associated with breastfeeding, but they also had the strategies needed to effectively manage the problem. Care of patients by CNMs has helped improve women's health overall and reinforced the fact that pregnancy is a normal health state for many women, easily managed by the CNM.

Certified Nurse Anesthetists

The number of CRNAs is reported to be about 32,523 nurses. They are generally registered nurses who have completed 2 to 3 years of higher education beyond a bachelor's degree (typically a master's degree), and national certification in the area of specialization is required to practice (HRSA, 2007). Most CRNAs have had previous experience in critical care, a criterion often used as part of admission requirements into graduate programs.

CRNAs are reported to administer more than 65% of the anesthetics given annually to patients. To date there are no studies that have demonstrated that patient outcomes are different based on the type of provider rendering the care (AANA, 2002). From its inception, the role of the CRNA focused on providing safe, effective anesthesia care to patients in the hospital setting. No particular groups of patients have been singled out (i.e., healthier, more stable, poor, ethnically diverse, rural, or inner city) as a specific focus of care. There has been an increasing demand for CRNAs, and this trend continues especially in poor and under served areas (AANA, 2002).

During the 1980s, there was an especially critical shortage of anesthesia providers. In response to this crisis, the American Association of Nurse Anesthetists (AANA) established the National

Commission on Nurse Anesthesia Education (NCNAE) to oversee all aspects of CRNA preparation and develop strategies that would enable nurses to respond in increasing numbers to this crisis (Mastropietro, Horton, Ouellette, & Faut-Callahan, 2001). The CRNA role has grown because of the talent and knowledge exhibited by these APNs. Surgeons in general, have recognized the CRNA as a team player, with an ability to solely attend to the patient during surgery. Although there have been attempts by anesthesiologists to undermine the quality of care of the CRNA and thwart their independence, the CRNA role has prevailed, especially in rural settings (AANA, 2002; Simonson, Ahern, & Hendryx, 2007).

Outcome studies associated with anesthesia administration have suggested that when anesthesia is provided by a specialist—whether it be a physician or CRNA—the outcomes are better than when care is provided by a nonspecialist. Despite these findings, physician anesthetists continue to regulate CRNA practice and limit their work as independent providers of anesthesia care. Comprehensive studies comparing the two groups of providers—anesthesiologists and CRNAs— report that the care provided by the CRNAs is comparable to care provided by anesthesiologists (Simonson et al., 2007). The literature also cites that the most common anesthesia accidents are related to hypoxia and intubation into the esophagus and lack of monitoring. These are general problems described and not linked specifically to a particular group providing anesthesia care. Attributes of the anesthesia providers that do affect patient outcome are related to careful monitoring, concentration, organization, and the ability to function as part of a team. A current shortage in anesthesia care providers continues to increase opportunities for the CRNA.

Nurse Practitioners

According to the HRSA (2007), there were an estimated 141,209 NPs in the United States in 2004. The majority of these nurses are master's prepared and nationally certified. Within all settings, the role of the APN has centered on direct comprehensive patient care. However, activities around support system development, research, and education along with professional development have been reported in the literature (Mick & Ackerman, 2000).

Traditionally, NPs in the primary care setting often practice in environments similar to that of the CNM. They often care for elderly, poor, ethnically diverse, and rural or inner city populations with otherwise limited, or no access to health care. Often settings such as churches, which are versatile and accessible to the population, are used as the site of care delivery. Pulcini, Vampola, and Levine (2005) report that the majority of NPs practice in the urban setting, as opposed to rural, and practice primarily in primary care settings. There is, however, a new and increasing trend toward NPs practicing in the acute care environment.

Studies focusing on the care provided by NPs as compared to that provided by physicians for a variety of primary care–related conditions (e.g., hypertension management, cardiovascular risk reduction, obesity, and sexually transmitted diseases) have demonstrated that NPs provide care that is as safe and as effective as that by physicians. Additionally, patients often report higher levels of satisfaction with NP practice, particularly in areas of increased communication and information gathering (Hayes, 2007; Hoffman et al., 2005).

Research comparing the work of the NPs with the practice outcomes of physicians in the primary care setting also yielded positive outcomes. In a randomized clinical control trial, primary care physicians were compared to NPs on the following dimensions: (a) length of time spent with the patient, (b) patient satisfaction, (c) health status, (d) return clinic visits at 2 weeks, and (e) costs. The research analyzed care given to 641 patients whose care was provided by a NP with 651 patients whose care was provided by a general medical practitioner. Findings suggest that NPs spent significantly more time with their patients (4.29 minutes more), and patients reported significantly higher levels of satisfaction with care rendered by the NP. There were no significant differences reported in health status or prescribing practices between the two groups of providers. NPs did have significantly more patient "return visits," but overall there was no significant difference in patient care costs between the two providers (Venning, Durie, Roland, Roberts, & Leese, 2000).

These results are consistent with the findings of Horrocks et al. (2002), who completed an extensive review of 34 clinical studies comparing NP practices with that of the general medical provider. Additional investigations have reported that although NPs may order more tests, they focus heavily on teaching, health promotion, and self-care. This in fact may be an important factor that contributes to decreased overall cost and return visits to the provider.

Studies support the fact that NPs prescribe less costly, but equally effective drugs and treatments than their physician counterparts (Erikson, 2000). NPs also come to know the patient in the context of overall sociocultural, financial, and life situations. This factor may significantly affect the NP's ability to provide care that is responsive to cost, quality, and effectiveness for both the organization and the patient.

As the NP role has developed, they have expanded their practice settings to include urgent care, emergency room, and acute care. Though there are limited studies to date on NP practice in these venues, the few that exist report no statistical difference in overall satisfaction with care or patient outcomes for diabetes or asthma when managed by the NP as compared to the physician. Further, NPs did demonstrate better outcomes in the management of hypertension (Mundinger et al., 2000; Hoffman et al., 2005).

Clinical Nurse Specialist

There are 69,071 CNSs who are registered nurses with advanced degrees in either master's or doctoral preparation and working with specialized populations in varied areas of clinical practice (HRSA, 2007). The CNS role developed as a result of fragmented health-care services and a lack of expert nursing care at the bedside and limited continuity in care across settings. The CNS has historically been prepared in master's programs. They are educated, knowledgeable, autonomous, independent, certified providers and work within a framework of nursing and advanced practice. Most CNSs work in conjunction and collaboration with multiple members of the health-care team, in settings in which they are recognized as the expert in a specialized area of care. Although this is also true of NPs, CNMs, and CRNAs, they often work under the supervision of, or in direct collaboration with, physicians, whereas the CNS is an autonomous practitioner, dependent on referral from other providers who may be physicians, as well as nurses (Naylor & Brooten, 1993 Oermann & Floyd, 2002; Urden, 1999). The psychiatric mental health CNS often works in collaboration with physicians but also has a high degree of autonomy and in many settings has prescription writing privileges. Although most APNs can write prescriptions, it is not a consistent part of the CNS's practice.

Functioning in hospitals, home, and transitional care environments, the CNS provides specialized care to patients with health problems such as diabetes, ineffective pain management, cardiovascular health care, wound care management, and oncology care. In recent years this role has been challenged in many institutions and responsive to budget cuts. This fact, along with a lack of outcomes research demonstrating the effectiveness of the role (Oermann & Floyd, 2002), has reduced the presence of the CNS in many clinical settings. With the increased visibility of the CNS through groups like the NACNS, there has been renewed attention to the role of the CNS: increased attention to evidenced-based practice, scrutiny of the outcomes of their care, and the contribution of this role to overall health care. It is essential that CNS conduct outcomes evaluation that clearly link cost savings, patient care effectiveness, and improved satisfaction to their role (Oermann & Floyd, 2002; Urden, 1999). Today there has been a trend to hire the CNS back into the practice setting to improve staff development, especially with novice nurses and to help educate staff, patients, and families on new information and technology needed to optimize health care in the 21st century.

Research conducted especially during the past decade, provides supportive evidence to link the contributions of the CNS to (a) reduced length of hospital stay, (b) reduced use of emergency rooms for care, (c) decreased hospitalization admissions and recidivism after discharge, (d) diminished cost and increased satisfaction with care received (Brooten, 1995; Brooten et al., 1995; Oermann & Floyd, 2002; Urden, 1999).

Despite this compelling evidence demonstrating effectiveness of the role, it remains a vulnerable APN role for nursing. Urden (1999) identified nurse-sensitive outcomes that CNSs should focus on to increase visibility and retention within the practice environment. These include symptom management as supported by NACNS, as well as indicators related to sleep, fatigue, satisfaction, quality of life, response to treatment regimens, and family coping. Urden also suggests measuring clinical outcomes in terms of symptom control, morbidity, mortality function, and fiscal and psychological gains and satisfaction. Additional emphasis on the role of the CNS in symptom management, staff development, collaboration, research, and patient education is critical in linking CNS practice to patient outcomes (Lyons, 2005; Kring, 2008).

PRACTICE CHARACTERISTICS AND REIMBURSEMENT

Research conducted by Pulcini et al. (2005) makes the case that it is essential for the APN to fully participate in direct patient care that includes prescription writing, as well as the ordering of treatments and procedures. In addition, APNs should have hospital admitting privileges, conduct patient rounds, and participate in urgent and emergency care.

The mean salary for the APN is varies significantly within regions of the United States and is influenced by years of practice and education. The salary of CRNAs remains highest of all APNs. In 2008, CRNA salaries ranged from a low of $116,670 for hospital practice to more than $180,455 in private practice (Pay Scale, 2008). Rollet and Lebo (2008) report that salaries for NPs have increased 8.8% from $74,812 in 2005 to $81,397 in 2007 reflecting 55% growth over the decade. NPs in California, and those with a doctorate, report up to $15,000 more in salary than those in other regions of the United States with only a master's degree. Recent data on salaries is limited, but the range for the experienced CNS is generally reported to be around the same as the NP, whereas the CNM is the lowest paid at an average of $65,000 yearly in 2008 (Simply Hired, 2008). Other benefits that are valued by APNs include health insurance, continuing education support, paid sick leave, and paid vacation.

Another consideration in regard to the compensation of all APNs is the critical need to document capability and contributions to care and patient outcomes. Data that links the work of the APN to improved patient outcomes, reduction in costs, increased patient/family satisfaction, and increased efficiency can be used to examine care and demand compensation that is consistent with the contributions of these nurse providers. This may be either direct reimbursement or salary.

The reimbursement rules detailed in the *Federal Regist*er (1996) revised Medicare reimbursement for physicians and included other health-care providers. Currently, Medicare payment is allowed for CNSs, NPs, and physician assistant services in certain situations (Minarik, 1997). In addition, the Balanced Budget Act of 1997 facilitated direct Medicare reimbursement for the NP (Richmond, Thompson, & Sullivan-Marx, 2000). Expanded Medicare reimbursement for acute care NPs continues to be reviewed. The ANA works with a variety of federal agencies to improve direct reimbursement for APNs, regardless of specialty and geographical location. Challenges associated with reimbursement in today's health-care environment are often linked to care outcomes and reimbursement policy established by insurers, mostly controlled at the state level.

FUTURE DIRECTIONS AND FUTURE CONSIDERATIONS

APN is a hybrid term that is broadly defined as master's prepared nurse practicing either as an NP or CNS. CRNAs and CNMs, although also increasingly mastered prepared, are not always included in this broad category of advanced practice nurse, which in itself underscores an issue. Is it the area of specialization and tasks associated with different roles that identify a nurse as an APN? Are some of these roles more complex than what has been described? Do nurses with master's preparation bring expert nursing knowledge to the patient care experience? Is what nursing offers to complement medical care clearly defined and valued? Is nursing able to link its contribution to care to cost efficiency and quality? Does the area of specialization define advanced practice?

Skills Versus Knowledge

Being master's prepared in nursing includes knowledge, skills, and the resultant competencies for a particular role and specialty population, plus advanced knowledge in the discipline of nursing itself. The graduate curriculum includes content on role preparation, research, health policy, as well as concepts that reflect disciplinary theory and concepts (e.g., holism and healing). In addition, specialty content related to medical diagnosis, procedures and treatments, and disease management enhances an APN's ability to minister to a specific patient cohort.

The ability to blend components of both medicine and nursing makes advanced practice unique. However, in many instances, the work of nursing becomes invisible as the nurse takes on more and more of the medical role while underusing all the domains unique to advanced practice nursing (Bryant-Lukosius et al., 2004). APNs may risk becoming invisible within such health-care settings despite their ability to legally and therapeutically care for the patient. APNs in these cases are not able to practice to the full extent of their potential, and ethically this raises issues of what is good nursing care (Grace, 2008). Often APNs are expected to be clinically competent and expert in medical knowledge, without being able to integrate nursing science into their work. Lack of time and autonomy are often reasons why there is this discrepancy in the reality of clinical practice. The struggle for a "lost nursing identity" continues to plague the NP, while the CNS is devalued as job opportunities diminish (Mick and Ackerman, 2002, p. 397).

Advancing the Discipline

The literature cites and specialty conferences continue to discuss the need for APNS to work together, increase their focus on cost-effective, outcomes-based practice, and demonstrate patient satisfaction (Mink & Ackerman, 2002; Oermann and Floyd, 2002; Prevost, 2002; Urden, 1999). Several issues continue to be troublesome in advanced practice nursing: (a) advanced nursing practice roles are consistently developed and morphed in a response to fill gaps in medicine, (b) APNs do not distinguish the uniqueness of their role—either in comparison to medicine or to each other, and (c) there is a continuing lack of evidence to support the contribution of APNs to personal health and well-being and to the delivery system.

Despite the need for evidence-based practice, research is not a priority in clinical settings, and when it does exist, the primary focus is to describe how the APN is "as good as" rather than unique and distinct from their physician counterpart. The role appears to be a response to shortages in physicians, rather than a complement or alternative in care, with clear distinctions about why a consumer would prefer one over the other. It is this lack of evidence, which has negatively affected the CNS in the past decade. Increases in health-care costs and ensuing budget cuts, combined with a lack of evidence supporting the value of the CNS in the practice setting, made them vulnerable to being eliminated in many settings. This resulted in academia reducing the number of CNS programs and shifting the focus toward NP preparation. It was originally thought that NPs would be able to satisfy the shortage of primary care physicians. Today, although primary care physicians remain in short supply, NPs are being increasingly used in more specialized practices, managing acute care patients and those with chronic illnesses (Pulcini et al., 2005).

Some of the NP roles in acute care are often in response to the cuts in the hours worked by medical residents, and evidence suggests that NPs are "as good as" or a welcome complement to physician care teams. But even where they are seen positively, APNs do not distinguish the uniqueness of their practice and knowledge, as compared to other providers (Hoffman et al., 2005; Steven 2004). The care provided by NPs in acute and chronic care settings reflects comprehensive specialty care and is sought for patients with complex medical and psychosocial problems. This role in many ways mirrors CNS practice and has led to a blurring of NP and CNS roles.

Naylor and Brooten (1993) in a state of the science paper, addressed the importance of research, practice, education, and administrative to the role of the APN. Consistently, all of these aspects are valued by the APN, but research is the least visible element. This finding is also consistent with studies of the CNS. Evidence suggests that the majority of CNSs spend their time in the practice setting, teaching staff, participating in educational activities, and fulfilling administrative obligations. As a result, there is much less time available to pursue research and other professional and scholarly activities. Education, research, and practice are fundamental to the role of the APN. Without research, however, the role of the APN will lack evidence to advance and could risk extinction.

Nursing studies that link nurse-sensitive quality indicators to patient care outcomes are essential to advancing the discipline. Doctorally prepared APNs in clinical settings are critical to this end, as well as increasing the practitioners' visibility. Sigma Theta Tau International (2002) recommends several steps to address the nursing shortage and nurse retention and satisfaction within the profession. They are listed in **Box 22-1.**

These ideas call for nurses, particularly those in advanced practice, to be clear about nursing as an art and science in the practice setting. Otherwise, nurses in advanced practice roles are at risk for being identified as technicians who perform medical tasks within a curative framework.

It is the mandate of the APN to visibly assimilate concepts of state-of-the-art nursing into their care that will stake our claim within a changing and dynamic health-care environment. Often the most critical element is the relationship between the nurse and patient (Flanagan, 2008; Grace, 2008; Jones, 2006; Newman et al., 2008) and its impact on individual choices, actions, life changes to promote health, and engagement in living and personal transformation. This holistic approach involves an intentional caring presence by the nurse in collaboration with other professionals, all working from their unique perspective to improve the human condition. In this scenario, nursing is seeking ways to uncover an individual's personal story and meaning and taking time to allow new possibilities to emerge and promote new actions; and the APN is doing this most artfully (Flanagan, 2008; Newman et al., 2008). Attending to this mandate can

---

BOX 22-1

Guidelines to Promote Retention in Professional Nursing from Sigma Theta Tau International*

■ Demonstrate to health-care leaders that nurses are the critical difference in the U.S.'s health-care system.

■ Reposition nursing as a highly versatile profession in which young people can learn science and technology, customer service, critical thinking, and decision making.

■ Construct practice environments that are interdisciplinary and build on relationships among nurses, physicians, other health-care professionals, patients, and communities.

■ Create patient care models that encourage professional nurse autonomy and clinical decision making.

■ Develop additional evaluation systems that measure the relationship of timely nursing interventions to patient outcomes.

■ Establish additional standards and mechanisms for recognition of professional practice environments.

■ Develop career enhancement incentives for nurses to pursue professional practice.

■ Evaluate the effects of the nursing shortage on the next generation of nurse educators, nurse administrators, and nurse researchers, and take strategic action.

■ Implement and sustain a marketing effort that addresses the image of nursing and the recruitment of quality students into nursing as a career.

■ Promote nurses of all educational levels to pursue higher education.

■ Develop and implement strategies to promote the retention of registered nurses and nurse educators in the workforce.

---

*Adapted from Sigma Theta Tau International. (2002). *Excellence in Clinical Practice*, Indianapolis, IN: Author, p. 1.

---

sustain new behaviors and ultimately influence health-care outcomes in a cost-effective, efficient, timely, and safe manner.

CONCLUSION

This chapter focused on the role of APNs and the contributions they have made to improve health care for all. Data points to patient care provided by NPs, CNMs, CRNAs, and CNSs as significant, safe, cost effective, and satisfying to patients and families. Trends in care suggest that both the practice settings and roles of APNs have changed greatly since their inception. It is important for nurses practicing in these roles to continue to document and research practice outcomes, so that when evidence is needed to support a role, it can easily be made available.

As health care continues to evolve, it is important that APNs reflect a clear image of professional nursing, as opposed to changing in response to the call of medicine. Loss of our disciplinary focus creates nurses who may be technically skilled and competent, but at a loss to believe or prove their own uniqueness. It is essential that an evaluation of the impact of the APN take into account those accomplishments that are often silent in a medically driven health-care system. These events may require the transition from "fix it" models of care delivery to frameworks guided by nursing knowledge to achieve personal changes and improved life for the patient.

References

American Association of Nurse Anesthetists. (2002). *Patients: Quality of care in anesthesia—section two.* Available from the American Hospital Association Web site: www.aha.org.

American Nurses Association. (1997). *Nursing facts—advanced practice nursing: A new age in health care.* Available from American Nurses Association Nursing World Web site: www.nursingworld.org.

American Nurses Association. (2000). *Certified nurses report fewer adverse effects: Survey links certification with improved health care.* Available from the American Nurses Association Nursing World Web site: www.needlestick.org.

American College of Nurse-Midwives. (2002). Resources and bibliography: Quality and safety of direct entry midwifery practice in the U.S. Available from the American College of Nurse-Midwives Web site: www.acnm.org.

Brooten, D. (1995). Perinatal care across the continuum: Early discharge and nursing home follow-up. *Journal of Perinatal and Neonatal Nursing, 9*(1), 38–44.

Brooten, D., Naylor, M., York, R., Brown, L., Roncoli, M., Hollingsworth, A., et al. (1995). Effects of nurse specialist transitional care on patient outcomes and costs: Results of five randomized trials. *American Journal of Managed Care, 1*(1), 35–41.

Bryant-Lukosius, D., Dicenso, A., Browne, G., & Pinelli, J. (2004). Advanced practice nursing roles: Development, implementation and evaluation. *Journal of Advanced Nursing, 48*(5), 519–529.

Cumbie, S., Conley, V., & Burman, M. (2004). Advanced practice nursing model for comprehensive care with chronic illness: Model for promoting process engagement. *Advances in Nursing Science, 27*(1), 70–80.

Davidson, M. (2002). Out comes of high-risk women cared for by certified nurse-midwifes. *Journal of Midwifery & Women's Health, 47*(1), 46–49.

Declercq, E. (2002). CNM birth attendance in the United States, 1999. *Journal of Midwifery and Women's Health, 47*(1), 44–45.

De Koninck, M., Blais, R., Joubert, P., & Gagnon, C. (2001). Comparing women's assessment of midwifery and medical care in Quebec, Canada. *Journal of Midwifery and Women's Health, 46*(2), 60–67.

Dexter, F., Macario, A., & Traub, R. D. (2000). Statistical methods using operating room information systems data to determine anesthetist weekend call requirements. *AANA Journal, 68*(I), 21–26.

Elsom, S., & Happel, B. (2006). The clinical nurse specialist and nurse practitioner roles: Room for both or take your pick? *Australian Journal of Advanced Nursing, 24*(2), 56–59.

Erickson, V. (2000). Prescriptive practices of nurse practitioners for acute otitis media. *Programs and abstracts of National Organization of Nurse Practitioner Faculties 26th Annual Meeting.* Washington DC. Session MR6.

Fawcett, J., Newman, D., & McAllister, M. (2004). Advanced practice nursing and conceptual models of nursing. *Nursing Science Quarterly, 17*(2), 135–138.

Flanagan, J. (2008). Ethical issues for advanced practice nurses caring for the adult health population. In P. Grace (Ed.), *Nursing ethics and professional responsibility in advanced practice.* Boston: Jones & Bantlett Publishers.

Fulton, J. (2002). Editorial: Defining our practice. *Clinical Nurse Specialist: The Journal for Advanced Nursing Practice, 16*(4), 167–168.

Grace, P. (2008). Nursing ethics. In P. Grace (Ed.), *Nursing ethics and professional responsibility in advanced practice.* Boston: Jones & Bantlett Publishers.

Gunn, I. P. (2000). Rural health care and the nurse anesthetist. *CRNA—The Clinical Forum for the Nurse Anesthetist, 11*(2), 77–86.

Hayes, E. (2007). Nurse practitioners and managed care: patient satisfaction and intention to adhere to nurse practitioner plan of care. *Journal of American Academy of Nurse Practitioner, 19*(8), 418–426.

Health Resources and Services Administration. (2007). *The registered nurse population: Findings from the March 2004 national sample survey of registered nurses.* Washington, DC: U.S. Department of Health and Human Services.

Hellings, P., & Howe, C. (2000). Assessment of breastfeeding knowledge of nurse practitioners and nurse midwives. *Journal of Midwifery and Women's Health, 4*(3), 264–270.

Hoffman, L., Tasota, F., Zullo, T., Scharfenberg, C., & Donaue, M. (2005). Outcomes of care managed by an acute care nurse practitioner/attending physician team in a subacute medical intensive care unit. *American Journal of Critical Care, 14*(2), 121–130.

Horrocks, S., Anderson, E., & Salisbury, C. (2002). Systematic review of whether nurse practitioners working in primary care can provide equivalent care to doctors. *British Medical Journal, 324*(7341), 819–823.

Ingersoll, E., McIntosh, M., & Williams, M. (2000). Nurse-sensitive outcomes of advanced practice. *Journal of Advanced Nursing, 32*(5), 1272–1281.

International Council of Nurses. (2002). *Definition and characteristics of the role.* Available from the International Council of Nurses Web site: www.icn-apnetwork.org.

Institute of Medicine. (1999). *To err is human: Building a safer health care system.* Washington, DC: National Academy Press.

Institute of Medicine. (2001). *Crossing the quality chasm.* Washington, DC: National Academy Press.

Jones, D. (2006). Are we abandoning nursing as a discipline. *Clinical Nurse Specialist: The Journal for Advanced Nursing Practice, 19*(6), 275–277.

Kring, D. L. (2008). Clinical nurse specialist practice domains and evidenced-based practice competencies. *Clinical Nurse Specialist: The Journal for Advanced Nursing Practice, 22*(4), 179–183.

Lyons, B. (2005). Getting back to autonomous practice. *Clinical Nurse Specialist: The Journal for Advanced Nursing Practice, 19*(1), 25–27.

Mastropietro, C. A., Horton, B. J. Ouellette, S. M., & Faut-Callahan, M. (2001). The National Commission on nurse anesthesia education 10 years later—Part I: The commission years (1989–1994). *AANA Journal, 69*(5), 379–385.

McGee, L. A., & Kaplan, L. (2007). Factors influencing the decision to use nurse practitioners in the emergency department. *Journal of Emergency Nursing, 33*(5), 441–446.

Mick, D., & Ackerman, M. H. (2000). Advanced practice nursing role delineation in acute and critical care: Application of the Strong Model of advanced practice. *Heart and Lung, (29)*3, 210–221.

Mick, D., & Ackerman, M. H. (2002). Deconstructing the myth of the advanced practice blended role: Support for role divergence. *Heart and Lung, 31*(8), 393–398.

Minarik, P. A. (1997). Federal reimbursement clarified: Issues of recognition shifts to the states. *Clinical Nurse Specialist: The Journal of Advanced Nursing, 11*(1), 12–13.

Mundinger, M., Kane, R., Lenz, E., Totten, A., Wei-Yann, T., Cleary, P. et al. (2000). Primary care outcomes in patients treated by nurse practitioners or physicians: A randomized trail. *Journal of the American Medical Association, 283*(1), 59–68.

Naylor, M., & Brooten, D. (1993). The role and functions of clinical nurse specialists. *Image: Journal of Nursing Scholarship, 25*(1), 73–78.

Newman, M., Smith, M., Pharris, M., & Jones, D. (2008). The focus of the discipline revisited. *Advances in Nursing Science, 31*(1), 16–27.

Oermann, M., & Floyd, J. (2002). Outcomes research: An essential component of the advanced practice nurse role. *Clinical Nurse Specialist, 16*(3), 140–144.

Paine, L., Johnson, T., Lang, J., Gagnon, D., Declercq, E., DeJoseph, J., et al. (2000). A comparison of visits and practices of nurse-midwives and obstetrician-gynecologists in ambulatory care settings. *Journal of Midwifery and Women's Health, 45*(1), 37–44.

Pay Scale. (2008). *Average nurse anesthetist salaries.* Retrieved July 21, 2008, from Pay Scale Web site: www.payscale.com/research/US/Job-Nurse Anesthetist.

Prevost, S. (2002). Clinical nurse specialist outcomes: Vision, voice and value. *Clinical Nurse Specialist, 16*(3), 119–124.

Pulcini, J., Vampola, D., & Levine, J. (2005). Nurse practitioner practice characteristics, salary, and benefits survey, 2003. *Clinical Excellence for Nurse Practitioners, 9*(1), 49–58.

Raisler, J. (2000). Midwives helping mothers to breastfeed: Food for thought and action. *Journal of Midwifery and Women's Health, 45*(3), 202–204.

Reiter, F. (1966). The nurse clinician. *American Journal of Nursing, 66*(2), 274–280.

Richmond, T. S., Thompson, H. J., & Sullivan-Marx, E. M. (2000). Reimbursement for acute care nurse practitioner services. *American Journal of Critical Care, 9*(1), 52–61.

Rollet, J., & Lebo, S. (2008). A decade of growth: Salaries increase as profession matures. *Advance for Nurse Practitioners.* Retrieved April 20, 2008, from Advance for Nurse Practitioners Web site: www.advanceweb.com/np.com.

Schober, M. (2006). Advanced nursing practice: An emerging global phenomenon. *Journal of Advanced Nursing, 55*(3), 275–276.

Sigma Theta Tau International. (2002). *Guidelines to create to promote retention and promote professional nursing.* Retrieved April 20, 2008, from the Sigma Theta Tau International Web site: www.nursingsociety.org/reflections.

Simonson, D. C., Ahern, M. C., & Hendryx, M. S. (2007). Anesthesia staffing and anesthetic complications during cesarean delivery: A retrospective analysis. *Nursing Research, 56*(1), 9–17.

Simply Hired. (2008). *Average nurse midwife salaries.* Retrieved July 21, 2008, from the Simply Hired Web site: www.simplyhired.com/a/salary/search/q-NURSE+MIDWIFE.

Steven, K. (2004). APRN hospitalist: Just a resident replacement? *Journal of Pediatric Health Care, 18*(4), 208–210.

Urden, L. (1999). Outcome evaluation: An essential component for CNS practice. *Clinical Nurse Specialist, 13*(1), 39–46.

U.S. Department of Health and Human Services. (2002). *Healthy People 2010: Understanding and improving health.* Washington, DC: Author.

Venning, P., Durie, A., Roland, M., Roberts, C., & Leese, B. (2000). Randomised controlled trial comparing cost effectiveness of general practitioners and nurse practitioners in primary care. *British Medical Journal, 320*(7241), 1048–1053.

World Health Organization. (2006). *Strengthening nursing and midwifery care.* Retrieved April 25, 2008, from the World Health Organization Web site: www.who.int/hrh/nursing_midwifery/resolutions/en/index.html.

23

Promoting Advanced Practice Nurses to the Public

Donna A. Gaffney

INTRODUCTION

At the dawn of the 21st century the U.S. public is not satisfied with health care—the system or individual providers. The average office visit time in a primary care setting is shrinking. Insurers and corporations are making decisions about services and coverage, often leaving consumers and providers out of the process. Acute care facilities are markedly and dangerously understaffed. Even the abundance of health-related information on the Internet and bookshelves is overwhelming to consumers. The lack of guidance and access to high-tech resources prevents consumers from getting the facts they need.

Hanging a shingle and waiting for the first phone call is both unrealistic and naïve. Although providers hope that the consumer will understand the intent of advanced practice nurses (APNs), the reception may be anything but welcoming. In fact, because most people do not even understand the role and responsibilities of the APN, few may think this "product" is necessary. Like it or not, APNs in this evolving health-care environment must rise to the challenge of creating a market for our services.

With such dissatisfaction, gaps, and inadequacies, how is it that APNs cannot gain a foothold in this fertile field? Although the answer is somewhat complicated, it is far from elusive. Simply stated, the nursing profession is using conventional methods to promote unique health-care services. The mistake is often made when health-care providers think they know what the public needs. We survey and question, but do not dialogue with the consumer. We are remiss in going the extra step.

This chapter explores how to promote APNs in ways that not only suggest thinking outside the traditional health-care box, but also by dismantling the box altogether. It will help germinate new ideas and new approaches. Read through these pages with pen and pad at your side. Abandon convention, disrupt the status quo, and realize a vision to bring APNs into the hearts and minds of the consumer.

> *Marketing today is not a function; it is a way of doing business. Marketing is not a new ad campaign or this month's promotion. Marketing has to be all pervasive, part of everyone's job description. It is to integrate the customer into the design of the product and to design a systematic process for interaction that will create substance in the relationship (McKenna, 1991, p. 69).*

403

A PRIMER IN THE PRINCIPLES OF MARKETING

Historically, the principles of marketing emanate from strategies used on the battlefield (Reis & Trout, 1986). Such hard-hitting approaches may be intense for the helping professions, but these are times of tough competition and limited health-care dollars. But are tactics of warfare the best approach? Do we need yet another linear and perhaps even outdated model?

Marketing is a business strategy that advertises information about a particular product or service, and it is built on a combination of demographic and sociological data, strategic planning, product design, pricing policy, advertising, sales promotion, and actual selling (Cunningham, 1982). However, the American Marketing Association reexamines the definition of marketing every 5 years in an effort to reflect on the state of the marketing field. The new definition reads:

> *Marketing is the activity, set of institutions, and processes for creating, communicating, delivering, and exchanging offerings that have value for customers, clients, partners, and society at large (American Marketing Association Board of Directors, 2007).*

Threaded throughout textbooks on marketing is a practical model composed of four critical elements that have withstood the test of time. The components of the model are better known as the "Four Ps": product, price, place, and promotion (Kotler, 1976).

The APN must have insight into his or her own practice and the needs of the consumer. In **Table 23-1** the traditional four Ps of marketing—product, price, place, and promotion—are expanded to include public relations and networking, which are all critical strategies for educating consumers (Gaffney, 1999).

To understand how these elements interact with each other, one must have an appreciation of a holistic, systems view of the world. A systems approach allows one to recognize the logical, organized way of viewing various phenomena. Although first applied to mathematics, physics, and engineering in the late 1930s, it was not until the late 1960s that von Bertalanffy (1968) and Buckley (1967) applied general systems theory to the behavioral sciences. The tenets of general systems theory support the idea that there is a dynamic interaction within multivariable systems (von Bertalanffy, 1968). It is this interaction among the parts, not one singular part, that determines a specific outcome. Simply put in marketing terms, it is not the product, price, place, or promotion that determines success, but the dynamic process that occurs among these factors (Gaffney, 1999).

For APNs there are more challenges to selling the product than simply deciding where to locate one's practice and how much to charge for each session. Promoting the APN in some specialty

TABLE 23-1	
The Five Ps of Marketing and Public Relations	
Product	An intangible service or material good that satisfies a need
Price	The amount of money a product will cost the consumer
Place	The location where the consumer can secure services or goods
Promotion	Potentially influential communication of information regarding the goods or services by the seller to the consumer
Public relations	The activities used by the seller to promote a favorable relationship with the consumer and the community

areas (e.g., mental health, gastroenterology, or infectious diseases) may be hampered by stigma or embarrassment. Beyond pediatric nurse practitioners (NPs) and nurse-midwives, satisfied customers rarely make public statements to promote the services of their APN. Testimonials to APNs are almost nonexistent in the media. In fact, the use of high-profile acknowledgments extolling the value of any health-care services has only emerged in the 1990s. Therefore, it is important to add one more element to the dynamic marketing process, another *P*, public relationships. This fifth component is more than public relations and service promotion. It includes personal, professional, and community networking and public service efforts that demonstrate the value of health-care services to various target populations. It is essential for the health-care professional to clearly identify each area and the related objectives and strategies necessary for success. The marketing plan is the instrument that serves to organize the health-care provider and monitor the practice's progress.

THE FRAMEWORK: A MARKETING PLAN

The elements of a comprehensive marketing plan include the steps of the marketing process. Traditionally, operationalizing the sequential steps in the marketing process allows one to refine the process and rehearse before the real thing. There is one problem; it is a linear model that does not allow for a feedback loop. **Box 23-1** illustrates how one can operationalize or visualize the distinct steps in marketing within the practice context. **Table 23-2** offers the same steps, but places them in a circular model.

The elements of the marketing feedback loop reflect the importance of the consumer in the development of health-care services. The most effective marketing plans are those that include thorough research, planning, and sending the right message to the consumer (Kennedy, 1991; McDonald, 2007). Kennedy calls this important message the ultimate selling point (USP). It is the service provider's number one secret weapon. The USP identifies the most important benefit of your service to the consumer. The goal of the USP is to find that "something" so unique about your practice

---

BOX 23-1
An Operational Definition of Marketing

The advanced practice nurse (APN) plans to offer a service.

The APN wants to ensure financial success from the sales of this service.

The APN researches and surveys the public.

The APN tailors product design and pricing of the service to fit the needs and preferences of the public.

The APN uses advertising, networking, and promotion strategies to convince the public to purchase the service.

The public becomes aware of a need or preference for the service and purchases it.

The APN gains a profit from sales of service to the public.

The APN regularly evaluates the service and strategies to maintain and increase future profits sales of the service.

Adapted from Barton, E. (1998). *An operational definition of marketing.* Unpublished manuscript.

TABLE 23-2
The Marketing Feedback Loop
The advanced practice nurse (APN) plans to offer a service.

The APN researches, surveys, and dialogues with the public.	The public becomes aware of a need or preference for the service and asks for it.
The APN tailors product design and pricing of the service to fit the needs and preferences of the public.	The APN regularly evaluates the service and strategies to maintain and increase future profits and sales of the service.
The APN wants to ensure financial success from the sales of this service.	The APN gains a profit from sales of service to the public.

The APN uses advertising, networking, and promotion strategies to convince the public to purchase the service.

Adapted from Barton, E. (1998). *An operational definition of marketing.* Unpublished manuscript.

that it will be undeniably identified solely with you and you alone. McDonald (2007) warns that believing that advertising will increase use of your services, irrespective of the message, is not only naïve but reflects a poorly researched marketing plan. Given the gaps and flaws in health-care service delivery, APNs could have a gold mine of unique messages that can only be identified with them.

The Foundation for Service: A Philosophy of Care and Mission Statement

The statement of philosophy is a clear declaration of the practice's approach to health-care services. It is based on the APN's values, those aspects of the human experience the APN deems the most worthy, desirable, and important attributes. It takes time, reflection, and journaling to reacquaint oneself to the goals and ideals learned through education and practice. If the APN is not clear on his or her own philosophy of nursing practice, the consumer will not understand the message. A professional must be passionate about his or her vision for practice. Articulating a philosophy is not done for the sole purpose of writing brochures and setting up a practice; rather it is the foundation for creating vision. Crafting a statement of philosophy is a shared experience in multipartner practices. It is a time for addressing differences and strengthening commonalties, and it must be done in the earliest stages.

The mission statement describes how and what services the APN intends to offer and to whom; in other words, it is the proposed function of the practice. The practice further defines its role with the purpose, also known as a statement of intent. Goals, objectives, and tasks delineate the specific aims through measurable actions and distinct activities to meet the objectives. There must be synchrony between values and beliefs of health-care services and measurable health-care objectives. If not, there is a strong possibility that the practice will fail because the goals do not meet the needs or the interests of the professionals.

The APN needs to engage in thoughtful discussions when writing a statement of philosophy. The most important step is to start by analyzing one's philosophy of health care. What factors promote health and influence illness? What treatment approaches are practiced? This exercise draws on early influences of those people and experiences that have shaped our lives and continue to feed the passion for our work. A philosophy of practice may change over time. Experience, education, and new information shape the way a professional views the human condition.

The mission statement tells the consumer what the APN plans to do. It is based on the philosophies, values, and beliefs of every person in that practice or agency. Simply stated, the mission is the assignment to be carried out. Whether the practice will generate written materials for service promotion, defining the mission of the practice and publishing a mission statement is just as important for the professional as it is for the consumer.

Writing the mission statement usually involves multiple brainstorming sessions and numerous drafts. A series of thought-provoking questions can stimulate discussion: What motivates the APN to provide this service? Is the practice willing to let the mission evolve, grow over time, and change with the practice? What does the APN want to provide to the public? What does the practice want to be to the consumer? Look to those admired in the health-care profession, as well as other professions or disciplines. Identify their philosophies. Learn from them.

The values of the practice are those entities found worthy, important, and useful in the acquisition of health care. As an example, the practice may value an individual family's time, either at home or at work, and therefore arrange hours of operation to avoid any conflict with client's family activities. This requires the APNs to work hours that may not be conducive to their own family lives.

Goals and objectives are the most specific elements of the marketing plan. The goals are broad and usually long-term in nature. The objectives are the means with which the practice will achieve their goals. They are the "steps" to the long-term goal. Objectives are measurable and observable, the end result the practice seeks to achieve. Relevant tasks are developed to measure the achievement of the objective. These tasks are critical to measuring quality and overall clinical effectiveness.

However, it is crucial to remember that the philosophy, mission, and goals are words that tell the public what an APN hopes to accomplish. It is far more important to show the public through actions and behaviors. However, traditional approaches may not be effective in a competitive health-care market. APNs need to take a new route to bring their message to the public. The next section explores how APNs can do just that.

MOVING BEYOND CONVENTION

Jean-Marie Dru (1996) coined the concept of *disruption* in the early 1990s. It was originally conceived by Dru and his associates at the international advertising agency, TBWA, to produce more "intrusive advertising strategies, and to give brands more substance and weight by making a clean break with the status quo, by creating a disruption" (Dru, 2002, p. 19). As explained further, disruption is "a means of questioning the established order" and "challenging tried and true approaches" (Dru, 2002, p. 20).

The disruption process begins by identifying the conventions, that is, the established approaches that have worked in the past. However, these activities are often limiting. The next step is to introduce a novel and unexpected idea. This new idea is conceived with full sense of vision. Vision refers to defining the future market space. It is also about taking a larger share of the market space. In fact, the APN is an illustration of the disruption process at work in the health-care system. The APN is a powerful example of several of Dru's maxims: "Be what others are not," and "Change the actors, not the script." Given such auspicious beginnings, the promotion of APNs to the public requires an equally bold marketing plan. The sequel to Dru's work, *Beyond Disruption: Changing the Rules in the Marketplace* (2002) brings together partners from across the globe and proposes even more forward-thinking ideas. Partnering with others and tapping the potential of their imagination is Dru's message.

Dialogue: Defining the Need and the Service

In health care, market research is often called a needs assessment: identifying what the client needs, how those services are best delivered, and in what form the service will be most used by the consumer. A common mistake is to assume the APN knows what a consumer needs or desires. Often a needs assessment or survey is designed without talking to the consumer first. Whether the product is health-care services or a new restaurant, most basic market data can be found in public, university, or hospital libraries, community and government offices, the Census Bureau, and on the Internet. (Pinson & Jinnett, 1996). The Cornell Institute for Social and Economic Resources provides a listing of valuable information (http://ciser.cornell.edu/info/datasource.shtml), and there are a multitude of sources for the best Web sites and blogs linked to this chapter on DavisPlus. Although this information is continually updated, it is collected at one point in time; and as such it is only a snapshot of the community. Dialogue allows the APN to interact with the public, listen and ask questions, follow up, and listen again.

Identifying the needs of a community may have a significant influence on the kinds of services an APN decides to offer and how the public will respond. The APN must know how the community can best support the health-care services the practice plans to offer. Naturally, it is imperative to complete the assessment well in advance of selecting the office site.

Listening First

Consumers are the best sources of information on their own health-care needs. A conversation provides the circumstances to further explore what and how they would use health-care services. This important first step in the research process also allows the APN to determine office or agency location. Ongoing dialogue facilitates service promotion and brand recognition; the APN is the brand, health care is the product.

However, maintaining ongoing dialogue is challenging. Dialogue requires active listening and responses that are genuine. Dialogue takes time, costs money, and gives the consumer power to determine health-care services (Godin, 1999). It also allows the public to share in the development of community health-care services.

Before the dialogue can begin, the APN collects demographic data. Demographics include age (and age distribution in the population); gender; ethnic, cultural, and religious background; educational experiences; occupation; income; developmental or family status; and geographical location. Much of this information can be obtained from governmental records. It is also possible to approach local town halls for real estate values (the town hall) and school districts for student data. The public library is a good starting place. Reference personnel can either provide the documents needed for the information or refer the APN to other sources. The reference librarian will prove useful in identifying other data as the practice develops. A consumer profile allows the APN to formulate the types of services essential to the practice. However, the dialogue provides the opportunity to fill in the details, as well as giving salient historical trends. For example, if a new postpartum depression prevention program is going to be offered by a particular agency, locating the program in a site populated by senior citizens or young singles may not attract new mothers (Gaffney, 1999).

The dialogue begins when the APN goes into the community and meets with consumers. Moving into the community not only gives the APN initial visibility, but also affords the all-important opportunity to make contact with a point person or persons. Malcolm Gladwell, author of *The Tipping Point* (2000), calls the point person a "Connector" (p. 38). This is an individual who has a special gift for bringing the world together. The Connector not only brings together a small number of the "right" people for dialogue but spreads the word as well. Connectors know lots of people, and they know people who "manage to occupy many different worlds, sub-cultures and niches" (Gladwell, 2000, p. 48). They are not necessarily the most powerful in their own right, but have contacts with those who are influential. Begin by asking a simple question or two: Who should I invite to be a part of this discussion? Who would be helpful for this conversation? Ask the question in different places—for example, shops, schools, and libraries—and the same names will emerge. Those names are your Connectors.

The dialogue is not just a time for the group to give feedback to the APN about the practice's plans, but an exploration of services the community members would like to see. Start with a blank slate. Invite their ideas and suggestions and listen to their concerns. Thank them. Offer follow-up and send letters of appreciation. Send them a summary of the session. Thank them again. Maintain relationships with this group.

Schools and colleges provide more opportunities for dialogue. Identify all schools, preschool and elementary through postsecondary, in the geographical area to be served by the agency. Talk to school administrators. Start at the library and school board office for information. Go to the parent teacher organizations as well. Many schools now have their own Web sites. Secondary schools publish reports that describe their student body and the courses of study in their schools. These documents also contain standardized scores, types of programs, and how students compare to other schools at the county, state, and national levels. However, it is critical to remember that it is not just the students who may require health-care services, but faculty and families as well. Listen to students, teachers, and families.

Pinson and Jinnett (1996) suggest that the developmental needs of the community are apparent through family life cycle stages represented in the demographics. Each phase of individual growth and development and family stage requires different services and approaches to delivering those services. A family with young children is more likely to use health-care services if there is drop-in child-care and prevention programs addressing child development and parenting skills. Families in midlife may be struggling with caring for older parents, as well as dealing with adolescent or college-bound children. The geriatric population is more likely to be facing issues of loss and retirement. Understand your consumer and target a particular group for your services. **Box 23-2** offers a set of questions that will help the APN describe the community. From this exercise, APNs can create the beginning of a plan for services.

Be mindful of culture. Cultural, ethnic, and religious considerations can change a marketing strategy. Understand your population and the community. Learn as much as possible about the various groups and religions and how they perceive health and illness. Create an advisory board or focus group with representation from all segments of the community. If possible, find resources in the community who can talk about traditions, health rituals, and taboos and cultivate an ongoing relationship with these people. Determine how clergy, ministers, and rabbis are seen in the community.

Go to other organizations and agencies. They are potential collaborators and also sources of referrals. Identify your competition and determine who else provides health-care services. Businesses may have workplace programs and refer their employees for services. Employee assistance program personnel many times recognize mental health professional resources for brief psychotherapy referrals.

Now go to the Yellow Pages of the telephone directory. The small local phone books are best; they are much more useful. Find the section titled "Clubs and Organizations." These resources are less traditional but may be just as important as those listed previously. Women's resource centers have already found their own membership, and women are the greatest consumers of health-care resources. Dialogue with this group and you will learn valuable information addressing women's and

---

BOX 23-2
Describing the Community

1. Who are my Connectors?
2. Who are my clients?
   Culture/regional influences
   Lifestyle/psychological make up
   Age range
   Sex
   Income level
   Buying habits
   Crime statistics
3. Where are my customers located?
   Where do they live?
   Where do they work?
   What are employment rates in the community?
   Where do they shop (obtain health care)?
   Where are the schools?
   What transportation services are available?
   Is there a corporate presence?
4. What is the projected size of the market (patients/year)?
5. What are the patients' needs?
   What are the information sources?
   Who are the community contacts?
6. How can this practice meet those needs?
7. What is unique about this practice?
   How do I offer services?
   Are the public's needs being met?

Adapted from Pinson, L., & Jinnett, J. (1996). *Target marketing* (3rd. ed.). Chicago: Upstart Publishing, p. 150.

---

family health-care issues. The Young Women's Christian Association(YWCA)/Young Women's Health Association and Young Men's Christian Association(YMCA)/Young Men's Health Association organizations include virtually every segment of the population. In addition to being a source of referrals the "Ys" are also potential program sites for pubic service offerings and physical advertising space. Community groups and clubs can provide additional access to consumers.

Law enforcement, the local and state police departments, and children's services may provide still more opportunities to define services and find potential consumers. Contact the department of social services in the community for more information on the needs of the community.

Research hotlines, help lines, rape crisis centers, child abuse advocacy centers, and domestic violence safe houses that are part of the community as well. Remember that the identification of violence in a client population is going to fall on the APN as the first line of defense. The best way to become acquainted with crisis services is to meet with a director or board member. Ask about the rate of calls and referrals they receive each month and annually. Seasonal variations hold an important key to your own scheduling of services and programs. A rape crisis program located in a community with five colleges and two junior colleges found that during the summer, when the colleges were not in session, the rate of sexual assault and subsequent need for follow-up services was virtually nonexistent. When the students returned to campus and the first fraternity party was held, the incidence of reported rape soared. This is important information for several reasons. It dictates assessment strategies for primary care settings, outreach to crisis centers and hospital emergency departments, and program development and consultation with colleges and the APN in the college health service.

Although potential consumers and community groups can be surveyed by telephone, questionnaire, or by reviewing annual reports, do not do research this way. The public needs to meet the APN and dialogue. Telephone interviews with administrators in community institutions are difficult to schedule. Mailed questionnaires take too long and have a low return rate. Meet people instead. Keep a journal of important Connectors and the key points made through dialogue; they will be invaluable for future networking and promoting the role of the APN to the public.

Health-care providers need to know who pays for services in the community. Ask your group how they pay for their health care. Identify the most popular plans used and the types of coverage. If there is a large corporation in the community, a call to personnel will identify employee health insurance plans.

If all of this seems too overwhelming, consider segmenting the population. Engelberg and Neubrand (1997) define market segmentation as the process of dividing up a health-care organization's total market into smaller groups based on similar needs and defining characteristics. Some forms of segmentation are based on demographics, regional or geographic variations, or behavioral or use factors. The APN can then focus on each one of those subgroups at a different time or in a different manner (Engleberg & Neubrand, 1997). The fruits of the dialogue process will give the most relevant information for segmenting the community. Sometimes the APN will attempt to target the largest segment; however, it may be more sensible to start with a smaller segment and approach it as a "pilot" for the practice.

Think beyond face-to-face contact as well. Technological advances allow us to reach out to people through chat rooms, discussion boards, text messages, and online surveys. Kumar and Ramani (2006) believe that customers thrive on personal contact, and they readily adapt to electronic communications. In fact, online relationships may have distinct advantages that human interactions lack, for example, a greater sense of privacy and more freedom in expressing viewpoints.

IF YOU BUILD IT, THEY MAY COME

Getting There

If the APN does not succeed in promoting himself or herself to the public, the place and price may not be relevant. Once the public understands the role of the APN and has seen where the agency, office, or program is situated in the community, the word will travel and the buzz begins—but only if the practice is located in a convenient, easy-to-access location. Take a tour; walking or driving the area allows one to appreciate the community as an inhabitant, not a visitor. The image, reputation of the area, physical appearance of the building, and its proximity to other services and facilities are critical to the ultimate success or failure of a practice.

Easy and accessible transportation for the city, free or reasonable parking for the suburbs, and office hours that have flexibility help the practice flourish. Having to take time off from work for a health-care visit will not endear the APN to his or her clients. Consider the characteristics of the community: the location of their homes and workplaces, the mode and length of their daily commute to and from work, and family status.

First Impressions

The physical environment is the first thing the consumer notices. Promote a positive image. Overcoming a negative physical space takes time. No matter how effective the professional is in providing services, a negative space can sidetrack the development of trust in the professional relationship.

Assess the affect of physical space on all five senses. Sound, in and outside of the space, can enhance or distract the consumer. Professionals can invest in full-spectrum lighting, which has been shown to promote a sense of well-being and act as natural sunlight. Florescent lighting can be annoying; it can flicker and emit high-frequency sounds. Does the space have its own smell or scent? Consider touch. Is the space comfortable, well maintained, and clean? Choose comfortable furniture that is pleasing to the eye and the touch, for both the professional and the consumer.

Send a message to consumers that adds to their comfort level. Give consideration to age and developmental factors. For children, place child-oriented toys, games, and books in the waiting room, as well as in the office. On the walls, place literature for the parents. Books and magazines should be available for every age-group. Provide light reading and more serious publications. The most important point to remember about providing publications is to keep them current.

Market research is a rigorous, time-consuming process. However, on completion of this intensive work, the health-care professional has focused on what is needed (the product or service), who needs it (the target market), and where it should be located (the place). The goal of market research is to answer the question, "Why will my health-care services fill a need or solve the problem?" Without adequate assessment information, the APN is operating on a best-guess approach or meeting his or her own needs and not those of the community.

ADVANCED PRACTICE NURSES: A GOOD VALUE FOR THE PUBLIC

Mac Stravic (1997) states, "[w]hile there is wide agreement on the importance of value, there are a wide variety of definitions" (p. 50). Although value is defined as quality for the cost of services, it is also the net outcome of the positive and negative effects from using those services. Quality, peace of mind, reliability, access, breadth of service, and compassion are significant considerations for the health-care consumer (Mac Stravic, 1997). Mac Stravic states, "[by]y looking for and finding ways to increase the value they offer, providers can avoid the all-too-obvious and self-defeating approach of reducing price" (p. 51). APNs should not be recognized or strive to be the lower cost alternative to health care; rather, they should seek to enhance services and therefore increase value. When promoting APN services to the public keep Mac Stravic's words in mind. Find out customary and reasonable fees in the region and then add value to your services. For the consumer these benefits can translate into a savings of time, money, and effort. Think bold, take risks, break with convention, think outside the box, and remember to disrupt the traditional. **Box 23-3** lists some activities APNs are using to promote their practices and provide added value to their services; some of them are traditional whereas others are a bit more "outside the box."

> **BOX 23-3**
> **Advanced Practice Nurse's Activities**
>
> ■ Immediate appointment scheduling
> ■ Printouts of health-care articles (e.g., New York Times *Science Times, Personal Health* by Jane Brody) with a response by the advanced practice nurse (APN)
> ■ Book reviews
> ■ A lending library
> ■ A computer available for health Web sites in the office waiting room (and a class on how to search the Internet for health-care information and a list of Web sites)
> ■ Telephone consultation hours
> ■ Consumer education fact sheets
> ■ A discount of 10% if the consumer has had a recent mammogram, dental visit, or other preventive health service
> ■ Early payment or scheduling incentives
> ■ A prehospitalization workshop for families

No matter how many payment options an APN offers, all systems must be operational as soon as the doors open. Consider the case of one NP-run practice. The group began an advertising campaign, resulting in many phone calls inquiring about their services. The practice intended to participate in 10 insurance plans, but only 3 were in place when their doors opened for business. Clients were lost when they called for appointments and learned their health insurance plan was not yet accepted. Impatience will only lead to false starts, ultimately damaging the budding reputation of the agency or practice (Gaffney, 1999).

Creating Buzz

Rosen (2000) states, "[b]uzz is all the word of mouth about a brand. It's the aggregate of all person-to-person communication about a particular product, service or company at any point" (p. 6). Buzz can occur within an industry or among customers. Industry buzz is a good thing for the APN, but to promote APNs in the marketplace there must be customer buzz as well; after all, it is the customer who will recommend the APN's services to friends and family (Rosen, 2000). The nursing profession recognizes that the APN is an excellent health-care provider, but just having a good product is not enough. For buzz to spread, two things are necessary: "a contagious product—one that has some inherent value that makes people talk—and someone who is behind the scenes who accelerates natural contagion" (Rosen, 2000, p. 129). The APN needs to give the consumer something to talk about. It is not enough to say, "My provider is an APN"; a more effective strategy is to give the consumer something to talk about: "My APN called me at home last night to ask if I had any questions about my medication," or "If I schedule my check up within 30 days of my reminder postcard, I will get a 10% discount." Talking about the benefits of your services is far better than talking about your provider's role. Keep on the consumer's radar screen.

Getting the message out to potential clients is a necessary step in the marketing process. Alward and Camunas (1990) identify eight categories of promotional strategies. Five of them specifically focus on communications: written materials, audiovisual material, corporate identity media, and the news. However, buzz is not written or presented through media channels; buzz travels through invisible networks (Rosen, 2000). As such, it may be the most potent form of promotion. Yet traditional methods of promoting the APN and his or her services have to be incorporated into the overall plan.

Crafting the Message

Written communications and publications must appeal to the consumer. Dense text in the form of letters and brochures are likely to go unread. Use appealing color, texture, and layout to get the reader to take notice. Before a mass mailing ask others for their reactions. Invite your "focus group" to respond as well. What do they see as the message? What is the feeling conveyed? Do not depend on professional designers or artists to make decisions on the printed materials. Get feedback.

Visual images, whether art or photography, convey the strongest, most powerful message. Consider a variety of formats, brochures, foldover notes, postcards, bookmarks, business cards, and stationery, and have them all carry the same images throughout the marketing campaign. The goal is to increase practice recognition. However, keep the design classic and uncomplicated; use solid figures or silhouettes for artwork and black and white for photographs. Color photography is prohibitively expensive, and when trying to sell health-care services, close-up facial expressions convey compassion and support in a much more sensitive fashion. For example, one agency started a new program for parents coping with sibling rivalry after the birth of a new child. The practice group used a black and white photograph of a young child holding an infant. It was a close-up photograph allowing the audience to see both the smiling face of the older child, arms cradling the newborn, and the angelic look on the baby's face. The picture represented every new parent's wish for sibling harmony (Gaffney, 1999).

Language must be clear and brief. Make sure the typeface is easy to read. Reading levels are a significant factor in written materials when it is important to appeal to the broadest audience; in fact, most newspapers are written to target a seventh-grade reading level. Language that is too technical or academic may alienate important parts of the market. Personal success stories and quotes so common in other product or service endorsements are just as important in marketing health-care services. Do not just list services; offer testimonials related to those services. Keep on the radar screen—through monthly newsletters, mailed or electronic, and other publications that promote the practice, as well as the profession.

Distribution of written materials can be accomplished in any one of several ways. Although mailing is expensive, it is also reliable. Placing written material in an envelope will help distinguish it from much of the "junk" mail that postal customers receive. Developing mailing lists and a professional resource guide should be ongoing and will ultimately serve future market needs. Think about creating buzz; develop materials that can stimulate word of mouth, for example, coupons that are for the consumer and a friend. The discount coupons can be used in health food stores, bookstores, or pharmacies. The message will stimulate buzz among the consumer group, as well as within the business community.

Written materials can be distributed to other programs and agencies who have goals similar to the APN's practice. For example, locations for distributing literature on parenting programs and services can include pediatric primary care services, children's specialty stores, day-care and child care centers, nursery schools, and church or synagogue newsletters. Create materials that go beyond advertising services, for example, a recommended reading list that can be placed in libraries or a list of suggested health-care Web sites placed in computer stores, schools, and libraries.

Electronic communications and the Internet are here to stay. The APN should strongly consider building a Web site to tie in with all of the other marketing materials. The design and text of the Web site should reflect the philosophy and mission of the practice. Brief articles providing helpful information for Internet surfers and links to other sites are quite useful. Registering the name of the Web site is inexpensive. Maintenance of the Web site is also reasonable, averaging $1 or $2 a day. Web site design services are much more reasonsable than 5 years ago when the costs of creating the look for a new Web site could reach thousands of dollars. Chat rooms, Q-and-A columns, and advice columns must be carefully considered because there may be potential legal challenges for medical professionals prescribing and treating over the Internet (Gaffney, 1999). However, Weblogs, or blogs, have become so popular that the APN may want to consider adding one to his or her Web site. At the very least, Web sites should always provide educational and organizational resources for consumers. Two new video additions to the cyber community are You Tube (www.youtube.com/) and iTunes U (www.apple.com/education/itunesu_mobilelearning/itunesu.html). iTunes U carries links to major university courses and continuing education programs, all at no cost to the public.

Television and radio advertising for health-care services is an expensive and high-risk venture. It is far better to receive publicity and television exposure about a new program or project. The APN should develop relationships with journalists. Become a resource for them, and they will call for comment, putting the APN's name in the news.

Outreach: Education, Events, and the Advanced Practice Nurse in Public

The fifth *P* of the marketing puzzle centers on two related concepts: community relationships and public service. One effective way to work toward this goal is to give the public a sample of your skills and approaches. Bring the consumer behind the scenes in health care, offer them useful strategies to help them navigate the health-care system, and give them questions to ask and suggestions for wellness. Offer a lecture, brief class, or demonstration on an issue focused topic, for example, how to read news articles on the latest studies, determining the difference between generic and trade medications, or how to find a provider the patient likes. One sage practitioner with years of experience informed this writer, "When you do something for free, you will receive its benefits about 6 months later" (Gaffney, 1999, p. 109). At the very least, good word-of-mouth will follow. Professionals can easily provide educational programs in community, adult schools, resource centers, elementary and secondary schools, and colleges and workplace settings.

APNs should familiarize themselves with the community in which their practice is located. The chamber of commerce is a good starting point. The APN will come to know the goals of the community, as well as its merchants or service providers. Excellent contacts and membership to the chamber of commerce serves to promote good will. The APN will be recognized as an interested and contributing member of the business community.

Giving time further enhances good will and money to important community causes (Alward & Camunas, 1990). The APN may not be able to financially support an organization, but it is possible to donate time, services, and expertise. The APN should strive to be a good citizen in the community. Benefits may not immediately pay off, but there will be positive results in the long run.

Building relationships and connections is essential for creating buzz about APNs. The adage "It's not what you know, but who you know" has much truth behind it. Networking is the foundation. There are four different network types: personal, organizational, professional, and strategic (Michelli & Straw, 1997). Some networks may be influential, providing an entry into a previously closed system. Consider a five-step plan to maximize the benefits of networking: recognize and map networks; identify people who inhabit each one of those networks and look for overlap and links; assess networking styles; clarify goals; and develop and enhance networking behaviors (Michelli & Straw, 1997). The "unwritten code of ethics" for good networking practice includes open-mindedness;

keeping commitments; treating others as one wishes to be treated; freely asking questions and seeking advice; giving without exception; and expressing appreciation. The final step is the act of securing benefits of networking. Buzz travels along networks and is influenced by network hubs, individuals who communicate with more people about a product or service than the average person (Balter & Butman, 2005; Rosen, 2000). Public awareness of the APN depends on the message and the networks accessed.

Evaluating Successes and Missteps

Evaluation and dialogue should be linked and integrated into every aspect of promoting the APN. Prepare a time frame for evaluation activities and stick to it. Continue to dialogue with the community and update with changing trends and consumer interests. The APN needs to keep current, read everything possible, and recognize controversies in health care.

The APN's reputation is established not only on successes but on missteps as well. APNs should not be afraid to ask the consumers if they are satisfied. If they are not, dialogue, seek solutions, and reevaluate. Acknowledge when things do not work well and ask for suggestions and ideas on improving services. Follow through and let the consumer know when things change and what spurred new directions. The APN's reputation will not only survive these missteps, but also actually thrive. See the examples in **Boxes 24-4** through **24-6.**

BOX 23-4
The Case for Adolescent Services: I Do Not Want to Talk to Some Old Guy!

While surveying high school students for a major mental health prevention program, a few unanticipated lessons were learned by the researchers and school administrators. Identification of depressed teens and referral to a health-care agency often failed. The teens did not follow through. When asked why, they complained that the office, which was within the confines of the school building itself, was far too public, "I do not want my friends to see me." A good point. They let the professionals know that their developmental need to be like their peers was virtually ignored by the practice.

In another community, high school students also underused health-care agencies requiring public transportation or a car ride. They could not get there, and the hours were a problem as well. The most successful referrals came from the experience of an agency located one block from the high school, in a building with a variety of services. They also have a policy whereby students could come for information on their own, without any referral. An APN would talk to them, give them information, answer questions, and ask them to return. It is not difficult to see the varying responses to these well-meaning programs.

A school-based office that is used solely for mental health services will not attract students because they will try to avoid being noticed by their peers. One school even advertised the program by painting a sign on the door, "Substance Abuse Counselor." Needless to say the program failed. However, school-based clinics may offer potential because they usually offer a variety of health-related services. Students feel comfortable and develop relationships with the APNs who can then treat them or refer them to other providers.

In a recent dialogue on mental health services with high school students, the facilitator asked, "Who would you talk to if you had a problem?" The students replied that their first choice would be a friend. The reasons were articulated by the teens with clarity and conviction: "They care for me and do not ask for money, they will always be there,

BOX 23-4

The Case for Adolescent Services: I Do Not Want to Talk to Some Old Guy!—cont'd

they will not judge me." They further explained that a coach might be a possibility, a point substantiated by numerous coaches for both men's and women's sports. The facilitator pressed them to identify who they would talk to if they needed to see a professional, and received the answer, "Not some old guy like that what's-his-name-Freud, some young cool guy like Dr. Seaver [the father-psychiatrist from the sitcom *Growing Pains*]. He was a good guy; he helped his kid's friends and even sat on the roof with a boy who was going to commit suicide. I'd talk to him."

The dialogue proved informative on a number of fronts. The most important being the firsthand information regarding how the teens wanted to access services. The underlying strength was the connection made with the adolescents.

BOX 23-5

Advanced Practice Nurse Success and Sex Education: A Program That Works

Advanced practice nurses (APNs) have been in school systems for a long time. They are often employed in school-based clinics or as consultants from outside health agencies. Several advanced practice school nurses shared programs they have used to help young teens learn how to communicate with their parents on the sensitive issue of sexual decision making. *Heart to Heart: For Girls Only* is a program for 9- to 11-year-old girls and their mothers (J. Metzger, personal communication, 1991). The focus of the program is to encourage communication between mothers and daughters. By giving families a shared, guided opportunity to talk about sexuality, they feel more comfortable talking about it at home. The programs are offered through the local medical center (with a group of 25 girls and 25 moms).

Julie Metzger, RN, MSN, is the architect of *Heart to Heart*. The program is two 2-hour sessions. In the first class physical changes are discussed. However, it is not a lecture—in fact, far from it. There are fun exercises, including playing a rendition of "Pictionary." The girls and their moms talk about messages from our culture, about how a woman's body "should" look. There is a discussion of cultural diversity and how women in different parts of the world hear different messages. The bottom line? There are choices about how we care about our bodies and listen to our bodies.

Menstruation is deemed "a human being experience," and therefore teasing someone does not fit. There is respect for the "pioneers" who experience these changes first! And there is talk about helping each other feel "important and included" (J. Metzger, personal communication 2002).

Heart to Heart addresses sexual decision making by defining and separating feelings, actions, and consequences. There are definitions given for sexual body parts and body responses. In some groups the leader asks the girls to "shout out" their answers at the same time and the room explodes in hysterical chaos, but then there is time to talk about their responses individually. Moms get a chance to talk, too. The questions stimulate a great deal of energy and discussion. One particular favorite is the "How old should you be when you have intercourse for the first time?" scenario. First girls respond, then moms, and then there is discussion. Exercises offer a chance for experiential learning. What is the best quality

Continued

BOX 23-5
Advanced Practice Nurse Success and Sex Education: A Program That Works—cont'd

in a friend? Everyone answers, then the group facilitator suggests the girls add these qualities together, and that is what a partner should be.

The second class focuses on "feelings, actions, and consequences." The class is offered several opportunities to role-play and discuss how they problem-solve through challenging, but not threatening, peer pressure scenarios using the feelings, actions, consequences model.

Metzger explains to the girls and their moms, "Feelings are emotions that come from within, actions are the result of choices we make, given our feelings and/or the consequences, but consequences are 'what we live with afterwards.'"

Metzger facilitates a final exercise "To bring it all together," using the feelings, actions, and consequences continuum. Through five different scenarios the girls struggle with their choices and their outcomes. Sometimes the results are hilarious.

The equation clicks for the girls; it makes sense that there are big consequences for their actions. The exercise always works and it gives parents a model they can use in other "real-life" scenarios at home.

The discussions generated by the groups are enlightening for both parents and the young teens. Course evaluations and repeat visits from parents with younger siblings validate that this course has helped mothers and daughters communicate in a fun yet informative way. For Metzger, the proof is in the registration—the course is always sold out.

However, Metzger did not stop with *Heart to Heart*. She captured the success of her program and built a Web site around it. *Great Conversations* (www.greatconversations.com/) offers classes, lectures, and resources on the topics of puberty, sexuality, and parenting. These services intend to promote communication and enhance family conversations in a way that is fun and factual.

BOX 23-6
Seller Beware: A Cautionary Tale from September 11, 2001

In the days and weeks following the terrorist attacks of September 11, 2001, we learned an important lesson about the mental health profession. What seemed to be the right approach for what we, the professionals, perceived as an enormous mental health need was not the right approach at all. Nor did we assess the mental health need accurately or in the context of a catastrophic event.

Clinicians and researchers anticipated soaring rates of posttraumatic stress disorder and a population permanently incapacitated by the horrors they witnessed and the losses they sustained. Mental health providers flocked to New York and Washington to offer their services to both citizens and first responders. Local professionals, themselves victims of the trauma, tried to educate each other in the intricacies of trauma and bereavement work. Hospitals prepared for screenings, clinics added hours, corporations brought in employee assistance personnel, and schools made crisis counselors available to their students and staff. At first the public's response was overwhelming, phones rang off the hook and walk-ins streamed through the doorways. Then it stopped. The calls dwindled and people no longer seemed interested in support groups or any other mental health services for that matter. Those already in treatment or those with a history of mental health concerns accessed the system

BOX 23-6

Seller Beware: A Cautionary Tale from September 11, 2001—cont'd

quite readily. So mental health providers, freshly infused with Federal Emergency Management Agency funding, hung their shingles for the "new people." They waited in offices, trailers, and at assistance centers. No one asked for help.

We did not anticipate the need for people to come together—for support, for prayer, and for food. During the immediate aftermath of the terrorist attacks, people sought out families and friends, and they embraced religion. They sought out familiar people and places to find comfort. They stayed home and cancelled plans. *Cocooning* is a good term for this process. We did not realize how people would access mental health services, and what their needs for self-care would be. We minimized the comfort and support from familiar faces and places.

Just steps from the train station in a New Jersey community there is a tiny cheese shop. Barely wide enough to accommodate a half-dozen customers, commuters coming from New York's financial district stream into the shop after work. The owners, a warm and welcoming husband and wife, work in tandem, learning the life stories of their customers while offering tastes of the newest cheese from France. On September 11th, 2001, they found themselves a refuge for travelers in the storm of terrorism.

Just after the first attack on the World Trade Center, a young woman who was a regular customer, came into the couple's store after missing her train. She told them the horrific news. Having calculated where she would have been if she had not been late, she stayed to talk to them. She did not buy any cheese. The shopkeepers thought about closing the store because they assumed people would be racing home to be with their families. In a moment of clarity, they decided that they would stay open to "be there" for their friends. And they were. All day long people streamed into the tiny store, ashen and covered with ashes. Sometimes they just talked. Sometimes they cried. Some customers bought sandwiches or cheese, one young man told them he could only think about eating [olives] for the entire ride home to New Jersey. Was this just a quest for comfort food or were these shopkeepers a meaningful effort to connect with others who could offer them comfort?

Within a week the Cheese Shop became legendary in the community. Not just for their food, but also for the service they gave to those who escaped the collapsing towers. In the year after the terrorist attacks, the widows and widowers of those who died have returned, and the travelers on that fateful day continue to visit. What can professionals learn from this small example? Allow people to gravitate to their own families and friends and places of support. We do not have to be the first line of defense; we need to support those in an individual's life who will be a sustaining source of comfort.

We did not identify the needs of grieving families. We sent in the proverbial grief counselors; we developed camps for bereaved children; we started programs, support groups and more support groups. Mary Ellen Salamone, the director of *Children of September 11th*, reacts to the blanketing of mental health services in a straightforward, no-nonsense manner, "You have to come to us." She suggested that support groups were useful only to a point. As families move beyond the 5-year mark they need to help their children integrate the tragedy and learn how to deal with the rest of their lives. She suggested that an educational approach might be far more useful: "Plan workshops, ask us what we need . . . we'll help make it happen and even raise funds to support the project." This was an opportunity too good to refuse. As a result, partnership building between parents, professionals, and nonprofits was initated. The first conference focusing on how children can learn and heal from the challenging lessons of the global community was held just before the 6th year commemorating September 11th, 2001.

EXEMPLARS IN PROMOTING THE ADVANCED PRACTICE NURSE: THIS IS JUST THE BEGINNING

With a multitude of marketing theories, methods, and approaches, the APN can be overwhelmed. Eventually, the APN will learn what works and what needs to be revisited. It is an exciting journey that harkens back to the days when the role of the APN was first introduced to the profession. There will be continued challenges educating the public and promoting the APN to consumers. Be creative, take risks, and think outside the traditional health-care "box." Talk to people; most of all dialogue with the consumer. Form collaborations. Take what APNs do best and advertise it, but *tell* the consumer first. Write about what you learn and tell others what you do. Every interaction is an opportunity to educate and promote the APN; turn those interactions into a chain reaction as information floods into the community. The APN is the best-kept secret in health care, but only if we want to keep it that way.

References

American Marketing Association. (2007). *New definition of marketing.* Retrieved May 1, 2008, from the American Marketing Association Web site: www.marketingpower.com/content4620.php.

Alward, R., & Camunas, C. (1990). Public relations, Part II, Strategies and tactics. *Journal of Nursing Administration, 20*(11), 31–41.

Balter, D., & Butman, J. (2005). *Grapevine: The new art of word-of-mouth marketing.* New York: Penguin.

Barton, E. (1998). *An operational definition of marketing.* Unpublished manuscript.

Buckley, W. (1967). *Sociology and modern systems theory.* Englewood Cliffs, NJ: Prentice-Hall.

Cunningham, R. (1982). Hospital marketing is no cure. *Hospitals, 56,* 73–75.

Dru, J. M. (1996). *Disruption: Overturning conventions and shaking up the marketplace.* New York: Wiley & Sons.

Dru, J. M. (2002). *Beyond disruption: Changing the rules in the marketplace.* New York: Wiley & Sons.

Engelberg, M., & Neubrand, S. (1997). Building sensible segmentation strategies in managed care settings. *Marketing Health Services, 17*(2), 50–51.

Gaffney, D. (1999). Marketing mental health services. In C. Shea, L. Pelletier, L. Poster, G. Stuart, & M. Verhey (Eds.), *Advanced practice psychiatric nursing in psychiatric and mental health care.* St. Louis: Mosby, pp. 95–112.

Gladwell, M. (2000). *The tipping point: How little things can make a difference.* New York: Little Brown.

Godin, S. (1999). *Permission marketing: Turning strangers into friends and friends into customers.* New York: Simon and Schuster.

Kennedy, D. (1991). *The ultimate marketing plan.* Holbrook, MA: Bob Adams, Inc.

Kotler, P. (1976). *Marketing management* (3rd. ed.). Englewood Cliffs, NJ: Prentice-Hall.

Kumar, V., & Ramani, G. (2006). Interaction orientation: The new marketing competency. In J. N. Sheth, & R. S. Sisodia (Eds.), *Does marketing need reform? Fresh perspectives on the future* (pp. 109–118). Armonk, NY: M.E. Sharpe.

Mac Stravic, S. (1997, Winter). Questions of value in health care. *Marketing Health Services,* 50–52.

McDonald, M. (2007). *Marketing plans: How to prepare them, how to use them* (6th ed.). Oxford: Butterworth-Heinemann.

McKenna, R. (1991). Marketing is everything. *Harvard Business Review, 69*(1), 65–79.

Michelli, D., & Straw, A. (1997). *Successful networking.* Happauge, NY: Barrons.

Pinson, L., & Jinnett, J. (1996). *Target marketing* (3rd. ed.). Chicago: Upstart Publishing.

Reis, A., & Trout, J. (1986). *Marketing warfare.* New York: Penguin Books.

Rosen, E. (2000). *The anatomy of buzz.* New York: Doubleday.

von Bertalanffy, L. (1968). *General systems theory: Foundations, development, applications.* New York: Braziller.

Starting a Practice and Practice Management

24

Judith Barberio

Advanced practice nurses (APNs) increasingly strive for greater autonomy in their practice. This desire to have control over their work environment has lead to the emergence of independent nurse-managed health-care practices. But are an entrepreneurial spirit, fine-tuned knowledge base and clinical skills, and the desire to provide quality health care enough? Over the past 15 years, individuals, as well as schools of nursing, have increasingly opened nurse-managed health centers, only to see their viability threatened because of lack of financial self-sufficiency (Vincent, MacKay, Pohl, Hirth, & Oakley, 1999). If nurse-managed practices are to survive, APNs must arm themselves with business acumen and financial know-how to make their practices efficient and fiscally viable.

ADVANTAGES TO INDEPENDENT PRACTICE

Independent practice sounds like a dream. The ability to maximize the care of the client and the time to provide the educational base is necessary to enable the client to become a true partner in the health-care regimen. An independent practice can provide the APN with many opportunities, such as those listed in **Box 24-1.**

BARRIERS TO INDEPENDENT PRACTICE

With all the advantages to independent practice, why do so few APNs consider this alternative? APNs have long been lauded in the literature with respect to the high quality of patient care and cost effectiveness (Carzoli, Martinez-Cruz, Cuevas, Murphy, & Chiu, 1994; Office of Technology Assessment, 1986; Spitzer et al., 1974). Their practice has been compared to physicians in primary care practices, and findings suggest that APNs provide comparable high-quality care with similar positive health outcomes (Mundinger et al., 2000). What barriers to practice are so prevalent that they dissuade this competent, highly educated, and cost-effective group of health-care providers from establishing independent practices?

Nationally, Pearson (2007) identifies the four major roadblocks to independent APN practice as:

1. The need for direct reimbursement from third-party payors
2. Statutory limitations to the APN's scope of practice
3. Inconsistent and restrictive prescriptive authority
4. The inability to obtain hospital privileges

BOX 24-1
Opportunities That Can Come with Independent Practice

1. The freedom to focus the practice and your energy on your interests, such as alternative therapy or acupuncture, or specialty populations such as women's health or geriatrics.

2. Time management becomes flexible. You have the ability to structure your workload and allow time to examine, counsel, and educate clients.

3. The quality of your practice becomes your responsibility and is under your control. You are able to include the preventive health care and education needed at each client encounter.

4. Multiple sources for reimbursement can be identified and pursued. Beside third-party reimbursement, contracts for service can be sought out in industry and community groups. Income can be tied to workload.

5. New opportunities and requests for service provide a challenge to expand services and promote the growth of the practice.

6. Staffing becomes your responsibility and provides the opportunity to work with people you respect and who share your philosophy of health care.

7. Enhanced problem-solving skills and self-esteem are positive by-products of independent practice for the entrepreneurial APN. Learning to constructively deal with change, resolve conflicts, and successfully implement strategies creates a profitable practice and enhances self-confidence and self-esteem.

Many factors contribute to the roadblocks that stand in the way of independent APN practice. Throughout the 20th century physicians have controlled health-care practice and health information, partially due to the fact that they were the first health-care providers to be granted legislative autonomy. This legislative autonomy and recognition enhanced the public's confidence that the actions of physicians were always directed for the good of the public and not for personal gain. Financial security, legislative strength, and a unified medical community also played a role in organized medicine's control of hospital policy and third-party reimbursement (Mirvis, 1999).

In addition to persuasive national barriers, common problems applicable to most new start-up businesses contribute to the demise of independent APN practices. Major obstacles to overcome with the start of most new businesses include:

1. Start-up costs for the practice
2. Cash-flow and financing an ongoing practice
3. Accounting practices, billing, and collection of receipts
4. Day-to-day management of the practice
5. Compliance with city, state, and federal regulations
6. General and malpractice insurance for the practice and individual providers
7. Hiring, training, and retaining competent, enthusiastic personnel

The obstacles inherent in starting a business coupled with the unique barriers confronting independent APN practice have provided a challenge to many individuals. This chapter acknowledges their struggles, learns from their mistakes, and provides guidance to the entrepreneurial APN who is about to embark on this journey.

FIRST THINGS FIRST

The decision has been made: you want to be your own boss and deliver health care *your* way. No more time clocks, overbooking clients, or cutting short the patient visit due to time constraints. But where do you go from here? Key considerations and decisions must be made to get your business up and running. The items listed in **Box 24-2** will focus your operation and provide the organizing details that determine start-up efficiency in the world of managed care.

KEY QUESTIONS

As you embark on the key start-up decisions to be made, pay attention to the questions that may arise. A major question to consider is the scope of independent APN practice in the state in which you practice. Forty states currently have statutory or regulatory requirements for physician collaboration, direction, or supervision. And only 11 states (including the District of Columbia) have independent prescriptive authority that does not require physician involvement or delegation (Pearson, 2007). If your practice is not located in one of these enlightened states, carefully read and clarify the policies regarding collaboration or supervision of your practice and the regulation of your prescriptive authority. Developing a collaborative agreement with a physician and creating appropriate protocols, including protocols for controlled dangerous substances (CDS), are other areas to investigate if this is a state requirement for APN practice.

Reimbursement is another major question to consider. Where will it come from and will it be enough to cover your expenses? Investigate how pervasive managed care is in your practice location and determine if APNs are admitted to managed care panels and are listed as primary care providers

---

BOX 24-2
Key Business Decisions

- Develop a clear-cut strategy
- Determine the area's need for the service
- Develop a time line for business start-up
- Determine licensing, tax, and insurance requirements
- Select your consultants
- Decide on the appropriate business structure
- Create the business name and image
- Select a practice location
- Develop a business plan
- Determine financing options
- Develop fees, reimbursement, and billing procedures
- Purchase equipment and select suppliers
- Hire and manage personnel
- Develop an organized documentation and quality assurance process
- Develop policies and procedures
- Develop marketing strategies

(PCPs). If APNs are accepted in your state as PCPs and practice independently, how do you deal with the patient whose condition exacerbates and needs hospitalization? Investigate the area hospitals to determine if APNs are given hospital privileges. Even if APNs are admitted to hospital panels in your area, you will need a collaborative arrangement or referral agreement with various physicians in the area for management of your patients when they are acutely ill.

These, as well as other questions, will arise as you carry out the myriad tasks needed to launch a new business. Pay attention to detail and carefully consider each question and decision you make. These decisions will structure your practice operations and ultimately enable you to attain your personal and professional goals.

DEVELOP A CLEAR-CUT STRATEGY

Strategy distinguishes your business. It tells the consumer what differentiates your practice from the competition. It is the foundation of your business plan and dictates the day-to-day operations of your practice. How does one develop a strategy? Look around you and consider the market, consumer needs, the competition, your practice's strength and weaknesses, and your philosophy of health care and personal goals.

Focus the nature of your practice and do not try to be all things to all patients. Competitive personal service businesses, such as a health-care practice, will commonly use the strategy of specialization. Specialization reduces competition and drives reimbursement. Initially, you may want to see any patient who elects to seek your help. As you begin to develop your practice, simultaneously begin to advertise, write articles for the local newspaper, and hold seminars on topics that focus on your expertise. This exposure will promote the area in which you wish to specialize and will allow you to phase out other aspects of your practice.

Specialize by developing a niche market, one that you know extremely well. A niche market is one with a unique service or product that services a particular clientele. You may decide that you want the focus of your practice to be on wellness. You can then tailor your practice to offer individual health risk assessments, counseling on behavior change, work site wellness programs, smoking cessation and weight loss programs, and countless other health promotion activities that may be needed in your location. One word of advice; know your service. Do not begin a practice marketing alternative therapy without an exhaustive knowledge of these services or competent, knowledgeable staff. Remember that your competition is already established and knows the business aspects of the practice better than you do. You want to present yourself as an expert in the field.

DETERMINE THE AREA'S NEED FOR THE SERVICE

Determine who the potential clients are and then attempt to ascertain their needs. If you decide that your practice will serve the health care needs of inner-city, low-income residents, then you must investigate the most prevalent reasons for health-care use and follow-up care. This information can be gathered from various sources. The state nurses association, state division of health, and county and local health departments may be helpful in providing important data. Topics you may want to explore include health provider demographics for an area, medically underserved areas, and health-care delivery systems in an area such as ambulatory care centers, urgent care centers, and family planning clinics. Local businesses, such as pharmacies and medical device companies, may also provide information about the health-care needs of the local population, as well as advertising and articles placed in the local newspaper.

DEVELOP A TIME LINE FOR BUSINESS START-UP

Organization is the key ingredient to developing a business plan and moving your practice from the planning stage into action. A minimum of 9 months should be allowed to complete this project. Designate yourself as the project leader and determine other individuals who may assist you with start-up tasks. The key undertaking of business start-up is persistence and attention to detail. A sample time-line for completing major tasks is presented in **Box 24-3.**

BOX 24-3
Practice Start-Up Time Line

NINE MONTHS BEFORE PRACTICE START-UP

1. Select a geographical location.
2. Obtain contracts from third-party payors and hospitals you wish to join.
3. Determine start-up costs of a practice and your net worth.
4. Develop a business plan.
5. Investigate sources of capital investment in your practice.
6. Obtain loan applications, speak to various loan officers, and submit applications.
7. Determine when telephone books are printed and list your practice.
8. Open a business checking account.
9. Obtain state nursing license, advanced practice license, and federal Drug Enforcement Agency (DEA) number.
10. Investigate potential physician collaborators if needed in your state.

SIX MONTHS BEFORE PRACTICE START-UP

1. Investigate practice locations for rent or purchase.
2. Inquire about zoning laws regarding your type of practice and signage requirements.
3. Determine utility requirements for your practice, sources, and cost.
4. Determine office layout, design, and necessary structural improvements.
5. Determine needed office and medical equipment and determine cost of lease versus buy.
6. Explore and select business consultants, specifically a lawyer, accountant, banker, insurance broker, and medical biller.
7. Determine form of the practice, such as solo practice, partnership, or corporation, and have your attorney draw up all legal documents for your signature.
8. Evaluate all contracts with your attorney before signing.
9. Investigate medical practice systems that contain scheduling, billing, and records.
10. Make application for federal Medicare, Medicaid, and national provider identifier (NPI) numbers and obtain fee schedules.
11. Obtain current procedural terminology book (CPT-4) and International Classification of Diseases Ninth Revision, Clinical Manual (ICD-9-CM) and the HCFA 1500 insurance claim forms.
12. Formalize a collaborative agreement with an area physician if required by law.

Continued

BOX 24-3
Practice Start-Up Time Line—cont'd

13. Apply for an office laboratory license or a Clinical Laboratory Improvement Amendments (CLIA) Waiver.

14. Apply for provider status to managed care provider panels.

15. Apply for hospital privileges to local health-care institutions.

THREE MONTHS BEFORE PRACTICE START-UP

1. Arrange for professional malpractice insurance for providers and liability insurance for the practice and equipment.

2. Arrange for health and disability insurance for yourself and employees.

3. Arrange for telephone service installation and an answering service for the practice, beeper service, and call forwarding service.

4. Order signage for the practice.

5. Investigate and arrange for the acceptance of credit cards as a payment option.

6. Design and order announcements for the opening of your practice.

7. Apply for your federal and state employer identification number (EIN) through your local Internal Revenue Service (IRS) office and state labor department.

8. Review federal and state tax requirements with your accountant and obtain booklets describing federal, state, and city tax withholding requirements.

9. Develop a policy and procedure manual for the practice.

10. Develop job descriptions for all employees.

11. Begin advertising and interviewing for office personnel.

12. Arrange for needed services such as biomedical waste management, specimen pick-up, janitorial services, laundry services, and ground maintenance and snow removal.

13. Order clinical supplies and set up an inventory control system.

14. Order business supplies such as state prescription pads (if mandated), appointment cards, business cards, letterhead stationary and envelopes, stationery supplies, deposit stamp for checks, petty cash vouchers, purchase order forms, telephone message pads, and patient referral forms and disposition forms.

15. Order office equipment and arrange for delivery.

16. Determine office hours.

17. Determine fee schedule.

18. Develop advertising information such as a patient booklet of services, press release, and introduction letters to local health-care providers, pharmacy and medical equipment suppliers, and pharmaceutical representatives in your area.

ONE MONTH BEFORE PRACTICE START-UP

1. Set up your office.

2. Arrange for utility start-up, including telephone, gas, electric, and water.

3. Hire a medical biller and obtain your Medicare, Medicaid, NPI, and managed care organization provider numbers.

4. Hire office personnel and train them with respect to office policies, telephone procedures, appointment scheduling and collection of fees, and use of the medical office system.

BOX 24-3
Practice Start-Up Time Line—cont'd

5. Establish the office cash flow procedures and a petty cash fund.
6. Install your office sign.
7. Accept patient appointments.
8. Place announcements, advertisements, and press releases in local newspapers and send to local community groups and area professionals.

OPENING DAY
Congratulations, you have started an independent APN practice!

DETERMINE LICENSING, TAX, AND INSURANCE REQUIREMENTS

To open an independent APN practice, a number of licenses must be obtained. After choosing a location for your practice, the process of applying for all state and federal licenses should be your next priority. Besides state licensure for nursing and advanced practice nursing, you must also obtain state and federal identification numbers and a federal Drug Enforcement Agency (DEA) number, as well as others to open your door and do business. The most commonly required licenses and tax identification numbers have been listed.

State Nursing License and Advanced Practice License or Certification

The state board of nursing will be able to provide information and a list of documents you need to apply for these licenses. Be aware that in some states the board of nursing and the board of medicine oversee the advanced practice nursing license or certification.

State Narcotics License

Check with your state concerning the requirement for a state narcotics license. This is not a requirement of all states, but if it is, it must be obtained before application for a federal narcotics license. Your state's board of nursing will be able to inform you if this license is necessary and the procedure to obtain this license.

Federal Narcotics License

APNs do not have legal authority in all states to dispense narcotics. You will be able to obtain the necessary information from the board of nursing in the state. DEA numbers are assigned for your lifetime; they will not be reassigned if you move to another location. If you move to another state, you are required to notify the DEA authorities of your new address. If you do not have a DEA number and can legally prescribe narcotics in your state, you can obtain this license from the Department of Justice at:

Registration Unit
Drug Enforcement Administration

PO Box 28083 Central Station
Washington, DC 20005
Drug Enforcement Administration (DEA), Office of Diversion Control, Registration Unit,
     toll-free number, 24 hours a day 1-800-882-9539

The DEA also has forms online for registration of APNs. The application form can be found on the Web at the Diversion Control Program Web site at www.DEAdiversion.usdoj.gov.

Medicaid Provider Number

Medicaid is a jointly funded, federal-state health insurance program for certain low-income people. The people covered include children, the aged, blind, disabled, and people who are eligible to receive federally assisted income maintenance payments.

You can apply for this provider number through the state Medicaid agency. Obtain a provider application for APNs from the provider relations department of your state health department. The state Medicaid agency is billed using the Centers for Medicare and Medicaid Services (CMS) 1500 form unless the client is enrolled in Medicaid managed care.

The number you receive from your state Medicaid agency will remain with you while you practice in the state. If you move within the state, you only need to notify the carrier of your new address. If you move out of state, you will need to obtain a new number in the new state.

Medicaid Managed Care

Some patients who have health insurance through the state Medicaid program will be covered under a managed care organization. To obtain a provider number for Medicaid managed care organizations (MCO), you must contact the provider relations for each MCO and apply for admission to the panel of providers. APNs are not admitted to provider panels in all MCOs. In some states, MCOs cannot discriminate among providers on the basis of type of license held. In other states, an MCO can accept or reject any provider. Check your state law concerning managed care and provider panels. If you are initially rejected, request a meeting to present your case. Pursue the MCO to reevaluate your application and go up the chain of command with your request.

Medicare

Medicare is a federal health insurance program for certain groups of people including the elderly over the age of 65 and the permanently disabled. This program covers hospitalization (Part A), home care and outpatient health care (Part B), and medication (Part D).

If you will be providing health-care services to this population, you need to apply for a Medicare number. This number will only be valid in the state in which you currently practice. If you move out of state, you will be assigned a new Medicare number for that state.

An insurer in each state that has contracted with the CMS manages the administration and payment services for Medicare. You can find the Medicare carrier for your state by going to the CMS Web site at www.cms.hhs.gov/ or Medicare at www.medicare.gov/. Once you are aware of the carrier for your state, you can obtain an application and apply for a provider number. Medicare is billed on a form called the CMS 1500. These forms can be found in many office supply stores, as well as through the American Medical Association. The preferred method of billing for Medicare is electronic funds transfer (EFT), and this can be elected when enrolling in Medicare for the first time or when making a change to your existing enrollment information. If a patient is enrolled in Medicare managed care, reimbursement is handled by an MCO, and the provider must be admitted to the MCO provider panel.

Universal Provider Identification Number

The universal provider identification number (UPIN) was assigned to health-care providers when they made application for a Medicare provider number. This number was a "legacy identifier" or identification number assigned to health-care providers. Other examples of legacy identifiers are provider identification numbers (PIN), national supplier clearinghouse (NSC) numbers and online survey certification and reporting (OSCAR) numbers. The CMS Web site states that the national provider identifier (NPI) will replace the legacy identifiers. For further information, go to the CMS Web site at www.cms.hhs.gov/.

National Provider Identifier

The NPI is a unique identification number given to each health-care provider and used in standard transactions, such as claims for reimbursement for health-care services. This number may be used to identify health-care providers on a number of documents including prescriptions, patient medical records, and coordination of benefits between health plans. Once assigned, the NPI is expected to remain the same regardless of change of name, change of address, or change of other information provided on the original application. The compliance date for all entities to use the NPI number on transactions is May 23, 2008. As of this date, the NPI will be the only health-care provider identifier that can be used for identification purposes in standard transactions including electronic billing.

Health-care providers may apply for an NPI number through the national plan and provider enumeration system (NPPES) available at https://nppes.cms.hhs.gov. Providers may also apply for the NPI number on a paper application by requesting form (CMS-10114) through the NPI enumerator or by downloading the paper application. The phone number for the NPI Enumerator is 1-800-465-3203, and the paper application can be downloaded from www.cms.hhs.gov/NationalProviderStand/ and mailed to the address on the form. There is no fee associated with obtaining a NPI.

If the health-care provider does not have a Medicare or Medicaid provider number, they are encouraged to apply for the NPI before enrolling in these programs. If the health-care provider already has enrolled in these programs, they are encouraged to include their Medicare identification number and legacy identifiers, Medicaid identification number and state, and any other provider numbers issued by health plans in which they are enrolled when applying for the NPI.

Clinical Laboratory License

CMS regulates all laboratory testing performed on humans in the United States through the Clinical Laboratory Improvement Amendments (CLIA). The objective of the CLIA program is to ensure quality laboratory testing. These amendments require that all health provider office laboratories must be licensed according to the types of tests they perform. Office laboratories are subject to federal and state inspection and approval. The more complex the testing, the more stringent the state and federal laboratory requirements. However, any laboratory testing done on site will require the facility to have a CLIA number.

Laboratory tests are divided into categories, and there are a number of waived tests that can be performed in the office setting. A practice that only performs waived tests can apply for an exemption from inspection and the requirement of a medical director to oversee the laboratory. Federal

CLIA regulations can be found on the Internet at www.cms.hhs.gov/clia/, and state CLIA regulations can be obtained from the state health department. The state will provide forms for the federal and state application for a CLIA number. Pay particular attention to the state regulations because many times the state regulations are more restrictive than the federal guidelines.

Employer Identification Number

The employer identification number (EIN) is a tax identification number and is needed for all communication with the Internal Revenue Service (IRS). Contact your local IRS office or Social Security office and request Form SS-4 to apply for an EIN. This number can also be applied for by phone with the local IRS Service Center. Once an EIN is obtained, the IRS will send a booklet of payment coupons (Form 8109) for depositing your withholding taxes. The EIN will also be used to report compensation from third-party payors such as private insurance companies, Medicare, or Medicaid.

State Tax Identification Number

Contact your state to confirm if there is an additional need to apply for a state tax identification number. The local phone number can be found in the white pages listed under United States or the name of your state. Your accountant will be able to inform you of all identifying numbers needed to satisfy federal and state regulations.

Professional Liability Insurance

There are many carriers that cover APNs, including traditional insurance companies, self-insured companies, and group purchasing programs. Not all companies conduct business in every state. Choose a company that has experienced claim adjusters and a formidable legal network. Inquire about the company's service orientation and its capacity to offer risk management and loss prevention assistance and advice. Consider a company who has been in business for at least 10 years and has a good financial standing. Litigation can take many years to come to fruition, and you want a company with the capability to remain in business to defend you.

Some points to consider when evaluating insurance policies:

1. How comprehensive is the policy? Make sure you read the policy thoroughly and note the inclusions, as well as the exclusions. Question anything you do not understand; it may save you a great deal of stress and money if litigation ensues.
2. What type of insurance should you purchase: "claims made" or "occurrence"? A claims made policy will cover the APN only when the insurance policy is active, no matter when the incident occurred. If you were to retire and cancel your insurance policy, you would no longer be covered for any prior incident if litigation ensues at a later date. An occurrence policy will cover the APN for any incident that occurred while the insurance policy was in place.
3. Are the limits of coverage adequate? Many APNs purchase insurance based on the minimal coverage of $1,000,000 per occurrence and $3,000,000 cumulative. We reside in a litigious society, and this amount of coverage can easily be exhausted. Consider purchasing cumulative insurance that is at least double to triple the occurrence amount.
4. Should you purchase "tail coverage"? Frequently, APNs may join a group practice that already has a group policy for professional liability coverage. If you currently have malpractice insurance that you plan on canceling, consider purchasing tail coverage. This policy will cover any prospective legal action from events before joining the group practice.

5. Do you own the practice? If so, you may want to name the practice on your insurance policy. If litigation ensues, usually the practice, as well as an individual, is named.

6. Is business malpractice insurance necessary? Absolutely! Cover the practice. Inquire with the insurance company about the rates for covering an independent APN practice. This coverage will be in addition to your individual plan and can prove quite cost effective in the event of litigation.

Conventional Commercial Insurance Policies

Besides professional and business malpractice insurance, consider purchasing insurance protection for your office, the employees, and the equipment you have purchased. Some types of insurance to consider:

1. *Equipment insurance:* The expenditure for medical and office equipment is costly. A reasonably priced property insurance policy will cover the cost to replace the tangible assets of the practice. This policy should cover all medical equipment and supplies, office equipment, and supplies, textbooks, and journals. Insurance premiums typically decrease as deductibles rise.

2. *Equipment malfunction insurance:* Many companies sell product warranties to cover equipment malfunction, repair, and replacement. Investigate commercial insurance companies for a blanket policy that covers all major equipment purchases. Many policies will also cover lost revenue for the time period that the equipment is unproductive.

3. *General liability coverage:* This is comprehensive insurance coverage that protects your practice in the advent of litigation by a third party. It does not cover the policyholder or other parties specifically excluded. This policy typically includes lawsuits for personal injury, equipment failure, contractual liability, and advertising liability.

4. *Office disability insurance:* If your office becomes inaccessible as a result of property loss, your practice could go out of business in a short period of time. This policy should include reimbursement for lost revenue and profit, continuous expenses such as the lease on the copy machine, funding to temporarily relocate your office, purchase supplies, and advertise your new location, and finally the cost to return to your office after it has been restored.

5. *Workers' compensation insurance:* Most states require this insurance for any business that has employees. The owner of the business is usually not covered by this insurance unless the business is a corporation. This policy can be purchased from a commercial insurance company, but the state will regulate the benefits and cost of the policy. Therefore, most policies are comparable.

SELECT YOUR CONSULTANTS

Starting a health-care practice requires knowledge of state and federal laws, as well as general legal and accounting procedures. It is highly advisable to consult with these professionals as you set up your practice. Seek recommendations from other APNs, colleagues, business associates, the state nursing organization, and the board of nursing.

Attorney services will focus on setting up the legal structure of your practice and provide legal advice and contract development and review. When you interview attorneys, pay particular attention to their health-care law experience, especially with respect to independent APN practice.

An *accountant* is another professional whose expertise can be cost effective for the short term, as well as the long term. Initially, consult with this professional to develop an accounting system, initiate internal controls, and establish an operating budget. As the practice develops, the accountant may suggest operating procedures that will provide for the best tax advantage and provide tax-planning consultation.

A *medical biller* is an essential component of any health-care practice that intends to receive reimbursement from third-party payors. Medical billers will be involved in all aspects of billing and collecting accounts receivable. They may set up and track a charge account with a major credit card company for patients that are self-pay and send billing statements to patients who have been extended credit by the health-care practice. Medical billers frequently make application to insurer provider panels for the health-care providers in the practice. Additionally, they will make application to NPI, Medicare, and Medicaid for provider numbers for the practice and all professional staff. Once avenues of reimbursement are established, the medical biller will ensure that the patient and medical information requested by the payer is completed and will submit the bill for payment. Tracking accounts receivable and questioning and resubmitting denial of payments is another aspect of the services provided by a medical biller. The scope of services from a medical biller will depend on the expertise and experience of this consultant. Many practices find it more cost-effective to hire a full-time medical biller, whereas smaller practices may hire an off-site independent service to handle the billing aspect of the practice. Judiciously assess the qualifications and reputation of the employee or service you are contemplating.

A *practice manager* might be just the person or service you need if you are taking over an established practice or have a large patient following. An experienced practice manager may provide accounting and bookkeeping services, as well as total practice management. Services offered can vary greatly by consultant, and fees will increase as services provided increase. Practice mangers may perform such services as hiring employees, maintaining bank accounts, paying practice bills, billing and account receivables for services rendered, staffing, payroll, tracking and ordering supplies, and contracting for laboratory, biomedical waste and janitorial services. Many practice management consultants will develop employee job descriptions, policy and procedure manuals, and fee schedules that are consistent with the local market. Always ask for local references, preferably with other health-care providers, especially other APN practices. Remember to always check references and qualifications to get an idea of the types of services provided by this consultant, his or her experience and expertise, and his or her ability to competently complete the project in a timely manner.

DECIDE ON THE APPROPRIATE BUSINESS STRUCTURE

There are basically four types of business structures for a practice: sole proprietorship, partnership, corporation, or a limited liability corporation. The legal differences between these forms of business are contained in three issues: liability, the number of owners, and tax ramifications.

Sole Proprietorship

This is the simplest form of business, where the owner of the business and the business are one and the same. All of the assets and liabilities of the business are also the personal assets and liabilities of the owner. The owner of an independent APN practice is personally libel for any debt or legal infractions of the practice. There are no explicit prerequisites to establishing a sole proprietorship. A sole proprietorship can have only one owner of the business and is established when you go into business by yourself. This gives the APN the advantage of "running her own show" and establishing a practice according to specific beliefs and preferences. A sole proprietorship is not taxed per se. Because the business and the owner are one and the same, the owner completes an individual tax return along with a Schedule C. A Schedule C is a "profit and loss from business" form, which is used to file the practice earnings and expenses. Year-end profits and losses from the practice will be added or subtracted from the owners' personal income.

Benefits from this type of business structure include autonomy, flexibility, and the ability to make practice decisions based on your individual philosophy. Any losses suffered by the practice, which is common in the start-up phase of a business, can be deducted from your personal income. Control of the profits is another benefit of this business structure along with a simplified tax return. A major disadvantage of a sole proprietorship is the total liability for all start-up and maintenance costs of the practice, as well as the negligence of any employees.

Partnership

A partnership is defined as the association of two or more people to carry on as co-owners of a business to make a profit. Although a partnership agreement is not required by law, most parties will spell out the relationship in a legal agreement. In a partnership there is a differentiation between the partnership and the partners. Partnerships cannot sue or be sued. However, all partners are personally liable for losses, wrongful acts, and omissions or commissions assumed by the partnership. Partners share in the profits, administration, decision making, and workload of the practice as defined in the partnership agreement. In this type of practice, earnings or losses pass through to the individual partners and appear on each partner's personal tax return.

A major benefit of this type of business structure is the shared financial and professional risks and responsibilities. Decision making remains fairly flexible, and it is generally easier to attract venture capital for financing the practice. The disadvantages of a partnership include the unlimited personal liability of each partner and the responsibility of each partner to pay taxes on business income.

Corporation

A corporation is an individual legal entity without ties to the individual business owner and is generally formed as a C corporation. It has the legal status to buy and sell assets and enter into contracts. It has its own tax identification number, as well as tax return. A professional corporation enjoys limited liability in that only the corporate assets can be used to satisfy judgments and thereby reduces the personal and financial risk of the APN owner and shareholder. In a professional practice, the APN is paid a salary, and as an owner or shareholder receives the profits of the corporation as dividends throughout the year. The downside of this arrangement is that the corporation is taxed on its profits and then the individual is taxed on the dividends. The owner of a small corporation can elect to be an S corporation that offers special tax advantages. All profits of an S corporation are taxable only as they are distributed as dividends to shareholders. Because of the intricacies of the law and the ever-changing tax laws, it is essential that the APN consults a tax professional.

Advantages of a corporate structure is the limited liability of the shareholders, centralized management, tax advantages for pension and profit-sharing plans, and a larger talent pool for decision making. Disadvantages of a corporation include the costs involved to establish and operate the corporation. There are also time-consuming federal, state, and local government requirements and filings to deal with, as well as the possibility of double taxation on corporate profits and shareholder dividends.

Limited Liability Corporation

A limited liability corporation (LLC) is another form of corporate structure that provides the best aspects of a partnership and a corporation. Income and losses pass through to the shareholders or owners as in a partnership, and there is no limit on the number of owners or shareholders. Legal liability is also limited, and members are not liable for the overall obligations of the LLC, although an individual would still be liable for professional malpractice. This type of corporate structure is also easier to set up and is subject to less government regulation. Be aware that LLCs are not recognized in all states, so be sure to check with your accountant or attorney.

Benefits of this type of corporate structure include limited liability and taxation only on the member's share of the LLC's income. There are an unlimited number of shareholders allowed, and the shareholders or an appointed manager can manage the LLC. Disadvantages include limited recognition of this corporation by individual states and limited legal precedent addressing this form of corporate structure.

CREATE THE BUSINESS NAME AND IMAGE

Image plays an important role in how your practice is perceived in the marketplace. Your image is reflected in the office environment, advertising materials, your personal presentation and that of your staff, and written communication. Determine what image you want to present to your patients and convey this in your business name and practice style.

Ascertain what image would generate a positive response from prospective patients. Would a warm, homey atmosphere or a high-tech, professional office create more appeal for your target population? Are you trying to convey the notion of alternative therapy or new concepts in health-care delivery? Investigate what the potential consumer expects in his or her health-care provider. Above all, project high quality in every aspect of your practice, from the service you provide to the image you present.

Carefully evaluate the image you project in every patient encounter. Pay attention to every detail of the practice even if you delegate responsibilities to staff or consultants. Make sure the staff conveys their commitment to patient care and service during each interaction with patients. Consider the advantages of consulting with experts for certain aspects of the practice. A graphic artist may be better able to create a logo or brochure for the practice. Perhaps a marketing expert can develop a more effective advertising strategy. Keep in mind that image considerations play a part in all your practice decisions and should be used as a guide for future decision making.

A business name should convey the image you want to present to the public and will basically take on one of two forms: your name or a name you have created for the practice. By selecting your name as the legal name of the practice, you are conveying a professional image and making the patient aware of the health-care provider in this practice. If you have been part of another practice in the area or are well known in this location, your name recognition may draw in a number of patients. The addition of "and Associates" to your name will convey the appearance of a larger practice with additional resources.

Professional practices do not always convey the names of the health-care providers. Many APNs prefer to project the name of what they do to reflect their business focus. Lois Brenneman of NPCEU (www.NPCEU.com) decided to market her product versus her name. NPCEU offers continuing education programs to APNs nationally. An individual was purposely not identified with this practice to project the image of large numbers of programs with a variety of speakers. *Elder Choices* is a health-care counseling practice that was developed by a group of APNs with expertise in gerontology and counseling. The name of this practice conveys the target population and the focus of the practice. Ultimately the choice is yours. Consider the image you want to project and use this as a guide in choosing a name.

SELECT A PRACTICE LOCATION

Location, Location, Location. This will be one of your most important business decisions. Think about your ideal geographical location, knowledge of the marketplace, professional relationships, and professional climate. Remember, health care is local not global. The highs and lows of the local economy will have an effect on the success of your practice. Several factors will play into your ultimate choice of practice location.

Geographical Location

When you consider your practice location, think about convenience for your patients and the niche market you want to attract. A pediatric practice located in a downtown business location will not be as appealing as a practice location in a growing suburb. Ascertain parking availability in your practice location and determine if it is adequate to meet the needs of your clients. If on-site parking is limited or unavailable, investigate the proximity of public transportation to your practice location. If you hope to attract walk-in patients, determine if your practice is located in a heavily used pedestrian area. Remember that your services must not only be high-quality, cost-effective and have public appeal, but they must also be convenient.

Economics

The demographic make up of your location will provide a snapshot of your market. The U.S. Census Bureau, local, county, and state governments, and private demographic services can provide the data necessary to evaluate a location. Pay particular attention to a few key factors.

1. *Male versus female population in a given area.* Women are the primary purchasers of health care and typically direct the health care of their families.
2. *The age distribution of the local population.* Age dictates the type of services chosen. New-age therapies might not be as eagerly accepted by a rural aging clientele as they would by upwardly mobile city dwellers. Age also influences the types of care used. Pediatric and midwifery services are sought after in a childbearing, child-rearing population, whereas wellness programs, health education, and chronic illness management may have a higher use among an older population.
3. *The income distribution in the local population.* Income influences the probability of and type of health insurance coverage, as well as disposable dollars for noncovered therapies and preventive programs. A stable or growing population is frequently associated with higher incomes and employment security.
4. *Cultural and language influences on the local population.* Cultural background, values, and practices of particular groups of people will influence their use of health care and wellness programs. Language barriers can be a significant factor to patient use of your services. Consider hiring personnel from the neighborhood who are familiar with the culture and speak the language of the local population.

Professional Relationships

Do not discount the professional relationships you have made along your professional career path. Prior employment, educational training, preceptorships, and professional associates are all sources of reference and referrals for your practice. These people already know you, your competence, and your skill. They can provide references or testimonials to your practice, as well as opportunities to expand the services provided by your practice.

Professional Climate

Consider the professional climate in the area you are considering opening an independent APN practice. What are the legal restrictions to practice in your state? How will the local medical and nursing community respond to your practice? Will collaborative protocols with an area physician and hospital privileges be difficult to obtain? Will physician consultation and referrals pose a problem? Do not abandon a location because of these obstacles, but know if they exist. When you are aware of potential barriers, you can address them and seek solutions.

DEVELOP A BUSINESS PLAN

A business plan is a written document that encapsulates the practice strategy for the future direction of the business and an action plan to achieve the practice objectives.

Formulating a business plan is an effective way to plan for the practice and anticipate business decisions. Business plans may be developed for several reasons such as a new business start-up, business expansion, financing of the business, or as an ongoing plan to manage the business. An effective business plan will describe the elements needed to run the business. Items should include a summary, business concept, market analysis, competition, competitive analysis, marketing plan, management team and personnel, operations, financial plan, and repayment projections. A business plan should give a clear picture of what is really required to start the business.

Summary

This should be a short and concise explanation of the major features of the practice. In one to two pages you should describe your practice strategy, practice development, financial objectives, and business organization. It is important to describe your service, and why it has promise. Describe the status of the practice with respect to a start-up timeline and marketing research. Include information about the business structure and the location of the practice, as well as financial projections, financing needs, and the projected return on investment. Be sure to focus on the key elements of the plan. Give the reader an overview of the practice not a reiteration of the business plan.

Business Concept

This section should contain a clear explanation of the practice strategy. What sets your practice apart from other health-care practices in the area? Focus on the individuality of the practice and how this compares to the competition. Include areas that might have a significant impact on your strategy such as unique services, marketing ploys, or management team.

Market Analysis

This is where you document the need for your practice in a specific location. Has your location been designated as a health professional shortage area (HPSA)? If so, you must include citations of the documentation that supports this statement. Describe the marketplace and your potential competition. Discuss the size of the potential market and where patients are currently obtaining health care. Assess your competitors with respect to the size of their health-care practice, the clientele, the types of insurance accepted, and their fee structure. Determine if the population of the area is generally growing or shrinking and if there is a segment of the population that is medically underserved. Learn all you can about the population of your targeted location and consider this information when developing your marketing plan.

Where do you obtain this information? Seek out reports from various area trade associations and the chamber of commerce, as well as city, county, and state government reports. Research published material distributed by your competitors and reports published by area nursing organizations, hospitals, medical associations, and health departments. Conduct focus groups of area residents to determine what residents identify as a priority and the extent of these types of services in the specific location.

Competition

Know your competition and exactly what threat they are to your practice. Do they have a better location or a more convenient public transportation network than your practice? How do the services they offer and the quality of care compare to those of your practice? What are their practice fees and insurance reimbursement arrangements? Explore the reputation and image of your competition and the appearance they present to the public. Research the stability of the other health-care practices in your area, paying particular attention to staff turnover, reorganizations, and the announcements and cancellations of new initiatives. Pay attention to the advertising and marketing efforts of your competition and new health-care practices that may open in your area within the near future.

Competitive Analysis

This section of the business plan deals with an analysis of the strengths and risks associated with your practice. Be sure to include in your business plan a strategy to address these risks. An example of a business risk might be two established family medical practices within a 10-mile radius of your practice, thereby contributing to the risk of an inadequate patient caseload to financially sustain your practice. You can address this risk by renting highly visible space in a heavily trafficked area and target your services to a segment of the health-care market. A suburban storefront operation with convenient hours and walk-in appointments located in a strip mall next to the grocery store and cleaners may appeal to a large segment of the busy, well woman population.

Marketing Plan

Develop and describe your overall promotional plan. What strategies will you use to reach your target population? Explain the reasoning behind your choice of advertising media, use of publicity, and other promotional plans and how they will enable you to get your message across to the target audience. Appear realistic in your determination of a marketing budget and advertising time line. Remember that effective marketing relies on repetition of your message. If your marketing budget is limited, concentrate your efforts on a smaller geographical area and the target population.

Management Team and Personnel

Focus your attention on key personnel. Describe the skills and competencies your staff and consultants bring to the practice. This is the section to highlight the relevant experience of your consultants, management team, and personnel. Stress the training and experience of your team and correlate their abilities to their role in your practice. Résumés of each team member should be included in the appendices. Include an organizational chart and job description for each member of your practice staff and any incentives for significant performance such as bonuses or potential ownership privileges.

Operations

Discuss the major business functions of your office, and describe how the work will get done. Note any services that are "special" for a practice that deals with your target population. For instance, your specialty area may be women's health care and your practice provides the services that are typically expected for this type of practice. However, you may also provide a special service such as bone density scanning, which is not typically offered in the area. This specialty service should be highlighted in the business plan. This could be the reason why your practice may be more effective in soliciting and retaining patients than the competition.

Financial Plan

In this section of the business plan you should discuss projected income, balance sheets, the income or profit-and-loss statements, cash flow projections, and the break-even analysis. You should plan to show financial projections for 3 to 5 years.

Projected income statements should describe the amounts and types of costs associated with the practice and the receipts and profits on both a monthly and annual basis for each year of the plan. Balance sheets should summarize the assets and liabilities of the practice and should be prepared for the practice start-up interval, then semiannually during the first year of operation, and annually for the remainder of your financial plan. The profit-and-loss statement will discuss the costs to run the practice and income projections. The projected income minus the practice costs will enable you to infer proposed profits. Cash-flow projections describe the management of the practice funds. These projections should be annually for the time period discussed in the financial plan and monthly for the first year of the plan. The break-even analysis identifies the amount of cash that will cover all practice costs. In the financial plan describe how you would reduce the break-even point if practice receipts fall short.

The financial plan should include all information that will assist potential lenders in understanding your revenue calculations. These projections will be as important as the assumptions on which they are based.

Repayment Projections

When preparing your financial plan, be sure to specifically discuss how and when the borrowed funds will be repaid. Discuss the sources that will provide the funds for repayment, as well as any collateral you propose to use to guarantee the loan. Most individual investors typically prefer short to intermediate loans with repayment of the loan within a 5-year period. Commercial lending institutions frequently consider longer term loans and lines of credit.

DETERMINE FINANCING OPTIONS

Setting up a health-care practice involves many anticipated and established costs regardless of the target population or practice use. The most common source of start-up capital is personal funds or an investment in the business by family or friends. Personal loans are another alternative for attaining funds to use in setting up a practice. Equity in a residence is frequently used as collateral to attain personal bank loans or establish lines of credit with a financial institution. Personal loans are generally easier to obtain through a bank than a business loan unless the business has a history of being profitable. Bankers may look at the hard assets of the practice, such as equipment as collateral for a business loan. Criteria for securing a business loan vary among lenders, as does the emphasis they place on particular factors like hard asset collateral, profitability, or years in business.

The Small Business Administration (SBA) offers many financial programs for the small business owner. The SBA frequently funds federally specified projects and objectives. Frequently the SBA will guarantee up to 90% of a bank loan for a small business rather than make a direct loan to the business. The amount of the loan that the SBA will guarantee depends on the business equity. This guaranteed loan protects the lender in case of default by the business owner and is made available to small businesses unable to secure funding from conventional lenders. Information about SBA programs and requirements for participation can be obtained on their Web site at www.sba.gov/financing.

State and local government agencies are other sources of assistance for the small business owner. These agencies have a vested interest in enhancing the economic well-being of the community, and many offer various services to the entrepreneur. Information about programs offered by government agencies can be obtained by contacting the local chamber of commerce or state and city government offices.

Foundations frequently provide grants to businesses that focus on a specific area or related project and are another good source of funding. Geographical limitations are not often imposed on foundation funding.

DEVELOP FEES, REIMBURSEMENT, AND BILLING PROCEDURES

Establishing Fees

In the managed care world in which we practice, fees for health-care services are usually set by MCOs. The usual, customary, and reasonable fees of indemnity insurers are largely being replaced by a contracted fee schedule of the MCO. The APN can charge anything he or she wants; however, the MCO will reimburse only up to the maximum contractual allowance determined by their fee schedule. Is it worth the time and effort to develop a fee schedule?

Definitely develop a reasonable fee for your services. In developing this fee, you will have to consider a multitude of factors, including the work performed, clinical skills required, time spent with a patient, practice expenses (e.g., rent, staff salaries and benefits, supplies, utilities, insurance, etc.), risk involved in treating the patient, as well as indirect care such as making referrals to other health-care professionals and reviewing and evaluating laboratory and x-ray results. Ultimately, your fees should reflect what you feel your services are worth. They should not vary according to the type of insurance plan a patient carries or an MCO's maximal allowable fees.

In determining reasonable fees, the practitioner can review the annual Medicare rules and regulations published in the end of the year edition of the *Federal Register*. This edition lists all current procedure terminology (CPT) codes and their CMS determined resource-based relative value scale (RBRVS). The more complicated a patient visit or a procedure, the greater the RBRVS attributed to the service.

Establish the relative cost of a visit and compare the RBRVS for appropriate CPT codes and then set your fees accordingly. Another yardstick for measurement of your fee schedule is the MCO allowance for the service. If your fee is less than that approved by the MCO, your fee is unreasonably low. Finally, consider your comfort in charging this fee to the self-pay patient. If you feel it is a reasonable cost for your services and you are not consistently writing off a percentage of the fee, it most likely is a reasonable fee.

Reimbursement

A 2006 U.S. Census Bureau report states that approximately 46.9 million consumers do not have health-care insurance (U.S. Census Bureau, 2007). Many of these consumers will seek out services on a self-pay basis. Approximately 15% of your patient caseload will be self-pay patients who are not covered by a health care insurer (Boehler & Hansel, 2006) or who go out of plan because of the service you provide or the convenience of your service. Many patients will pay the fee for service in a walk-in, fast-track, health-care center, for example, because of the convenient location or extended hours. The best opportunity you have to collect a fee for service is while the patient is still in your office. Set up and publicize your policy that payment is expected at the time of service. Initial paperwork given to the patient on the first visit should include a financial policy that explains your payment expectations, any financial arrangements available, and your policy on filing insurance claims. Consider the acceptance of credit cards for payment of your fee for service. This provides a convenient method for your patient to pay your bill in full and transfers the risk of nonpayment to the credit card company. Most banks will process credit card transactions for a fee, and many credit card companies will electronically transfer funds to your bank for immediate access to the money.

Reimbursement from third-party payors varies according to the type of provider and usually requires specified billing forms with illness and procedure coding. Medicare and Medicaid insurers, as well as many indemnity insurers and MCOs, require the CMS 1500 insurance form to submit a claim for payment. This form can be purchased at local stationary stores and is contained in most medical management software. The coding required on the claim forms refers to nationally accepted, standard billing and coding systems. The most commonly used are the American Medical Association's CPT codes, the International Classification of Disease, 9th Revision, Clinical Modification (ICD-9-CM), and CMS' Healthcare Common Procedure Coding System (HCPCS) for durable medical equipment, medical supplies, and drugs. Indemnity insurers are the traditional insurance companies who usually have no relationship with the health-care provider other than paying the bill for service for a covered patient. These insurers typically require an annual deductible paid by the patient and then they pay 80% of the health-care provider's bill with the remaining 20% being the responsibility of the patient. Be aware that these insurers pay "usual and customary reimbursement" (UCR), which is rarely equal to the fee you charge for your service. The patient is responsible for any charges not covered by their insurance in addition to their 20% copay.

MCOs contract with health-care providers for patient services. Contracts may set specified fees for services provided to the patient or may be based on a monthly capitated fee, regardless of patient use. In either case, the health-care provider cannot bill the patient for the difference between the contracted or capitated fee and the provider's regular fee for service. The exception is patient copayment requirements for each MCO plan. Copayments may be different for each plan and is based on many factors, including the family's annual income level, the frequency of multiple encounters with the practitioner, or the nature of the health-care problem.

To contract with MCOs, the APN must apply and be accepted to each individual MCO provider panel.

Billing

There is a variety of medical management software that will automatically submit insurance claim forms. However, monitoring the claims submitted and tracking the date and amount of payments received requires an organized system. Controlling reimbursement will ensure the success and continuation of your practice. A billing protocol such as that shown in **Box 24-4** will allow you to track the timeliness of insurance payments and the number of insurance reductions and denials.

PURCHASE EQUIPMENT AND SELECT SUPPLIERS

Weigh the pros and cons of leasing versus buying equipment. Keep in mind that although leasing does not require the large up-front outlay, it does entail monthly payments with interest. Vendors typically have varied leasing options with opportunities to purchase the equipment at a lower price at the end of the lease. Look at the total cash investment requirements for practice start-up, the capital you have available, current equipment costs, and interest rates on loans versus equipment leasing.

A phone system is the communication system of your practice. Choose a system that will meet your needs and one that has expansion capabilities for the future. Besides front office phone lines, consider phone lines for the examination rooms and your office, as well as dedicated lines for the computer modem and the facsimile machine. Typically, six lines are the minimum needed in a health-care practice, with costs for a basic system in the $3,000 range. Other phone costs you might incur include Yellow Pages listing and an after-hours answering service.

A computer system is another essential need for your office. Consider the number of computers needed for the medical biller and front office staff and the need for laptops for the providers to access patient files, document clinical encounters, formulate treatment plans, and prepare referral and consultation reports. Many health-care offices have multiple computers attached together to form a local area network (LAN). This allows multiple staff members to access and share patient files, printers, hard disk drives, and CD-ROMS. A computer consultant will be able to recommend and install a system that will meet your practice needs.

Practice management software focuses on two basic areas for health-care practices. The medical care areas have a patient-driven management focus. They typically include copies of all front office forms, have the ability to generate insurance claims, assist in patient scheduling, bill insurance companies, and

---

BOX 24-4
Billing Protocol

- File claims daily or at least twice per week.
- Check all claims for accuracy and completeness prior to submission.
- Develop a "claims pending" report and revise and print it daily. Most insurers guarantee payment within 30 days of filing an accurate and complete claim.
- After 30 days, call all insurance companies about unpaid claims and make a notation.
- Refile the claim if it has not been received by the insurer.
- Develop and print an "aged accounts" analysis for each insurance company to track payment patterns longer than 30 days.
- Contact the plan administrator of habitually poor payers and request an explanation. This could be a sign of a financially troubled insurance plan.
- Periodically review the explanation of benefits (EOB) sent by the insurers that explains reductions or denials of claims.
- Contact the insurer to discuss reductions or denials of claims, and revise and refile the claim if appropriate.

have a complete electronic charting and clinical documentation system. The management focus is profit based and provides managerial and cost accounting information to maximize time and profits. Items contained in this section include the general ledger, accounts payable and receivable, monthly and annual financial reports and ratios, capitation disbursements and utilization rates, and the detection and tracking of trends for each patient encounter.

CTS (Computer Training Services) *Guide to Medical Practice Management Software* is a software evaluation program that reviews and analyzes the strengths and weakness of the leading medical management systems available in the marketplace. CTS has been publishing managed care software selection tools since 1983 and enables the practitioner to make an educated choice of a management system that best fits their individual needs. Information about this software can be obtained at www.ctsguides.com. Before purchasing any medical management system, contact several vendors and request a demonstration of their product. It is also wise to obtain references and contact local practices that use a particular system and ask about ease of use and satisfaction with the system.

Durable equipment, such as office furniture, examination tables, electrocardiogram machines, and so on, can be obtained from vendors such as durable equipment companies and medical supply companies. Investigate the purchase of secondhand medical equipment through brokers or through advertising in nursing and medical journals. Occasionally you may find office and medical equipment for sale due to the retirement or death of a practitioner or the downsizing of a health-care facility. If you purchase equipment through a vendor, be sure to compare costs by obtaining quotations on equipment, warranties, and services offered. Be sure to include "hidden" costs, such as termination fees if leasing, federal, state, and local taxes if applicable, shipping charges, installation charges, postwarranty maintenance charges, and interest costs for installment purchases.

The purchase of disposable medical supplies and periodic reordering of supplies is another financial consideration. Establish an organized purchasing system by centralizing the ordering process. Consider assigning one person in the practice to be responsible for tracking and ordering supplies. The designated person will be the one to talk to sales representatives and will become familiar with suppliers and prices to comparison shop for the best-quality supplies at the cheapest price. Centralized ordering will enable the purchaser to ascertain the quantity of supplies used per month, which will assist in the development of an inventory process. This will decrease unnecessary inventory, prevent running out of needed supplies, and avert higher prices due to "emergency" ordering.

HIRING AND MANAGEMENT OF PERSONNEL

APNs who open an independent practice and hire employees must have a working knowledge of the laws and statutes regulating a health-care practice, as well as a working knowledge of how to develop internal personnel guidelines for hiring and managing personnel. Human resource management incorporates all the federal, state, and local laws and regulations that must be complied with by the health-care practice. These laws govern how employees must be treated and paid and they protect the rights of the employees in the workplace. The components of human resource management include:

1. *Administration:* Activities include developing and updating employee handbooks, guides and regulations, and posters. Developing procedures for recruiting, hiring, review, discipline, and termination and having labor law expertise or a consultant.
2. *Labor and liability Issues:* Knowledge and compliance with a multitude of government regulations such as the Civil Rights Act of 1964 and the Equal Employment Opportunity Commission (EEOC), Federal Age Discrimination in Employment Act (ADEA), Americans with Disabilities Act (ADA), and the Fair Labor Standards Act (FLSA). These laws deal with

wrongful termination, unemployment, discrimination, sexual harassment, and employee rights and the practitioner additionally must deal with immigration regulations and other government rules such as personnel recording keeping (W4, I-9 etc).

3. *Payroll information and processing:* Knowledge and management of activities that include employer tax administration, record keeping, reporting, payroll calculations and deductions, paycheck imprinting and distribution, W2 and W4 and quarterly reports, unemployment administration, management reports, and time-off use and accruals.

4. *Workmen's compensation:* Knowledge of state law requirements and purchase of insurance from a qualified carrier, state insurance fund, or becoming self-insured according to state law regulations. Activities include claims filings, management and administration, fraud investigation and defense, audits and loss control, communication with injured employees, and return to work procedures.

5. *Safety:* The Occupational Safety and Health Administration (OSHA) regulations require that employees have a workplace safe from recognized hazards. Employer activities include the establishment and implementation of an illness and injury prevention program that includes general and specific safety training and required protective equipment.

6. *Benefits:* Knowledge and compliance of mandatory benefits that include overtime pay, unemployment insurance, and work breaks. Development and management of optional benefits such as health insurance, pension plans, vacation time, sick time, personal time off, continuing or advanced education credits, travel, bonuses, and so on.

There are many government regulations and time-consuming human resource responsibilities that must be dealt with before you open up your practice. Some practitioners hire an experienced office manager and rely on outside service providers such as a payroll service, insurance agent, and bookkeeper, as well as the expertise of an accountant and lawyer on retainer. This still leaves the responsibility of developing the employee handbook and job descriptions and advertising, interviewing, hiring, training, and evaluating personnel to the APN or their designee.

An innovative alternative to in-house human resource management is to outsource this responsibility to a professional employer organization (PEO). The PEO specializes in labor management and cost control and handles all of the human resource issues while the APN maintains functional control of the employees. The PEO becomes the "employer of record" for your workplace employees and by combining your employees with the employees of many other practices, the PEO is able to offer the employees better benefits such as health insurance, retirement plans, credit unions, and so on. As the owner, the APN benefits because the PEO has relieved the APN of the liability of compliance and administration of mandated government regulations and payroll administration and management. The PEO has no financial interest or ownership in the practice and only deals with employee issues. An example of a company that is a PEO is Medical Management Consultants, Inc., which can be accessed at www.mmchr.com.

DEVELOP AN ORGANIZED DOCUMENTATION AND QUALITY ASSURANCE PROCESS

Documentation

Organizing documentation for a health-care practice will facilitate the smooth flow of business activity. In addition to the front office forms such as patient intake forms, patient rights forms, and release of information forms, the APN must develop and organize the medical record, patient educational materials, and patient authorization forms such as the "informed consent to treat" forms. One of the most important documents of an APN practice is the medical record. A well-documented, legible, and structured medical record will facilitate claims processing and may serve as a legal document to substantiate patient care. The medical record is confidential and can only be released to third parties with patient consent. Frequently in the consent to treatment includes a "release of records" statement allowing records to be sent to third-party payors, if requested. Key elements of an effective medical record are:

1. *Organizing format:* All medical records should be uniform with separate sections for patient information, annual screening list, problem list, medication list, test results, consultations, daily encounter or progress notes, and other forms necessary for your particular practice. Information contained in these sections must be adequately secured and in chronological order. All coding on the charts, such as allergies or chronic health problems, must be uniform and the interpretation of the coding must be well known to all personnel.

2. *Timeliness:* Medical notations must be written at the time of the patient encounter. Always include the date and time of the patient contact in the progress notes. If notes are dictated, this should be at the time of the patient encounter and must be proofread and signed by the health-care provider, preferably before it is entered into the medical record.

3. *Accurate records:* Record all information using a concise and accurate format. Many APNs use a SOAP format to concisely record the patient's **s**ubjective statements and the provider's **o**bjective findings, **a**ssessment, and **p**lan of care. Hand written progress notes must be legible to prevent misinterpretations and clinical errors.

4. *Corrections:* Alteration of a medical record is unlawful. If an error has been made, draw a single line through the entry and add the correct information. Be sure to include the date, time, and your signature next to the correction or in the margin of the record. An addendum is also acceptable and can be added at the end of the record and cross-reference to the original note. The date and time of the addendum is noted and signed by the author.

5. *Telephone conversations:* Document all patient calls in the record with time, date, nature of the conversation, actions taken, and signature of the provider.
   Calls or conversations with family should also be included in the progress notes with the date, time, nature of the conversation, and provider signature. If calls were placed for consultations, appointments, or equipment rentals for the patient, this should also be recorded in the progress notes, dated, and signed.

6. *Treatment plan and instructions:* Record your plan of treatment for your patient including important instructions, educational information given verbally or in writing, and warnings about interactions or complications that may occur. A well-written and organized medical record will be your first line of defense against a malpractice claim and will facilitate accurate and timely claims processing.

Quality Assurance

MCOs, insurers, and the public are increasingly asking health care providers to demonstrate the value and improve the quality of their services. If outcomes management (OM) and performance improvement (PI) processes are put into place when the practice opens, then data collection about the quantity, quality, and cost effectiveness of the practice will be built into the foundation of the practice. OM is the process by which you measure, track, modify, and achieve the best clinical outcomes (quality), while incurring the fewest overall costs such as economic, intellectual, technical, and time spent (cost effectiveness). PI involves the measurement, evaluation, and improvement in the quality of the services of the practice and the patient care received, through a systematic and collaborative examination of the practice's entire operation (quality and quantity).

The initial step of OM is to determine what outcomes are to be measured (up-to-date immunization status of children under the age 6) or what change in functional status will be noted (maintain fasting blood sugar less than 130 for the diabetic patient). Outcome measurements vary between what is valued by the patient and what provides information to the health-care provider to improve care and reduce cost. The diabetic patient values a good quality of life free from complications of diabetes mellitus, such as decreased vision, peripheral neuropathy, fatigue, and polyuria. The health-care provider values 100% immunization coverage of the pediatric patients to prevent unnecessary illness and complications that could lead to serious injury and costly health care. Both of these examples represent appropriate areas to monitor outcomes of patient care.

In addition to monitoring clinical outcomes measuring the effects of treatment and the functional status of patients receiving treatment, other areas to monitor include patient satisfaction and financial and economic factors. Patient satisfaction evaluates the patient's satisfaction with the services provided by the practice staff and the health-care provider. Although not an indicator of the clinical quality of the provider, it does measure the provider quality. A review of the literature suggests that patient satisfaction highly correlates to clinical outcomes. A patient who feels they are respected by the staff and informed, educated, and considerately treated by the health-care provider is more apt to follow a treatment regimen and return for follow-up care.

To maintain cost effectiveness while offering quality services, financial and economic factors must be evaluated. Measuring the cost of resources consumed to produce a clinical outcome will evaluate these factors. Patients diagnosed with diabetes mellitus frequently require large amounts of time to educate them about the disease and possible complications, treatment plan, and medications. Measuring the time the health provider spends to maintain the health of these patients and the costs involved might justify the purchase of additional patient education materials or hiring a RN who is also a diabetic educator.

PI integrates the concepts of outcomes management by evaluating the data received from the patient and the provider and using the findings to improve patient care and practice services. The benefits of PI include continuous monitoring of health-care delivery, effective use and cost containment, and the development of practice guidelines for your health-care practice. Performance improvement processes should permeate all facets of the practice to ensure high-quality health care at the lowest cost.

Primary accrediting bodies in health care and third-party payors are increasingly using and requiring outcomes management data from providers to accredit or evaluate their performance. Insurance companies use this information to evaluate the retention of practitioners on their provider panels, as well as to sell services to employers. Health-care providers are increasingly subject to clinical and economic profiling by MCO plans, insurance companies, and consumer groups.

The National Committee for Quality Assurance (NCQA) has included in its health plan employer data and information set (HEDIS), the monitoring of additional quality criteria such as access and availability of care, health plan stability, use of selected services, patient orientation, and translation services, to name a few. The NCQA is the primary accrediting body of MCOs and health maintenance organizations and is a major organization looking after consumer interests and rating health plans and providers. Annually, the NCQA requests that all of the managed care plans submit information about themselves and publishes a report card titled "Quality Compass," which rates the health plans. This document is sold to medical plans, employers, and various other health-care consultants. For information about this report or to obtain a copy of this document, visit the NCQA Web site at www.ncqa.org.

Performance standards will become increasingly more important in the years to come as health-care providers are asked to document the value and improve the quality of their services. Strategies for complying with performance criteria must be a top priority for health-care practices. Delegating responsibility for continuous quality improvement monitoring and implementing tracking systems for compliance will greatly improve the use of performance standards for the practice. Revising practice services based on data from the performance standards and rewarding staff and providers for compliance and high scores will improve the practice's entire operation and increase the value and reputation of the practice.

DEVELOPING POLICIES AND PROCEDURES

Practice policies, procedures, and protocols should be written in great detail and should be part of every employee's orientation. Employees are expected to know these guidelines to ensure the smooth functioning of the practice. Additionally, important procedures and protocols should also be outlined in this manual such as a protocol for handling a medical emergency, a policy on confidentiality or annual equipment maintenance, and a procedure for handling patient complaints or termination of the professional relationship. Because this manual is essential to providing organized, high-quality services, each employee should sign a written acknowledgement that the practice manual has been read and this form should become part of their personnel record.

Specific office policies, procedures, and protocols that should be developed are listed in **Box 24-5.** Responsibility for the initial development of the practice policy manual should be the APN. However, updates and maintenance of this manual can be delegated to the office manager or another employee after the manual is established.

DEVELOP MARKETING STRATEGIES

Marketing can take many forms from word of mouth to high-priced television appearances. These external marketing strategies are tangible ways of reaching your target population to advertise the location of your practice and the services you provide. There are also internal strategies that you can employ to retain your patient base and increase your patient loyalty. For example, the internal strategies of competence and concern can be expressed through efficiency and friendliness of the staff and health-care provider.

A marketing budget should be an essential part of your start-up operational budget. Marketing is your practice's form of communication to the target population. This is how you inform patients about your location and what you can do to help them maintain their health or resolve a health problem. Marketing is not an optional expense.

A marketing plan helps you to organize your activities and prevents "lost opportunities" to showcase your practice or high-cost, "emergency" printing of practice brochures or appointment cards. Opportunities to showcase your practice can be found in many areas. Contact your local chamber of commerce to see if there is a "Welcome Wagon" service for new residents in your town and inquire about including your practice brochure for distribution to these consumers. Join community organizations to become known in your area and volunteer to offer free seminars on health-care topics. Inquire about membership in local speakers bureaus in your community or through professional organizations like the state nurses association or the state board of nursing. Offer to participate in community and organizational health fairs and screenings that are being planned in your area. Repetition is the name of the game. Your name, location, and services need to be repeated many times before it is remembered.

BOX 24-5
Necessary Policies, Procedures, and Protocols

- Communicating practice fees
- Office collection procedures
- Billing policies and follow-up
- Release of records procedure
- Registering a patient
- Source of patient referral log
- Setting up the patient record
- Completing the superbill
- Scheduling patient appointments
- Closing and reconciling daily cash collections and disbursements
- Cleaning laboratory equipment
- Performing an electrocardiogram
- Scheduling a laboratory test
- Handling test results and consultation reports
- Referring patients for consultation
- Arranging services for patient care
- Protocols for purchasing equipment and supplies
- Equipment maintenance policy
- Handling a medical emergency protocol
- Confidentiality policy
- Protocol for handling patient complaints
- Procedure for termination of patient care

Before opening your practice, be sure to order stationary, appointment cards, brochures, and announcement cards with your practice name, address, and telephone number engraved. Also order an inscribed stamp to imprint the name, address, and phone number of your practice on educational materials or any other forms of information that may be distributed to patients in your office or potential patients at speaking engagements and health fairs. Develop and submit articles that highlight health topics to local newspapers and community bulletins, being sure to briefly describe who you are, where you are located, and what services your offer. Before opening your doors, submit practice announcements to local media services such as cable television bulletin boards, community radio programs, local newspapers, and community bulletins, brochures, and calendars. Lastly, be sure to educate your staff about your credentials and what services you offer. Your staff is marketing your practice every time they answer questions or speak to a potential patient. Be sure they know about your education, experience, and specialty training, as well as what services you offer.

References

Boehler, A., & Hansel, J. (2006) *Innovative strategies for self-pay segmentation*. Available from the Healthcare Financial Management Web site: www.hfma.org/hfm.

Carzoli, R., Martinez-Cruz, M., Cuevas, L., Murphy, S., & Chui, T. (1994). Comparison of neonatal nurse practitioners, physician assistants, and residents in the neonatal intensive care unit. *Archives of Pediatric and Adolescent Medicine, 148*(12), 1271–1276.

Mirvis, D. (1999). The behavior of physicians. In J. Johnson & A. Kilpatrick (Eds.), *Handbook of health administration* (pp. 439–460). Boston: Marcel Dekker.

Mundinger, M., Kane, R., Lentz, E., Totten, A. M., Tsai, W. Y., Cleary, P. D., et al. (2000). Primary care outcomes in patients treated by nurse practitioners or physicians: A randomized trial. *Journal of the American Medical Association, 283*(1), 59–68.

Office of Technology Assessment. (1986). Nurse practitioners, physician assistants, and certified nurse-midwives: A policy analysis. Washington, DC: Author.

Pearson, L. (2007). The Pearson Report. *The American Journal of Nurse Practitioners, 11*(2), 10–101.

Spitzer, W., Sackett, D., Sibley, J. Roberts, R. S., Gent, M., et al. (1974). The Burlington randomized trial of the nurse practitioner. *New England Journal of Medicine, 290*(5), 251–256.

U.S. Census Bureau. (2007). *Income, poverty, and health insurance coverage in the United States: 2006.* Retrieved April 2008, from U.S. the Census Bureau Web site: www.census.gov/prod/2007pubs/p60-233.pdf.

Vincent, D., MacKay, T., Pohl, J., Hirth R., & Oakley, D. (1999). A tale of two nursing centers: A cautionary study of profitability. *Nursing Economics, 17*(3), 257–262.

25

The Advanced Practice Nurse as Employee or Independent Contractor: Legal and Contractual Considerations

Kathleen M. Gialanella

Kammie Monarch

INTRODUCTION

Advanced practice nurses (APNs) need to be clear about whether they are practicing as employees or as independent contractors. The difference between an employee and an independent contractor is a legal one based on common law or statutory definitions (Internal Revenue Service [IRS], 2008a). In general, if the individual or entity for whom the APN performs services controls what the APN does and when and how he or she does it, the APN is an employee. If, however, the individual or entity oversees only the result of the APN's work and not the manner or method in which the work is done, then the APN may be considered an independent contractor (IRS, 2008b). The distinction between the two has significant legal, tax, and financial implications. This chapter explores these implications and includes a discussion of the various contractual issues that apply to employment and independent contrator agreements. Pertinent case law is discussed as well.

EMPLOYEE OR INDEPENDENT CONTRACTOR: WHAT DIFFERENCE DOES IT MAKE?

An APN's status as an employee or independent contractor is a significant factor when considering issues pertaining to professional liability and other legal, tax, financial, and contractual situations.

Professional Liability Considerations

With regard to liability exposure, employees alleged to have engaged in negligence or malpractice will likely find a safe harbor in the doctrine of respondeat superior. This doctrine holds that an employer is responsible for the acts of its employee. Thus, if an employee is acting within the scope of his or her employment and is sued for negligent treatment of a patient, the employer is vicariously liable for the damages sustained by the patient. Although this doctrine is not an absolute bar to

449

suing an employed APN individually, it does give the employee a level of protection that is unavailable to APNs that function as independent contractors. An in-depth discussion of these considerations and the liability insurance implications attendant thereto can be found in Chapter 27.

Financial and Tax Implications

APNs who practice as employees receive paychecks that have monies withheld by the employer. The monies that are withheld include state and federal income tax payments, payments to Social Security and Medicare, and unemployment and disability taxes. In addition, the employer is responsible for paying its share of any Social Security, Medicare, and unemployment and disabilty taxes due on that employee's wages. The employer is responsible for forwarding any amounts withheld from the employee's paycheck, as well as its share of such payments to the government. The employer must also issue a Form W-2 statement to each of its employees showing the total amount of taxes that were withheld from the employee's pay during the previous year.

Employees may deduct unreimbursed business expenses (e.g., dues for professional organizations, subscriptions to professional journals, and premiums for professional liability insurance) on their tax returns, but only if the deductions are itemized and the unreimbursed expenses exceed 2% of the employee's adjusted gross income (AGI). For example, if an employed APN had an AGI of $100,000 in 2007, the APN could deduct unreimbursed employee expenses that exceeded $2,000 (2% of AGI). If the APN spent $3,500 that year on profressional dues, subscriptions and liability insurance, the APN can deduct only $1,500—the amount that exceeds 2% of the APN's AGI.

If the APN practices as an independent contractor, the organizations to whom he or she provides services must issue a Form 1099-MISC showing the total amount of money it paid to the APN during the previous year. Unlike the employee, the independent contractor is responsible for paying his or her income and self-employment taxes. The organization is not required to withhold any taxes or make any Social Security or Medicare payments that an employer of an APN would be required to make. The savings in time and money that independent contractor arrangments present to the organization make it an attractive alternative.

If the APN is an independent contractor, his or her business expenses are reported annually on the income tax return. Unlike the unreimbursed business expense threshold of 2% that an employee must meet before being allowed to take a deduction, business expenses incurred by an independent contractor do not have to amount to any specific percentage of AGI to be deducted. Thus, in the example previous given, the APN would be able to dedcut the full expenses incurred of $3,500.

The APN must keep other trade-offs in mind when contemplating employment versus an independent contractor arrangement. Employers often provide certain benefits to their employees (e.g., health insurance, pension plans, and paid personal time off for holidays, vacations, illnesses, etc.). These benefits are not made available to independent contractors. Some organizations prefer to offer an independent contractor arrangment to an APN to avoid the cost of providing such benefits. If an APN wants or needs these kind of benefits, then an independent contrator arrangement is not advisable.

Factors Used to Determine Status

Because the liability, financial, and tax implications of one's work status can be significant, it is important for APNs to understand the factors that are considered to determine whether an APN is an employee or an independent contractor. The Internal Revenue Service (IRS; 2008b) considers common law and looks at the degree of control asserted by the organization versus the degree of independence maintianed by the worker. To determine whether an APN is an employee or an independent contractor from a federal tax perspective, the IRS would evaluate behavioral and financial controls and the type of relationship that exists between the APN and the organization for which the APN provides services.

Questions the IRS would pose to evaluate the status of the arrangement include the following:

■ What instructions does the organization give to the APN? If the organization instructs the APN about when and where to work, the equipment and supplies to be used, who will assit the APN, what work must be performed (or even the results that the APN is to achieve) these are factors that indicate the APN is employed by the organization.

■ Does the organization educate and train the APN to perform services in accordance with certain policies and procedures, or does the APN have his or her own protocols for providing services? The former arrangement points to an employer-employee relationship. The latter would indicate the APN is an independent contractor.

■ Does the APN have significant fixed unreimbursed business expenses (e.g., office rent, telephone and computer services, professional dues and support staff to pay) in connection with providing services to the organization? If so, this generally indicates that the APN is an independent contractor.

■ Does the APN advertise and are his or her services available to more than one organization or to individuals? If so, the APN is likely to be considered an independent contractor.

■ How is the APN paid? Does the APN receive a set amount of pay over a certain period of time and receive benefits from the organization or is the APN's compensation based on a flat fee without the provision of benefits? The former arrangement indicates an employment situation, whereas the latter arrangement would suggest the APN is an independent contractor.

■ Does the APN realize a profit or take a loss? If so, it indicates the APN is an independent contractor.

■ What type of relationship exists between the organization and the APN? Is it for an indefinite period or will it end on completion of a particular project? Is there a written contract that describes the type of relationship that exists? (If the contract is an employment agreement, the employer-employee relationship is obvious.) Does the APN receive benefits such as health insurance, a retirement plan, and paid time off? If so, it indicates the APN is an employee.

State taxing authorities make similar inquiries for state tax purposes. The factors relied on by these taxing authorities can differ from the IRS and vary from state to state. Some states are more stringent than the IRS and other states when classifying workers as employess versus independent contractors. Thus, it is important for an APN to be familiar with the federal bases used to distinguish between employee and independent contractor arrangements, as well as the bases used by the states in which the APN practices. APNs should seek out sound legal and accounting advice to address these issues.

Failure to properly classify the work status of an APN can be costly to the APN if he or she is treated as an independent contractor but is, in fact, an employee. A case filed by individuals who had been classified as independent contractors rather than employees at Microsoft illustrates this. *Vizcaino v. Microsoft Corporation* (1997) arose out of a tax audit of Microsoft conducted by the IRS. The audit concluded that a number of individuals classified as independent contractors needed to be reclassified as employees, and the requisite taxes paid. The IRS concluded that the individuals were employees because Microsoft controlled the manner and way in which the individuals performed their services for the company. Microsoft ended up paying the required taxes and overtime that resulted from the reclassification, and it reclassified some of the individuals as permanent employees. Eight of these reclassified individuals demanded that they receive all of the employment benefits they did not receive during the time they were considered independent contractors, including participation in Microsoft's employee stock purchase plan. Microsoft refused to issue these benefits, so the individuals sued the company. The Ninth Circuit Court of Appeals in *Vizcaino* ordered Microsoft to provide employment benefits to its employees for the periods of time that those individuals had been erroneously classified as independent contrators. The financial impact on the company was significant, as were the financial gains realized by the reclassified workers. Although the workers in *Vizcaino* were not health-care providers, the findings and results of that case would apply equally in the health-care industry.

The Advanced Practice Nurse as Employee

Employees working without a contract guaranteeing a specific position for a definite time at a designated pay rate are referred to as employees "at will." Until the late 1970s this kind of employment arrangement allowed employers to terminate any at-will employee for any reason or for no reason. Although the general rule that an employee can be hired or fired for any reason or no reason continues to exist, there now are many exceptions in place. These exceptions include public policy concerns, antidiscrimination laws, and whistleblower statutes. Thus, employers no longer enjoy the unbridled latitude the general rule of law previously afforded them.

Although the absence of job security continues to be an issue for at-will employees, federal and state statutes have been enacted and judicial decisions have been made to ensure that employers treat employees more fairly, regardless of the employee's status as a contract or at-will employee.

One of the key limitations on an employer's ability to terminate an employee at-will is called the "public policy" exception. It is a judicially mandated exception that permits a terminated at-will employee to pursue a wrongful termination claim against the employer in cases in which the employee has a reasonable basis to believe he or she was terminated in violation of a clear mandate of public policy. *Kirk v. Mercy Hospital Tri-County* (1993) is an example of such a case. Pauline Kirk worked as a registered nurse (RN) at the hospital until she was terminated. She was an at-will employee who reportedly told a family member that the death of one of the patients for whom she cared was hastened by the actions of the physician. She offered to assist the family with obtaining a copy of the patient's medical record. When hospital officials learned of Ms. Kirk's actions, she was terminated. Ms. Kirk filed a lawsuit claiming wrongful termination by the hospital. The case was dismissed by the trial court, but Ms. Kirk filed an appeal with the Missouri Court of Appeals. That court reversed the decision of the trial court and sent the case back for hearing. It agreed that Ms. Kirk had a right to pursue her wrongful termination lawsuit because of her claim that she was terminated for reporting serious misconduct that could constitute a violation of the law. The Court of Appeals recognized that Ms. Kirk's actions warranted protection under the public policy exception.

APNs practicing as employees have the opportunity, like Kirk, to pursue wrongful termination causes of action when they believe that adverse employment action was taken against them in violation of public policy. Many states and the federal government have adopted strong whistleblower statutes that enhance the common law public policy protections available to employees. Some of those laws have specific protections for health-care professionals. An example of such a statute is the New Jersey Conscientious Employee Protection Act (1986, as amended 1989, 1997 and 2005). It specifically prohibits employers from taking retaliatory action against heatlh-care professionals, such as APNs, who disclose information about employers who provide improper patient care.

Other statutory protections include a variety of antidiscrimination laws. There are a number of federal laws, and many states have their own laws as well, that protect workers from discrimination based on race, sex, ethnicity, religion, and disabilty. The most recent antidiscrimination statute to be enacted by the federal government is the Genetic Information Non-Discrimination Act of 2008. It protects individuals in the workplace from discrimiation based on their genetic information.

Employees are afforded additional protections under federal and state laws that provide benefits for unemployment, injuries on the job, the need for family and medical leave, and continuation of health-care benefits. APNs who work as employees should be aware of their many rights under these laws.

Some APNs may have written employment contracts that provide them with additional rights. Contractual issues are discussed in greater detail later in this chapter.

The Advanced Practice Nurse as Independent Contractor

An APN who is an independent contractor has a contract, which may be verbal, written, or implied, with another party to provide specific services. The contract does not stipulate a level of behavioral and financial controls over the APN that would be associated with an employer-employee relationship. If an APN is working as an independent contractor, he or she is not entitled to benefits that the organization provides to its employees. The APN also would not be able to obtain unemployment compensation, workers' compensation, or family and medical leave protections through that organization if the need arose. This is because the legal relationship is not an employment relationship. Of equal concern is the impact potential professional liability claims would have on the APN. For example, an APN who is not an employee at a hospital, but has privileges there, would be individaully responsible for his or her negligent acts that occur in the hospital.

The case of *Hansen v. Caring Professionals, Inc.* (1997) is illustrative. Although it does not involve an APN, it does involve a nurse and the issues presented in the case also would apply to APNs who work as independent contractors. The case examines whether the nurse, who was retained by Caring Professionals to provide temporary nursing services to a local hospital, was an employee or independent contractor of that agency. The distinction was fundamental in determining whether or not the agency could be held liable for the alleged negligent acts of the nurse. Mr. Hansen, the plaintiff in the case, claimed that a malpractice occurred when a central venous catheter that had been inserted into his wife's jugular vein became dislodged. It was alleged that air entered the intravenous line and created an embolus that caused Mr. Hansen's wife to sustain severe brain damage and total disability.

Eileen Fajardo-Furlin, RN, was named as a defendant in the case because she cared for Mrs. Hansen while she was in the hospital. Furlin was working at the hospital on temporary assignment through Caring Professionals. Caring Professionals also was named as a defendant. The patient's husband sought to hold Caring Professionals responsible for the alleged negligence of Furlin. Caring Professionals sought to be removed from the case, asserting that there was no employee-employer relationship, but rather an independent contractor relationship, thereby absolving Caring Professionals from any liability for Furlin's actions. The trial court agreed and dismissed Caring Professionals from the case. An appeal followed, but the appellate court agreed with the trial court. Caring Professionals succeeded in getting removed from the case because Furlin was an independent contractor. Furlin remained in the lawsuit as an individual defendant. This case illustrates how the type of working relationship an APN has with an organization could have significant impact on the outcome of a negligence or malpractice case.

CONTRACT ISSUES FOR APN EMPLOYEES AND INDEPENDENT CONTRACTORS

APNs should have a basic understanding of contract law. It is often advisable and sometimes a requirement for APNs to have written agreements in place to address certain work and practice issues. The remainder of this chapter introduces the APN to these types of considerations.

Types of Contracts

Contracts are promises or sets of promises that outline the rights and responsibilities of the parties. They are legally binding, and if valid, they can be enforced. When one or more parties fails to perform in accordance with articulated rights and responsibilities, that failure is termed a *breach*. When a breach occurs, remedies outlined in the agreement or contract are available to the nonbreaching party. In addition, when an agreement-related dispute is tried in the civil justice system or the subject of binding arbitration, the nonbreaching party can obtain damages if a breach is found to have occurred.

Contracts are usually categorized by the way in which they are formed. They can be express contracts, implied contracts, or quasi-contracts. Express contracts are promises or sets of promises to which the parties agree either verbally or in writing. Implied contracts are promises or sets of promises that are derived from the conduct of the parties to the contract. Quasi-contracts are not considered contracts per se, but they are used by courts in some jurisdictions to allow one or more parties to the quasi-contract to avoid unjust enrichment at the expense of the other party or parties. This is known as *equitable relief.*

Some contracts, whether express or implied, are considered invalid for various reasons. An invalid contract will not be enforced by the courts. An example of an unenforceable contract is one that is illegal because fullfilling its terms would be considered a crime. For instance, if an APN enters into a contract which provides that he or she would receive financial incentives for referring patients to a health-care facility, this would be an antikickback violation. Taking kickbacks for patient referrals is a crime and a court would not enforce such a contract. The contract is considered to have been void at its inception. Some contracts can be considered voidable. For example, if one of the parties to the contract is a minor or has a level of mental illness or dementia that prevented him or her from understanding the terms of the contract, then the contract is considered voidable by that party. Unenforceable contracts are those that may be valid but not enforced because of some defense that may be asserted by one or more parties to the contract. An example would be if a party was tricked into signing the contract or entered into the contract by mistake.

For any contract to be enforced, the parties must have reached a "meeting of the minds" about its terms. When the parties have reached a meeting of the minds, the result is called *mutual assent.* Mutual assent is achieved when one party makes an offer and the other party unequivocally accepts the offer. In addition to offer and acceptance, there must be an exchange of consideration for the contract to be valid. For example, an APN can enter into an employment contract with a physician practice. The consideration received by the APN is monetary compensation. The consideration received by the physician practice is the services that the APN provides to the practice.

Contracts can be unilateral or bilateral. A unilateral contract is one in which there is no opportunity for negotiation. An example of such a contract is a professional liability insurance policy. The insurance company promises to defend an APN in a malpractice case pursuant to the terms of the insurance policy in exchange for the payment of premiums by the APN. The terms of the policy (contract) are not negotiated. Once the APN pays the premium, the policy becomes effective.

A bilateral contract is one in which the parties negotiate the terms. APNs often negotiate the terms of their employment contracts to obtain compensation and benefits that are acceptable to them.

Common Contractural Terms Included in Written Agreements

Agreements can be struck with a handshake or with the stroke of a pen. Agreements struck with a handshake, although honorable, may prove to be frustrating, unworkable, and largely unenforceable because many of the issues that are addressed in written agreements are not addressed in verbal agreements. In addition, it is much easier to prove the terms of an agreement that has been reduced to writing. Written agreements can help the parties avoid the misunderstandings that may arise with implied or verbal contracts. Thus, it is recommended that APNs who enter into employment and independent contractor agreements do so in writing whenever possible.

Written agreements can be brief, limited to just a few pages, or they can be lengthy, detailed documents. The length and terms of the agreement depend on the specific arrangements contemplated by the parties, as well as their needs and preferences. Regardless of the length of an agreement, there are certain terms that routinely are included in employment and independent contractor agreements for APNs. Among them are the scope of the contract; its effective date; the relationship and responsibilities of the parties; confidentiality; conflict of interest; compensation; indemnification and subrogation; dispute resolution; term, renewal, and termination; remedies for breach; notices; modification and assignment of the agreement; severability; conflict of laws; legal authority; force majeure; covenant not to compete; and signatures. Each of these provisions will be discussed.

Scope

The section of a written agreement addressing scope recites the activities governed by the agreement. In this section the services provided by the APN are identified. The services may be stated quite broadly, or they may be listed individually. A broadly written scope statement for an APN might state that he or she agrees to render services that are consistent with the scope of practice articulated in his or her state's nurse practice act and in accordance with all applicable national practice standards, such as the American Nurses Association's (ANA's) *Scope and Standards of Advanced Practice Registered Nursing* (2004). A more specific scope statement might identify the APN's specific job responsibilities and list the individual services to be provided. In either event, it is important to verify that the services contemplated by the agreement fit within the APN's scope of practice as defined by the state.

Effective Date

The section of a contract addressing the effective date will specify the date on which the agreement begins. It is also the date against which time frames identified in the agreement may be measured. For example, if the effective date of the agreement is July 1, 2008, and the APN is required to provide a certain report to the other party every 90 days, the first report is due on October 1, 2008.

Relationship of the Parties

In the relationship of the parties section of the contract the APN is identified as either an independent contractor or an employee. If the APN is going to be considered an independent contractor, it is important to keep that status in mind as other contractual provisions are written. Classifying an individual as an independent contractor but prescribing when, where, and how services will be performed may subject an organization to having that independent contractor reclassified as an employee.

As previously discussed, this could expose an organization to liability for unpaid taxes and employment benefits, as well as governmental penalties.

In situations in which an APN is going to function in an independent contractor role, the contract should specifically state that the APN is not eligible for paid sick leave or vacation time, health insurance, retirement plans, and other benefits extended to the organization's employees. An employee contract, on the other hand, should specifically include all of the benefits to which the APN is entitled.

Responsibilities of the Parties

Once the relationship of the parties has been established, the responsibilities of each party can be more easily identified. Like other provisions, this section may be brief, or quite lengthy, comprehensively listing what the expectations are of each party. In situations in which an APN is going to work as an independent contractor, it is imperative that the APN maintain the decision-making ability with regard to the manner and means by which services will be provided to patients. In addition, the APN should contemplate adding a provision that he or she be consulted about any existing and future clinical practice guidelines the organization may have or consider and be permitted to provide appropriate changes, if necessary, before implementation.

Should an APN be identified as an independent contractor in the agreement and then be required to operate in a controlled manner proscribed by the other party, it is likely that the APN will be considered an employee, not an independent contractor. If, on the other hand, the agreement being executed is an employment contract, it is reasonable to identify when, where, and how the APN is to function.

Typically, APNs practicing as independent contractors have the responsibility to ensure that they are and remain properly credentialed, that they have adequate liability insurance, and that they perform contractual services in a manner that complies with professional practice and ethical standards, as well as all applicable local, state, and federal regulations, statutes, and case law. However, APNs might consider including a contractual requirement that the organization with whom they are contracting assist with the credentialing and recredentialing process for area hospitals, managed care organizations, third-party payors, and regulatory agencies. In addition, APNs, whether practicing as employees or independent contractors, may be asked to promptly disclose any disciplinary actions taken against them. If a contract contains this type of provision it is imperative that the APN understand his or her obligation to report and act promptly when the need arises. Otherwise, the failure to report may be an event identified in the agreement that would permit immediate termination of the APN.

Usually, the organization with whom the APN is contracting requires the APN's assistance and cooperation with the collection of data to confirm the APN's competency and proper credentialing. Required data may include confirmation of educational preparation, specialty certifications, licensure, prior employment, status of existing and past practice privileges, liability insurance, malpractice claims, criminal background information, membership in professional associations, and compliance with the Drug Enforcement Agency. In addition, APNs practicing as independent contractors may be asked to provide information regarding the types of client populations previously served, charges per encounter, visits per hour, visit frequency, incidence of diagnostic procedure use, admission and readmission rates, complication and mortality rates, outcomes, accessibility and availability history, appointment waiting times, and after-hours coverage history.

The responsibilities of APNs are delineated in written agreements and organizations with whom they contract should have their responsibilities delineated in the agreement as well. In that regard, it is the organization's responsibility to execute contracts that are consistent with the organizational bylaws. The APN may explicitly require that the organizational bylaws be incorporated into the agreement by reference and that he or she be provided the most current edition of the bylaws. The APN may also negotiate involvement on the bylaws committees or other organizational committees or panels.

It is also the organization's responsibility to have sound corporate compliance programs in place and to provide the APN with the information he or she needs to provide the agreed-to services. These and other organizational responsibilities can be stated broadly or can be delineated specifically and in detail with set deadlines and penalties for failure to meet those deadlines.

Confidentiality

The confidentiality section of a contract usually deals with information and documents that the parties wish to protect as confidential. The responsibilities of the parties with regard to this information and these documents is also outlined. Some confidentiality provisions simply state that confidential, proprietary, and trade secret information shall not be disclosed to third parties, without describing what information is considered to be confidential, propietary, or a trade secret. If there are questions about what specific information is protected, it is prudent to clarify this so that potential breaches of confidentiality are minimized.

With regard to the privacy and confidentiality of protected health information, many contracts now address the requirements of the Privacy Rule and Security Rule adopted by the federal government in 2003 and 2005, respectively. These rules are commonly referred to by health-care providers as "HIPAA"—an acronym for the Health Insurance Portability and Accountabiltiy Act of 1996. APNs must be fully familiar with the requirements that apply to them under these rules, as well as the HIPAA policies and procedures of the organizations with whom they contract.

Conflict of Interest

Conflict of interest provisions are contained in written agreements in an effort to ensure that both parties are acting in the best interests of each other and promoting the mutual success of the relationship. Potentially conflicting loyalties can be problematic and should be avoided. Typically, conflict of interest provisions require the party who becomes aware of a potential conflict to promptly disclose it to the other party. When these provisions are included in a an APN's written agreement, it is important for the APN to act in a manner that avoids potential conflicts and is not contrary to the contractural requirements, such as always acting in the best interest of the patients and not in the best interest of any other third party. For instance, an APN's prescribing habits ought to reflect what medication is most effective for the patient, not an interest or investment the APN has in a specific drug or drug company.

Compensation

Compensation provisions in written agreements delineate the payment that will be rendered once agreed-to services are provided. The sum may be listed as a total amount of money that will be paid over the course of the contract, or it may be listed as an incremental amount, paid according to established benchmarks. Caps may be identified that limit the total amount of money that will be paid, as well as any bonus payments. With regard to bonus payments, it is important to decide whether bonus payments will be based on profit that is generated from the services provided by the APN, the productivity of the APN, the quality of care given by the APN, or some combination thereof. Not only does the APN need to decide whether or not bonus payments are going to be incorporated into the written agreement, a great deal of attention needs to be paid to the formula used to calculate bonus payments. It is important to be sure the formulas used are reasonable, are regularly audited, and do not benefit one party more than the other. Care should be taken to avoid financail incentives that may be viewed as kickbacks or otherwise illegal.

In addition, health-care organizations, plans, and practice groups will likely include a statement conveying that it is the responsibility of the APN practicing as an independent contractor to pay all taxes associated with contracted services.

APNs executing written agreements need to consider adding specific dates on which payments will be made. When those payments are not forthcoming, a late fee can be imposed so long as it is included in the agreement. Additionally, when the compensation for the APN is based on billing receipts, the APN should be provided with ongoing documentation tracking the billing process and reimbursement levels from each payer, including secondary sources and previously denied claims. Time frames within which claims will be processed should be set, and penalties for failure to meet those time frames should be negotiated.

Indemnification and Subrogation

Indemnification and subrogation issues are typically addressed in written agreements. Indemnification is a promise between the parties to hold each party harmless for the wrongdoing of the other party. For example, an APN may enter into a contract with a physician practice as an independent contractor. The contract will contain language that says the APN is responsible for his or her own wrongdoings. If a malpractice occurs for which the APN is solely responsible, it is the APN who must bear the loss associated with that claim. The APN must indemnify the physician practice. The contract will also contain language that requires the APN to carry his or her own insurance coverage. It is important to ensure that an indemnification provision is reciprical so that both parties are extended the same level of protection. The APN should be indemnified by the physican practice if someone other than the APN is responsible for a malpractice or other type of claim.

Subrogation, on the other hand, permits the substitution of one party for another. In health-care matters, the doctrine of subrogation has been used by health-care facilities to recover from the APN the monetary losses sustained after the health-care organization is found liable for the negligence or malpractice of the APN or other individual to whom the APN delegated any aspect of care or treatment. Like indemnification, a subrogation provision will likely be included in certain contracts. If it is, the APN should be sure the provision is reciprocal so that both parties to the contract have a right to subrogation.

Dispute Resolution

Dispute resolution provisions describe the process to be used when the parties disagree about any aspect of the contract. Usually, this provision states that both parties will use their best efforts to promptly resolve all disagreements. In situations in which the disagreement cannot be resolved there may be a requirement for the parties to submit the dispute to mediation or arbitration as alternative dispute resolution mechanisms. The parties to the contract may negotiate terms that require either binding or nonbinding dispute resolution. If there is binding arbitration, for example, the parties to the contract are waiving their rights to file a lawsuit in the event one of the parties is dissatisfied with the arbitrator's decision. If the parties agree to a nonbinding dispute resolution process, it is important to state that the process must be concluded before filing a cause of action in court.

Term, Renewal, and Termination

Term, renewal, and termination provisions in written agreements specify the length of the contract, usually in months or years, and the process to be used to renew and terminate the agreement. Renewal clauses typically require one or both parties to notify the other party within a certain period of time of their intention to renew the contract. Some written agreements approach the issue differently by providing for automatic renewal for a specific period if one party does not notify the other of its intent to *not* renew the agreement.

Termination provisions in written agreements usually require the terminating party to notify the other party within a specific period, usually 60 or 90 days, of that party's intent to terminate the agreement. Agreements may be terminated with or without cause, and severance payment may or may not be incorporated into the agreement. Termination without cause provisions permit the APN to be terminated for any reason or no reason, so long as the termination is not unlawful. Sometimes courts consider termination without cause provisions in written agreements to be insufficient or unenforceable, thereby permitting the terminated party to pursue a wrongful termination in violation of public policy. This is especially true if the terminated party is characterized as a whistleblower who reported an allegedly illegal practice and was subsequently notified of the termination of the agreement.

If a "termination without cause" provision is going to be included in the written agreement, it needs to be reciprocal, permitting the APN to terminate the agreement for any reason or no reason within a comparable period. APNs, like other parties to written agreements, need to be sure that their decision to terminate an agreement is lawful.

Not only may agreements be terminated without cause, they may be terminated with cause. An event giving rise to termination with cause usually results in the immediate dissolution of the contract. Terminations for cause are typically limited to instances in which the APN commits a crime, breaches his or her fiduciary duty to the organization, is disciplined by his or her professional board, or acts in a manner that potentially compromises the standing of the organization in the community. These provisions may also be stated more broadly by permitting "for cause" termination with any illegal occurrence. Like termination without cause provisions, termination of the agreement "for cause" may be exercised by an APN, so long as an identifiable "for cause" event has occurred and the agreement permits termination. It is, therefore, important to ensure that termination clauses are reciprocal and for the APN to articulate the occurrence of those events that would permit the APN to terminate the agreement, as well as the financial consequences for the party with whom the APN has executed a written agreement.

Remedies for Breach

Written agreements usually identify the remedy or consequence of breaching or failing to perform the services, as indicated in the agreement. In an attempt to limit the circumstances that can give rise to a breach, and to minimize the amount of money to be paid because of a breach, one party may attempt to limit the definition of breach to a specific provision in the agreement. In situations in which a limited definition of breach is acceptable to the APN, it is important to ensure that the limited definition is reciprocal.

Notices

The notices clause in written agreements identifies the individuals who are to receive notice from the other party. The clause contains specific contact information for each of the individuals listed. The provision also outlines the process, such as certified mail, to be used when notifying the other party of any occurrence requiring notification. It is important that the notification information be current so that the proper individuals are apprised of any communication between the parties to the agreement.

Modification

Modification provisions in written agreements permit the parties to modify the terms of the agreement without having to execute a new contract. For multiyear contracts, modification clauses are important because they permit an APN to renegotiate the compensation package or any other aspect of the agreement on an annual or other agreed-to basis. Any specific term of the contract may be modified so long as the modification provision states that the contract may be modified at any time and as long as both parties agree to the modification. Modifications invariably must be in writing and signed by all parties to the contract. Sometimes modification provisions will specify only certain components of the agreement that can be modified. Before executing an agreement, it is important for the APN to understand which terms of the agreement are subject to modification and, if necessary, negotiate for the right to modify additional terms before signing. Typically, modifications that occur throughout the term of the contract accompany the agreement in written form and are attached to the agreement as addendums.

Assignment

Assignment provisions in written agreements either permit or prohibit the assignment of the contract from one of the parties to another individual or entity. When assignment is permitted, one party may pass a contract on to a third party. That third party then assumes the responsibility for performing in accordance with the terms of the contract. On the other hand, when assignment is prohibited the agreement cannot be sold or transferred to another party. Often, if an APN is contracting with an entity, the entity will want the ability to assign the contract to another entity or subcontract (such as a hospital or group practice), but will be unwilling to allow an APN to assign the contact to another APN.

Severability

Severability clauses help to keep noncontested and enforceable provisions of the written agreement in effect. Sometimes one specific provision of an agreement is disputed and deemed unenforceable. The severability clause permits the rest of the contract to remain in full force.

Conflict of Laws

The conflict of laws clause in a written agreement identifies the jurisdiction within which the agreement was executed and the jurisdiction that governs contractual disputes that may arise. It is important for APNs to know which jurisdictions apply. For example, if an APN is contracting with a health-care faciltiy that is owned by a company located in another state, the APN may be subject to another state's laws if a dispute arises. Sometimes this clause will require the APN to seek relief in another state's court system rather than the court system of the state where the APN is located. These types of provisions can make it quite difficult for the APN to obtain remedies if there is a breach of the contract.

Legal Authority

The legal authority section of a written agreement states that the parties to the agreement have the authority to enter into the arrangement. This provision ensures that only the individuals with the authority to bind the parties are participating in the negotiation and execution of the written agreement.

Force Majeure

The force majeure clause of a written agreement ensures that the contract will not be considered to be breached in situations in which an "act of God" prohibits one party from performing in accordance with the terms of the agreement. "Acts of God" include natural disasters like floods, earthquakes, tornados, and hurricanes, as well as human disasters such as wars, terrorist acts, and riots. A force majeure clause has the effect of putting the performance requirements of the contract on hold until performance can be reasonably resumed.

Covenant Not to Compete

Covenants not to compete limit an APN's ability to enter into other ventures that would compete with the interests of the organization, plan, or practice group with whom he or she is contracting. Typically, covenants not to compete are time limited and may contain geographical limitations. That is, an APN may be prohibited from entering into other ventures that directly or indirectly compete with the other party for a certain period of time, such as 2 years after the contract terminates. The prohibition also may be limited to a certain geographical radius, such as a 10-mile radius from the location of the other party. This type of limitation is meant to protect the organization or practice group from direct competition by the APN, who could otherwise open a practice in the same general location and take business from the other party.

When a covenant not to compete is included in an independent contractor agreement, it is important for the independent contractor to know what organizations or entities the other party considers to be within the scope of the covenant not to compete. It is also important to clarify what the other party means by the use of the term *interests,* to limit the applicable period to as narrow a time frame as possible, to limit the geographical restraints, and to include a specific sum of money that will be received by the APN for agreeing not to compete.

Also, in exchange for retaining this covenant in an agreement, an APN should give serious consideration to requiring the other party to execute an exclusive agreement that would not allow the other party to contract with other APNs. Alternatively, the APN might ask for the right of first refusal on all projects and referrals for which the APN is qualified. An example might be the closure of a pain service and termination of the APN who functioned as staff, with subsequent reopening of the same service on receiving new grant monies.

Signatures

The signatures section of a written agreement is the place where the parties sign and date the document. After the parties sign the agreement, it is considered to be executed. An agreement that is executed signifies that the parties have reached a meeting of the minds and that both parties intend to interact with each other in accordance with the terms of the contract.

Other Provisions to Consider Included in Written Agreements

Although most written agreements contain some combination of the provisions previously identified, there are contemporary issues that need to be addressed by APNs. Those issues include the proprietary rights of the parties and incentives, as well as the frequency with which clinical practice guidelines and collaborative practice agreements will be negotiated.

Proprietary rights of the parties should be discussed by the parties considering entering into a contractual business relationship. Who owns what tangible and intangible property is important to clarify at the beginning of the business relationship so that royalty arrangements can be explored and restrictions on use, if any, can be articulated. Tangible personal property might include equipment, supplies, or furnishings. Intangible property, on the other hand, includes things like intellectual property and good will. In situations in which these issues have been addressed during the negotiation period, the parties are clear about what property they each own and the expectations regarding the use of the proprietary property once the agreement expires or is terminated.

With regard to incentives, it is important for APNs to avoid agreeing to participate in any incentive arrangement that is based on the denial or rationing of care or schemes to acquire new patients in which the APN knowingly receives inducements. Incentive arrangements that fit into this category include any limitations on the numbers of diagnostic tests that can be performed, admissions ordered, patients seen in clinic settings, or drugs prescribed within any specific period. Engaging in these kinds of activities subjects health-care professionals to fraud and abuse allegations and to breach of fiduciary duty causes of action. Health-care providers are experiencing the consequences associated with these problems. Monetary penalties imposed by the U.S. Department of Health and Human Services/Office of Inspector General (HHS-OIG) are illustrative of this. Penalties imposed during the first half of 2008 for alleged kickbacks and false and fraudulent claims exceeded $2.2 million (Health Industry Washington Watch, 2008). It may be appropriate, however, for APNs to consider including legal incentives that are based on the achievement of quality outcomes. Quality outcomes that might be used as incentives include, but are not limited to, patient satisfaction, length of stay, mortality, readmission rate, and adherence to recommended clinical regimens.

Avoiding Legal Pitfalls Associated with Written Agreements

Written agreements are executed in an effort to establish the ground rules the parties agree to follow. Sometimes, however, these agreements are the subject of litigation. Usually, in litigation arising out of a written agreement executed between two parties, one party alleges that the other has breached the contract. In other instances, one party may attempt to argue that the contract should be deemed illegal or that certain provisions of the contract should be disregarded.

In 1999, juries in two Florida cases awarded health-care professionals significant damages for breach of contract by the health-care organizations with which the professionals had been working. In the first case, a jury awarded $22.8 million to two oncologists, Jerome J. Spunberg and Bruce W. Phillips, who had their practice agreements wrongfully terminated by Columbia/JFK Medical Center in Atlantis, Florida (*Spunberg v. Columbia/JFK Medical Center,* 1999). In the second case, a jury awarded Ho Chung Tu, a neonatologist, $2 million in damages after it determined that Mount Sinai Medical Center of Greater Miami breached its contract with the doctor by directing patients to other physicians (*Tu v. Mount Sinai Medical Center,* 1999).

Some agreements entered into by health-care professionals are not only unenforceable, but they are also considered illegal. When that occurs, health-care professionals or the organizations they contract with may be subject to civil and criminal sanctions. In December 2006 HHS-OIG reached a settlement with Murray-Calloway County Public Hospital in Kentucky. The hospital agreed to pay a civil monetary penalty of $175,000 for, among other things, leasing space in its medical arts building to physicians at less than fair market value (OIG-HHS, 2008). These types of arrangements are considered to be kickbacks from the hospital for patient referrals from the physicians. APNs need to be vigilant and avoid these and other types of arrangments that may be characterized as kickbacks.

The case that follows is illustrative of some of the contractual terms previously discussed in this chapter, as well as some problems APNs may encounter in situations involving written agreements. *Washington County Memorial Hosptial v. Sidebottom* (1999) involved a nurse practitioner (NP) who entered into an employment agreement with the hospital in 1993. The employment agreement contained a covenant *not to compete* during the term of the agreement and for 1 year following the termination of the agreement. The covenant applied to the geographical area within a 50-mile radius of the hospital. The NP could not "directly or indirectly engage in the practice of nursing [elsewhere] without the express direction or consent" of the hospital. In February 1994, the NP was still employed at the hosptial and asked for permission to provide prenatal care elsewhere. The hospital was not providing prenatal care for its patients at the time and allowed the NP to provide the care elsewhere. However, the hospital reserved the right to rescind its permission if it offered prenatal services in the future.

The employment agreement terminated in 1996, and the NP and the hospital entered into a new employment agreement that had a term of 2 years. The second agreement contained the same covenant not to compete. It also provided for an additional 2-year term, unless either party provided written notice of termination, at least 90 before its expiration in 1998. The agreement also gave the parties the right to review the NP's compensation at set intervals.

During the course of the second employement agreement there were some discussions between the parties about increasing the NP's compensation. In January 1998, the hospital unilaterally gave the NP a 3% salary increase, which the NP considered to be unfair, although she did sign a modification to the agreement concerning the increase. The NP resigned a few months later and immediately began employment with a physician practice that was located within the 50-mile radius of the hosptial. The hosptial went to court and obtained an order prohibiting the NP from practicing within the 50-mile radius for 1 year from the effective date of her resignation.

The NP appealed and argued the court should not enforce the covenant "because there was no threat of significant patient loss" to the hospital. However, the appellate court found the geographical limitations and time frame of the covenant to be reasonable and protective of the hospital's patient base, which was the source of its revenue. The court noted that the hospital had helped the NP get established in the community by setting up two clinics, advertising her services, and providing her with the support necessary to maintain her practice.

The NP also argued that the hospital materially breached the employment agreement by unilaterally amending the contract with a salary increase without the NP's review or any negotiations. The appellate court rejected this argument as well and found the hosptial had acted in good faith by giving the NP an increase equal to a cap it had imposed on salary increases at the time. Had the court agreed that the hospital breached the employment contract, the NP would *not* have been subject to the covenant not to compete.

CONCLUSION

Traditionally, nurses have practiced as employees and not independent contractors. However, this trend is changing as more and more APNs embark on private practice careers and pursue entrepreneurial opportunities. Because executing written agreements governing the working relationship between the APN and another party is relatively new, it is important to understand the basic, foundational issues that need to be addressed in written agreements. This chapter has identified a number of those issues.

Although written agreements can provide APNs with great flexibility and autonomy, they can also result in the APN, rather than the health-care organization, being held liable for alleged acts of negligence. In addition, the terms included in written agreements may be the focus of litigation themselves. Cases discussed in this chapter demonstrate how some courts have addressed these issues.

In light of the principles discussed in this chapter, it is important for APNs to ensure that agreements regarding their status as employee or independent contractor be memorialized in writing. In addition, these written agreements need to be carefully reviewed for compliance with federal and state laws and regulations and to ensure that the written agreement accurately reflects the mutual assent of the parties.

References

American Nurses Association. (2004). *Scope and standards of advanced practice registered nursing.* Washington, DC: American Nurses Publishing.

Hansen v. Caring Professionals, Inc., No. 1-95-2346 (appeal from the Circuit Court of Cook County, February 20, 1997).

Health Industry Washington Watch. (2008). *Annual OIG safe harbor, fraud alert proposal solicitation.* Retrieved July 8, 2008, from the Health Industry Washington Watch Web site: www.healthindustrywashingtonwatch.com/tags/oig/.

Internal Revenue Service. (2008a). *Publication 15.* Washington, DC: Department of the Treasury, Internal Revenue Service.

Internal Revenue Service. (2008b). *Publication 15A.* Washington, DC: Department of the Treasury, Internal Revenue Service.

Kirk v. Mercy Hospital Tri-County, 851 S.W.2d 617 (Missouri 1993).

New Jersey Conscientious Employee Protection Act. (1986, as amended 1989, 1997 and 2005).

OIG-HHS. (2008). *Kickback and physician self-referral.* Retrieved December 1, 2008, from the OIG-HHS Web site: http://oig.hhs.gov/fraud/enforcement/cmp/kickback_archive.asp.

Spunberg v. Columbia/JFK Medical Center, Inc., No. CL-97-008937 (Florida 1999).

Tu v. Mount Sinai Medical Center of Greater Miami, Inc., No. 93-03552 (Florida 1999).

Vizcaino v. Microsoft Corporation, 120 F.3d 1006 (Ninth Circuit 1997).

Washington County Memorial Hospital v. Sidebottom, No. ED75301 (Circuit Court of Washington County, Missouri, 1999).

The Law, the Courts, and the Advanced Practice Nurse[1]

Virginia Trotter Betts

David Keepnews

Kammie Monarch

INTRODUCTION

Health care is experiencing a rapid and somewhat chaotic change in which the guiding rules of the game are being developed in a variety of arenas that have not been the usual focus of attention for nurse professionals. Among the most important arenas for developing the rules for nursing and health care are: government, public policy, and the law. When thinking about nursing and the law, nurses have tended to focus on issues of liability and malpractice that of course are of great concern and are addressed in Chapter 27. Advanced practice nurses (APNs), perhaps more than their generalist counterparts, have recognized the importance of the law to acknowledge their authority for practice in each state and have frequently relied on federal and state initiatives to facilitate APN practice and provide reimbursement for APN services. By affecting the law through legislation, regulation, and the courts, advanced practice nursing can gain a greater range of effective strategies to achieve its preferred outcomes. APNs must become increasingly comfortable, proficient, and well prepared in all arenas of the law, and at all levels of government.

The purpose of this chapter is to highlight, from the perspective of the APN, several areas of the law that have a day-to-day affect on the role and practice of APNs. It gives an overview of the sources of law in the United States; how the branches of government as set out in the U.S. Constitution work, especially in the courts; and some specific areas of law that guide all APNs in their daily practices.

THE BROAD CONTEXT FOR LAW

When many people hear a reference to "the Law," they think immediately of a courtroom with opposing attorneys, a presiding judge, and a jury listening attentively and waiting for their opportunity to render a verdict. To be sure, the courts are an essential part of the legal system in the United States, and no discussion of the relationship between advanced nursing practice and the law is complete (or even especially useful) without an explanation of their role. However, it is likewise essential

---

[1]The views expressed in this chapter are those of the authors and do not represent the official position of the American Nurses Credentialing Center.

to understand the context in which the courts operate—for instance, the different sources of the law that the courts enforce and interpret.

Sources of Law

The legal environment for nursing practice is derived from a number of sources, including *legislation* that governs and otherwise affects practice; *regulations* that implement legislation and specifically shapes nursing practice; and the *actions* of courts that interpret and enforce laws, including both legislation and regulation.

Legislation

Much of the legal context for advanced nursing practice originates in statutes; that is, in legislation that is passed in Congress and in state legislatures. Legislation defines the legal authority for practice, legal responsibilities of practitioners, many of the penalties for failing to live up to those legal responsibilities, and other critical aspects of practice, including reimbursement.

Different responsibilities fall to the state legislatures and to Congress. Congress votes on legislation that involves the use of federal funds, relates to issues that spans across state boundaries, or affects commerce between states. For instance, the Medicare program was created by federal legislation in 1965, and Medicare funding, financing, eligibility, coverage, and payment are all governed by federal statute. Although state laws may have some indirect affect on Medicare (e.g., by defining the scope of practice of health professionals in the state), Medicare is a federal program, and Congress has the power to define and shape that program.

A large number of health-care issues are the responsibilities of the states. State legislatures define licensure requirements for health-care professionals and for hospitals and other health-care organizations. States also determine issues related to the scope of practice of APNs and other health-care professionals—major issues such as whether APNs must practice in collaboration with physicians or the scope of and limits on APN prescriptive authority.

In theory, Congress passes laws that deal with national or federal issues, whereas most health-care issues are "reserved" for the states to address. In reality, this demarcation is becoming harder and harder to distinguish. For instance, states are responsible for regulating hospitals and other health-care organizations. However, to participate in the Medicare program—that is, to be able to receive Medicare payments—a hospital, skilled nursing facility, or home-health agency has to be in compliance with Medicare requirements, including Medicare conditions of participation (COP). In turn, the federal government has deemed accreditation by The Joint Commission or the Community Health Accreditation Program for home-health agencies as meeting these COP. The states have traditionally been responsible for regulating health insurance, but as national concern has grown about quality and use controls under managed care, Congress has debated federal legislation establishing patients' rights in relation to health insurance and managed care plans.

Generally speaking, when Congress acts in a given area, it occupies the field as under the doctrine of *preemption,* federal legislation overrides states' actions in the same area. For instance, the federal Employee Retirement Income Security Act of 1974 specifically preempts any and all state laws insofar as they may now or hereafter relate to any employee benefit plan, including employer-provided health insurance. This provision in the law has had the effect of exempting self-insured plans (in which employers bear their own insurance risk directly) from state regulation (Keepnews, 1999.) It also has had the effect of preempting state courts' ability to try damages suits based on damages allegedly caused by the actions of an employer-provided health plan (Keepnews, 1999).

Federal legislation (the National Labor Relations Act) defines the rights of private sector employees to engage in collective bargaining and concerted activity related to wages, hours, and working conditions. If a state legislature passes laws regarding the rights of private sector employees to unionize, those laws are subject to being challenged based on the fact that they are preempted by federal law.

In some instances, however, both Congress and the states may act—either because Congress explicitly allows the states to act or because Congress and the states address different aspects of the same issue. For example, the federal Occupational Safety and Health Act addresses health and safety issues of employees, but it allows states to pass more stringent laws and regulatory mechanisms to protect the health and safety of employees within the state. Both the Congress and many state legislatures have enacted antitrust laws, which address anticompetitive marketplace activity. Although Congress has strengthened and broadened federal laws on health-care fraud and abuse, including fraudulent and abusive activities directed against private health insurers, states also have laws that address health-care fraud and abuse, as will be discussed.

Rule-Making

The affect that regulatory agencies' actions have on health-care and professional practice is often overlooked and underestimated. In fact, regulatory agencies have a critical role to play in health care, including the practice of APNs. In many respects, their actions are as important as the actions of Congress and the state legislatures because the rules and regulations they issue have the force of law.

Readers may remember—from a high school civics class or later courses in public policy—that the U.S. government is divided into three branches: legislative, executive, and judicial. Under this scenario, the legislature passes laws, the executive branch implements them, and the judicial branch interprets and enforces them when controversies arise.

The executive branch is headed by a chief executive—either the president (at the federal level) or the governor (at the state level). It includes a number of different agencies that administer the day-to-day workings of the government; these are headed by officials who report directly or indirectly to the president or governor, and who (generally) are appointed by he or she. These agencies cover a broad range, addressing not only health care, but public safety, financing, natural resources, education, labor relations, consumer protection, and so on.

For the most part, these agencies act only based on the authority given to them through Congress (for federal agencies) or the state legislatures. Thus, a common explanation of these agencies' responsibilities is that they implement legislation. This description is not inaccurate, but it is deceptively simple. "Implementation" may involve a range of activities, from simply operationalizing a clear legislative mandate to filling in complex details in a legislatively developed program to acting spontaneously based on a long-standing, broad grant of legislative authority.

A few examples may help illustrate the differences between each of these types of executive agency action. In one hypothetical state, following intensive lobbying efforts by nursing organizations, the state legislature passes legislation authorizing APNs with specified coursework in pharmacology to prescribe drugs without physician supervision. The relevant part of this legislation reads as follows:

1. *An Advanced Practice Nurse (APN) shall be authorized to write prescriptions for drugs, regardless of class of drug, if that APN:*
   (a) *Is certified by the Board of Nursing as an APN; and*
   (b) *Has successfully completed 90 hours of coursework in pharmacology offered by an accredited School of Nursing, either as part of an educational program leading to preparation as an APN or subsequent to completing such program.*

2. *The Board of Nursing shall provide a mechanism for ensuring that APNs have completed required coursework prior to prescribing drugs.*
3. *The Board of Nursing shall maintain a list of APNs who are qualified to prescribe drugs and shall make this list available to the Board of Pharmacy.*
4. *A licensed pharmacist, upon being presented with a valid prescription written by an APN who is qualified to prescribe drugs, shall fill such prescription in the same manner as a prescription written by any other qualified prescriber.*
5. *Nothing in this section shall be construed as requiring physician supervision of APN prescriptions or prescribing practices.*

To implement this change in the law, the state board of nursing (BON) and state board of pharmacy must then propose amendments to their regulations. The BON's regulations include a process for tracking and verifying completion of required pharmacology coursework and for maintaining a list of APNs who are authorized to prescribe. This is the simplest form of implementation—providing a mechanism to operationalize a clear legislative mandate. Imagine that the law was written a little differently and instead reads as follows:

Advanced Practice Nurses shall be authorized to prescribe drugs, provided that they have completed coursework in pharmacology, and in accordance with standards and mechanisms as determined by the Board of Nursing.

This law is much less precise. How much coursework do APNs need to take to prescribe? Where can this coursework be offered? What other standards are appropriate—should there be restrictions based on the APN's area of expertise or certification? Are pharmacists required to fill prescriptions written by APNs? What role (if any) will physicians have related to APN prescribing? These are all issues that are left to the government agency (in this case, the BON) to answer when it proposes and issues regulations.

Why would a state legislature adopt a law that is so sparse on details? Perhaps it was the result of a compromise—an inability among interest groups and legislators to reach agreement on the details and an agreement to let the details be worked out in regulation. Or, as is often the case, perhaps legislators preferred to leave some of the important details to the government agency that is expected to have the expertise to set appropriate standards, based on the belief that legislators lack the expertise (or time) to debate whether 60, 90, or 120 hours of pharmacology coursework is appropriate, but that the government agency charged with regulating nursing practice is in a better position to make such a determination.

This type of scenario—the legislature enacting legislation that leaves it to a government agency to determine major details—is fairly common. When Congress passed the Health Insurance Portability and Accountability Act (HIPAA) in 1996, it included requirements for safeguarding the privacy of medical records. It was left to the U.S. Department of Health and Human Services (USDHHS) to develop and promulgate rules that spell out the mechanisms for implementing and enforcing standards for doing so. When Congress expanded the scope of Medicare reimbursement for APNs as part of the Balanced Budget Act (BBA) of 1997, it was up to USDHHS (and, specifically, to the Health Care Financing Administration, now the Centers for Medicare and Medicaid Services [CMS]) to address important questions such as who would qualify for reimbursement and how statutory requirements that APNs work in collaboration with a physician would be implemented. When the California legislature passed legislation calling for nurse staffing ratios in acute care hospitals, it did not adopt specific ratios; instead, it mandated the California Department of Health Services to adopt ratios after further study.

Sometimes government agencies act under a broad scope of authority that has been granted to them in a specific area by Congress or a state legislature, rather than in response to a specific legislative mandate. A state health department may be granted the authority to establish licensing standards for hospitals, for instance. After initially establishing regulations containing standards for licensure, the agency may subsequently decide to revise those standards as part of its broad mandate to provide for licensure standards that adequately protect the public's health.

The Court System

What Courts Do

In the United States, courts function to publicly administer justice by applying laws to controversies. Facts are determined, the law is applied to those facts, and a decision is rendered. In civil matters, civil courts adjudicate controversies between individual parties or ascertain the enforcement and redress the rights of the parties. Parties in these matters are referred to as *plaintiffs* and *defendants.* Plaintiffs are the suing party, and defendants are the party defending the cause of action filed against them.

Criminal courts, on the other hand, are charged with the administration of criminal laws and the punishment of wrongs against society. In some states, criminal and civil courts are separate, whereas in others a court of general jurisdiction exists. In these states, courts of general jurisdiction have unlimited trial jurisdiction with civil and criminal matters. These courts of general jurisdiction are typically referred to as Superior Circuit, District, or Common Pleas Courts.

Historically, APNs have had more interaction with the civil court system. However, with the stepped-up enforcement of criminal statutes that seek to eliminate fraud and abuse in health care, APNs, as well as other health-care professionals, must be prepared to face criminal prosecution in cases in which the facts suggest that wrongdoing has occurred.

Structure of the U.S. Court System: Federal and State

In the United States, there are 52 court systems—one in each state and the District of Columbia and the federal court system. It is in the state court systems that most lawsuits are tried in what is commonly referred to as "trial courts." In state-based civil proceedings, breach of contract, negligence, and malpractice causes of action are typically heard, as well as domestic relations, real estate, probate, and other state-specific matters. These trials may or may not be heard by a jury, but they are always overseen by judges who are appointed or elected.

In most states, the party losing the case at the trial court level has the opportunity to appeal the matter to an appellate court. States use differing names for this level of court, but they all are considered intermediate appellate courts. Generally, these courts are referred to as *courts of appeals.* In these courts, the appealing party is referred to as the *appellant,* and the other party is the *appellee.* Cases coming before a court of appeals are not retried. Rather, appellate judges determine whether or not the trial was properly conducted from a procedural point of view. After reviewing the trial court record, the court of appeals may affirm, modify, reverse, or remand the judgment made at the trial court level. Affirming the trial court decision upholds the original determination made in the matter. Modifying the trial court decision changes the decision in some substantive way. Reversing the decision of the trial results in an opposite determination being made, whereas remanding the decision results in the case being sent back to the trial court for retrial in whole or in part.

The losing party at the appellate court level has the opportunity to appeal the matter to the state supreme court. Many state supreme courts have the discretion to determine which cases it will and will not hear. Once the state supreme court renders a decision, that decision is final, with the exception of those cases that raise federal constitutional claims. Cases raising federal constitutional issues may be appealed to the U.S. Supreme Court. Those cases that state supreme courts refuse to hear are concluded. The decision rendered at the appellate court level is final.

Unlike the varied and fragmented nature of the state court system, the federal court system is uniform. Every state is divided into federal districts. Some larger states like California, New York, and Texas are each divided into four districts. In total, there are 94 federal district courts. These district courts are presided over by appointed federal district judges. Federal district judges hear both civil and criminal matters. Cases tried in federal district courts include those cases in which the United States is a party, disputes between states, between a state and a citizen of another state, between citizens of different states, between a state or its citizens and a government abroad, disputes affecting foreign ambassadors, cases arising under federal law and the U.S. Constitution, and admiralty and maritime cases.

After a judge in a federal district court has rendered his or her decision in the case, the losing party may appeal that decision to 1 of 13 circuit courts of appeal. The losing party at this level may appeal the decision to the U.S. Supreme Court.

The U.S. Supreme Court is located in Washington, D.C., and is composed of nine justices. One of those justices is the chief justice; the other eight justices are associate justices. Supreme Court Justices are nominated by the President of the United States and confirmed by the U.S. Senate.

Why Court Opinions Matter: The Role of Precedent

Courts, whether state or federal, state supreme court or U.S. Supreme Court, attempt to decide cases based at least in part on decisions reached in previous cases. Cases, previously decided, having similar facts or legal principles are called *precedents*. It is these precedent setting cases that judges use to render decisions in subsequent cases.

Why Many Issues Never Result in Legal Opinions

Daily, courts across the United States render decisions in civil and criminal cases. However, many of those decisions do not result in the judge issuing an opinion for publication. That is because the judge is simply following the law as it has already been clearly delineated. There are instances, however, when the law used in a given case is interpreted in a new way, or with a different perspective, and it is these decisions that are released for publication. Typically, these types of cases are considered landmark cases, signifying that precedence related to a point of law raised by the case has changed.

SELECTED LEGAL ISSUES

Legal Scope of Practice Issues

The framework within which a health-care professional must practice is articulated as the scope of practice for that health-care profession. Nurse-attorney Ginny Wacker Guido (2001) defines scope of practice as "the permissible boundaries of practice for a health care professional . . . which defines the actions and duties of nurses in these roles" (p. 35). The scope of practice statements for APNs can be found in the nurse practice act for each state and the District of Columbia. Typically, scope of practice statements are written broadly and do not involve the delineation of specific tasks. For instance, the Arkansas State BON (State of Arkansas, 1998), in its rules and regulations, define the scope of practice for the APN as follows: "The advanced practice nurse (APN) may provide health care for which the APN is educationally prepared and for which competence has been attained and maintained" (p. 2). In that state, advanced practice nursing is defined as the delivery of health-care services for compensation by professional nurses who have gained additional knowledge and skills through successful completion of an organized program of nursing education that certifies nurse anesthetists, certified nurse-midwives (CNMs), and clinical nurse specialists (CNSs; State of Arkansas, 1998, p. 7).

State laws and rules provide the legal authority for nursing practice, including advanced practice nursing. However, the nursing profession itself plays a crucial role in setting forth the context of practice and the standards of practice on which legislatures, government agencies, and courts often base their actions. Recognizing that APNs have acquired significant knowledge and clinical skills, the American Nurses Association (ANA), in *Scope and Standards of Advanced Practice Registered Nursing* (1996), observe that APNs exercise a high degree of independent judgment, conduct comprehensive health assessments, formulate clinical plans to manage acute and chronic illness, promote wellness, and deliver health-care services to clients in various settings and throughout the life cycle.

To provide more guidance to APNs and the elements of the legal system, the ANA has published standards of care and professional performance for APNs. It is these standards that more definitively outline an APN's scope of practice. According to the ANA, standards of care for advanced practice nursing incorporate the nursing process and are delineated in **Table 26-1.**

These standards of care identify the client care areas within which the APN must be competent. (The use of the term *client*, rather than patient recognizes that in fact the APN may be caring for an individual, family, community, or other group.). There are interventions that are unique to certain

TABLE 26-1	
American Nurses Association Standards of Care for Advanced Practice Nurses	
The advanced practice registered nurse:	
Standard I: Assessment	Collects comprehensive client health data.
Standard II: Diagnosis:	Critically analyzes the assessment data in determining diagnoses.
Standard III: Outcome identification	Identifies expected outcomes derived from assessment data and diagnoses and individualizes expected outcomes with the client, and with the health-care team when appropriate.
Standard IV: Planning	Develops a comprehensive plan of care that includes interventions and treatments to attain expected outcomes.
Standard V: Implementation	Prescribes, orders, or implements interventions and treatments for the plan of care.
Standard Va: Case management/care coordination	Provides comprehensive clinical coordination of care and case management.
Standard Vb: Consultation	Provides consultation to influence the plan of care for clients, enhance the abilities of others, and effect change in the system.
Standard Vc: Health promotion, health maintenance, and health teaching	Employs complex strategies, interventions, and teaching to promote, maintain, and improve health and prevent illness and injury.
Standard Vd: Prescriptive authority	Uses prescriptive authority, procedures, and treatments in accordance with state and federal laws and regulations to treat illness and improve functional health status or to provide preventive care.
Standard Ve: Referral	Identifies the need for additional care and makes referrals as needed.
Standard Vf: Evaluation	Evaluates the client's progress in attaining expected outcomes.

specific advanced practice roles, and these standards of care suggest that APNs practicing in those roles must also maintain competence with regard to those specialty-specific interventions.

Although the ANA's standards of care outline what can be expected from APNs with regard to the client for whom they are caring, they do not address expectations associated with the professional role of the APN. As a result, the ANA has also issued standards of professional performance for the APN. **Table 26-2** identifies those standards.

To practice in accordance with the scope of practice, APNs must integrate the state nurse practice act, the national standards of care, and professional performance standards in daily practice. To do that with precision, APNs must know the activities in which they are authorized to engage. That legal authority is determined by state legislatures and government agencies. Prescriptive authority, relationships with physicians such as physician supervision, collaborative practice agreements, and practice protocols are addressed in a variety of ways. Across the 50 states it is imperative for the APN to know what a particular state's nurse practice act proscribes about these issues before engaging in the practice of advanced practice nursing. Failure to act in a manner that is consistent with the scope of practice and the standards of care can subject the APN to litigation. In some instances, litigation may arise because the actions of an APN are alleged to be infringing on the scope of practice for another health-care discipline. The following cases illustrate how the courts have addressed these thorny matters that are an ongoing matter of tension especially between organized medicine and APNs.

Advanced Practice Nurses in the Courts

In 1936, for the first time, scope of practice issues between nurses and physicians were addressed in a published opinion. The case was *Chalmers-Francis v. Nelson* (1936). This was a case involving a nurse's administration of anesthesia over the objection of a physician and one of his associates. In that case, the physician asserted that administration of anesthesia by a nurse was a violation of the

TABLE 26-2

American Nurses Association Standards of Professional Performance for Advanced Practice Nurses

The advanced practice registered nurse:	
Standard I: Quality of care	Develops criteria for and evaluates the quality of care and effectiveness of advanced practice registered nursing.
Standard II: Self-evaluation	Continuously evaluates his or her nursing practice in relation to professional practice standards and relevant statutes and regulations and is accountable to the public and to the profession for providing competent clinical care.
Standard III: Education	Acquires and maintains current knowledge and skills in the area of specialty practice.
Standard IV: Leadership	Serves as a leader and a role model for the professional development of peers, colleagues, and others.
Standard V: Ethics	Integrates ethical principles and norms into all areas of practice.
Standard VI: Interdisciplinary process	Promotes an interdisciplinary process in providing client care.
Standard VII: Research	Uses research to discover, examine, and evaluate knowledge, theories, and creative approaches to health care.

California Medical Practice Act and should be immediately stopped. The case was eventually heard by the California Supreme Court. In reviewing the matter, the justices of the California Supreme Court concluded that anesthesia administration by nurses did not constitute diagnosing or prescribing within the state medical practice act. In other words, nursing prevailed in this case and it became an important precedent in years to follow,

Fein v. Permanente Medical Group (1981) was decided 45 years later. In this case, a nurse practitioner (NP) was alleged to have been negligent when she diagnosed chest pain as a muscle spasm rather than as a myocardial infarction. At trial the patient was awarded almost $1 million in damages. The case was appealed to the California Supreme Court, where the justices reviewed a number of issues that had been raised in the appeal. One of the issues raised was the appropriate scope of practice for NPs. With regard to that issue, the justices concluded that the activity engaged in by Cheryl Welch was within her scope of practice even though that activity overlapped with activities engaged in by physicians. Again, the court ruled in favor of advanced practice nursing. *Sermchief v. Gonzales* was decided in Missouri 2 years later in 1983. In that case, the Board of Registration for the Healing Arts threatened to file unauthorized practice of medicine charges against two nurses and aiding and abetting the unauthorized practice of medicine charges against five physicians, all of whom practiced at East Missouri Action Agency (EMAA). In an attempt to resolve the issue, the seven health-care professionals asked the civil justice system in Missouri to grant them an injunction, prohibiting the Board of Registration for the Healing Arts from taking action and to declare that their actions were lawful. At EMAA, nurses performed family planning, obstetrics, and gynecology services using standing orders and protocol that were approved by physicians. The case went to the Missouri Supreme Court, where the justices affirmed the right of the nurses to practice as APNs. In reaching this decision, the state's highest court reviewed the definition of the professional nurse and noted that the scope of practice for nurses had been expanded and that the nurses in this case were practicing consistently with applicable statutory provisions. As a result, the activities engaged in by these two nurses were deemed to be authorized. Because these nurses were acting consistent with the nurse practice act, they were not engaging in the unauthorized practice of medicine.

Bellegre v. Board of Nurse Examiners was decided 2 years after *Sermchief* in 1985. In this case, physicians challenged the validity of rules promulgated by the Texas Board of Nurse Examiners concerning advanced nursing practice. The case went to the Third District Court of Appeals in Austin, Texas, where the justices ruled that the Texas BON had the statutory authority to make and issue rules pertaining to advanced practice nursing.

Planned Parenthood v. Vines (1989) was decided by a Court of Appeals in Indiana 4 years after *Bellegre.* In this case, a patient sued Planned Parenthood after an NP, Debra Pasternak, allegedly inserted an intrauterine device (IUD) negligently. One of the issues addressed by the court was the standard of care required of the NP. After considering the matter, the court concluded that the NP was a specialist and should be held to the standard of care for a person with superior knowledge and skill and thus must practice consistent with others with superior knowledge and skill. At trial, expert testimony asserted that the standard of care for inserting IUDs was the same for nurses and physicians. As a result, the NP was required to insert the IUD using the care and skill of others, including physicians, performing that same skill. *Berdyck v. Shinde and HR Magruder Memorial Hospital* was decided by the Ohio Supreme Court 4 years later. In this case, the justices determined that the standard of care applicable to any other health-care professional was the same, regardless of the particular health-care professional performing that skill. Here, a nurse and physician were both accused of negligence with regard to recognizing the signs and symptoms of preeclampsia. One of the issues the justices dealt with on appeal was the duty of care owed to the patient. In rendering its decision to affirm the lower court's denial of the hospital's motion for summary judgment, the justices noted that just because a physician owes a particular duty of care to a patient does not mean that the nurse is exempt from executing care in accordance with that same duty of care. The court observed that the same act may be within the practice standards for both nurses and physicians and that both groups of health-care professionals must embark on the completion of that act in a way that is consistent with their respective duties of care to their clients.

The Ohio Supreme Court's determination in the *Berdyck* case was reiterated in *Ali v. Community Health Care Plan, Inc.* (2002). The plaintiff, Rabia Ali, sued Community Health, an HMO that employed a nurse-midwife. The plaintiff alleged that she was treated negligently during her pregnancy, thereby causing her to lose her baby. Ali reported the development of a vaginal discharge to the HMO's nurse-midwife during a telephone conversation approximately 2 weeks after having an amniocentesis. Ali claimed the nurse-midwife failed to direct her to see a doctor. The nurse-midwife countered that the character of the vaginal discharge reported by the patient was not indicative of a loss of amniotic fluid. The nurse-midwife's documentation supported her position. The case was tried and the judge instructed the jury to apply a certain standard of care—what a reasonable and prudent nurse-midwife practicing obstetrics and gynecology would have done under the same circumstances. The jury rendered a verdict in favor of the HMO. The plaintiff appealed and argued the trial judge should have directed the jury to apply a different standard—what a reasonable and prudent *professional* practicing obstetrics and gynecology would have done under the same circumstances. The plaintiff contended the nurse-midwife standard was a lower standard. The appellate court disagreed and determined that any professional practicing obstetrics and gynecology would be required to direct a patient to be seen if the patient reported signs and symptoms consistent with loss of amniotic fluid. The verdict rendered by the trial court was affirmed.

Professional Discipline

Boards of nursing govern the practice of nursing in every state and in the District of Columbia. It is the responsibility of the BON to protect the public within its jurisdiction from any nursing practice that poses a threat to the health, safety, and welfare of the citizens of that jurisdiction. To protect its citizens, the BON can take disciplinary action against any nurse who does any of the following (Monarch, 2002):

- Makes false representations of fact to the BON
- Commits acts of negligence
- Is habitually intemperate or addicted to substances
- Engages in unprofessional conduct
- Jeopardizes a patient's life, health, or safety
- Fails to satisfy licensure requirements
- Is convicted of a crime or pleads no contest to a crime that adversely affects the practice of nursing
- Engages in unethical conduct
- Practices beyond his or her scope of practice

In 1980 an APN was disciplined because he was found to have violated the Nurse Practice Act in Florida. The case was *Hernicz v. State of Florida, Department of Professional Regulation.* Hernicz's license was suspended because he was alleged to have treated two patients without physician supervision. Disciplinary action was taken in this case because the state of Florida required that APNs have sponsoring physicians.

In this case, the Florida Court of Appeals concluded that the disciplinary action taken was proper because the Florida Department of Professional Regulation presented credible and substantial evidence that the NP did not have a supervising physician when he treated two patients.

When an APN is accused of violating the nurse practice act, he or she must be notified in the complaint of the specific violations of the nurse practice act. The disciplinary action process will be held in accordance with the administrative procedures act (APA). It is the provisions of the APA that ensure that individual disciplinary action proceedings occur in a manner that respects the constitutional rights of the nurse. Of particular concern are the nurse's rights to due process. This constitutional right requires that the nurse have a meaningful opportunity to respond to the complaint and to be meaningfully heard. When that is provided, the BON will be found to have complied with the nurse's right to due process.

Following disciplinary proceedings, boards of nursing are required to issue final agency orders. This document describes any disciplinary action that was taken, outlines the finding of facts, as well as the conclusions of law that were relied on in rendering the decision. Disciplinary action may include reprimand, suspension, or the revocation of licensure. Once a final agency order is issued by a BON, the matter is concluded, unless one of the parties elects to appeal the decision. In the case of an appeal, the matter may be heard by a district court, or in many states, the state supreme court.

Although courts are reluctant to overturn decisions rendered by boards of nursing, there are instances in which BON action is reversed. Typically, reversals occur in the following situations (Monarch, 2002):

- Constitutional rights are violated.
- The BON acted beyond its statutory authority.
- The procedure used by the BON was unlawful.
- There was an error of law.
- The BON reached a clearly erroneous decision.
- The BON made an arbitrary and capricious decision.
- Findings of facts or conclusions of law were not made by the BON.

Hogan v. Mississippi Board of Nursing (1984) is an example of a case in which a BON decision involving a nurse anesthetist was overturned by a court. Hogan was investigated by the Mississippi Board of Nursing for misappropriation of narcotics from the hospital where she worked. The BON conducted a hearing, found her guilty, and revoked her license. Hogan appealed. Although a lower court agreed with the decision rendered by the BON, the Mississippi Supreme Court reversed the lower court's findings and held that the BON failed to prove Hogan misappropriated narcotics. The court determined that the allegations against Hogan were penal in nature, which would have required the BON to find clear and convincing evidence of misappropriation. The court determined that the BON failed to do this and directed it to restore Hogan's license.

FRAUD AND ABUSE

Responsibility and accountability are not new concepts for APNs or, for that matter, for any professional nurse. As APNs have expanded their practice and as their roles in health care have become wider, the areas of potential legal risk have grown. Many of the issues that were formerly of primary concern to other health-care professionals are now much more clearly relevant to APNs as well.

Today, APNs are recognized as providers under Medicare. They are able to receive Medicare provider numbers and to bill Medicare directly for covered services. Increasingly, APNs are also recognized as independent providers by many group and private health plans as well. Along with increased financial autonomy for APN practice has come an increased responsibility (and need) for APNs to understand the requirements for sound, legal billing practices.

At the same time that APNs' role as independent providers (and billers) of services has grown, the federal and state governments have sharpened their focus on fraudulent and abusive practices by all health-care providers. Government agencies have concentrated increasing resources on investigating and prosecuting fraud and abuse. Recent federal legislation has expanded not only the scope of billing practices that may be considered illegal, but it also has increased the penalties that violators may face.

As independently accountable professionals, it is in APNs' interests to understand what is expected of them as providers under Medicare, Medicaid, and other health-care programs and plans. In this as in many other areas of law, ignorance of the law does not excuse violations. Importantly, ignorance of fraudulent billing practices within a practice is likewise a violation if the APN should have known about these practices. In other words, the fact that a practice may use billing staff or an outside billing specialist does not mean that providers are not expected to know, and to be responsible for, claims and documentation submitted in their name and under their provider numbers.

Most APNs are prudent, conscientious, law-abiding, and ethical professionals who would never purposely commit fraud or abuse. Regrettably, these qualities by themselves do not offer sufficient protection from violating fraud and abuse laws. APNs need to have some familiarity with reimbursement laws and what they are expected to do to avoid legal or regulatory violations. Some common examples of conduct that may be considered to violate fraud and abuse laws are the following:

- Billing for services that were not actually furnished to the patient
- Misrepresenting the patient's diagnosis—providing a false or more severe diagnosis to justify payment or increase the amount of payment
- Misrepresenting the services provided—billing for more complex or intense services than those that were actually furnished to the patient ("upcoding" to a more expensive service)
- Billing for services that are not covered
- Misrepresenting the medical necessity of services provided
- Billing for services under circumstances in which requirements for payment have not been met (for instance, billing for services "incident to" the services of a physician when the physician is not present—this will be described)

The federal government has been stepping up investigation and enforcement activities related to fraud and abuse for several years. However, in the last few years, Congress has not only provided greater resources for these activities but also has expanded the circumstances under which certain activities will be subject to federal antifraud laws (Abood & Keepnews, 2002). The federal HIPAA (1996) is widely known for expanding portability of health-care coverage and for calling for new standards for protection of health information. In addition, HIPAA created new penalties for defrauding (or attempting to defraud) virtually any health plan—federal, state, or private. HIPAA prohibits making knowing and willful false statements in connection with the delivery or payment of health-care services. Those who violate these provisions may face criminal penalties, including fines and imprisonment.

In addition, however, HIPAA created a broader standard for determining violations of the law. A provider may be liable for submitting a claim that she or he knows or should know is false. This is a concept known as "constructive knowledge." For instance, a provider is presumed to know what was included in a claim submitted under his or her name. If the claim included services that were not actually delivered, or which were "upcoded" to yield higher payment, the fact that the provider never knew what was being billed under his or her name and provider number is generally not a strong defense against allegations of fraud.

Although HIPAA has significantly expanded the scope of federal law on fraud and abuse, other important antifraud laws preceded it and remain in effect. The Medicare and Medicaid Patient Protection Act (1987) identifies six types of conduct that, under this law, are treated as felonies and that are punishable by fines (up to $25,000) and/or prison (up to 5 years). One such category of conduct is "knowingly and willfully mak[ing] or caus[ing] to be made any false statement or representation of a material fact in any application for any benefit under a Federal health-care program" (Medicare and Medicaid Patient Protection Act, 1987). This broad language applies not to false claims, but any kind of misrepresentation associated with benefits or payment under Medicare or Medicaid. The statute also provides for penalties for other conduct connected with fraudulent claims or other misrepresentation related to benefits or payment under Medicare or Medicaid.

Another law, known as the Federal Anti-Kickback Statute (1980) provides for fines of up to $25,000 and imprisonment of up to 5 years for "knowingly and willingly solicit[ing] and receiv[ing] any remuneration (including any kickback, bribe or rebate) directly or indirectly" in exchange for making referrals to other providers or for ordering, purchasing, or leasing goods, facilities, services, or items under Medicare or Medicaid (Federal Anti-Kickback Law & Regulatory Safe Harbors, 2008) The clearest application of this law is to prohibit fees for referrals—such as a psychiatric NP paying a family NP for each patient the family NP refers. (In this case, both NPs are violating this law). Other arrangements are also prohibited, including discounts, rebates, or other reductions in fees. The Office of the Inspector General of the USDHHS has issued a list of "safe harbors"—arrangements that are not considered a violation of the antikickback law (Safe Harbor Provisions, 1999). The idea behind providing a list of safe harbors is to provide a degree of prospective guidance—to help avoid violations of the antikickback laws by identifying activities that are normally considered within the law. That list is periodically updated and should be regularly reviewed by the APN.

The federal False Claims Act (1986) is another important statute relating to fraud and abuse in health-care payment. The law applies to federal programs far beyond the Medicare and Medicaid programs. In fact, it long predates those programs, having been first enacted during the Civil War to address fraudulent activity by military contractors. In 1986, Congress enacted amendments to the False Claims Act to strengthen it and to make explicit its application to the Medicare and Medicaid programs. The law creates civil liability for anyone who is found to have submitted a false or fraudulent claim that has been paid by the government.

Under the False Claims Act, a private individual with knowledge of fraud against the federal government can bring suit in federal court on the federal government's behalf. Such an individual is known as a *qui tam relator* (or more simply as a financial whistleblower). The qui tam relator is entitled to a share of any damages that the government may recover either in court or in an out-of-court settlement.

Other federal laws (known as Stark I and Stark II, after their chief sponsor in Congress) limit a physician's ability to refer patients to various health services (including clinical laboratories) in which the physician or an immediate family member has a financial interest (Omnibus Reconciliation Act, 1989, 1993). These laws are intended to ensure that referrals are made based on patients' actual health-care needs rather than the referring physician's financial self-interest.

The laws are written to apply to physicians. They do not address referrals by APNs. The final Stark II regulations issued by the CMS make clear that these laws do not apply to referrals by nonphysician practitioners—NPs, CNSs, certified registered nurse anesthetists (CRNAs), CNMs and physician's assistants (PAs)—unless a physician "controls or influences" the referral. In other words, if the APN is not exercising independent judgment in making a referral, but is essentially acting as a proxy for the physician, then the self-referral laws apply (CMS, 2008).

Even though the laws do not, for the most part, directly affect them, APNs should be aware of the self-referral laws. The laws express a clear intent by Congress to avoid referrals based on a provider's self-interest. Thus, it is possible that these laws may be amended in the future to include self-referrals by APNs.

Assessing Risk and Avoiding Fraud and Abuse

The climate for fraud and abuse enforcement has changed for all clinicians, not just APNs. Whether in their own practices, in physician-based practices, or in hospital-based practices, APNs should be aware of programs in place to ensure compliance with applicable laws on billing for services. APNs should not assume that billing practices that have been in place for some time must be okay because "we have always done it this way." Many offices may have adopted billing practices long ago that are inappropriate or sloppy, but they have not had the misfortune of being audited—yet. Innocent mistakes occur. Enforcement agencies are not generally interested in going after isolated incidents or errors; they are usually concerned with *patterns* of inappropriate, illegal billing practices over time.

Billing, coding, and payment policy are complex. Most APNs are not experts in this area, although the authors strongly believe that all APNs should have a general understanding of coding, billing, and payment. In most instances, working with a billing specialist—either one employed by the practice or an external consultant—is highly advisable. However, each APN must have sufficient knowledge to work with these specialists to ensure their accuracy. This is because, as we have stressed in this section, APNs are responsible for claims submitted in their names and because ignorance of the content of these claims is not a defense against allegations of fraudulent billing.

One specific area in which APNs (and the practices in which they work) must be extremely careful is the area of "incident to" billing. Since its inception, Medicare has paid not only for "physician services," but also for services and supplies furnished incident to the services of a physician. (Abood & Keepnews, 2002). Among other things, this provision has allowed physician practices to bill for services provided by employees—not just APNs, but also other nurses, medical assistants, and other office personnel. For years, this was the only way that services provided by APNs were covered under Medicare. As APNs won Medicare reimbursement for eligible services—first in rural areas and skilled nursing facilities as a result of the Omnibus Budget Reconciliation Act of 1990 and later in all areas and practice settings as a result of the BBA of 1997—more and more APNs have been billing Medicare directly for their services.

However, many practices have chosen to continue billing APN services under the "incident to" provision. When APNs bill Medicare directly (under their own names and provider numbers), Medicare pays for their services at 85% of what it would pay a physician. Incident to services are billed under the physician's name and number and are paid at 100% of the physician rate—in essence, they are treated as if the physician personally performed the service. Thus, many physician practices that employ APNs see a financial incentive in billing under incident to. Incident to billing, however, comes with several requirements. These include the following (CMS, 2008):

- The physician must initiate the case. This means that the physician must see each new patient. It also means that the physician must also see for the first visit each established patient who presents with a new problem.

- There must be evidence of ongoing physician involvement in the case.
- The physician must be present (in the office suite, not necessarily in the same room) when the APN is providing services to the patient.

These requirements reflect the fact that incident to payment was not designed as a payment mechanism for independent providers of care, but rather for office staff who act as an extra pair of hands for the physician. As noted previously, services by any office staff acting within the scope of activities allowed under the law—including medical assistants and other unlicensed staff—can be billed under incident to when all other conditions are met. Incident to billing long predates the widespread use of APNs to provide comprehensive health-care services.

The potential for inappropriately billing for services is increased when practices depend on incident to billing for services provided by APNs. Is there a physician on the premises and available at all times, or do APNs cover for the physician during lunch, hospital rounds, or at other times when the physician is out of the office? Are there ever times when a new patient is seen by an APN? Are there times when an established patient is seen by an APN and reports a new health-care problem? Moreover, even if the practice complies with all of the conditions for incident to billing, are the details of such compliance adequately documented?

Incident to billing presents risks for the practice and the APN—risks that are largely not present if billing for services provided by APNs are billed under the APN's name and provider number. It should be noted that none of the restrictive conditions that apply to incident to billing apply when an APN is billing under his or her own name and number. The APN need not be an employee; he or she can initiate a new patient or a new problem for an established patient, and there is no requirement for a physician to be present when the APN provides services. In addition, billing under the APN's name and number means that those services are no longer "invisible" (i.e., services billed under incident to are reflected in Medicare data as having been provided by the physician, not the APN). APNs should be aware of the inherent risks involved in incident to billing. Quite frankly, some practices rely on this type of billing because it pays 15% more for services provided by the APN without balancing the costs of compliance—and the considerable risk (and immense potential cost) of noncompliance.

ANTITRUST LAW

Antitrust is another area of the law that has an important bearing on APNs and other health professionals' practices. It is an area in which the courts have played a significant shaping role.

Antitrust laws apply much more broadly than just to health care. The first federal antitrust statute, the Sherman Act, was passed by Congress in 1890, followed by the Clayton Act and the Federal Trade Commission Act, both in 1914.

Congress's goals in enacting these statutes was to ensure free competition by countering business practices and transactions "which tended to restrict production, raise prices or otherwise control the market to the detriment of purchasers or consumers of goods and services" (*Apex Hosiery Co. v. Leader,* 1940). When competitors work together to restrain competition by others, this deprives consumers of the purported benefits of a free economic market—it removes incentives to lower prices and improve quality. Some activities that had been undertaken by large industries at the end of the 19th century—dividing up economic markets, agreeing on minimum prices, boycotting other competitors—were seen as inherently injurious to consumers. However, the antitrust laws represented more than an attempt to make some adjustments in certain economic practices. As part of a populist reaction to the "robber barons" in industries, like steel and oil, the antitrust laws were seen as an effort to reclaim the free enterprise system as the United States had previously known it. For instance, in describing the Sherman Act, the Supreme Court has stated that this statute was designed to be a comprehensive charter of economic liberty aimed at preserving free and unfettered competition as the rule of trade. It rests on the premise that the unrestrained interaction of competitive forces will yield the best allocation of our economic resources, the lowest prices, the highest quality, and the greatest material progress, while at the same time providing an environment conducive to the preservation of our democratic, political, and social institutions. However, were that promise open to question, the policy unequivocally laid down by the act is competition (*Northern Pacific Railway v. United States,* 1958).

These broad goals may be hard to discern from the relatively sparse text of the antitrust statutes. Section 1 of the Sherman Act, for instance, simply prohibits contracts, combinations of conspiracies in restraint of interstate trade or commerce. Section 2 prohibits monopolization, attempted monopolization, and conspiracies to monopolize. Section 7 of the Clayton Act prohibits mergers and acquisitions that may lessen competition or tend to create a monopoly. Section 5 of the Federal Trade Commission Act prohibits unfair methods of competition. The U.S. Department of Justice and the Federal Trade Commission (FTC) share federal enforcement responsibilities for these antitrust statutes; in addition, state attorneys general and private parties may also bring suit under these laws. Most states also have their own antitrust laws, generally with provisions parallel to the federal laws.

The antitrust laws are written broadly and not are not especially descriptive. The application of these laws has been shaped by decades of judicial interpretation. For instance, the courts have developed two distinct approaches to assessing the anticompetitive affect of business activities. Some activities—price-fixing, group boycotts, and market allocation (dividing up markets among competitors)—are considered per se violations. This means that once it has been established that a competitor has engaged in one of these activities, the courts do not inquire as to its anticompetitive effects, such as whether and how it has harmed competition or injured consumers. Other activities are analyzed under a *rule of reason* approach. Under this approach, the court analyzes an alleged restraint on competition, weighing the procompetitive effects of an agreement against its anticompetitive effects (Swearingen, 2000). This means that the court carefully examines the industry involved, the history and purpose of the restraint, the relevant market, and any special circumstances that exist in that market (Swearingen, 2000; *United States v. Topco Associates,* 1972). Meeting this standard is clearly a much more involved, costly and time-consuming analysis than that required for activities that are considered per se violations.

For decades, the antitrust laws were considered by the courts to be inapplicable to the activities of many professionals. "Learned professions" like law and medicine generally were considered sufficiently different from other businesses for concerns about anticompetitive conduct to be relevant. Any exemption for learned professions is, at this point, long gone. In 1975, in *Goldfarb v. Virginia State Bar,* the U.S. Supreme Court found setting minimum attorneys fees to be a Sherman Act violation, rejecting the defendant bar association's argument that they were exempt because the law is a learned profession. Subsequently, the U.S. Supreme Court made the application of the antitrust laws to medicine explicit in *Arizona v. Maricopa County Medical Society (1982).* In that case, local physicians had agreed on maximum fees that could be charged. This decision indicated that such acts were price fixing and effectively eliminated any belief that physicians were outside the reach of antitrust laws.

Price-fixing—a per se antitrust violation—remains an important potential area of enforcement within health care. Attempts to set minimum or maximum fees charged to consumers are a prime example. Price-fixing can also involve agreeing on rates to charge insurance companies. Physicians (or other health-care professionals, including APNs) cannot work together to determine acceptable payment rates for insurers, including managed care companies.

Another per se violation with important relevance for health care is the group boycott. In general, a group boycott occurs when a group of competitors organizes to refuse (or encourage others to refuse) to patronize a competitor or another business entity to advantage themselves. One example would be if a group of physicians or APNs jointly decides to refuse to contract with a specific managed care organization because of its reimbursement rates.

Another example would be if a group of physicians organizes to disadvantage another group of health-care providers. In *Wilk v. American Medical Association* (1990), the American Medical Association (AMA) was found to have engaged in a boycott of chiropractors. The AMA's code of ethics had declared it unethical for physicians to associate with unscientific practitioners, and later determined that chiropractic practice lacked a scientific basis. The effect of these determinations was a pronouncement that any physicians who referred patients to chiropractors, accepted referrals from chiropractors, or taught at a chiropractic school would be committing an ethical violation. A group of chiropractors sued the AMA, alleging that the AMA was attempting to eliminate chiropractic care through an illegal boycott. The U.S. Court of Appeals for the Seventh Circuit eventually determined that this AMA policy (which had subsequently been changed) was, in fact, a per se violation of the Sherman Act.

Because the goal of antitrust laws is to eliminate anticompetitive practices that injure (or may injure) the interests of consumers, the focus of enforcement and interpretation is on the effect on consumers (not on competitors) of allegedly anticompetitive activities. The aim of enforcement is to protect consumers' interests, not to ensure fairness among competitors. This means that unfair or even anticompetitive actions against APNs may not be antitrust violations if a harmful effect on consumers cannot be demonstrated. Thus, proving that allegedly anticompetitive behavior is a violation of antitrust law can be a heavy burden to bear because the determination of whether consumers have been harmed is highly fact-specific, depending heavily on the industry involved, the definition of the competitors' market, and the evaluation of the actual effect of the conduct in question. Therefore, individuals or enforcement agencies seek to demonstrate that anticompetitive behavior fits within the category of per se antitrust violations to eliminate the need to prove the actual effects of such behavior.

In one of the few antitrust cases involving APNs, a group of CNMs, brought suit against hospitals, a physician-owned insurance company, and several physicians. The CNMs charged that the defendants had engaged in concerted actions to prevent them from gaining hospital privileges, required physician supervision, and the ability for their collaborating physician to secure liability insurance. Their thriving practice was eventually forced to close. Eventually the CNMs won settlements against some of the defendants, and the U.S. Court of Appeals for the Sixth Circuit ruled against the remainder of the defendants (*Nurse Midwifery Associates v. Hibbett*, 1990).

Oltz v. St. Peter's Community Hospital (1994) is an antitrust case that involved a nurse anesthetist whose billing contract with the hospital was cancelled after the anesthesiologists with whom he competed obtained an exclusive contract with the hospital. Oltz, the nurse anesthetist, had previously entered into a billing contract with the hospital. The hospital was located in a rural community in Montana, and it provided 84% of the surgical services rendered in the area. The anesthesiologists did not want to compete with Oltz, who charged a lower rate for anesthesia. The hospital cancelled Oltz's contract after it entered into the exclusive agreement with the anesthesiologists. Oltz was effectively put out of business and had to relocate to find suitable employment. Oltz sued the doctors and the hospital and claimed their actions constituted a violation of the Sherman Act. Oltz agreed to settle with the physicians for $462,500 before trial. The case proceeded against the hospital, and the jury awarded over $400,000 to Oltz for lost income. The trial court deemed the jury award excessive and ordered a new trial on damages. The issue was resolved by summary judgment on the basis that Oltz could not prove his damages exceeded the settlement amount he had received from the doctors. Appeals followed and ultimately the Ninth Circuit Court of Appeals remanded the case for a new trial on the issue of damages. The Circuit Court noted Oltz presented ample evidence to support his claim that the hospital and doctors conspired to eliminate him as a competitor.

Enforcement of the Antitrust Laws

The FTC and the U.S. Department of Justice, through its Antitrust Division (ATD), share federal responsibility for enforcement of antitrust laws, although the ATD has exclusive responsibility for criminal prosecution of antitrust violations. Recently, the FTC and the ATD announced a Memorandum of Understanding regarding responsibility for antitrust enforcement in different agencies. Under this agreement, the FTC is designated as the lead agency for civil enforcement of antitrust laws in the health-care industry.

In 1993, the ATD and the FTC first issued their *Statements of Antitrust Enforcement Policy in Health Care* (ATD & FTC, 1993). This joint document discusses a variety of arrangements among and between hospitals and physicians and outlines several important safe harbors—activities that normally are not considered antitrust violations. (This is similar to the concept of antikickback safe harbors, discussed previously). For example, although price-fixing and group boycotts are illegal, the FTC and ATD recognize a safe harbor for health-care providers who collectively provide current or historical information about their fees to purchasers, as long as that information is not provided for the purpose of setting fees. Such information must be provided through a third party (e.g., a purchaser, government agency, health-care consultant, academic institution, or trade association); it must come from at least five providers and be at least 3 months old. This represents an attempt by these two agencies to demonstrate a degree of flexibility in antitrust enforcement in health care, particularly during a period of rapid transformation within the industry.

States and private individuals may also seek civil action for alleged violations of the antitrust laws. The cost of such litigation can be considerable, however, and is a significant barrier to private individuals who contemplate taking legal action to address anticompetitive practices.

Over the last decade, organized medicine has made "reform" of antitrust laws a major legislative priority. The AMA and other physician groups have pushed legislation (thus far without success) that would allow physicians to enter into joint negotiations with insurance companies to set fees and other contractual arrangements (Quality Health-Care Coalition Act, 1999). The FTC opposed this legislation (Pitkofsky, 1999), as did nursing organizations and insurers. A more recent attempt at antitrust "reform," the Health Care Antitrust Improvements Act (2002) would have changed the standard of review under the antitrust laws when two or more physicians or other health-care professionals attempt to negotiate with a health plan over contractual terms or plan policies. The bill would have applied a "rule of reason" approach to judicial analysis of such conduct (rather than the per se analysis currently applied to price-fixing and group boycotts), taking into account all relevant factors affecting competition, including access to care, quality of health-care services, and actual or proposed contract terms. Nursing organizations, including the ANA, opposed the bill on the grounds that it would increase health-care costs and could result in limitations on APN practice (ANA, 2002).

CONCLUSION

Laws, regulations, court decisions, and other arenas of public policy continue to ever increasingly affect health care and nursing, both positively and negatively. From Medicare, Medicaid, and direct reimbursement at the federal level to scope of practice, health plans and insurance development, and mental health services at the state level to public health preparedness, addressing homelessness, and providing school health programs at the local level, governments and the law are an everyday presence in the lives of APNs. Knowing the current law is critical to success as an APN. However, just as important for the APN's and nursing's future is the need for organized nursing to make a difference in shaping the laws of tomorrow. Through organizational membership and focused activism, APNs can provide leadership to nursing and demand through participation "nurse-friendly" legislation, regulation, and judicial decisions that serve to advance the profession and secure quality health services for our clients. Involvement in law-making and law-shaping should become an expected part of the APN role and self-image. Where laws, regulations and declaratory decisions are contrary to our favor, much of the fault lies in our inability to protect our own interests.

References

Abood, S., & Keepnews, D. (2002). *Understanding payment for advanced practice nursing services. Volume II: Fraud and abuse.* Washington, DC: American Nurses Publishing.

Ali v. Community Health Care Plan, Inc., 801 A.2d 775 (Ct. 2002).

American Nurses Association. (1996). *Scope and standards of advanced practice registered nursing.* Washington, DC: American Nurses Publishing.

American Nurses Association. (2002). *ANA activities and accomplishments.* Retrieved December 10, 2002, from the American Nurses Association Nursing World Web site: www.nursingworld.org/about/lately/2002/ceomay02.htm.

Antitrust Division & Federal Trade Commission. (1993). *Statement of antitrust enforcement policy in health care.* Washington, DC: Author.

Apex Hosiery Co. v. Leader, 310 U.S. 469 (1940).

Arizona v. Maricopa County Medical Society, 457 U.S. 332 (1982).

Bellegre v. Board of Nurse Examiners, 685 SW 2d 431 (Texas Appellate Court, 1985).

Berdyck v. Shinde and H.R. Magruder Memorial Hospital, 613 NE 2d 1014 (Ohio, 1993).

Centers for Medicare and Medicaid Services. (2008). *Medicare learning network.* Retrieved July 13, 2008, from the Centers for Medicare and Medicaid Services Web site: www.cms.hhs.gov/MLNMattersArticles/.

Chalmers-Francis v. Nelson, 6 Cal. 2d 402 (California, 1936).

Employee Retirement Income Security Act. (1974). P.L. 93-406.

False Claims Act. (1986). 31 U.S.C. Sec. 3729.

Federal Anti-Kickback Law and Regulatory Safe Harbors. (2008). Retrieved July 14, 2008, from the Office of Inspector General Web site: www.oig.hhs.gov/fraud/docs/safeharborregulations/safefs.htm.

Federal Trade Commission Act. (1914). U.S.C. Sec 44–48.

Fein v. Permanente Medical Group, 121 Cal. App. 3d 135 (California, 1981).

Goldfarb v. Virginia State Bar, 421 U.S. 773 (1975).

Guido, G. W. (2001). *Legal and ethical issues in nursing* (3rd. ed.). Upper Saddle River, NJ: Prentice Hall.

Health Care Antitrust Improvements Act. (2002). HR 3897 in 107th Congress.

Health Insurance Portability and Accountability Act. (1996). P.L. 104-191.

Hernicz v. State of Florida Department of Professional Regulation, 390 So. 2d 194 (Florida Appellate District Court, 1980).

Hogan v. Mississippi Board of Nursing, 457 So.2d 931 (Miss. 1984).

Keepnews, D. M. (1999). The scope of managed care liability. In S. H. Altman, U. E. Reinhardt, & D. Shactman (Eds.), *Regulating managed care: Theory, practice and future options.* San Francisco: Jossey-Bass.

Medicare and Medicaid Patient Protection Act. (1987). 42 U.S.C. Sec.1320a-7b(a). Retrieved July 9, 2008, from Cornell University Web site: www.law.cornell.edu/uscode/42/1320a-7b.html.

Monarch, K. (2002). *Nursing and the law: Trends and issues.* Washington, DC: American Nurses Publishing.

Northern Pacific Railway v. United States, 356 U.S. 1 (1958).

Nurse Midwifery Associates v. Hibbett, 918 F.2d 605 (CIR.6, 1990).

Oltz v. St. Peter's Community Hospital, 19 F.3d 1312 (9th Cir. 1994)

Omnibus Reconciliation Act. (1989). P.L. 101-239.

Omnibus Reconciliation Act. (1993). P.L. 103-166.

Pitofsky, R. (1999). Testimony before the Committee on the Judiciary, United States House of Representatives concerning H.R. 1304, the Quality Health-Care Coalition Act of 1999. June 22, 1999. Retrieved October 10, 2008, from Federal Trade Commission Web site: www.ftc.gov/os/1999/06/healthcaretestimony.htm.

Planned Parenthood v. Vines, 543 NE 2d 654 (Indiana, 1989).

Quality Health-Care Coalition Act. (1999). HR 1304 in 104th Congress.

Safe Harbor Provisions. (1999). 42 CFR Sec. 1001.952.

Sermchief v. Gonzales, 660 SW 2d 683 (Missouri, 1983).

State of Arkansas. (1998). *Arkansas State Board of Nursing Nurse Practice Act—Rules and regulations* (p. 4-1). Little Rock: Author.

Swearingen, M. J. (2000). Applying antitrust law to nonprofit health entities: Arguments for a greater attention to detail. *Journal of Health and Hospital Law, 33*(1), 57.

United States v. Topco Associates, 405 U.S. 596, 621 (Illinois, 1972).

Wilk v. American Medical Association, 895 F.2d 352 (Illinois, 1990).

Malpractice Insurance 27

Sharon E. Muran

Amy Muran Felton

Marie Infante

INTRODUCTION

Professional liability is a recognized risk for advanced practice nurses (APNs) that must be addressed seriously as a matter of professional responsibility. With this increased responsibility and autonomy comes increased risk. These risks include the possibility that the nurse will be held legally accountable for errors or omissions that result in harm to a patient or for noncompliance with a growing array of state and federal laws and regulations that provide the framework for advanced practice nursing and direct reimbursement for the services rendered. The purpose of this chapter is to provide some basic information about the increasing legal accountability of APNs and an overview of the current health-care practice climate with increasing risks that affect malpractice insurance and other methods of risk management. Finally, the chapter discusses additional ways to minimize the risk of being sued for malpractice. These approaches include (a) maintaining current clinical skills and knowledge, (b) documenting clear supportable reasons for taking or not taking diagnostic and therapeutic actions, as well as the patient's response to the interventions, and (c) retaining optimal professional and business relationships that are a part of advanced practice nursing.

NURSING TRADITION AND THE PARADIGM SHIFT

Advanced practice nursing is a challenging arena for the nursing profession, one that is quite independent in nature, and as described previously, one that is associated with risks quite different from those of nurses in traditional practice settings. Historically, nurses were perceived to be protected against malpractice liability because most were employed in hospitals (Shinn, 1998). As "charitable organizations," hospitals were generally exempt by statute or common law from malpractice liability. In these settings nurses were assumed to be a "one-size fits all caregiver" held in high esteem by the public.

Although nurses became more aware of their ethical and legal responsibilities with the evolution of state licensing of nurses, nursing practice was largely defined by employers and directly controlled by physicians. Independence and autonomy were discouraged. Compliance with employer policies was perceived as tantamount to safe practice under the law. As charitable immunity statutes were eliminated and institutions began to insure against liability, nurses assumed they were likewise protected under the hospital's insurance policy by virtue of their employment relationship. This misapprehension too often persists to this day (Shinn, 1998).

In the 1960s and 1970s, state and federal laws began to change in response to citizen, employer, and insurance carrier demand for containment of health-care costs and equitable access to health care. APNs evolved to meet the need for midlevel providers focused on promotion of health and pro-vision of primary care services for all citizens, including underserved and vulnerable populations.

Since then, APN educators and practitioners have defined and tested standards of care. State nurse practice acts have changed to encompass increased independence for APNs in the delivery of nursing service. Access to third-party reimbursement continues to grow at the federal and state levels (e.g., Medicare and Medicaid, Civilian Health and Medical Program of the Uniformed Services [CHAMPUS], and so on) and among private insurance companies such as Blue Cross/Blue Shield.

These events coupled with public acceptance increase the visibility of APNs, a desirable effect that has increased over time. However, as societal awareness of the roles of APNs in the provision of health care expands, so does the APNs' ever-growing accountability for the delivery and outcomes of their professional practice. Consequently, as APNs gain recognition as prominent, independent members of the health-care team, they become vulnerable, as are physicians, dentists and other professionals, to any sway in the malpractice insurance markets and to the growing trend in our society toward litigation as the solution to any life disappointment.

Whether employed, engaged in collaborative and consultative practice, or in independent prac-tice, the reality is that APNs are becoming more recognized as targets in the medical malpractice world, a situation unlikely to abate in the near future. Proactively, the best defense is a good offense. Thus, APNs must actively and continuously engage in effective risk management strategies such as professionally responsible behaviors and use of malpractice insurance to guard against the risk of new legal exposures and professional liability.

THE RISKS OF ADVANCED PRACTICE NURSING

There are at least three types of exposure that APNs should seek to avoid: (a) financial exposure in terms of judgments or settlements from a civil lawsuit, (b) licensure or certification actions by the relevant state agencies or private associations, and (c) civil or criminal sanctions and exclusion from participation in the federal health-care programs for fraud or abuse.

Civil Lawsuits

The first type of exposure is liability for professional malpractice. Malpractice is a type of profession-al negligence that results when the practitioner fails (by act or omission) to exercise due care and use the degree of skill and learning, under the circumstances, that a reasonably prudent APN would use (Black, 1979). The failure to follow the appropriate standard of care results in harm to the patient and financial exposure to compensate the patient or the patient's family. This exposure is the typical risk that most malpractice insurance policies cover.

Licensure or State Certification Exposures

There are other types of direct or indirect financial exposures that arise from breaking state or fed-eral laws or regulations that control advanced practice nursing and direct reimbursement for the services rendered. For example, an overpayment or false claim in the Medicare, Medicaid, or other federal health program can result in licensure action or loss of certification. State regulatory actions or actions by private associations generally are taken against the license or certification of the indi-vidual practitioner. Substance abuse, fraud, unprofessional conduct, or failure to have a written col-laborative agreement with a physician where one is required are other examples of charges that can result in licensure sanctions by a state board of nursing. These same behaviors may result in loss of a professional certification. Failure to maintain essential professional credentials in good standing can abruptly end a promising career. These types of risks may or may not be covered by a professional liability insurance policy. The wise APN will shop around to locate the liability insurance that will cover the costs of defending against such licensure actions.

Federal Health Program Exclusion

Another type of legal risk is noncompliance with laws and regulations of the federal health-care programs that provide direct reimbursement for the services of APNs (Buppert, 2002; Infante, 2000). The penalties can be both criminal and civil. A conviction for fraud is referred by the courts to the state board of nursing for appropriate action with respect to license of the guilty nurse (Bureau of National Affairs, 2002). The most severe civil penalty for breaking these laws is exclusion from federal health-care programs based on the authority of the Secretary of the U.S. Department of Health and Human Services (DHHS) to ban practitioners from receiving payments from any federal health-care program when they have violated certain laws. These risks are generally not covered in a typical professional liability insurance policy.

There are mandatory exclusion laws that require the secretary to exclude a practitioner if, among other things, the person is convicted of a crime related to the delivery of an item or service paid for by a federal health program. Medicare, Medicaid, TriCare, Federal Employee Health Benefits Program, the Veterans' Administration, and CHAMPUS are the most common federal health-care programs that reimburse for the services of eligible APNs.

The secretary of DHHS also has permissive authority to exclude an individual practitioner or entity if he or she has committed fraud or has been otherwise sanctioned for reasons related to professional competence, performance, or financial integrity. Under the "permissive exclusion authority," for example, an APN who is sanctioned by the state board of nursing can then be excluded by the secretary from participation and from receiving reimbursement for services from any federal program. Additionally, all providers (e.g., hospitals, health maintenance organizations [HMOs], home health agencies, nursing homes, and others) and all other practitioners (e.g., physician, group practices, and others) who themselves participate in federal health-care programs are banned from hiring the excluded APN at risk of losing their own federal reimbursement. Therefore, program exclusion is a career-ending event for most individuals.

Although a thorough discussion of these statutory risks is beyond the scope of this chapter, APNs must know the laws that control their practice and reimbursement, develop behaviors to ensure compliance with these laws, recognize the risks associated with noncompliance with these laws and regulations, and use risk prevention strategies to manage their professional practices and minimize those risks (Infante, 2000).

MALPRACTICE AND THE ADVANCED PRACTICE NURSE

How frequently are APNs sued for malpractice? There is no reliable way to gather information on the number of lawsuits filed on a national basis. There is also little to stop a patient from bringing a malpractice lawsuit regardless of the ultimate merits of their allegations against the practitioner. However, there are reliable sources that report on verdicts and settlements resulting from malpractice claims from which some inferences concerning the actual risk of a malpractice lawsuit can be assessed and monitored on a state-by-state basis.

The National Practitioner Data Bank and Healthcare Integrity and Protection Data Base

The National Practitioner Data Bank (NPDB) was established by Congress in 1986 (NPDB, 2008). The U.S. DHHS is responsible for implementing and maintaining this databank. The NPDB is intended to improve the quality of care by restricting the ability of incompetent practitioners to move from state to state without disclosure of previous malpractice payments or adverse actions.

In 1996, Congress created a second data repository. The secretary of the U.S. DHHS, acting through the Office of Inspector General (OIG), was directed by the Health Insurance Portability and Accountability Act (HIPAA) of 1996 to create the Healthcare Integrity and Protection Data Bank (HIPDB) to combat fraud and abuse in health insurance and health-care delivery (HIPDB, 2008). The HIPDB collects, reports, and discloses information regarding licensure and certification actions, program exclusions, criminal convictions, and other adjudicated actions and decisions against both individual practitioners and institutional providers. Although there is some overlap between the NPDB and the HIPDB, only the NPDB reports malpractice judgments and settlements.

State licensure boards, hospitals, and other eligible entities access these databanks to assess an individual practitioner's (including APNs') responsibility for errors and professional misconduct when considering applications for state license, employment, staff privileges, or other affiliations. A report on the NPDB, however, should not be the sole determinant of a credentialing or licensure decision. According to the NPDB fact sheet, the data contained in the NPDB repository is only one indicator among many (e.g., evidence of current competency through continuous quality improvement studies, peer recommendations, health status, verification of training, and experience and relationships with patients and colleagues) that should be considered when evaluating a professional's credentials (NPDB, 2008b).

The NPDB collects information on all malpractice payments made by insurance companies on behalf of individual health-care practitioners. Payments must be reported to the NPDB no matter how small the amount, whether or not the case is settled before filing suit, and whether or not the payment was the result of a confidential settlement. Reporting of malpractice payments is mandatory for all types of licensed health-care practitioners. The NPDB also collects information about adverse licensure or professional sanctions imposed on health-care practitioners. Reporting of adverse licensure actions, clinical privilege actions, and professional society actions are mandatory for all physicians and dentists in this country. Adverse actions against APNs and other health-care practitioners may be voluntarily reported to the NPDB.

Trends in Malpractice Claims

The NPDB began collecting and analyzing data on malpractice claims in 1990 and issues annual cumulative reports of its findings. The most recent data is from the 2006 Annual Report (NPDB, 2008a). Before March 2002, the NPDB classified nurses into four categories: professional (registered) nurses (RNs), certified registered nurse anesthetists (CRNAs), certified nurse-midwives (CNMs), and nurse practitioners (NPs). A fifth category, advanced nurse practitioners, subsequently amended to advanced nurse practitioner/clinical nurse specialist, was added in 2002.

Based on inquiries made to the NPDB, interest in nurse malpractice payments is growing. The average annually from 1990 to 2000 was 320 payments; the average from 2001 to year end 2006 was 501 payments annually, an increase of 37%. Despite this, the NPBD indicates that malpractice payments for nurses are relatively rare. From September 1, 1990 to December 31, 2006, 6,208 payments were made for all nurses, with 61.6% of payments made for nonspecialized RNs. In total, payments made for all nurses represented only 2.1% of all payments reported to the NPDB (2008a).

There continues to be little in the scant claims experience or research to explain why APNs are sued so much less than physicians. In light of substantial evidence that many more medical errors are made than lawsuits filed, it appears that little is known about why malpractice claims are filed in some circumstances but not in others, regardless of the type of health-care provider (Schmidt, Heckert, & Mercer, 1992; Weiler, et al., 1993).

The rarity of malpractice claims against nurses in general may in part be explained by a continuing public perception that nurses are the most honest and ethical of professionals. There is also a lingering belief by some lay public and lawyers that the physician is the "captain of the ship" and bears full legal responsibility for bad outcomes. However, as practice patterns change to include more independent advanced nursing practice, this principle is rapidly becoming obsolete (Jenkins, 1994). Some liability for errors made by employed APNs is imputed to the hospital, institutional, or physician employer under the legal theory of respondeat superior ("let the master respond"), but in other circumstances in which the relationship between the professionals is not an employment relationship, each practitioner's actions are judged on their own merits.

Some preliminary evidence suggests, however, that certain practitioner characteristics—such as being female, the amount of time in practice, and the average length of office visit—may be inversely related to claims experienced for physicians (Schmidt et al., 1992). Another study found that better communications by physicians with patients, particularly about adverse outcomes, may also reduce the possibility of a claim (Lefevre, Water, & Budetti, 2002; Sloan & Hsieh, 1995). These same characteristics may be applicable to the study of claims experience for APNs, and as such, they suggest an agenda for future research.

For claims or judgments reported in the NPDB Annual Report (2008a) against nurses themselves, almost two-thirds of the malpractice payments were made on behalf of RNs, not APNs **(Table 27-1)**. Of the 6,208 payments reported for APNs for September 1990 through December 2006, CRNAs were the most frequently sued, accounting for 19% of the reported payments. CNM and NP payments were 9.6% and 9.6% of the total, respectively. Anesthesia problems were responsible for 82.4% of payments for CRNAs. Adverse obstetrical outcomes were responsible for 81% of the CNM payments; 44.9% of NP payments were for diagnosis-related problems; and treatment-related problems accounted for 24.9% of payments.

For calendar year 2006 only, the number of payments for all nurses was 645 with a mean value per claim of $277,431 and a median value of $112,500. When adjusted for inflation, the cumulative mean payment for nurses ($322,463) was $50,092 larger that the inflation-adjuested mean physician payment of $282,371. This variation is likely attributable to the fact that there are far fewer nurse payments than physician payments so that one large payment for APNs negatively affects the mean. Because the inflation-adjusted median nurse payment ($106,924) was $29,858 less than that a physician's ($136,782), the median amount is more representative of the typical payment **(Table 27-2)**.

The NPDB also reports on payments by state. The highest number of claims against nurses from September 1990 to December 2006 was in New Jersey with 667 and Texas with 478 **(Table 27-3)**. Vermont and Delaware had the lowest number of suits, seven and three, respectively. This data is of limited interpretive value for APNs because it is reported for all nurse categories. Additionally, the number of payments in any given state is affected by the number of APNs and may represent a reflection of the professional opportunities in that state. The numbers are also a function of the specific provisions of the malpractice and evidence laws in each state.

TABLE 27-1

Nurse Malpractice Payments by Reason and Type of Nurse

Malpractice Reason	Number of Malpractice Payments					Total
	Registered Nurses‡	Nurse Anesthetists	Nurse-Midwives	Nurse Practitioners	Advanced Practice Nurse/Clinical Nurse Specialist*	
Anesthesia related	137	973	1	10	1	1,122
Behavioral health related†	6	1	0	1	1	9
Diagnosis related	253	17	43	267	2	582
Equipment or product related	60	6	0	6	0	72
Intravenous line and blood products related	172	14	0	2	0	188
Medications related	605	31	4	73	1	714
Monitoring related	776	21	19	29	0	845
Obstetrics related	428	7	483	32	1	951
Surgery related	399	69	9	13	1	491
Treatment related	761	36	36	148	6	987
Miscellaneous	227	6	1	13	0	247
All reasons	**3,824**	**1,181**	**596**	**594**	**13**	**6,208**

This table includes only disclosable reports in the National Practitioner Data Bank (September 1, 1990–December 31, 2006) as of the end of the current year. Voided reports have been excluded. Medical malpractice payment reports, which are missing data neccasary to determine the malpractice reason (eight reports for RNs) are excluded.

*Reporting using the "Advanced Nurse Practitioner" category began on March 5, 2002. The advanced nurse practitioner was changed to clinical nurse specialist on September 9. 2002. Before March 5, 2002, these nurses were included in the "RN (Professional Nurse)" category.

†The "Behavioral Health" category was added on 01/31/2004. Reports involving behavioral health issues filed before 01/31/2004 used other reporting categories. Cumulative data in this category include only reports filed after 01/31/2004.

‡A professional nurse is an individual who has received approved nursing education and training, holds a BSN degree (or equivalent), an associate degree (or equivalent), or a hospital program diploma, and who holds a State License as a Registered Nurse. This definition includes Registered Nurses who have advanced training as nurse-midwives, nurse anesthetists, advanced practice nurses, and so on.

TABLE 27-2

Mean and Median Malpractice Payment Amounts (Actual and Inflation Adjusted) for Nurses by Malpractice Reason, 2006, and Cumulative Through 2006—Professional Nurses‡ (Registered Nurses, Nurse Anesthetists, Nurse Midwives, Nurse Practitioners, and Advanced Practice Nurses/Clinical Nurse Specialists)

Malpractice Reason	2006 Only			Cumulative Through 2006				
				Actual			Inflation Adjusted	
	Number of Payments	Mean Payment ($)	Median Payment ($)	Number of Payments	Actual Mean Payment ($)	Median Payment ($)	Inflation Mean Payment ($)	Adjusted Median Payment ($)
Anesthesia related	76	290,001	175,000	1,122	284,102	100,000	320,811	133.184
Behavioral health related‡	3	328,633	30,000	9	194,122	30,000	197,932	30,000
Diagnosis related	78	321,367	187,251	582	294.398	125,000	345,385	150,000
Equipment or product related	7	89,831	35,000	72	149,280	38,250	190,482	41,116
Intravenous line or blood products related	11	124,084	100,000	188	216,646	75,000	266,889	83,604
Medications related	64	195,331	75,000	714	260,909	82,500	308,375	73,581
Monitoring related	95	274,086	112,500	845	295,401	100,000	350,615	111,606

Continued

TABLE 27-2—cont'd

Mean and Median Malpractice Payment Amounts (Actual and Inflation Adjusted) for Nurses by Malpractice Reason, 2006, and Cumulative Through 2006—Professional Nurses‡ (Registered Nurses, Nurse Anesthetists, Nurse Midwives, Nurse Practitioners, and Advanced Practice Nurses/Clinical Nurse Specialists)

| Malpractice Reason | 2006 Only | | | Cumulative Through 2006 | | | | |
| | | | | Actual | | | Inflation Adjusted | |
	Number of Payments	Mean Payment ($)	Median Payment ($)	Number of Payments	Actual Mean Payment ($)	Median Payment ($)	Inflation Mean Payment ($)	Adjusted Median Payment ($)
Obstetrics related	127	394,306	200,000	951	514,553	235,512	593,095	270,603
Surgery related	45	118,745	100,000	491	145,969	50,000	175,218	61,323
Treatment related	120	284,476	87,500	987	181,904	50,000	208,731	64,614
Miscellaneous	25	99,985	82,500	247	223,327	40,000	262,203	51,640
All reasons	**645**	**277,431**	**112,500**	**6,208**	**282,297**	**95,000**	**322,463**	**106,924**

This table includes only disclosable reports in the National Practitioner Data Bank (September 1, 1990–December 31, 2006) as of the end of the current year. Voided reports have been excluded. Medical Malpractice payment reports that are missing data necessary to determine the malpractice reason (eight reports cumulatively) are excluded.

†See Behavorial Health note in Table 27-1.

‡See Professional Nurse note in Table 27-1.

TABLE 27-3

Nurse (Registered Nurses, Nurse Anesthetists, Nurse-Midwives, and Nurse Practitioners) Malpractice Payments by State

State	Number of Reports	Adjusted Number of Reports	Ratio of Adjusted Nurse Reports to 100 Adjusted Physician Reports
Alabama	42	42	7.09
Alaska	8	8	4.30
Arizona	46	46	2.09
Arkansas	26	26	3.84
California	125	125	0.76
Colorado	49	49	3.06
Connecticut	21	21	1.44
Delaware	3	3	0.91
Florida	219	219	2.28
Georgia	97	97	3.90
Hawaii	7	7	2.06
Idaho	22	22	7.17
Illinois	138	138	2.08
Indiana*	16	12	0.60
Iowa	18	18	1.55
Kansas*	51	34	2.97
Kentucky	43	43	2.93
Louisiana*	116	100	5.27
Maine	9	9	2.18
Maryland	60	60	2.64
Massachusetts	198	198	7.31
Michigan	77	77	0.93
Minnesota	19	19	1.61
Mississippi	33	33	3.02
Missouri	136	136	5.05
Montana	7	7	1.10
Nebraska	26	26	4.87
Nevada	8	8	1.03
New Hampshire	25	25	4.36
New Jersey	392	392	7.06
New Mexico*	60	59	7.55
New York	173	173	0.89
North Carolina	48	48	2.16
North Dakota	4	4	1.66
Ohio	117	117	1.71
Oklahoma	45	45	4.66
Oregon	21	21	2.24
Pennsylvania*	97	88	0.98
Rhode Island	9	9	1.36
South Carolina*	15	14	1.66
South Dakota	10	10	4.41

Continued

TABLE 27-3—cont'd

Nurse (Registered Nurses, Nurse Anesthetists, Nurse-Midwives, and Nurse Practitioners) Malpractice Payments by State

State	Number of Reports	Adjusted Number of Reports	Ratio of Adjusted Nurse Reports to 100 Adjusted Physician Reports
Tennessee	82	82	4.80
Texas	305	305	2.94
Utah	11	11	1.05
Vermont	1	1	0.32
Virginia	49	49	2.28
Washington	44	44	1.78
West Virginia	19	19	1.33
Wisconsin*	26	24	2.38
Wyoming	8	8	3.02
Washington, DC	22	22	3.81
All reports	**3,208**	**3,158**	**2.22**

This table includes only disclosable reports in the National Practitioner Data Bank (September 1, 1990–December 31, 2006). The "All Reports" row includes jurisdictions not listed (Puerto Rico, Virgin islands, Guam).

*The "Adjusted" column excludes reports from state patient compensation funds and other similar funds that make payments in excess of amounts paid by a practitioner's primary malpractice carrier. When payments are made by these funds, two reports are filed with the National Practitioner Data Bank (one from the primary insurer and one from the fund) whenever a total malpractice settlement or award exceeds a maximum set by the state for the practitioner's primary malpractice carrier. States marked with asterisks have these funds. Thus, the adjusted columns provide an approximation of the number of incidents resulting in payments rather than the number of payments.

Malpractice Lawsuits and State Laws

Malpractice lawsuits, with rare exceptions, are filed in state court under state law rather than federal law. State laws pertaining to filing a malpractice claim vary widely and may make it easier or more difficult for patients to sue for malpractice and obtain a judgment or settlement. For example, differences in statute of limitations (the time from discovery of an injury to filing of a lawsuit), burdens of proof, caps on noneconomic damages (e.g., pain and suffering), attorneys' fees, and use of mandatory medical review panels or arbitration to resolve issues, make a great difference in the frequency of malpractice lawsuits in a given state and the amount of a judgment or settlement.

Advanced Practice Nurses and the Malpractice Crisis

Periodically the country experiences a "crisis" in professional liability fueled by, among other things, the economic downturns in society, societal expectations, the cyclical business of professional liability, and perceived increases in both the number of claims filed and the amounts of judgments or settlements paid on behalf of health-care professionals (Council of Economic Advisors, 2002; Freedman, 2002; U.S. DHHS, 2002). Malpractice crises occurred in the 1970s, the 1980s, in 2002, and again in 2004 (Thorpe, 2004).

Often, the stakeholders seek state or federal legislation to solve the problems of too many lawsuits and too little access to affordable insurance. Commonly referred to as *tort reform,* these proposed laws seek to make it more difficult or less profitable to file claims against health-care professionals. The intended results are (a) to create a more favorable market for malpractice insurance carriers to continue to provide coverage and (b) for health-care practitioners to continue to provide services. In every session of Congress there are legislative proposals and political calls for national tort reform at the federal level (Bureau of National Affairs, 2004; Congressional Budget Office, 2004; U.S. DHHS, 2002). Although there are strong policy arguments to support Congress taking such action, malpractice litigation is a matter of state law and state legal practice. National tort reform, although repeatedly proposed, remains unlikely any time soon.

Realistic prospects for meaningful state tort reform as of this writing have been passed in 2005 and 2006 in Arizona, Connecticut, Iowa, Missouri, South Carolina, Utah, Virginia, Washington, and Wisconsin (National Conference of State Legislatures [NCSL], 2007).

In general these reforms focus on (a) limits to noneconomic damage awards, (b) allocation of plaintiff attorney fees as a percentage of a damages award, (c) expert witness standards, and (d) the inadmissability of apology statements by health-care practitioners. However, as of 2006 there was also an increasing focus on insurance company accountability by requiring reports from medical malpractice insurance providers and state control on insurance premium rates. This development, along with the cap on noneconomic reforms and inadmissability of apology statements as evidence of liability, are common elements of several jurisdictional proposals and should be closely followed by APNs in their respective practice jurisdictions, especially those in New York, New Jersey, Virginia, and Wisconsin (NCSL, 2007; Silverman, 2004).

There is growing evidence that some tort reform initiatives have little effect on the number and amount of malpractice judgments or settlements (American Society for Healthcare Risk Management [ASHRM], 2002; Office of Technology Assessment [OTA], 1993; Viscusi & Born, 1995). A more productive reform may be the increasing attention that the Congress, federal agencies, and The Joint Commission (TJC, formerly The Joint Commission for Accreditation of Healthcare Organizations) are devoting to prevention of medical errors (Bovgjerg, Miller, & Shapiro, 2001; Institute of Medicine, 2000; TJC, 2008).

Notwithstanding their historically low incidence of claims, APNs can expect to find themselves increasingly affected by situations that arise in a "hard" malpractice insurance market. The effects are escalating insurance premiums, coverage limitations, insurance company insolvencies, or decisions by carriers to stop covering medical malpractice altogether, limiting access to whatever liability insurance is available (America Association of Nurse Anesthetists [AANA], 2002a; ASHRM, 2002; Silverman, 2004). As a result of prohibitive insurance costs or complete lack of insurance, some practitioners have taken drastic actions, including early retirement, closure of high-risk practices such as obstetrics, or relocation to a state where the claims experience is more reasonable and insurance is available (Freedman, 2002; Silverman, 2004). In another response, associations such as the American College of Nurse-Midwives (ACNM) and other professionals, including a number of physician groups, have formed their own insurance companies to ensure insurance access to their members in the periodic downturns of the insurance business.

Although the aggregate claims history for APNs may seem modest, a hard market for malpractice insurance affects APNs, as well as physicians and all licensed health-care practitioners. The best advice is for APNs to engage in a form of risk management called *risk prevention* and make every effort to reduce errors. APNs need to incorporate error reduction principles into their daily practice.

APNs must also remain informed in changes in the legal landscape in the states in which they practice that potentially could have a profound impact on their legal and financial well-being.

PRACTICE SETTINGS AND SPECIALTY PRACTICE RISKS

Recognizing that APNs have a significant responsibility to practice sound risk management in the clinical areas of their practice, they must also understand that the risks associated with advanced practice differ according to the business relationships within which APNs practice. This does not lessen the imperative to manage clinical risks but strongly indicates that each specialty practitioner must consider the uniqueness of practice risks in their own setting and protect themselves and their patients accordingly.

As an initial legal principle, each person is always individually accountable for his or her own torts (wrongs). As demonstrated by the NPDB statistics, APNs can and do get sued in their own right. Liability in all cases turns on whether the APN exercised due care under the circumstances. This conclusion is determined by examining the duty owed to the patient, the professional standards that apply to a reasonable APN practicing under similar circumstances, and the causal effect of any act or omission of the APN to the injury suffered by the patient. Whether anyone else, such as collaborating physicians, are accountable and can be sued for the harm caused by substandard acts or omissions of the APN depends on the relationship between the parties and on the facts and circumstances of the incident.

EMPLOYED ADVANCED PRACTICE NURSES

As noted previously, RNs historically have been employees of hospitals, physicians, or other health-care entities. There are many in today's world, including health-care systems, physicians, lawyers, judges, and lay persons, who still view all nurses as subservient to a hospital or physician employer. However, the development of advanced practice nursing has given rise to other types of professional opportunities and relationships that differ from the traditional employee role of the RN.

APNs such as NPs and clinical nurse specialists (CNSs) are often employed by health-care systems, as well as by acute care, extended care, home care, and managed care organizations, to name just a few. As employees, APNs are presumed to be covered by the employer's malpractice program because under the concept of "vicarious liability" the employer is held responsible financially for harm caused to a patient by its employee. The Latin term for this principle of imputed responsibility is respondeat superior. It applies only in an employment situation because the employer effectively controls the manner in which the care is rendered (i.e., the employer has legal control over the actions taken by the employee that are within the scope of the employee's job description). When hospitals or health-care systems are sued, it is typically a result of errors or omissions committed by employees such as physicians, technicians, nurses, and APNs. From an economic perspective, employers have more assets to pay a settlement or a judgment, and therefore, are better able to bear the risk.

When an APN is in a true employment relationship, liability for negligence continues to flow through to the employer as a consequence of this traditional principle of tort law. The insurance rates charged to the employer reflect the risks associated with the entire pool of employees. However, this allocation of risk also provides the employer with the best opportunity to manage the risk through direct payment of claims. Many health-care employers are self-insured, meaning they personally "retain" risk or fund the settlement of claims to a given dollar ceiling. In effect, they are settling with their own money, thus avoiding the higher insurance premium costs. Self-insured employers are thus strongly motivated to keep claim settlements below their self-insured limit. To achieve this objective, it is common to agree to a settlement without disputing which of the named health-care employees were actually liable.

The danger to the employed APNs is twofold. First, if named individually in a lawsuit, the APN can be found jointly and severally liable or liable for contributory negligence as an individual, not just an employee. If, under these circumstances, the APN relies only on the employer's malpractice insurance to cover the claim, the hospital defense counsel could decide to settle the case and leave the remaining liability to the APN individually. Second, an APN without individual malpractice insurance coverage is subject to the decisions of the one hospital lawyer, which may not be in the APN's best interest. Moreover, if the APN is at the mercy of the hospital insurer, a settlement of a suit on behalf of any named health-care practitioner must be reported to the NPDB as required by law. Such a settlement could be negotiated without knowledge or consent of the APN. With the APN's professional reputation and financial well-being at stake, the APN cannot afford to abdicate responsibility to an employer. It is advisable to carry sufficient amounts of individual malpractice insurance to maintain control and to avoid these types of conflicts (CMF Group, 2002). With individual malpractice insurance coverage, the APN has separate counsel who is not conflicted by the interests of the hospital and can zealously represent the interests of the APN.

INDEPENDENT PRACTICE

The APN, subject to state nurse practice acts, is increasingly likely to become an independent practitioner who controls his or her own professional judgments and actions. However, with greater autonomy comes greater individual accountability for actions. In this type of practice arrangement the APN may deliver health-care services in any one or more of several settings, including traditional employer settings. Independent practice is usually accomplished through solo practice, group practice with other APNs, or business arrangements in which the APN and the health-care system, HMO, physician, or group practice structure their relationship as one of "independent contractor" or as a credentialed member of a hospital's medical staff with defined privileges.

As an independent contractor, the general rule is that no vicarious liability flows from the APN to the institution, physician, or other third party (Ingram, 1993). In real life, however, circumstances are seldom that clearcut. Even when the APN is not the employee of the institution, a lawyer may still argue that the institution is responsible because ostensibly the APN and the hospital or practice encourages patients to believe the nurse is employed by the institution. This type of ostensible agency theory is frequently argued in emergency room and anesthesia cases or whenever the lawyer wants to get to the (presumably) "deep pocket" of the hospital as a source of money for the patient. Or the lawyer will argue that responsibility is shared by all who were involved in the events leading to the claim of injury, including the institutional provider and any physician (or APN) involved in the care of the patient at the time under legal theories of joint and several or contributory liability (Silverman, 2004).

However, whether vicarious liability on any theory is imputed to the hospital, group practice, HMO, physician, or other party turns on the specific relationships and the degree of control exercised by one professional or party over the APN. A hospital, for example, is not held liable for the professional negligence of nonemployed medical staff members regardless of whether they are physicians or APNs. Although courts take many factors into account, the final decision in any case depends on the facts and circumstances particular to that situation (Jenkins, 1994; Silverman, 2004).

To illustrate this, consider the experiences of CRNAs. These independent APNs provide 65% of all anesthesia care in the United States annually, are the sole providers in two-thirds of rural hospitals in the United States and the primary provider for the military. According to the American Association of Nurse Anesthetists, the laws of every state permit CRNAs to work with physicians or other authorized health care practitioners without being supervised by an anesthesiologist (AANA, 2002b). CRNAs have long been recognized by TJC and Medicare as independent practitioners. Additionally, there are multiple court decisions that support the conclusion that surgeons, dentists, and health-care centers working with CRNAs do not face increased liability. These others are not liable for the actions of the CRNA because they do not control the CRNA (AANA, 2002b). In fact over the past few years 14 states have "opted out" of the of the anesthesia care rule published in 2001 by Centers for Medicare and Medicaid Services in the *Federal Register* [66 FR 5672-56769] (AANA, 2005, 2007). This rule required that CRNAs practice under the supervision of a physician. CRNAs, their institutions, and their colleagues remain challenged by this form of imputed liability. This is a lesson for all APNs: To manage the risks associated with independent practice, regardless of specialty or business relationships, APNs must be armed with adequate professional liability coverage.

COLLABORATIVE PRACTICE

Collaborative practice settings are rapidly increasing. For example, nurse-midwife practice trends indicate a continual shift from practice as an employee in acute care (hospital) settings to collaborative practices with physicians (American Nurses Association, 1998; K. Fennel, personal communication, August 6, 2002; Silverman, 2004). In a true collaborative practice, the CMN, or any APN, is an independent practitioner and not an employee. This business arrangement is a prudent form of risk management for all parties because accountability rests with the individual provider. No one practitioner controls or is liable for the activities of another. This risk control strategy does not ensure an APN will not be sued, but it does appreciably diminish the chances of unprotected and unwarranted vicarious liability for all parties.

The specific issue of legal exposure of the physician collaborator for the acts of the APN has received a great deal of attention over the years. Jenkins (1994) reported that certain insurance companies have been known to place an automatic surcharge on the insurance premiums of any physician who collaborated with CNMs or for that matter physicians who collaborated with an NP (Silverman, 2004). These insurance practices were based on the premise that any physician practicing with an APN was at greater risk of a malpractice action. Although it is true that the physician who employs an APN can be liable, like any employer, for the negligence of their employees under the theory of respondeat superior, if another type of business relationship exists between the physician and the nurse, there is no legal basis on which to impute liability automatically to the physician.

It should be noted that over time, surcharges or practice restrictions have increased in some jurisdictions as the independent stature of CNMs continues to expand under most state practice laws, altthough overall there is a caveat that the practices may wax and wane as the market for malpractice insurance changes. Although progress in this area was noted in surveys conducted by the American College of Obstetricians and Gynecologists (1992, 1999), reporting that insurance carrier surcharges declined from 59.7% of physicians in 1992 to 38.5% in 1999 as the number of collaborative practices increases, the similarity of liability claims demonstrates a growing public perception that liability can now be shared equally by physicians and APNs. For example, physicians and midwives parallel one another in the incidence of common claims, such as in the case of dystocias and adverse caesarian section outcomes when a midwife is involved in patient management. Accordingly, as Fennel (personal communication, August 6, 2002) reports, malpractice premiums for CNMs rose dramatically (21% in 2002 versus 7% in 1999), and as of 2004, premiums for nurse-midwives in states such as New York and New Jersey doubled (Silverman, 2004). Midwives with a history of malpractice suits are being denied insurance, and the majority of claims are the greater risk and more costly "claims made" policies as opposed to the preferred lower risk "occurrence" claims still available for NPs (K. Fennel, personal communication, August 6, 2002; J. O'Sullivan, personal communication, May 5, 2002; Silverman, 2004).

MALPRACTICE INSURANCE AS A RISK MANAGEMENT TOOL

A critical element of preparation for advanced practice is the ability to manage the risks associated with the specialty and the intended practice setting. Liability for individual acts or judgments as a professional cannot be transferred, but financial responsibility for damage awards (indemnity) and legal (defense) fees incurred in arriving at damages may be transferred. The objective is to limit the financial effect "should you cause or be accused of causing injury to another" (Shinn, 1998; Silverman 2004). Purchasing professional liability coverage involves thorough investigation and selection of insurance with a regular review of coverage to be sure it continues to meet practice risks. A suggested process includes the following steps.

Identify the Carriers

Professional liability carriers differ from one specialty to another. APN professional associations and their websites are a reliable source of information. Practicing colleagues with coverage are another source of information.

Coverage Selection Criteria

In investigating forms of coverage, expect to find some standard elements in most policies. Carriers generally provide legal defense if the insured is named in a claim resulting from an adverse event, pay defense legal fees, and if the APN is found negligent or the case settles for any number of reasons, pay damages up to the limits of coverage. However, importantly, how an insurer defines these elements and carries out these common responsibilities can vary greatly. This information should be requested and disclosed before purchase to make an informed decision about which policy to buy.

Develop a clear understanding of the policy coverage limits. For example, $1,000,000 each occurrence/$5,000,000 annual aggregate means the most paid for any one claim is $1,000,000 and the number of claims at that amount that can be paid in 1 year is five. Find out exactly how legal costs are treated in the policy. Are they included *within* the limits of liability or *in addition* to the limits? If legal fees and expenses are within the limits, then on resolution (settlement or judgment), legal costs and damages must fall beneath the ceiling. If they do not, the extra costs are the responsibility of the APN. For example, assume a policy limit of $1,000,000/$5,000,000 with legal costs of $300,000 and damages of $1,000,000. In this example, if legal costs were *within* the limits of liability, the APN would be responsible to pay the $300,000 shortfall not covered by the policy (CMF Group, 2002).

"Occurrence" and "claims-made" coverages are two different forms of coverage the APN must understand. They are equivalent in terms of the insurer's obligation to defend claims and pay damages, but differ with regard to which policy applies at the time a claim is made (Shinn, 1998). With occurrence coverage, the older of the two forms, the policy that was in effect at the time the adverse event occurred is the policy that applies for that claim. For the nurse there is some comfort in knowing coverage is available for claims that may not be filed for years. Traditionally, NPs and CNSs have occurrence coverage, whereas CNMs and CRNAs have claims-made coverage. With the exception of NPs, occurrence coverage is becoming exceedingly rare in the malpractice marketplace.

If occurrence coverage is available at all, the APN must carefully consider that protection purchased now may not be adequate for a claim in the future because the terms and conditions and limits of coverage may not be adequately indexed to account for inflation.

Claims-made coverage is a more recent form of coverage. Adverse events must occur *and* the claim must be made during the policy period. The benefit is that current terms, conditions, and coverage limits are contemporaneous with the claim. The problem is that there is a need to purchase extended reporting period coverage to continue coverage to ensure future protection for today's events if the policy is canceled or not renewed, or if the health-care professional retires. Experts suggest purchase of adequate "tail-funding" insurance that provides extended reporting period coverage that is not a financial burden, especially in the early years of practice (Shinn, 1998).

Policy settlement provisions are an important insurance policy element and require careful consideration. Although all policies require the insurer to pay for defense and damages, how they honor these duties varies from carrier to carrier. Some insurers retain the right to settle a claim without input or approval of the insured. Through this practice settlement, decisions may be predicated solely on monetary considerations, thus avoiding the costs of defending against the claim.

This practice may be inconsistent with the facts of the case and often inappropriately places the interests of the insurance company above the interests of the insured. Negotiate or locate another policy that provides an acceptable degree of control over important decisions in the case, such as choice of lawyer and whether or not to accept a settlement. Become actively involved. Look only for an insurer who agrees to consult, will permit choice of counsel, and will not settle without written consent.

The carrier should have extensive experience in the health-care insurance industry and even in the segment of advanced nurse practice coverage and representation. Established insurers usually work with panels of lawyers and health-care provider experts in the defense of malpractice claims. They are likely to have handled similar claims and can better advise you in the wisest course of action. Claims of expertise need to be validated independently. Financial stability is a critical factor in selection of an insurer because malpractice liability claims tend to have a long "tail," meaning a claim may not be made until years after an adverse event has occurred. Statutes of limitations, the period following an event in which the injured party can make a claim, vary from state to state and cannot be counted on to prevent the filing of a claim. For many reasons a judge may elect to "toll" the statute, thus allowing filing after the expiration of the statute of limitations. Birth injuries, delayed events resulting from improper delivery of anesthesia, and deliberate concealment of injury by the provider delivering care are but a few of the reasons to toll a statute.

Risk retention groups, a form of self-insurance usually used by professional associations, and small boutique carriers should be carefully evaluated for financial solvency and stability. In an environment of runaway awards, these insurance options may not be financially solvent when the practitioner needs them—that is, if they are still in business at all. Financially sound carriers are more likely to be around to provide protection if needed far into the future, particularly in an unstable insurance marketplace. Information about the financial status of an insurance company is readily available. For example, industry rating is a good indicator of an insurer's financial health. A.M. Best & Company rates all insurance companies by assigning a letter grade. A++ is the best rating (A.M. Best & Co., 2002).

Costs of Malpractice Insurance

Insurance premiums for APNs are increasing, a reflection of the costs carriers incur in defending against claims, the reduction of carriers available to underwrite claims in a given state and the of paying damages in the current litigation environment. For example, CNM premiums rose 7% in 2000 after more than 5 years without an increase. As of 2004, premiums doubled from 2003 (Silverman, 2004). Additionally because some obstetricians/gyneocologists choose to work with NPs, liability claims for NPs are also increasing. This situation is also an illustration of the differences among APN specialties because NP rates remained fairly stable (J. O'Sullivan, personal communication, May 5, 2002). In actuality, there is not a wide variability in premiums among the various carriers for any of the APN specialties. This information can easily be verified through professional association Web sites. Ironically, insurers consider APN premiums low compared with the exorbitant costs incurred by physicians and some other professionals. Yet APNs consider them high (J. O'Sullivan, personal communication, May 5, 2002; Silverman 2004).

CONTRACTUAL OBLIGATIONS

Know your coverage. In addition to the duties the insurer has to you, there are limitations of which the APN needs to be aware. All policies have specific exclusions under which the insurance does not apply. All policies exclude criminal acts or events that are "against public policy." In general, the broader the coverage, the higher the premiums. The best protection from unpleasant surprises is to be an informed self-advocate. Take the time to read the policy carefully to determine what is covered and what is not covered. One of the first steps to take when considering a change in specialty practice or in the practice setting is to review the terms of liability coverage with the insurer and make necessary changes when appropriate.

Maintaining professional liability protection is a partnership. The insured also has obligations to the insurer that must be honored if professional risks are to be successfully managed. Truthfulness when applying for insurance, timely premium payments, and complying with the conditions of coverage as stated in the policy are essential. Key among all policy conditions is notification of the insurer as soon as possible if an adverse event occurs (Shinn, 1998).

What Happens When a Lawsuit Is Filed

Being sued is one of the most traumatic experiences an APN can have. In health care, education is a tool that is frequently used to reduce stress and promote informed decision making. The same approach applies here. Forewarned is forearmed! Know what to do if the lawsuit appears. Patients bring lawsuits against nurses with the belief that the nurse, or the nurse's insurance company, can pay the damages that the patient alleges were caused by the nurse's negligence (Sloan & Hsieh, 1995). As a practical matter, the lawyer for the patient or the patient's family makes a case assessment before filing the lawsuit to determine whether the case has merit. For a malpractice lawyer who takes cases on a contingency basis (i.e., the lawyer is paid a percentage of any award, but only if the patient wins), the golden rule is to go after only the "live fish." In other words, malpractice lawyers only sue professionals, including doctors or nurses, who have the money or insurance to pay any judgment or settlement. To ensure there will be someone at the end of the lawsuit to pay an award, lawyers for patients frequently name any and all entities or individuals who could possibly have something to do with the claim of injury.

By the time a malpractice action is filed against an APN, most of the defense attorney's key cards have been dealt. The lawyer representing the nurse is not able to change what the nurse did or failed to do, what happened to the patient and family, and attitudes toward the nurse, including training, qualifications, and history. The attorney's ability to defend the lawsuit depends in large part on whether the APN has taken steps to maintain current professional skills, knows and consistently practices within the applicable standard of care, delivers quality care, and documents those actions.

As plaintiff's (patient's) attorneys develop standardized methods for identifying, evaluating, and litigating advanced practice nursing malpractice cases, APNs must also pursue comprehensive and equally standardized strategies for limiting their exposure to such cases. As regards APN practice and liabilities, these attorneys are learning how to review clinical records to identify negative patient outcomes that can be blamed on the APN rather than on the patient's age or preexisting medical problems. The patient's clinical record survey reports often provide a "road map" for the plaintiff's liability case at trial, and for the recovery of compensatory damages. At the same time, plaintiff's attorneys are learning that the real money in malpractice cases is in punitive damage awards. Thus, when evaluating cases, they focus on factors that will make a jury want to punish the APN, not just compensate the victim. These factors include evidence that the APN consistently failed to maintain skills and continuing education, treated patients or hospital staff poorly, allowed or even practiced falsification of medical records, or failed to address significant changes in condition and obtain timely physician assistance when the need became apparent.

When a suit is filed, the APN should anticipate the following activities:

- The APN is served with copy of the suit that includes the summons and complaint filed by the plaintiff (patient).
- The professional liability coverage must be activated by immediately notifying the insurance agent or the insurance company.
- The specifics of the claim and the date of notification are recorded. The insurance agent or insurance company is notified verbally. Conversation must be thoroughly documented, including the next steps each party is to take.
- One copy of the summons is retained; one copy is sent to the insurance agent and one to the employer, if applicable.
- Anecdotal documentation is prepared (i.e., all that can be recalled about the incident: who, what, when, where, how and why). If possible, the patient record should be consulted. Dates, times, and people involved should be noted.
- If employed, the APN is to notify the risk manager verbally and in writing, again documenting everything.
- The temptation to discuss the suit with others should be avoided. Discussions should be limited to the insurance agent, claims representative, attorney, and if applicable, the employer's risk manager. Do not discuss the case with anyone related to the plaintiff, anyone who might be a witness for the plaintiff, or the news media.
- Do *not* assume any financial obligation or pay any money without the insurance company's consent. If this occurs, the APN cannot expect the costs to be covered by the liability policy (Shinn, 1998).

Insurer's Response

- Within 24 to 48 hours from the time of notification of the filing of a claim, the APN should be contacted by the insurer's claim representative whose skills have been matched with claim specifics to ensure the best qualified person manages the claim.
- The insurer will have determined whether other providers covered by the insurer are being sued or have been sued by the same patient. If so, the insurer will determine whether there is

any conflict in having one person manage the lawsuit for all the insured providers. The assignment of a single claims representative occurs when all the insured agreed with the carrier that no one is at fault or fault lies with someone not insured by the liability carrier.

- The claim representative interviews the APN by phone and explains what the insurance policy covers. In addition, the claim representative contacts any other carriers (e.g., the employer) that should or might be providing coverage for the APN (Shinn, 1998).

Legal Counsel

- Once coverage is confirmed, the APN is advised by the claim representative what law firm will be providing counsel. Attorneys are usually from local or regional firms who have negotiated fee arrangements to handle the insurer's claims and have medical malpractice experience related to the specific claim.
- The assigned lawyer interviews the APN. The objectives are for the lawyer to become more familiar with the case while the APN becomes comfortable with the lawyer. To facilitate this process the APN should ask for (a) the lawyer's credentials, (b) the number of cases of this type previously litigated, (c) the number of cases that have gone to trial, and (d) the outcomes.
- The APN should contact the claim representative immediately if he or she is dissatisfied with the assigned attorney and request that a change be made.
- Once the lawyer is agreed on, the APN should receive a written outline from the insurer's claim representative stating what law firm will provide defense, as well as any investigative firm that will be used, and explaining how the claim will be handled. Coverage issues should be described along with current status and detailed resolutions.
- The APN's counsel and the plaintiff's lawyer then engage in discovery (i.e., investigation of the facts of the claim). Written questions called *interrogatories* are served by both sides, followed by written responses and the appearance of the plaintiff, defendant, and witnesses at depositions where a court reporter will take their testimony under oath. In the end all information gathered is used to settle or ready the case for trial (Shinn, 1998).

Settlement

- Although each case should be evaluated on its merits, it is possible for settlements to be reached regardless of whether the APN has some fault or not. In the first instance, variables include some degree of fault, social climate, plaintiff socioeconomic factors, local statutes, previous jury verdicts for similar claims, the APN's ability to pay the claim, and the potential for a verdict in excess of the liability limits. Reasons for settlement even when the APN is not at fault include economics, medical records that do not support APN actions, impracticality of having the APN testify in his or her own defense, or the desire to avoid the unpredictability of a jury trial (Shinn, 1998).
- In the end the best rule for the APN is never to agree on a settlement until having had the opportunity to express personal opinions about the case, have them seriously considered, and conclude personally that a settlement is the best resolution of the matter (Shinn, 1998).

TRIAL

Risks Inherent in Witness Testimony

In a trial, the patient has the burden of proof. Evidence must be sufficient to meet the four elements of negligence to be successful: duty, breach of duty, causal connection, and damage. The plaintiff's attorney typically presents his case with as many types of witnesses as possible. Witnesses may include the patient, aggrieved family members, APN experts, medical experts, hospital employees, or economic experts. Each of these witnesses plays a different role in the plaintiff's case.

The patient allegedly injured by the APN is often the most powerful witness. If possible, the injured party describes firsthand what he or she thinks occurred, as well as the bad effect caused by the APN's actions or omissions. Family members are effective witnesses because they serve to personalize the patient, demonize the APN, evoke jury sympathies, and inflame jury passions. Their role is to describe the decline in the patient's condition while under the APN's care or as a result of the care provided by the APN, any promises that the APN made (whether orally or in its written educational materials) about the care that the APN would provide, and all problems that the patient experienced while under the care of the APN or subsequently. Their testimony is based on personal observations, particularly subjective impressions or statements made by others (which often are comments made by the APN's own colleagues, medical staff, or hospital employees).

The testimony of nursing and medical experts is crucial to a plaintiff's case because it provides a clinical perspective on the problems described by the patient and the patient's family members. The plaintiff's APN experts explain how the APN breached the standard of nursing care owed to the patient. They do so by pointing out problems found in the APN's own clinical records and other ways in which the care was allegedly substandard. They also challenge the adequacy of the APN's continuing education.

Medical experts testify about the nature and extent of the patient's injuries and describe the pain and suffering, disability, or additional health risks resulting from these injuries. In addition, the experts opine on the manner in which the APN's breach of the standard of care directly caused these injuries and point out any ways in which the APN, and often, the collaborating physician failed to comply with the applicable standard of care. Finally, they explain why the patient's injuries were *not* a natural and unavoidable result of the individual's medical condition, known risks associated with the procedure or treatment, aging process, or of a preexisting health problem.

It is not unusual to see experts attack the qualifications, training, and continuing education of the APN. Perhaps of greatest importance are their attempts to increase the opportunity to have the judge or jury assess punitive damages by linking a lack of qualifications to a wanton or reckless disregard for the welfare of the patient. Finding evidence in memos and e-mail files of shortcuts, failure to respond to telephone calls, or undue financial controls is usually not difficult. "Putting profits or self-interest before patients" is a common mantra of the plaintiff's bar.

Testimony of current and former colleagues and employees of a hospital on behalf of the plaintiff presents a danger to the APN because they will claim that the APN treated them badly, was unprofessional, unreliable, and consistently put his or her own self-interests ahead of patient care by consciously not responding when needed, or simply not knowing the appropriate thing to do. They will point out examples in which patients did not have access to adequate consultations from physicians or specialists. They may allege that the APN attempted to hide evidence of substandard care by creating false clinical records or not charting at all. They will claim that they or other employees were discouraged from bringing patient care concerns to the attention of the collaborating physician or administration. Employee testimony is orchestrated to increase the APN's punitive damages exposure by showing a pattern of callous behavior toward both patients and employees.

In the trial process, the plaintiff's witnesses are questioned by the plaintiff's attorney and cross-examined by the APN's counsel. Once the plaintiff concludes, the APN's counsel has the opportunity to present witnesses to rebut the plaintiff's allegations. The APN may or may not testify, depending on the specifics of the suit (Myers & Fergusson, 1989).

Trials may end with the successful defense move for a directed verdict against the plaintiff. This means the APN's lawyer asserts and succeeds in arguing the plaintiff failed to meet the burden of proof or has not made a valid case for malpractice. Shinn (1998) states, "Should the court not agree, the trial continues; jurors are presented with any additional evidence and closing arguments; and the jury deliberates and renders a verdict" (p. 95). If the trial is a bench trial, the judge rather than a jury decides on the verdict (Aiken, 2004). Most plaintiffs demand a jury trial. If the verdict is against the APN, then the APN, counsel, and insurer determine the next steps (Shinn, 1998). One option following an unacceptable verdict is to file an appeal to the next highest court.

Managing Risks by Fostering Positive Relationships

Strategies for limiting exposure to a significant malpractice case must focus on neutralizing the factors that are favorable to the plaintiff's case or on turning them to the APN's advantage. In the best of all circumstances, these interventions and practices are put into action to prevent a lawsuit from being filed in the first place.

Specifically, APNs must find ways to foster a positive relationship with all patients and their families, improve the delivery and documentation of all care rendered, understand and manage the patient's medical issues, maintain professional competence by continuing participation in clinical skills training and professional education, maintain positive professional relationships with colleagues and institutional staff or employees, and manage the business aspects of the practice to minimize legal exposure for the APN and collaborating physicians. Efforts to pursue these strategies should be thoroughly documented to provide evidence of the APN's good faith in the event of litigation.

The Patient and Family

APNs must manage expectations by providing the patient and family with a realistic depiction of care and treatment needed, as well as expected outcomes. This message should be reinforced consistently in clinical records and written materials, including educational materials and all one-on-one communications. If a big gap exists between what is promised and the actual capacity to deliver care and services, there is a high risk that the patient and the family will be disappointed.

In addition, when discussing any aspect of care and services, particularly any aspect of informed consent, the APN should present the information in easy-to-understand lay person's terms that take into account the patient's condition and the limitations of treatment. Finally, the APN should explain issues typical to all patients in similar circumstances and encourage the patient and family to work with the APN to identify and prevent problems.

In the event of a poor outcome or adverse reaction, every effort must be made to disclose the events to the patient and family to respond to their concerns and to ensure resolution at the most accessible levels. Even if this means giving patients an apology with admission that an error was made and discussing the need for compensation of the victim at some level, current thinking indicates that full disclosure mitigates the risks in the long run and may be part of the ethical duties of an APN (Reckling & Welsh, 1998). The good faith effort of this practice standard should be noted by APNs as it is now recognized and protected in many states (NCSL, 2007).

In these days of instant communication, maintaining an appropriate level of accessibility to both patients and institutions is a must. It is far better for patients to contact the APN directly at any time than for them to feel they must call an attorney or a government agency to report substandard care or medical errors. These efforts should continue throughout the patient's course of treatment. Office and hospital staff members should be encouraged to get to know the patients. Staff members who know their patients' names and individualized care needs and preferences make better caregivers and poorer litigation targets than staff members who do not take the time to develop such relationships. Emphasize this point to staff whenever possible. It seems too obvious to state, but everyone wants to be treated with dignity and recognition of their individuality. No one wants to be the "backache in room 3" or the "elderly primip down the hall." Positive relationships may be one of the primary reasons why people decide *not* to sue a health-care professional.

APNs must pay particular attention to the patient's medical history and understand the patient's underlying medical conditions and concurrent treatment and drug therapies to meet their medical needs. In a lawsuit it may be necessary for the APN to address medical progress by explaining how that patient's underlying medical conditions affected any negative outcome experienced by the patient. At the beginning of evaluation and treatment it is prudent, if not always practical, for the APN to obtain from the patient or a legal representative an authorization to release medical information from all other facilities where the patient has been treated and to obtain these materials and review them. This activity not only assists the APN to appreciate and understand the patient's full medical and behavioral picture, but also provides a wealth of information in the event of a subsequent lawsuit.

In turn, the patient's medical history is essential for determining the patient's prognosis, rehabilitation prospects, and medical risks; for developing and carrying out an effective care plan; for providing a context in which to evaluate the patient's progress; and for providing possible medical explanations for negative outcomes experienced by the patient while under the APN's care.

Developing positive relationships with the patient's friends and family also is important because they are the patient's chief support system. To develop positive relationships with family and friends, they should be encouraged to participate, with the approval of the patient, in the care and treatment plan. Staff should be responsive and courteous to the patient's family and friends whenever they visit with the patient. Adequate communication with the patient's family member is crucial. The APN should invite family members to appointments, care planning conferences, and any other meetings involving the patient's care. If the family comes to these meetings, then the chances for identifying and resolving potential problems early on are increased. If the family does not take advantage of these opportunities, it may lose jury sympathy in a subsequent lawsuit.

APNs should make family members feel they are part of the care team. Staff should candidly discuss treatment options, or the lack thereof, with family members. The family should be made to understand, when appropriate, that many treatment options also have a downside. Whenever possible, avoid making significant treatment decisions without including as many family members as necessary or appropriate. Keep the patient and family advised of all changes in the condition, incidents, accidents, or other significant developments. Encourage patients and their families to provide feedback early and often. Whenever possible, allow family members to participate as much as they wish in caring for the patient. This all assumes that the patient has no objection to including his or her family.

Staff Relationships

To cultivate office and hospital staff, the APN should acknowledge and respect them. To the extent possible, APNs should ensure that their own office staff are paid and treated as well as their counterparts at other offices. Acknowledging caring behavior early and often is important. Employees appreciate the opportunity to participate in decisions that affect their work environment. Feedback should always be encouraged on issues of importance to staff. Staff training not only is the key to improving the delivery of care but also may be presented as a benefit, particularly to employees of the hospitals and nursing home where the APN practices. It helps to have employees and staff members improve their business, administrative, and clinical skills. In many ways the APN depends on them for carrying out orders. All training efforts by the staff should be encouraged and rewarded.

Collaborating Physician and Medical Staff Colleagues

Maintaining open lines of communication with collaborating and attending physicians in the community and on the medical staffs is also essential to minimizing the risks of future lawsuits. As for the professional relationship with the collaborating physician, the APN must be informed about the requirements, if any, under the state nurse practice act for advanced practice nursing. The state laws on the required nurse-physician relationship vary greatly from nothing at all to the need for written agreements and protocols that must be submitted and approved by certain state boards or committees of the state boards. Although the trend in both state and federal law is toward independent practice for APNs, the picture remains mixed.

Approximately half of the states provide the right to practice independently. For CRNAs the right is provided by all the states (AANA, 2002a). Even in states where physician supervision remains a requirement, the physician often does not have to be present. Congress recognized the independence of APNs in 1997 by eliminating the need for physician supervision to receive Medicare reimbursement in nonhospital settings (Sox, 2002).

APNs must also manage the business relationships between themselves and their physician colleagues and institutions. It is essential to review all written agreements and institutional credentialing procedures and bylaws to be sure they do not create the impression of an employee relationship or impute vicarious liability on the physician or the institution unless that is what both parties intend. Requirements for unnecessary controls, such as supervision or practice restrictions, should be addressed because they could actually increase rather than decrease exposure to legal liability for both the physician and the institution.

APNs should keep collaborating physicians informed of developments in the practice or the care of a specific patient that might create the risk of a lawsuit. The physician-APN team should confer and decide whether changes in care are indicated and whether both need to more closely monitor care delivery systems and identify potential areas of concern. APNs should seek the collaborating physician's help in resolving any concerns about a patient's course of treatment.

CONCLUSION

The key to developing a comprehensive, concrete, and workable plan to manage the risks of liability is to engage in a deliberative and comprehensive thought process. Maintaining current clinical knowledge and skills are essential. Contemporaneous clinical documentation that articulates the rationale for therapeutic decisions and the patient's response to treatment is also critical. A working knowledge of the laws that affect advanced nursing practice is an essential element of a risk management plan. APNs should rely on only original source documents to know what the law actually requires, regardless of whether the issue is of one of state practice or of Medicare or Medicaid reimbursement. It is unwise to rely only on secondary sources or someone else's interpretation of what is legal. APNs must read the laws and regulations and make practice decisions on how to comply with the law. Remaining within the appropriate scope of practice and recognizing when changes in a patient's medical condition require additional support and consultation are sound guidelines to follow. Understanding and maintaining appropriate, comprehensive malpractice insurance coverage is an effective way to manage the risks of advance practice nursing. Finally, evaluating and maintaining positive relationships with patients, their friends and family members, office and hospital staff, caregivers, and others are also part of an effective risk management approach. With the increased professional responsibilities, independence, and prestige of advanced practice nursing comes increasing public and private accountability.

In an increasingly litigious society in which education and public access to information fuel ever higher expectations for only good outcomes of care, it is realistic to accept the premise that all health-care professionals, including APNs, are at risk of exposure to financial consequences for providing substandard care. As a matter of professional responsibility, APNs must act prudently to identify the rights, minimize or avoid the risks when possible, and manage those risks by both professionally responsible behavior, and in anticipation of the lawsuit, by use of appropriate malpractice liability insurance that transfers the risk to insurance institutions qualified to act on your behalf.

References

Aiken, T. D. (2004). *Legal, ethical and political issues in nursing* (2nd. ed.). Philadelphia: F.A. Davis.

A. M. Best & Company. (2002). *Rating insurers*. Retrieved July 2, 2008, from the A. M. Best & Company Web site: www.ambest.com/ratings/about.asp.

American Association of Nurse Anesthetics. (2002a). *CRNA malpractice update*. Retrieved July 3, 2008, from the American Association of Nurse Anesthetics Web site: www.aana.com/insurance/insur042302.asp.

American Association of Nurse Anesthetists. (2002b). *Legal issues in nurse anesthesia practice*. Retrieved July 3, 2008, from the American Association of Nurse Anesthetics Web site: www.aana.com/crna/prof/legal.asp.

American Association of Nurse Anesthetists. (2005). *Gov. Rounds removes physician supervision for South Dakota CRNAs*. Retrieved July 3, 2008, from the American Association of Nurse Anesthetics Web site: www.aana.com/news.

American Association of Nurse Anesthetists. (2007). *Wisconsin medical examining board dismisses WSA petition*. Retrieved July 3, 2008, from the American Association of Nurse Anesthetics Web site: www.aana.com/news.

American College of Obstetricians and Gynecologists. (1992). *American College of Obstetricians and Gynecologist's survey on professional liability*. Washington, DC: Author.

American College of Obstetricians and Gynecologists. (1999). *American College of Obstetricians and Gynecologist's survey on professional liability*. Washington, DC: Author.

American Nurses Association. (1998). Collaboration and independent practice: Ongoing issues for nursing. *Nursing Issues and Trends, 3,* 1–12. Retrieved July 2, 2008, from the American Nurses Association Nursing World Web site: nursingworld.org/readroom/nti/9805nti.htm.

American Society for Healthcare Risk Management. (2002). Perspectives on the state of the insurance market and answers to health care risk managers' million-dollar questions. *Monograph of the American Society for Healthcare Risk Management*. Retrieved July 2, 2008, from the Hospital Connect Web site: www.hospitalconnect.com/ashrm/resources/files/monograph.pdf.

Black, H. (Ed.). (1979). *Black's law dictionary* (7th ed.). St. Paul, MN: West.

Bovgjerg, R. R., Miller, R. H., & Shapiro, D. W. (2001). Paths to reducing medical injury: professional liability vs. patient safety. *Journal of Law, Medicine and Ethics, 29*(3-4), 369–380.

Buppert, C. J. (2002). Steering clear of medicare fraud. *NSO Risk Advisor, 11,* 1–2. Retrieved July 2, 2008, from the Nurses Service Organization Web site: www.nso.com/newsletters/newsletters.php#archives.

Bureau of National Affairs. (2004). Nurse-anesthetist sentenced to probation, restitution for fraudulent health care billing. *BNA Health Fraud Report, 6*(4), 424.

CMF Group. (2002). *Don't make mistakes when buying your malpractice insurance*. Retrieved July 2, 2008, from the NP Jobs Web site: www.npjobs.com/malpractice/buying.mistakes.shtml.

Congressional Budget Office. (2004). *Limiting tort liability for medical malpractice, economic and budget issue brief,* 01/08/2004. Retrieved July 2, 2008, from the Congressional Budget Office Web site: www.cbo.gov/doc.cfm?index=4968&type=0.

Council of Economic Advisors. (2002). *Who pays for tort liability insurance claims: An economic analysis of the U.S. tort liability system*. Washington, DC: Author.

Freedman, M. (2002, May 24). The tort mess. *Forbes,* 90–98.

Healthcare Integrity and Protection Data Bank. (2008). *Fact sheet*. May 2008 Washington, DC: Author. Retrieved July 2, 2008, from the Healthcare Integrity and Protection Data Bank Web site: www.npdb-hipdb.hrsa.gov/pubs/.

Infante, M. C. (2000). Legally speaking: Malpractice may not be your biggest risk. *RN, 63*(6), 67–71.

Ingram, J. D. (1993). Liability of medical institutions for the negligence of independent contractors practicing on their premises. *Journal of Contemporary Health Law and Policy, 10,* 221–231.

Institute of Medicine. (2000). *To err is human: Building a safer health system.* Bethesda, MD: National Academy of Sciences.

Jenkins, S. M. (1994). The myth of vicarious liability: Impact on barriers to nurse-midwifery practice. *Journal of Nurse Midwifery, 39*(2), 98–106.

Lefevre, F. V., Water, T. M., & Budetti, P. P. (2002). A survey of physician training programs in risk management and communication skills for malpractice prevention. *Journal of Law, Medicine and Ethics, 28*(3), 258–266.

Myers, K., & Fergusson, P. S. (1989). *Nurses at risk.* Des Moines, IA: HealthPro & Kirke Van-Orsdel.

National Conference of State Legislatures. (2007). *Medical malpractice tort reform: 2006 state introduced legislation.* Retrieved July 2, 2008, from the National Conference of State Legislatures Web site: www.ncsl.org/standcomm/sclaw/medmalrefrom06.htm.

National Practitioner Data Bank. (2008a). *2006 Annual report.* Washington, DC. Retrieved June 26, 2008, from the National Practitioner Data Bank Web site: www.npdb-hipdb.hrsa.gov/annualrpt.html.

National Practitioner Data Bank. (2008b). *Fact sheets.* Washington, DC. Retrieved June 26, 2008, from the National Practitioner Data Bank Web site: www.npdb-hipdb.hrsa.org.

Office of Technology Assessment. (1993). *Impact of legal reforms on malpractice claims.* Washington, DC. Retrieved July 2, 2008, from http://scholar.google.com/scholar?q=Office+of+Technology+Assessment+(OTA).+(1993).+Impact+of+legal+reforms+on+malpractice+claims&hl=en&client=firefox-a&channel=s&rls=org.mozilla:en-US:official&hs=gKv&um=1&ie=UTF-8&oi=scholart.

Reckling, J. B., & Welsh, R. (1998). *Ethics and managing risk. The nursing risk management series.* Retrieved July 2, 2008, from the American Nurses Association Nursing World Web site: www.nursingworld.org/mods/archive/mod312/cerm3ful.htm.

Schmidt, W. C., Heckert, D. A., & Mercer, A. A. (1992). Factors associated with medical malpractice: Results from a pilot study. *Journal of Contemporary Health Law and Policy, 7,* 157–182.

Silverman, J. (2004). Premiums doubled since last year: Nurse-midwives feel sting of rising premiums, lawsuits; Professional collaboration increases ob.gyns,' litigation exposure, vulnerability. *OB/GYN News. 6/15/2004.* Retrieved July 2, 2008, from International Medical News Group Web site: www.imng.com/titles/OBGYN/index.html.

Shinn, L. J. (Ed.). (1998). *Taking control: A guide to risk management.* Chicago: Kirke Van-Orsdel, Inc. & Chicago Insurance Company

Sloan, F. A., & Hsieh, R. (1995). Injury, liability and the decision to file a medical malpractice claim. *Law and Society Review, 29,* 413–438.

Sox, H. (2002). Screening mammography for younger women: Back to basics. *Annals of Internal Medicine, 137*(1), 361–362.

The Joint Commission. (2008). *2008 Patient safety goals.* Retrieved July 2, 2008, from The Joint Commission Web site: www.jointcommission.org/PatientSafety/NationalPatientSafetyGoals.

Thorpe, K. (2004). The medical malpractice 'crisis': Recent trends and the impact of tort reforms. *Health Affairs* Web Exclusive, January 21,2004. Retrieved June 20, 2008, from the Health Affairs Web site: content.healthaffairs.org/cgi/gca?ck=nck&allach.

U.S. Department of Health and Human Services. (2002). *Confronting the new health care crises: Improving health care quality and lowering costs by fixing our medical liability system.* Washington, DC: Author.

Vicusi, W. K., & Born, P. (1995). Medical malpractice insurance in the wake of liability reform. *The Journal of Legal Studies, 24,* 463–495.

Weiler, P., Hiatt, H. H., Newhouse, J. P., Johnson, W. G., Brennen, T. A., & Leape, L. I. (1993). *A measure of malpractice: Medical injury, malpractice litigation and patient compensation.* Cambridge: Harvard University.

28

Ethics and the Advanced Practice Nurse

Gladys L. Husted

James H. Husted

One day two nurses in a jungle village passed under a coconut tree. As they passed, a coconut fell from the tree to the ground. An argument arose between them as to who had a right to possession of the coconut. Finally, they decided to do what seemed the only fair and ethical thing to do. They would split the coconut in half and each nurse would take one half of the coconut. They shook hands and each prepared to go on her[1] way.

Nurses (and everyone else) sometimes make unfortunate decisions without ever realizing it and without learning anything from it (Tuckett, 1999). This is especially likely to occur when we do not engage ourselves in a process of discursive thought.

Fortunately, before the nurses parted, a colleague passed them. She was an advanced practice nurse (APN) whose years of well-examined experience had developed in her the habit of seeking out reasons and relevance. When she asked them what they were going to do with the coconut, each was surprised by the answer of the other. One wanted the shells to use as cups for holding water and was not interested in the meat of the coconut. The other only wanted the meat and had no interest in the shells. As a result of the APN's intervention, one nurse now has twice as much coconut meat as she would have had otherwise and the other nurse has two cups instead of one.

Responsible ethical decision making and action in health-care is very much like the division of coconuts. It requires awareness and understanding of the context in which the decision to be made is to be made. All health-care professionals should assume the responsibility of seeking out what ought to be done and *why* it ought to be done. None of the contemporary ethical systems, as we will discuss, consistently recommends attention to these distinctions. An APN has come to a state of development wherein she can interweave the ethical and professional aspects of her practice.

A patient is dying, death is imminent, and the physician has left an order for the patient to go to physical therapy. A nurse is allowing a family to talk about funeral arrangements in front of a patient who may still be able to hear and comprehend. Ethics is not only about difficult dilemmas; it is also about everyday occurrences. "Although ethical issues in health care receive much publicity, attention is rarely given to the non-dramatic, everyday ethics of health care" (Smith, 2005, p. 32). If an APN faces a choice between following present convenience and the welfare of her patient, she, hopefully, will choose her patient's welfare.

---

[1]We use the pronoun she for the nurse or any health-care professional and he for the patient. This convention is for the reader's ease of understanding and to keep understanding in context. The singular is preferred to the plural or indeterminate because professionals and patients are individuals, and a practice-based ethic is, and ought to be, an individualistic ethic.

A practice-based ethical system attends to practice. The welfare of her patient is the focus of a nurse whose ethical practice is mature and advanced.

PRACTICE-BASED BIOETHICS

A practice-based, symphonological (*symphonology* from *symphonia,* a Greek word meaning agreement) approach to ethical interaction is an approach from professional responsibility. Symphonology defines ethics as a system of standards to motivate, determine, and justify actions directed to the pursuit of vital and fundamental goals.[2] Ethics is not convenience; it is not etiquette, and it is not that which brings on a state of self satisfaction. Symphonology is a *practice-based bioethic* derived from, and intended to be appropriate to, the self-determination of a patient, the purposes of a health-care setting and the role of a health-care professional.

A practice-based bioethic aims to relate professionals and patients internally (to bring them into the same ethical context), to make human values its focus, and to make the health-care setting maximally purposeful.

A practice-based bioethic is based on interactions between a professional and a patient who relate themselves through agreement and understanding. When a nurse strengthens a patient's confidence in his recovery or supports him in dealing with a morbid prognosis, she is nursing within a practice-based ethical system.

The measure of success for a practice-based bioethic is a patient's vital objective that he shall retain or regain his power to initiate and sustain actions. An ethic that is not skillfully exercised and harmoniously interwoven with practice cannot justifiably be the ethic of a health-care professional. It is the ethic of a nurse who is merely "going through the motions."

The nurses who passed the coconut tree made a valuable discovery. The best action to take depends on the nature of the context, the motivations of the persons involved, and what it is possible to do in this context. The best professional actions depend precisely on the same realities—and on respect for individual rights. These produce relevant, appropriate, and justifiable ethical actions.

RIGHTS

Individual rights belong to each human individual by virtue of his membership in the human species. In becoming a patient, an individual does not lose either his membership or his rights. Traditionally, the concept of "rights" has been viewed as entitlements, options to which one has a rightful claim. Symphonology, on the other hand, holds rights as a singular concept (Scotto, 2008).

Rights[3] is the product of an implicit agreement among rational beings made and held by virtue of their rationality, not to obtain actions nor the product or conditions of actions from one another, except through voluntary consent, objectively gained.

It is freedom from aggression—an agreement not to aggress (Husted & Husted, 2008a). See **Table 28-1.**

In any society to the extent people recognize and are faithful to this agreement, its members possess human rights. When this is lacking, they do not. Every human being possesses human rights. "When ethical agents live and interact together, the benefit of the rights agreement is so great and

---

[2]All definitions, unless otherwise stipulated, are taken from the text by Husted and Husted, 2008a.
[3]Rights is a singular term denoting a single, noncomplex agreement.

TABLE 28-1

Individual Rights

Individual rights	The state of nonaggression that results from this agreement
Among rational beings	One who can think, a quality of all humans
Made and held by virtue	Made because of their rationality and the fact that being rational, they can see the advantage to it
Not to obtain actions	For example, by coercion
Nor the product of actions	By theft of another's property, money, etc.
Conditions of actions	By changing the circumstances of the person's life for the worse, for example, through kidnapping
Through voluntary consent	One is not coerced—the agreement establishes the terms of interaction
Objectively gained	One is not deluded or deceived, but is fully informed

Adapted from the digital supplement for educators accompanying G. L. Husted & J. H. Husted. (2008a). *Ethical decision making in nursing and health care: The symphonological approach* (4th ed.). New York: Springer.

so obvious, the detriment of not having this agreement is so manifestly ruinous, that the agreement literally "goes without saying" (Husted & Husted, 2008a, p. 23).

Ethical practice does not allow a professional to violate the rights of a patient. A dedication to human values is internal to the ethical nature of the health-care setting. This presupposes respect for the rights of patients.

The practice of nursing, ideally, goes beyond respect for rights. However, a professional, practice-based ethic must *begin* with the recognition of a patient's rights. Through this recognition, a nurse provides a bridge between a patient's present condition and situation and the realization of the values her profession promises.

The reality of individual rights is not complex. It is present whenever two or more people are together. Each has a right not to be aggressed against by the other. Rights surround every human interaction, however insignificant. Rights is a reality so familiar and all encompassing that, in normal circumstances, it is the last thing with which one has to be concerned.

The rights agreement is the ethical foundation for all explicit agreements. It is the already preestablished implicit agreement that explicit agreements will be kept.

The rights agreement structures and defines *human* interaction and the pursuit of human values. The recognition of rights produces interaction according to the standard of reciprocity—a voluntary process of give and take, without force or deception, noninterference with another person's pursuit of values.

ADVANCED PRACTICE AND A PRACTICE-BASED BIOETHIC

Rapid advances in technology make many demands on the character, education, and abilities of the advanced practice nurse. The emphasis on scientific developments throughout the past several centuries has caused ethics to take a quantitative rather than a qualitative approach. Science has sought to separate itself from concerns about human values and values systems (Callahan & Mannino, 1998, p. 282).

Again, an APN has come to a state of development wherein she can interweave the ethical and professional aspects of her practice. She may well have shaped her practice in harmony with some aspects of a practice-based ethic. Nothing does more to produce effective advanced professional practice. She can master skill in ethical decision making by attending to what is important in her patient's life. In doing this, she will establish pride in what she is and what she is doing (Husted & Husted, 1998). Few APNs can remain unaffected by this on some level.

Whenever the need for an ethical decision arises in the health-care setting (and this is daily), it is confined within a specific, radically limited, yet complex context. The more complex the context, the more valuable are the ethical attitudes of a nurse who makes decisions that are based on this context—a nurse who makes practice-based decisions.

All of a nurse's experience that is relevant to her ethical competence is, ultimately, experience with individual human beings. The health-care setting is defined by the nature and purposes of human beings. A practice-based ethic is defined by the same realities. Each follows and enhances the other.

There is no such thing as being competent without being competent in ethical analysis. Ethical reasoning and clinical judgment share a common process, and both serve to teach and inform the other. The importance, therefore, of attention to clinical practice, regardless of how far removed an APN is from the clinical setting, cannot be overemphasized (Solomon et al., 1994). A person does not graduate from nursing school already skilled in bioethical decision making. A nurse does not enter graduate school taking with her an already perfected ethical judgment. Just as clinical expertise requires experience and attention, so does ethical expertise. As one gains experience in her ethical interactions with patients, many, hopefully most, APNs discover the inadequacies of contemporary ethical theories.

THE CONTEMPORARY ETHICAL THEORIES

Skillful ethical comportment will deteriorate to a merely competent level if we apply norms and principles to complex practical situations where we have the potential for skillful recognition of patterns. . . . Strategies of adjudication and the search for certitude through the application of norms and principles, though comforting, do not produce skillful ethical comportment (Benner, Tanner, & Chelsa, 1996, pp. 276–277).

Yet this is exactly what the contemporary ethical theories demand **(Table 28-2).**

TABLE 28-2

Contemporary Ethical Systems

Systems	Defining Characteristic	View on Consequences
Deontology	Following the rule	Not important
Utilitarianism	Doing the greatest good for the greatest number	Consequences to the greatest number
Social or cultural relativism	Beliefs of a particular society, culture, or religion are paramount	Only consequences to the group matter
Emotivism	If I believe it is right, it is right	The individual determines consequences for self; consequences to others are irrelevant

If professional nursing practice is to be shaped by bioethical concerns, the ethic of nursing, of necessity, must be derived from, and relevant to, the profession and its practice. Attention to the context and careful thought and analysis are the essence of any competence, let alone advanced practice competence. Contemporary ethical theories do not lend themselves to the health-care professions or to ethically defensible decisions in health-care practice. None of the dominant ethical theories could be discovered in, or derived from, the profession of nursing. None can be made relevant to nursing practice.

Things are seldom what they seem. Skim milk masquerades as cream. — *Gilbert & Sullivan, 1885*

A young woman or man entering the profession has every reason to believe that the purposes of nursing are shaped by the deepest and most vital human concerns—those concerns that are related to the life, health, and well-being of those who are sick and disabled. At the same time, no one entering into nursing has any objective reason to believe that any contemporary ethical theory is relevantly related to these purposes.

The dominant ethical theories of today that nurses are taught are deontology, utilitarianism, and cultural or social relativism. The result always involves an element of emotivism.

Deontology is the theory that actions in conformance with formal rules of conduct are obligatory regardless of their results (Angeles, 1992). Deontology requires a nurse to attend to out-of-context duties. It makes intention the overriding ethical concern and holds *consequences* to be irrelevant. It makes the individual motivations and character-structures of a patient secondary, or more often, *unrelated* to the ethics of nursing practice.

There is nothing inherent in the practice of nursing that implies that in a clash between the requirements of a patient's welfare and the demands of deontology, a nurse ought to choose deontology. Van Hooft (1990) states, "The idea that we are following rules when we act morally is a tired hangover from the days when the lives of people were controlled by religious and secular absolute rulers who accorded no respect or independence to ordinary people" (p. 211). "Deontology is entirely concerned with an agent's actions. It is unconcerned with consequences. It is also indifferent to the agent's intentions, except his intention to do his duty" (Husted & Husted, 2008a, p. 211).

Utilitarianism is the theory that one should act so as to promote the greatest happiness (pleasure) of the greatest number of people (Angeles, 1992). Utilitarianism requires a nurse to pay attention to consequences, but consequences to a larger number than one patient. It is impossible for a nurse to give her concern to the largest number possible, and at the same time, provide optimum care for her individual patients. Only optimum care—the best care a professional is capable of—is ethical care.

There is nothing in nursing as a profession that justifies the idea that, once a nurse has accepted a patient, she ought ever to abandon concern for her patient in favor of pursuing the greatest good for the greatest number. The profession of nursing is incompatible with such a demand. Utilitarianism is a theory in which the end is said to justify the means (Gibson, 1993). It would, all too often, make the patient a means, and the desires of the patient's family, for example, an end. The purposes of individual patients, and not the whims of a greater number, are the reason for being of professional nursing. Nothing in the principle of utility (i.e., the greatest good for the greatest number) establishes the principle of individual justice (Sarikonda-Woitas & Robinson, 2002).

Social or cultural relativism is the theory that what is ethical and what is unethical is determined by the customs, beliefs, and practices of a society or a culture (Angeles, 1992). There is nothing in the traditions of nursing to suggest that, in a clash between the requirements of a patient's welfare and the demands of one's society or culture, a nurse should choose the sentiments of the society or culture. This would turn a nurse's attention onto the views of a society or culture and away from her patient. Relativism undermines professional practice and the well-being of patients.

A patient's culture may be important, but it can be of no greater importance than the importance given to it by a patient. Barnes and Boyle (1995) state, "Unfortunately, the emphasis on shared patterns has rather rigidly defined nursing's perceptions of people from specific cultures and has not allowed for personal variations [of individual persons] within a given culture" (p. 414). Communication between patients and cultures is, at best, a figure of speech. Cultures, as such, have no tongues, no ears, and no ability to evaluate another's circumstances. Only individuals have this (Kikuchi, 1996).

"While cultural factors are a valuable blueprint to caring for a patient, there can be no justification for failing to allow for the patient's personal evaluation of the beliefs or her culture to serve as the standards of culturally congruent care. Otherwise one is caring for the culture and not the patient, and the concept of 'care' will have been subjected to a radical change in meaning" (Zoucha & Husted, 2000, p. 326). A flawed definition of a human being is more virulent than a plague.

Emotivism is the doctrine that holds that feelings or emotions are forms of ethical knowledge. The doctrine states that every ethical judgment and decision is simply a disguised description of a person's feelings (Angeles, 1992). The irrelevance of the contemporary ethical systems inevitably leads ethical agents to depend on emotions, rather than objective awareness.

There is nothing in the nature of nursing to suggest that in a clash between the requirements of her patient's welfare and the demands of her present emotional state, a nurse should guide her actions by her feelings—quite the contrary. Emotivism turns a nurse's attention into herself and away from her patient. It replaces her professional responsibility with an obsession onto her ever-changing emotional moods. It makes ethical interaction between a professional and her patient entirely illusory.

"Knowledge" of all these theories is gained by cultural osmosis and expressed in largely unverbalized feelings. None of these theories produce a concern for a person in one's care. Close attention to the appropriate context, or careful analysis based on the nature and purposes of nursing, is what defines nursing.

The Rational Form of Bioethical Decision Making

The ethic that is intrinsic to a profession is structured by a process of discovering facts, causes, and motives. The contemporary theories demand that a nurse evade her objective, contextual awareness and the discovery and recognition of immediately given facts relevant to her patient's situation. The theories project discovery and recognition away from a patient's values onto her first emotional responses, or onto the sentiments and opinions of others. For a practice-based ethic, answers to a dilemma that a nurse and patient share is one that is independent of out-of-context beliefs and attitudes. Ideas based on one or more of these theories strengthen views such as the following:

- Ethics is constituted of issues—euthanasia, harvesting organs from anencephalic infants, research on the incompetent, cloning, medical use of marijuana, and so on.
- Unanalyzed individual or cultural opinions are ethical facts.
- Ethical action, in certain circumstances is important, but the circumstances requiring ethical action are unimportant.
- What is true or false in any circumstance is true or false in every similar circumstance.
- Rights are alienable. I would not let you decide for me, but I will decide for you.
- It is the role of a professional to make ethical decisions for her patients, but these roles are not reversible.

In fact, these views are either misleading or entirely false. A practice-based ethic, and *nursing itself,* is intrinsically and directly related to the unique needs and circumstances of individual human beings. If ethics is not so related, then *nothing* is. If bioethics is not, then nursing is not. Ethical facts concern that which motivates, determines, and justifies actions taken in relation to the human realities discovered in an individual context. In health care, this structures the nature of professional practice.

Maintaining adherence to one or more of these theories while developing professional practice through experience is equivalent to placing one's hand on a table and walking across a room without removing one's hand from the table.

THE IMPORTANCE OF CONTEXT

Ethics is concerned with the good of the individual. What is the good for an individual can only be discovered in a context. A professional ethic assumes that a professional's strength of character is appropriate to produce the flourishing of her patients. So do her patients (Guido, 2006).

This is basic and the defining end of a professional ethic.

A professional ethic aims at a single end—the end that is the reason for being of the profession. This reason for being establishes and structures the APN's professional context. It relates an APN and a patient internally within this context.

Gastmans (1998) states, "The nurse functions both as a professional and as a human being within a variety of contexts. These contexts influence directly or indirectly the way in which the nurse performs caring tasks" (p. 126).

When a nurse, as an ethical agent, learns how to identify the various parts of an ethical context and their interrelations, she has developed a significant practical skill. When she is able to understand the individual human values that make each context what it is, she has developed an advanced practice competency. The ancient Greek philosophers described this ability as "practical wisdom." The great Chinese thinkers (whose benign influence in the West, although largely unacknowledged, was enormous) called it the *Way*—acting in harmony with the nature of things.

"Context is complex and comprehensive, dynamic, and interactive. Despite how tempting and how much easier it is to resort to the general, the abstract, and the theoretical, any form of bioethics that does not put moral [ethical] problems in their myriad contexts is, in many senses of the word, unreal" (Hoffmaster, 2006, p. 40).

There are three elements of every context that guide objective awareness and action **(Table 28-3).** First is the *context of the situation.* This is the interwoven aspects of a situation that are fundamental to understanding the situation and to acting effectively in it. These are the facts that are necessary to act on to bring about a desired result.

The second is the *context of knowledge.* This is the agent's awareness and understanding of the aspects of the situation that are necessary to an understanding of the situation and to acting effectively in it. In other words, this is the knowledge one has of how to deal with these facts most effectively. These resources of knowledge enable a nurse to identify and interweave the two sides of the context into a coherent plan of action.

The third is the *context of awareness.* This is the agent's present awareness of the relevant aspects of the situation and of her present knowledge. An agent's context of awareness includes her awareness of those aspects of the situation that invite action. Every decision that an agent makes, if she acts in (or according to) the context must be made according to:

- Her knowledge
- That which is appropriate to the situation

TABLE 28-3	
The Three Elements of the Context	
Of knowledge	The relevant knowledge that a health-care professional brings to the situation
Of the situation	The interwoven aspects of the situation that are fundamental to understanding and to acting effectively in it
Of awareness	The agent's present awareness of the relevant aspects of the situation and of her present knowledge

■ Her present awareness of what she knows, and of what is relevant in the situation (Husted & Husted, 2008a, p. 89; also see Table 28-3)

A person's context is the interweaving of these three elements. A context is that which provides the resources for making a justifiable decision. Reigle (1996) states, "Knowledge of facts is insufficient if not tempered with the contextual features of each case. Only after the unique conditions of the case are considered can an ethically acceptable solution be identified" (p. 275).

Everything relevant to a context is contained within the context. A multitude of factors that surround that context are irrelevant. These are the factors that play no part in the nature of the dilemma. They neither cause the dilemma nor can they help to resolve it. The resources of the context are resources because they provide *relevant* criteria for ethical decision making.

Here is a simple example: A nurse discovers that a patient is allergic to a certain medicine and acts accordingly. The fact that he is allergic is one part of the context of the situation. Her discovery of this fact, made by virtue of her past experience and her present thinking processes, becomes one part of her context of knowledge. Her purpose is to protect him. This is made possible by her context of awareness.

A context always forms itself around a purpose. One discovers a change to be made or a goal to be achieved and sets about to learn how, in the circumstances, this is to be done. The key to this is to be able to know the difference between the relevant and the irrelevant. The relevant is any factor in the context that will enable a profession to bring about a change in the context and facilitate the achievement of a purpose. The irrelevant is that which does neither. The inappropriate is that which threatens to frustrate the purpose.

Wurzbach (1999) states that although persons seek certainty in their decisions, "ethical certainty can provide [unwarranted] comfort for the ethical decision maker . . . and stifle dialogue and in-depth discussion of the [situation]" (p. 287). All the certainty that one has in any given context is the certainty that the context allows. One can have contextual and contingent certainty but never final and immutable certainty.

The Levels of a Context

There are a number of levels to every context. The first level is the split second, immediate present—the sensory level of awareness. This is all the objective factors composing the situation at any given moment taken in isolation from one another but without the awareness of their vital influence and relationship. This is the level of the contemporary ethical systems.

The second level is brought into being by a cognitive level of awareness. This level is provided by one's grasp of the nature and relationship of the objective factors as they exist in the present. This is the level of a nurse whose sole concern is the well-being of her patient.

The third level is produced by foresight. Foresight provides the awareness of relationships, events, and causal sequences as they have evolved out of the past into the present and how they are relevant to the future. This is the level of a professional bioethic.

The higher the level of a context and the more an APN relates herself internally to the context, the more appropriate her decisions and the more effective her actions will be. A nurse is "the agent of a patient doing for a patient what he would do for himself if he were able." Her patient is the center of the context. She is acting internally to the context when the values and motivations that produce decisions and actions on her part are her patient's values and motivations. Values and motivations that are not her patient's, but demanded by the contemporary ethical theories, are external and irrelevant to the context. They produce externally related, out-of-context actions, and very often, tragic examples of injustice.

That which is relevant to a practice-based professional ethic is not a matter of tradition or social convention. In the health-care setting, ethical decisions and actions begin with a grasp of those things that are crucially important in the life of a human individual. An APN is a human individual and is capable of understanding and dealing with this.

THE FLOURISHING OF AN APN

Decision-making is that which most characterizes advanced practice. . . . Underlying decision-making are clinical judgments, scholarly inquiry, and leadership. . . . The work of the advanced practice nurse is practice, the product is patient care; therefore, leadership in the advanced practice role supports the scientific process by:

- *Interpreting the context of practice*
- *Demonstrating influences on care*
- *Leading changes in practice (Erickson & Sheehy, 1998, p. 244)*

That ethical decision-making skills are part of the core competencies of all APNs is a basic tenet and central to the definition of advanced nursing practice (Reigle, 1996). Ideally, the ethical aspects of her practice will have developed along with the clinical aspects.

A practice-based ethic aims to relate professionals and patients internally, to bring them into the same ethical context, to make human values its purpose, and to make the health-care setting maximally purposeful and intelligible. An APN can master the art and science of ethical decision making and interacting with what is important in her patient's life. In doing so, she increases her patient's well-being, strengthens the profession of nursing, keeps the practice of nursing contextually intelligible, and establishes for herself the conditions of pride in herself and her profession.

Only by following the definition of her profession, can a nurse make her profession intelligible to her patient and to herself. Being the agent of her patient defines her profession. She takes actions for a patient—a person who has been formed by a lifetime of unique experiences and unique reactions to these experiences. In doing this, she develops pride in herself and in her practice. To allow a relatively helpless person to decide for himself is the hallmark of a nurse's pride in her profession and her self-esteem.

She takes actions that a patient cannot take for himself. Yet, although she takes these actions, they are his actions. In coming under her care, he does not give up his right to self-determination—his right to think, decide, and act for himself. He is in a health-care setting to gain the power of expressing himself in action. He is there so that health-care professionals can take the actions that he would take if he were able. These are actions that he has lost the power—but not the *right*—to take.

Every action of an APN is an interaction, whether the action is a cause that results in an immediate effect or a cause whose intended effect occurs farther on down a chain of causal sequences. All cooperation requires interaction.

The noblest action a nurse can take, without which no justifiable action is possible, is her act of accepting her patient as a human being as real as she is. Without this, the context is unintelligible and no real interaction is possible.

THE NURSE/PATIENT AGREEMENT

Interaction requires intelligibility. Interaction is not possible unless each party to the interaction knows what they are doing, why there are doing it, and what they intend to accomplish. All of this requires a prior agreement. An agreement is a shared state of awareness on the basis of which interaction occurs.

A nurse agrees that, for a time, she will be part of a patient's world. Her skills make her a vital part. Decisions can be made and actions can be taken based on an ethical agreement between a professional and her patient. The nature of these decisions and actions are limited by the terms of their agreement. Non–practice-based ethical theories demand that in her ethical decisions and actions she abandon her patient and his world. Her patient is protected by nothing. He cannot rely on his nurse's dedication. To a greater or lesser extent, his rights and human dignity—his very reality—has been dispensed with.

An APN has the resources for appropriately meeting the demands of the context. An effective health-care setting encourages her in discernment and discovery. Hardt (2001) states: "The . . . [APN] cannot practice successfully in an environment that does not foster context-driven decision making. If [caring nurses] . . . are not able to apply the knowledge they have gained from patients, related to their patient's preferences, then the patient's context is not honored" (p. 45).

A professional, through her open declaration that she is a professional, takes on various obligations as part of the nurse-patient agreement. Through these obligations a patient can rightfully expect the nurse to act ethically within the context. These obligations and these expectations are an integral part of the agreement between a nurse and her patient (Husted & Husted, 2008b).

If a patient's context is not honored, the APN's agreement, in whatever form it takes, is not honored. If the APN-patient agreement is not honored, then the professional is not practicing a profession, but a sham. All APNs have moved beyond the point at which their ethical decisions *must* be irrelevant to their professional practice.

Professional practice is sufficient to establish a health-care professional-patient agreement. One human recognizes another. They recognize the human values that are the basis of their interaction and the attitudes appropriate to guiding these interactions. Because of this, the agreement between them can be formed spontaneously and on an implicit level. Under the circumstances, the human nature of each guides their awareness, the forming of an implicit agreement to interact, and their interaction. Even with an incompetent, comatose, or very young patient, the nurse's responsibility remains the same. There is a professional agreement in place. She does not have an explicit agreement with this patient. But, she does have an implicit agreement.

Even APNs who are not practicing in the arena of direct patient care, still have the nurse-patient agreement in place. Educator, administrator, and researcher are ultimately responsible for patients and their well-being. The role of the educator is for the benefit of the patient. There is a teacher-student-patient agreement. A nurse administrator is ultimately responsible for patients and their well-being. There is an administrator-staff-patient agreement. A researcher must have the well-being of her subjects uppermost in mind, and thus, there is a researcher-subject agreement. The research cannot come before the welfare of persons.

THE AGREEMENT ONE HAS WITH ONESELF

Socrates, the first systematic ethicist of the Western world (470–399 BC), is known to have observed that the unexamined life is not worth living. Every nurse, every APN, ought to examine her life, at least to the point at which she comes to an agreement with herself that she will be a nurse. To the extent that a nurse has not made this agreement with herself—a commitment to be a nurse—she resembles a patient more than she resembles what she would be if she were a nurse.

A nurse who directs her long-term actions guided by her awareness of what is needed for her to keep that agreement embraces her profession. A nurse who is inspired by it, and who is dedicated to it, is far less likely to experience burnout. She experiences joy in taking action . . . and pride and confidence in acting as she does.

. . .a nurse [who] tries to avoid taking those long-term actions that constitute her professional life breaks the agreement she made with herself to be a professional. She becomes indifferent. She undermines herself as a professional and as a person. If she has replaced her confidence and pride with indifference, she has done this because she abandoned herself when she abandoned her profession.

If one is a nurse and is likely to continue to be a nurse, one ought to take the actions [nursing] calls for. At worst, this will make life far less boring. At best, it may restore one to the confident expectations and the pride that she began with at the beginning of her career.

Dedication to what one professes—acting on that which one affirms and believes—is sometimes difficult to do. Adversities and frustrations arise. And these attack one's desire and one's sense of self (Husted & Husted, 1999, p. 17).

Overcoming adversities through dedication produces pride in oneself as a professional. A patient could not reasonably ask for more and should not find less. He needs a rational agent to do for him what he would do for himself simply because his well-being depends on someone using reason.

THE ADVANCED PRACTICE NURSE AND THE ETHICAL AGREEMENT

To the extent that an APN acts without regard for her patient's needs and values, she assumes that his decisions and actions have no ethical standing. To the extent that an APN acts for a patient—according to his motivations—she shares her patient's rightful authority over himself. His rightful authority over himself is absolute.

Many agreements require detailed, explicit discussion. For obvious reasons, the agreement between an APN, or any nurse and patient, cannot require this. A nurse's interventions, quite often, must begin immediately. What will be discovered during the course of treatment is unpredictable.

An implicit agreement can be formed immediately. This is made possible by the fact that the role of nurse and patient are firmly settled in rational human expectations. Reflection on herself and on her needs gives a nurse a clear idea of a patient's needs and values. Although it is not possible for any person to know fully and completely the lived reality of another, it is the nature of human understanding to draw on common experiences and images to form agreements.

BIOETHICAL STANDARDS

The bioethical standards (autonomy, freedom, objectivity, self-assertion, beneficence, and fidelity) signify properties inherent in the nature of every human person **(Table 28-4).** They are the innate and defining properties of a human life. As guidelines they prevent "contradictions," actions or interactions that conflict with a patient's power to act—his agency.

There are certain individualized characteristics that every patient brings into the health-care setting and retains by right. Any human characteristic—any virtue—that is necessary to his successful interaction, first as a human and then as a patient, is a resource that cannot, in any way, be justifiably violated.

It greatly increases an APN's efficiency if she understands the functions of these characteristics to exercise and to interact with them. The bioethical standards signify these characteristics. They are the resources without which no interpersonal agreement or interaction would be possible, without which a patient's recovery would be inconceivable, and without which a nurse could not function. These are the following characteristics of a patient:

- **Autonomy**—The individual uniqueness of each patient. This uniqueness is the structure of his individual nature, the liaison of his character structures.

His autonomy is structured by the way he uses his mind, the decisions he has formed, his view of his life, his purposes, and the powers and disabilities of his agency. His autonomy includes his power of reason and his animal nature. As a consequence of his rational animal nature, his ethical equality with all other rational agents is established. Primarily, however, autonomy refers to a person's uniqueness. No two people develop identically. There is no alternative to a human person being unique. Therefore, his uniqueness is a person's innate right. It is a nurse's guidepost to her professional actions.

There is no possibility of one's being and sustaining the excellence of the person he is, unless he sustains who he is. Thus, autonomy is a basic virtue.

- **Freedom**—Self-directedness. An agent's capacity, and consequent right, to take independent, long-term, actions based on his own evaluation of his present situation.

It is the responsibility of a nurse to enable a patient to exercise his freedom. The ability to foresee, plan, and act effectively in his future is a value to, and an excellence of, any human being as such.

- **Objectivity**—The ability to focus one's attention onto an objective context.

Objectivity is a person's need and right to achieve and sustain his exercise of objective awareness. This standard calls for a nurse to sustain this in her patient and in herself.

TABLE 28-4	
The Bioethical Standards	
Autonomy	Uniqueness and independence
Freedom	Right to direct the course of one's life
Objectivity	Ability to deal with the reality of one's situation
Self-assertion	Right to control of one's time and effort
Beneficence	Right to judge benefit and harm for one's self
Fidelity	Faithfulness to the terms of an agreement

To the extent one fails to exercise objectivity, he cannot act to enhance his life. The complete absence of this would destroy the ability to sustain his life. Objectivity is a necessary element of human excellence.

■ **Self-assertion**—The power and right of an agent to control his time and effort.

This power produces each person's self-ownership. It establishes the right of an individual to be free of undesired or undesirable interaction; the right to initiate individual actions. On a nurse's part, it is her actions in nurturing and sustaining this power.

No human excellence would be possible without the power to control one's time and effort. This is a basic value.

■ **Beneficence**—The natural inclination of a person to act to achieve that which is beneficial and to avoid that which is harmful.

A nurse's actions assist this effort. This standard establishes the right of a patient (or professional acting as the agent of a patient) to act for his benefit. It is established by the necessity he faces to act, insofar as possible, to acquire the benefits he desires and the needs his life requires.

The ability to achieve benefits is what makes life worth living. The ability to avoid harms is a correlate of this.

■ **Fidelity**—Adherence to the terms of an agreement. More generally, an individual's faithfulness to his autonomy.

For a nurse, fidelity is a commitment to the obligations she has accepted as part of her professional role—her professional role being a significant part of her autonomy.

The dedication to continue on courses of action that are appropriate to enhancing life and well-being—this is fidelity. This is essential to human excellence. It is a most desirable virtue.

A nurse ought to recognize these virtues, not as obstacles to be overcome, but as character resources to be nurtured. She ought to recognize these virtues as her own. A person's life would be a woebegone affair without them.

There is a saying from Lao Tzu, "A picture is worth a thousand words" (**Fig. 28-1**).

THE NECESSITY OF THE AGREEMENT

Every APN is, at least, implicitly aware of a patient's possession of these virtues. She cannot escape awareness of them. Without these virtues, their agreement would not be possible. Without agreement, their interaction would not be possible. If their interaction is not possible, then professional actions are not possible. If the virtues are violated, the nurse-patient agreement cannot be sustained. If the agreement is not sustained, interaction, properly so called, is impossible. If interaction is not possible, the practice of a profession is not possible. This is the source of the importance of the bioethical standards to professional practice. Their irreplaceable importance arises in the very first moment.

The Virtues of an Advanced Practice Nurse

Here we are using virtue in its original Greek and Chinese sense: the excellence of a person in performing his role. Thus, the virtue of a farmer is to farm well, of a tailor is to make excellent clothing, and of a nurse is to nurse well. The virtue of every human being is to *live* well, to sustain and enhance his life. Thus, virtue is the excellence of a human being in being human.

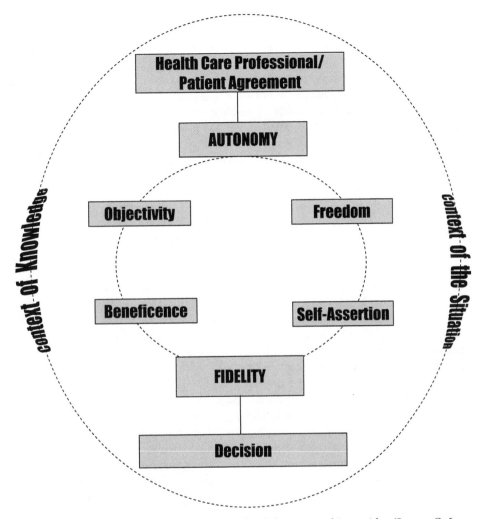

FIGURE 28-1 Husteds' symphonological bioethical decision making guide. *(Source: G. L. Husted & J. H. Husted. (2008a.)* Ethical decision making in nursing and health care: the symphonological approach *(4th ed.). New York: Springer. Used with permission of Springer Publishing Company.)*

Aristotle states, "Now fine and just actions . . . admit of much variety and fluctuation of opinion, so that they may be thought to exist only by convention, and not by nature" (as cited in McKeon, 1941, p. 936). However, fine and just action follow from characteristics that are fundamental aspects of human nature and the virtues of a human person.

The standard of autonomy includes the inescapable fact (that is too often evaded), that every member of the human species—every rational animal—derives his ethical dignity from his nature as a member of the human species. This produces the fundamental ethical reality. Every ethical agent is the ethical equal of every other. No ethical agent can rightfully aggress against another for the benefit of that second ethical agent (Mill, 1988). Infidelity to, and aggression against, another can never arise from the virtues.

An APN is much more able to take direction from her patient's *autonomy*—his uniqueness—because she is not as engrossed in her own uniqueness as she would be if she were relatively new to the profession. If she is new to the profession, she is more focused on herself because she is, quite rightly, unsure of the requirements and techniques of her profession.

An APN is much more capable of allowing and fostering the *freedom* of her patient because she, herself, has mastered the skills that an advanced beginner must still acquire. Therefore, she is free to act within her patient's entire context. Every APN has taken independent and long-term actions to become an APN. Now she can assist her patient to take the independent and long-term actions that will restore him to a state of agency. Here, her experience is her best teacher.

An APN has a much greater ability to observe a context and to form *objective,* meaningful patterns of action because her body of knowledge is greater. She has had to exercise objective awareness to acquire the skills of an APN.

An APN has been able to gain more control over her time and effort because she can now sort out the relevant and the irrelevant aspects of her profession. She can focus on her patient's individual and vital needs. An APN is aware of a person's *self-assertion*—the right to control his own time and effort. In becoming an APN, she has exercised this right. An advanced beginner may be aware of this but may be unable to act on it.

An APN has exercised a greater than average *beneficence* toward herself in achieving the benefit of becoming an APN. She has also made herself better able to assist her patient in pursuing his values. She sees the patient as the beneficiary of her actions and has, hopefully, automatized this in her practice. This is the ethical foundation of her practice.

An APN has had the opportunity to develop a personal and professional integrity to the point that she understands that fidelity to her patient is *fidelity* to herself, to her professional practice, and to her life. As a nurse, she does not see this fidelity as separate from herself.

Because an APN does not have to think solely about the technical aspects of her professional practice, she is free to see the agreement as reciprocal (given the differences in their roles) and necessary.

An APN's knowledge is comprehensive and elaborately organized so that information storage and retrieval is easy. Her clinical knowledge is linked into networks of concepts and relationships, which are then compiled into a higher order knowledge structure that links intricate mental networks into a scheme of relationships and interaction.

Through experience, an APN has become capable of discovering much that an unexperienced nurse is incapable of discovering. Progress in an APN's development will move through, and be structured by, her experience to the extent that she has capitalized on her experience. Retaining her experience of ethical situations will increase her context of knowledge. It will enable her to structure and integrate it. As her context of knowledge becomes greater, the context of every situation can become clearer to her. If she deliberates about the meanings of her experiences, this produces a relationship between her context of knowledge, the context of each individual situation that leads to an increase in her professional competence, and her context of awareness. This is also true of her ethical competence generally.

The big picture and its meaningful details will become evident through an increase in her knowledge and its attendant power to increase her awareness of present facts and future conditions. The increased acuity of her awareness will form an ever-greater body of knowledge with its power to clarify and sharpen her awareness of her patient's context. This is the source of her ethical competence.

This process of an APN's discovery and learning can never be complete. Learning that makes further learning seem impossible or unimportant has destroyed itself as a biological instrument in human life. The nature of every new situation must be learned. It can only be learned through contextual analysis of each situation. By its nature and its function in human life, learning can never be complete.

Ethical efficiency requires that every situation be approached without one's mind being enclosed in a handful of out-of-context-assumptions. Out-of-context truths also work *against* ethical judgment.

Even the knowledge that character and motivations are produced by the dynamic complex of relationships among one's virtues (the bioethical standards) is a dead-end to practice if knowledge stops there. This knowledge of the bioethical standards is not sufficient to ethical decision making. It is not knowledge of self-sufficient rules. Through analysis, the bioethical standards are simply sufficient to guide the awareness that they can produce practice-based resolutions to every *individual* dilemma. *The standards must always be applied in context.*

If there is any reason why nursing diagnosis and treatment is centered on her patient, there is no reason why her ethical decisions and actions should not be. Each serves the same values. To be faithful to the context, an APN cannot turn her back on anything in the context, most especially on her patient. If her patient cannot "call out" to her, then nothing in the context can.

A context-based model actualizes the concept of treating persons as individuals, and therefore, selecting individualized interactions based on a unique patient's needs and circumstances. It is a nurse's awareness of the patient's perceptions of his situation that assists her in understanding her patient's needs and desires. Symphonology theory is not just another compilation of traditional cultural platitudes. Symphonology presents a method of helping the nurse determine what is practical and justifiable regarding those aspects of her practice. Further, the theory of Symphonology recognizes that the context guides what is possible and desirable in the agreement (Scotto, 2008).

ABOUT CASE STUDY ANALYSIS

When analyzing a case study, a difficulty arises in that, in practice, one would want more information—more pieces of data, answers to a greater number of questions. However, in a case study one has to work with what one has. In an actual situation one ought to collect as much data as necessary or as time allows. However, in a case study, the dilemma must occur entirely within the given context. Now consider the case presented in **Box 28-1.**

Notice that in analyzing this case we did not once use the term *ethics* nor did we name the bioethical standards. Nonetheless, our process was one of ethical decision making from a practice-based perspective. In a more complex case, analysis through each standard would be desirable to arrive at the most appropriate decision within the context.[4]

In a study done by Irwin (2004), when patients had an ethical decision to make, it was found that in talking about the decision and in trying to reach a conclusion, patients used all the bioethical standards (albeit not the words) in arriving at their conclusions.

As we have demonstrated through the contemporary ethical theories, ethics means different things to different people. By concentrating on decision making and speaking in human terms, terms that everyone can understand, you can probably avoid the chaos that results when, for instance, the head of a societal expectation bumps into the head of a plan for the greatest good for the greatest number. Or either bumps into the head of an irreconcilable rule.

---

[4]For examples of more complex cases in which the analysis is done through the bioethical standards see Husted and Husted, 2008a.

BOX 28-1
Case Study

Lois Ott, a 58-year-old, is suffering from end-stage renal disease. She can no longer do anything that gives her pleasure, and she is exhausted all the time. She has decided to forego dialysis and let the disease take its course. She has given this decision careful thought. Her family disagrees with her decision and has tried to talk her out of it. They are even thinking about trying to have her declared incompetent on the basis that the toxins in her blood system are making her thought process erratic. Roger, a family nurse practitioner, has been seeing Lois in the dialysis clinic for years. Lois has discussed her plans with Roger. Her family has tried to elicit Roger's help in getting her declared incompetent. With the dialysis, Lois could probably live another 6 to 9 months. In supporting Lois, Roger can argue as follows:

Lois has had a lifetime of experiences. She has made a lifetime of choices and decisions and formed her life and *herself* according to her experiences and choices. If we, as professionals, have a right to ignore this, then the rights in the health-care system are displaced by force. What we have become through our experiences and choices does not entitle us to erase out the person that Lois is and treat her as one object among other objects in the health-care system. There is nothing in this situation that would, objectively, justify our stripping Lois of the right to determine her own life. On the surface, it seems that Lois' family is acting in her place and trying to think and decide with her. However, what Lois needs most is help in convincing her family that they are abandoning her and leaving her all alone in the experience of dying. Lois should not be all alone.

The course of action that Lois has chosen will injure no one and violate no one's rights. If we join her family in making her the instrument of what they desire, we will be harming her and violating her rights. However we go about the business of violating Lois's rights, we cannot make our actions right. We cannot make our actions appropriate and justifiable. It is not appropriate that Lois spend another 6 or 9 months alone, abandoned by the health-care system and her family and suffering during this time.

If we take control of her life and actions, her life will not belong to her. It will belong to us. We will act as though she is not the one living her life. We would not be content for someone else to choose the level of suffering we should endure and the way we should end our life. By the same token, we should not choose for her.

Lois has expressed her individual desires. Many people would not desire this, but many would, and Lois does. If, in every difficult decision, we were determined that those who disagree with us must accept our perspective, we would simply be acting as terrorists. These arguments can be offered in support of Lois. No comparable arguments can be made against Lois' position.

We made an agreement with Lois that we would act as her agent. Now we are entertaining the justifiability of breaking that agreement. This will make us unfaithful to Lois and unfaithful to our profession. There is no earthly way we can justify this.

MUSINGS

Each patient entering the health-care system hopes to derive some benefit. He hopes to regain his competence to perform his normal functions and to live his life as he chooses. He wishes to enter again into the pursuit of his happiness. At the very least, he expects to come out better able to live than when he went into the health-care system. Each of the bioethical standards is appropriate to these purposes:

1. The *standard of autonomy* enables a patient to maintain his way of understanding himself and his world. (In a psychiatric setting, objectivity replaces autonomy as a goal. Objectivity—an awareness of the facts of the external world—is a necessary precondition of autonomy. An autonomous being is autonomous in his relation to the external world.)

    Sara is a timorous 82-year-old lady. Roseanne, her nurse practitioner, relates to her in a manner that implies that it is all right to be a timorous 82-year-old lady. When Sara leaves the health-care setting she will have a sense of her autonomy as strong as, or stronger than, when she entered.

2. The *standard of freedom* supports a patient's right to function as an independent being. It is the freedom to make the ethical decisions that affect his life.

    Billy is a curious 6-year-old boy. Jane, his pediatric nurse practitioner, talks to him. She explains things to him. She asks his opinion. She allows him to make appropriate choices. Billy leaves the hospital as independent and self-confident as he was when he entered, or more so. In relation to his sense of freedom, Billy's hospital stay has had a positive effect.

3. The *standard of objectivity* is a patient's ability to function as a reasoning being. To do this, he must have access to the understanding of his situation.

    Jeff has been put on a low-salt, low-fat diet. Robert, his nurse practitioner, takes the time to explain to Jeff why he ought to stay on the diet. He motivates Jeff to stay on his diet by appealing to his understanding (his reason). He makes Jeff an active participant in his plan of care. He does not depend only on a passive emotional motivation that, in a few weeks, would probably fade away.

    As Oscar Wilde (1989) observes, "The only difference between a caprice and a life-long passion is that the caprice lasts a little longer" (p. 27).

4. The *standard of self-assertion* demands recognition of a patient's self-ownership. Leah is careful not to do anything that would interfere with her patient's control of his time and effort.

    Ronnie is a 7-year-old child who is dying. He comes to the clinic every week for a transfusion. One day he says to Leah, his pediatric nurse practitioner, "I don't want this anymore." Leah explains what will happen if he does not get the transfusion. Ronnie says that he knows and he still does not want the transfusion. Leah gets the parents, physician, and other consultants together and tells Ronnie's story. Ronnie takes control of his life with Leah's help (Woods, 1999).

5. The *standard of beneficence* protects a patient's reasonable expectation that he will derive some benefit from the health-care system. It is also a recognition of a person's right *not* to be harmed.

    A patient is dying of metastatic cancer. His family believes that he is going to recover and has made him a full code, despite the evidence of his suffering. He has expressed not wanting to live while he was conscious. He is now semiconscious and cannot make his wants known. The only thing he has to look forward to is avoidance of suffering. Barbara, his nurse, arranges to discuss the situation with the family. If she is unsuccessful, she will request an ethics consult.

6. The purpose of the *standard of fidelity*—faithfulness to the nurse-patient agreement is, very simply, to enable everyone to know what he and she are doing.

    A child has wet the bed. He begs his nurse not to tell his parents. She promises that she will not. Fidelity establishes a predictable universe for the nurse and for her patient.

The agreement, with the bioethical standards as preconditions, is designed to enable a patient to bring his virtues into a biomedical setting, retain them while he is there, and have them intact when he leaves.

Bioethical analysis and interaction guided by the standards is not possible, in any objective sense, apart from the patient's purposes and attitudes. A patient is passive. His entire ethical purpose is to become an agent, to act, to once again take charge of his life. The best thing that can happen to him is to encounter a nurse whose purpose is the same.

Through her progress as a nurse, an APN has, if only potentially, come to a greater understanding and experience of herself, of who she is, and, hopefully, she has come to appreciate the importance of this. Through her experience, she has come to understand the difference in the uniqueness in individuals and has gained a clearer insight into the meaning of this to an individual's progress toward a better life.

Through her experience, she has developed a greater than average skill at pursuing long-term goals guided by her objective awareness and an understanding of the importance and joy of this. Because of this she is able to lead her patient down a version of the same path she has taken.

References

Angeles, P. (1992). *Dictionary of philosophy.* New York: Harper Collins

Barnes, D. M., & Boyle, J. S. (1995). *Transcultural concepts in nursing case* (2nd ed). Philadelphia: Lippincott.

Benner, P., Tanner, C. A., & Chelsa, C. A. (1996). *Expertise in nursing practice.* New York: Springer.

Callahan, L., & Mannino, M. J. (1998). Legal aspect of advanced nursing practice. In C. M. Sheehy, & M. C. McCarthy (Eds.), *Advanced practice nursing* (pp. 281–302). Philadelphia: F.A. Davis.

Erickson, R., & Sheehy, C. M. (1998). Clinical research in the advanced practice role. In C. M. Sheehy & M. C. McCarthy (Eds.), *Advanced practice nursing* (pp. 241–263). Philadelphia: F.A. Davis.

Gastmans, C. (1998). Challenges to nursing values in a changing nursing environment. *Nursing Ethics, 5*(3), 236–245.

Gibson, C. H. (1993). Underpinnings of ethical reasoning in nursing. *Journal of Advanced Nursing, 18*(12), 2003–2007.

Gilbert, W. S., & Sullivan, A. (1885). *The mikado.* Retrieved June 9, 2007, from the Boise State University Web site: http://math.boisestate.edu/ gas/mikado/webopera/operhome.html.

Guido, G. W. (2006). *Legal and ethical issues in nursing* (4th ed.). Upper Saddle River, NJ: Prentice Hall.

Hardt, M. (2001). Core then care: The nurse leader's role in "caring." *Nursing Administration Quarterly, 25*(3), 37–45.

Hoffmaster B. (2006). 'Real' ethics for 'real' boys: Context and narrative. *The American Journal of Bioethics, 4*(1), 40–41.

Husted, G. L., & Husted, J. H. (1998). Ethical decision making and the role of the nurse. In G. Deloughery (Ed.), *Issues and trends in nursing* (3rd ed., pp. 216–242). St. Louis: Mosby.

Husted, J. H., & Husted, G. L. (1999). Agreement: The origin of ethical action. *Critical Care Nursing, 22*(3), 12–18.

Husted, J. H., & Husted, G. L. (2008a). *Ethical decision making in nursing and health care: The symphonological approach* (4th ed.). New York: Springer.

Husted, G. L., & Husted, J. H. (2008b). The nurse as ethical shield: The symphonological approach. *Perioperative Nursing Clinics, 3*(3).

Irwin, M. (2004). Application of symphonology theory in patient decision-making: Triangulation of quantitative and qualitative methods. Ph.D. dissertation, School of Nursing, Duquesne University.

Kikuchi, J. F. (1996). Multicultural ethics in nursing education: A potential threat to responsible practice. *Journal of Professional Nursing, 12*(3), 159–165.

McKeon, R. (Ed.). (1941). *The basic works of Aristotle.* New York: Random House.

Mill, J. S. (1988). *On liberty.* New York: Penguin. (Original work published 1819).

Reigle, J. (1996). Ethical-decision making skills. In A. B. Hamric, J. A. Spross, & C. M. Hanson (Eds.), *Advanced nursing practice: An integrative approach* (3rd ed.). (pp. 273–295). Philadelphia: Saunders.

Sarikonda-Woitas, C., & Robinson, J. (2002). Ethical health care policy: Nursing's voice in allocation. *Nursing Administration Quarterly, 26*(4), 72–80.

Smith, K. V. (2005). Ethical issues related to health care: The older adult's perspective. *Journal of Gerontological Nursing, 31*(2), 32–39.

Scotto, C. (2008). Symphonological bioethical theory. In A. M. Romey & M. R. Alligold (Eds.), *Nursing theorists and their work* (7th ed.). St. Louis: Mosby.

Solomon, M. Z., Jennings, B., Guilfoy, V., Jackson, R., O'Donnell, L. Wolf, S. M., et al. (1994). Toward an expanded vision of clinical ethics education: From individual to the institution. *Kennedy Institute of Ethics Journal, 1*(3), 225–245.

Tuckett, A. (1999). Nursing practice: Compassionate deception and the good Samaritan. *Nursing Ethics, 6*(5), 383–389.

Van Hooft, S. (1990). Moral education for nursing decisions. *Journal of Advanced Nursing, 15*(2), 210–215.

Wilde, O. (1989). *The complete works of Oscar Wilde.* New York: Harper and Row.

Woods, M. (1999). A nursing ethic: The moral voice of experienced nurses. *Nursing Ethics, 6*(5), 423–433.

Wurzbach, M. E. (1999). Acute care nurses' experiences of moral certainty. *Advanced Nursing, 30*(2), 287–293.

Zoucha, R. & Husted, G. L. (2000). The ethical dimensions of delivering culturally congruent nursing and health care. *Issues in Mental Health Nursing 1*(3), 325–340.

Index

Note: Page numbers followed by an "f" indicate figures, page numbers followed by a "t" indicate tables, and page numbers followed by a "b" indicate boxes.

A

AACN. *See* American Association of Colleges of Nursing
AANA. *See* American Association of Nurse Anesthetists
AANM. *See* American Association of Nurse-Midwives
ABNS. *See* American Board of Nursing Specialists
Absolute risk reduction, 253t
Accountability
    for quality, 172
    reporting, 157–158
Accountant services, for independent practice, 431–432
Accreditation, 59, 133, 466
    for APNs in cultural competence, 376–377
ACNM. *See* American College of Nurse-Midwives
ACOG. *See* American College of Obstetricians and Gynecologists
ACP. *See* American College of Physicians
Acquired immunodeficiency syndrome (AIDS), 90
ACT. *See* Anesthesia care team
Acute care nurse practitioner, 33–36
    adult, 35
    of elderly, 36
    in pediatric setting, 34–35
    profile of, 34b
    on specialty services, 35–36
ADA. *See* Americans with Disabilities Act
ADEA. *See* Federal Age Discrimination in Employment Act
Administrative procedures act (APA), 475
Adolescent services, communication aiding, 416b–417b
ADR. *See* Alternative dispute resolution
Advanced nurse practitioner (ANP), 161
Advanced nursing practice (ANP)
    global perspectives on, 73b, 79–97
Advanced practice license, for independent practice, 427
Advanced practice nurse (APN). *See also* Certified nurse-midwife; Certified registered nurse anesthetist; Clinical nurse specialist; Nurse practitioner
    accreditation in cultural competence for, 376–377
    acute care nurse practitioner, 33–36

ADR, exercises for, 386–387
ADR, observations of, 384–386
advantages of using, 377–378
advocacy by, 261–274
attributes for research role of, 296–297
autonomy, 76
behavior for research of, 298–302
billing options and, 105–109
case management by, 277–292
change agency of, 302
clinical relationships and, 216–217
from "cognitive dissonance," 144
collaborative practice's status for, 146–150
community outreach of, 415–416
conflict and, 382
continuous quality improvement with, 288–289
contract issues for, 454–463
core competencies and, 211–214, 212f
in courts, 472–474
credentialing, 76–77, 131–133, 131b
cultural competence and, 355–357
dialogue with consumers for marketing of, 408–411
disease management with, 287–289
education and, 390
education program quality, 76, 77b
as employees, 452–453
ethical agreement and, 520
evolution of, 393–394
financial/tax implications for, 450
future of, 42
health-care policy and, 367
HMO with, 287
identity challenges for, 398
identity uncertainty, 74
impact of, 393
as independent contractor, 453
knowledge's value to, 371–373, 373b
lack of recognition and, 75–76
learner, assessment of, 331–337
legalities concerning cultural competence for, 375–376
maintaining data about performance, 140–141
malpractice and, 487–496
malpractice crisis and, 494–496
managed care with, 288–289
marketing problems of, 403
marketing promotions for, 412–413, 413b

marketing's operational definition for, 405b
in MCPs, 174–175, 178–180, 186–188
Medicare reimbursement and, 239–240, 397–398
models of collaboration and, 214–216, 214f, 215t
numbers of, 24t
nurse anesthetist, 39–41
partnership of, 378
patient empowerment and, 368, 368b
patient's perspective imagined by, 357, 369
philosophy of, 298–302
physicians' relationship with, 152
practice-based bioethics of, 518–519
prescriptions and, 77–78
professional liability considerations, 449–450
professional nursing connections and, 220–221
proliferation of titles, 74–75
in quality initiatives, 181–186
reforms impacting, 392
regulation, 76–78
regulatory standards of, 78b
reimbursement for, 109–115, 110b
removing barriers to research by, 302–304
research by, 295–306, 375, 398–399
risks of, 486–487
role as educator, 349
roles of, 23–24, 221b–228b, 352, 390–391
    development of, 47–53, 50b, 51b, 52b
    theoretical perspective on, 46–47, 47b
salaries of, 194–195, 206, 397
scholarship, 304
scope of practice, 24–41, 25t, 470–472
second licensure models of, 141–142
self-assessment process for, 174–175
sex education, successful programs for, 417b–418b
standard setting, 76–78
stress and strain on, 53–56, 54b
Sunrise Model for, 358f
teaching plan, development of, 337–349, 339f

testimonials for, 405
therapeutic prescriptions, 77–78
"titling" of, 161
value increased by, 412–413
virtues, 522–525
work status determination factors for, 450–452
Advanced practice professional nurse (APPN), 161
Advanced practice registered nurse (APRN), 161
regulation of, 25–26, 26t, 27, 27t
Advanced registered nurse practitioner (ARNP), 161
Advocacy, 261–274, 359
case management skill of, 284t
Community Choice Counseling involvement with, 268–271
consumer-driven systems-level of, 271–273
definitions of, 263
evidence base for, 262
family court system involvement with, 264–266
family level of, 263–266
individual level of, 263–266
individual/family exemplar, 264–266
levels of, 263
NJDHSS involvement with, 269–270
nurses learning of, 273–274
nursing home involvement with, 267–271
nursing roots of, 261
suicide prevention, 271–272
systems-level of, 267–273
Affective domain, learner, assessment of, 337
Africa, global perspectives on ANP, 79
AFT. *See* American Federation of Teachers
Agency for Healthcare Research and Quality (AHRQ), 161, 257, 352–353, 361
health literacy defined by, 362
AHA. *See* American Hospital Association
AHNA. *See* American Holistic Nurses Association
AHRQ. *See* Agency for Healthcare Research and Quality
AIDS. *See* Acquired immunodeficiency syndrome
Ali v. Community Health Care Plan, Inc., 474
Allied health professional, 134
Alternative dispute resolution (ADR)
APN exercises for, 386–387
APN observations regarding, 384–386
development of, 383–384
health care and, 381
narrative mediation for, 384
self-assessment for improving, 387
transformative practice for, 384
Alternative medicine, research on, 313–315

Alternative therapies, 310t
AMA. *See* American Medical Association
AMA-PCPI/Consortium. *See* AMA-Physician Consortium for Performance Improvement
AMA-Physician Consortium for Performance Improvement (AMA-PCPI/Consortium), 181
activities of, 184
for development, 185
performance measures for, 185b–186b
Ambulatory cardiology clinic, blood pressure measurement in, 305–306
American Association of Colleges of Nursing (AACN), 59, 295
American Association of Nurse Anesthetists (AANA), 8–9, 394–395, 495, 498
American Association of Nurse-Midwives (AANM), 6
American Board of Nursing Specialists (ABNS), 58, 113
American College of Nurse-Midwives (ACNM), 6, 147, 148, 495
American College of Obstetricians and Gynecologists (ACOG), 147, 148
American College of Physicians (ACP), 254
American Family Physician, 145, 165
American Federation of Teachers (AFT), 165
American Holistic Nurses Association (AHNA), 310
American Hospital Association (AHA), 144. *See also* Patient Care Partnership
cultural competence products of, 372–373
Patient's Bill of Rights by, 360
American Medical Association (AMA), 481
collaboration and, 168
CPR against, 179–180
CPT codes, 440
single standard of obstetrical care, 5
American Nurses Association (ANA), 143, 355–356, 393, 455
Code of Ethics of, 261
on restrictive legislation, 159
Scope and Standards of Practice by, 295–296
American Nurses Credentialing Center (ANCC), 113, 302
case management definition by, 278
American Psychiatric Association (AAP), 144–145
American Psychological Association (APA), 373
American Society for Healthcare Risk Management (ASHRM), 495
American Society of Superintendents of Training School for Nurses, 5

Americans with Disabilities Act (ADA), 442
Americas, global perspectives on ANP, 82–84
America's Health Care Safety Net: Intact but Endangered (IOM), 362
ANA. *See* American Nurses Association
ANA code of 1950, on nurse-physician relationship, 145
Analytic process, 248, 250f
ANCC. *See* American Nurses Credentialing Center
Anesthesia care team (ACT), 40
ANMC. *See* Australian Nursing and Midwifery Council
Annual Review of Medicine, 165
ANP. *See* Advanced nurse practitioner
Antibiotics, 10
Antifraud laws, 476
Antitrust Division (ATD), 482
Antitrust laws, 479–482
enforcement of, 482
APA. *See* Administrative procedures act; American Psychiatric Association; American Psychological Association
Apex Hosiery Co. v. Leader, 479
APN. *See* Advanced practice nurse
Appellant, 469
APPN. *See* Advanced practice professional nurse
APRN. *See* Advanced practice registered nurse
Arizona v. Maricopa County Medical Society, 480
ARNP. *See* Advanced registered nurse practitioner
Aromatherapy, 319
ASHRM. *See* American Society for Healthcare Risk Management
Asian Americans, health literacy and, 364
Assessment
ADR improvement through self-, 387
CCHPA tool for self-, 367–368
communication's importance to, 374–375
of diabetes using BMI, 370
health literacy and tools for, 360–361, 361t
NCCC's tool for self-, 369
for nursing and cultural congruent care, 359
spiritual, 377b
Assignment, of contracts, 460
Association of American Medical Colleges, 144
ATD. *See* Antitrust Division
Attestation page, in career portfolio, 140
Attitudes, toward teamwork, 162
Attorney services, 431
Australia, global perspectives on ANP, 91–92

Australian Nursing and Midwifery Council (ANMC), 91
Autonomy, bioethics and, 521, 521t, 527

B

Bachelor of science in nursing (BSN), 62, 65, 280
Bahrain, global perspectives on ANP, 85
Balanced Budget Act (BBA), 104, 176–177, 468
Ballard, Martha, 3
Bankert, Marianne, 7
Barton, Clara, 3
BBA. *See* Balanced Budget Act
Bellegre v. Board of Nurse Examiners, 473
Bellevue School for Midwives, 5
Beneficence, bioethics and, 521, 521t, 522, 527
Berdyck v. Shinde and HR Magruder Memorial Hospital, 473
Bernard, Sister Mary, 7
Best Evidence (BMJ publishing group), 258
Beyond Disruption: Changing the Rules in the Marketplace (Dru), 407
Billing
  direct, 203
  options and, 105–109
    health maintenance organizations, 107–108
    incident-to-billing, 108–109
    indemnity insurance companies, 109
    managed care organizations, 107–108, 108t
    Medicaid, 107
    Medicare, 106–107
    physician-hospital organizations, 107–108
    preferred provider organizations, 107–108
    provider sponsored organizations, 107–108
    shared visits, 109
    TRICARE, 109
  volume's measurement for, 203
Billing procedures, for independent practice, 440–441, 441b
Bioethical decision making guide, Husted's symphonological, 523f
Bioethics, 511. *See also* Ethics; Practice-based bioethics
  autonomy and, 521, 521t, 527
  beneficence and, 521, 521t, 522, 527
  fidelity and, 521, 521t, 522, 527
  freedom and, 521, 521t, 527
  objectivity and, 521, 521t, 527
  self-assertion and, 521, 521t, 522, 527
  standards, 521–522
Biological remedies, 318–319
Blinding, 254

Blood pressure measurement, 305–306
BMI. *See* Body mass index
Board of Nursing (BON), 468, 470
Boards of nursing (BON), state, 313
Body mass index (BMI), diabetes assessment using, 370
BON. *See* Board of Nursing
Botswana, global perspectives on ANP, 79
Breach of contract, 454
Breach remedies, in contracts, 459
Breckenridge, Mary, 147
Breckinridge, Myra, 5, 6–7
Brown, Esther Lucile, 10
BSN. *See* Bachelor of science in nursing
Budget(s)
  breakeven for, 199–200, 199f
  capital, 198
  cash, 199–200
  long-range, 197
  operational, 197–198
  program, 198–199
  types of, 197–200
Budgeting process
  DRG in, 200
  implementation with evaluation in, 201–202
  interventions in, 200
  output v. input for, 202
  projected workload volume for, 200–201
  resource drivers in, 200
  total revenue in, 201
  variable supplies projection for, 200–201
  workload measures in, 200
Bunker Hill/Massachusetts General Nurse Practitioner program, 16
Business. *See also* Organization
  community transportation considerations for, 411–412
  office environment impacting, 412
Business concept, for independent practice, 436
Business decisions, for independent practice, 423b, 424
Business location, for independent practice, 435
Business name/image, for independent practice, 434
Business plan, for independent practice, 436–438
Business start-up time line, for independent practice, 425b–427b
Business structure, for independent practice, 432–434

C

CAM. *See* Complementary-alternative medicine
Canada, global perspectives on ANP, 82–84, 82b

Canadian Nurses Association (CNA), 82–83
Cancer Awareness Network for Immigrant Minority Populations (CANIMP), 365
CANIMP. *See* Cancer Awareness Network for Immigrant Minority Populations
CAPC. *See* Center to Advance Palliative Care
Capital assets, 195
Capital budgets, 198
Care. *See also* Cultural congruent care
  CNM and outcome of, 394
  CNS and outcome of, 396–397
  CRNA and outcome of, 394–395
  NP and outcome of, 395–396
  nursing's central mission of, 357–358
  teamwork impacting, 381
Career portfolio, 137–140
  attestation page, 140
  credentials component, 140
  practice-based evidence component, 138, 139f, 140
  practitioner contact information, 138
Carrier identification, in malpractice insurance, 499
Case management, 277–292
  advocacy skill for, 284t
  ANCC definition of, 278
  assessment for, 284t
  associations for, 290–292
  CCMA's five care domains for, 285
  certification for, 290–292
  chronic disease in, 280
  Civil Rights Movement influencing, 279
  Community Chest Movement influencing, 278
  community-based model for, 282t
  confidentiality for, 284t
  coordination of care for, 285
  cost-benefit analysis for, 284t
  CPT codes for, 289
  critical thinking for, 284t
  differentiating levels of nurse practice in, 280–281
  discharge planner for, 284t
  disease management v., 287–288
  education for, 290, 291b
  education levels for nurses in, 280–281, 281b
  follow-through for, 284t
  good process in, 286
  good structure in, 286
  historical background on, 277–279
  HMO with, 279
  hospital-based model for, 282t
  hospital-to-community-based model for, 282t
  insurance structures/benefits knowledge for, 284t

interpersonal skills for, 284t
manager role competitors for, 279–280
models, 282–283, 282t
negotiation for, 284t
NIC for, 285–286
NOC for, 285–286
organizational skills for, 284t
outcomes management for, 284t
patient adherence for, 285
patient empowerment for, 285
patient involvement in care for, 285
patient knowledge for, 285
PPO with, 279
professional skills for, 284t
reimbursement with, 289
responsibilities for, 283
RN with bachelor's degree in, 280–281
Saint Peter's College's Master of Science program in, 291b
skills for, 283–284, 284t
tools/strategies for, 284–287
Villanova University College of Nursing program on, 290
Wald's work with, 277–278
Case Management Society of America (CMSA), 278
CCMA of, 285–286
curriculum sponsored by, 290
reimbursement of services requested by, 289
Case study
of practice-based bioethics, 525, 526b
teaching plan, development of, 344
Case Western Reserve University, inaugural doctor of nursing practice program, 63t
Cash budgets, 199–200
Cayman Islands, global perspectives on ANP, 92–93
CCC. *See* Community Choice Counseling
CCHPA. *See* Cultural Competence Health Practitioner Assessment
CCMA. *See* Council for Case Management Accountability
CCNE. *See* Commission on Collegiate Nursing Education
CDS. *See* Controlled dangerous substances
Center for Case Management, certification from, 292
Center to Advance Palliative Care (CAPC), 373
Centers for Medicare and Medicaid Services (CMS), 146, 177, 428, 468, 498
Central venous line securement, 306
Certified midwife (CM), 147–148
Certified nurse anesthetist. *See* Certified registered nurse anesthetist
Certified nurse practitioner (CNP), 161
Certified nurse-midwife (CNM), 5, 6, 23, 391, 471, 495. *See also* Nurse-midwives

care outcomes and, 394
leadership with, 236–238
nurse-physician collaboration in, 146, 147–148
practice settings for, 232, 232t
reporting relationships for, 230–241
Certified registered nurse anesthetist (CRNA), 8, 23, 152, 498
care outcomes and, 394–395
in nurse-physician collaboration, 146–147
practice settings for, 232, 232t
reimbursement in, 240–241
reporting relationships for, 230–241
role of, 391
Cesarean section, nurse-midwives and, 39
Chalmers-Francis v. Nelson, 472
CHAMPUS. *See* Civilian Health and Medical Program of the Uniformed Services program
Child health, education impacting, 355
Children of September 11th (Salamone), 419
Chloroform, 7
CHNPs. *See* Community health nurse practitioners
Chronic disease, 280
Civil lawsuits, 486
Civil Rights Act, 375–376, 442
Civil Rights Movement, 279
Civil War, 3
Civilian Health and Medical Program of the Uniformed Services program (CHAMPUS), CNS and NP reimbursement under, 238
Clayton Act, 479, 480
CLIA. *See* Clinical Laboratory Improvement Amendments
Clinic, collaborative practice model in, 167
Clinical competence, teaching and, 332t
Clinical conference, teaching plan for, 343–344
Clinical Evidence Handbook, 256–257
Clinical judgment, 245–257
analytic processes for, 248, 250
clinical reasoning v., 246
clinician's background influencing, 246
context of patient care in, 247–248, 250
defined, 245
evidence-based practice in relation to, 245–250
intuition for, 248, 250f
model of, 250f
narrative thinking for, 248–249
patient knowledge in, 247
patterns of, 248–249
problem solving and, 245
reflection on practice following, 249, 250

relationship with patient in, 247, 250
research evidence to improve, 251–257
Clinical Laboratory Improvement Amendments (CLIA), 429, 430
Clinical laboratory license, for independent practice, 429–430
Clinical nurse leader (CNL), 12
Clinical nurse specialist (CNS), 9–12, 23, 152, 390, 471
ambiguity and, 28–29
care outcomes and, 396–397
case management by, 281
critical care, 31b
incremental/opportunity costs for, 196–197
merge with nurse practitioner, 12
in nurse-physician collaboration, 148–149
population-based, 30b
practice settings for, 232, 232t
prescriptive authority and, 122
promoting, 393
psychiatric, 28, 29b
reimbursement for, 238–240
reporting relationships for, 230–241
research by, 295
role expansion of, 10–11
role/development of, 391–392
Clinical practice guidelines, 161
Clinical practices, inefficiency in, 206
Clinical reasoning, 246
Clinical relationships, 216–217
CM. *See* Certified midwife
CMS. *See* Centers for Medicare and Medicaid Services
CMSA. *See* Case Management Society of America
CNA. *See* Canadian Nurses Association
CNL. *See* Clinical nurse leader
CNM. *See* Certified nurse-midwife
CNP. *See* Certified nurse practitioner
CNS. *See* Clinical nurse specialist
Coalition for Patients' Rights (CPR), 179–180
Cocooning, 419
Code of Ethics for Nurses (ANA), 355–356
Cognitive dissonance, 144
Cognitive domain, learner, assessment of, 336, 337t
Cognitive readiness, of learner, 333–334
Collaboration, 230, 234
AMA and, 168
definition of, 150
future for, 168–169
language of, 158–159
models of, 214–216, 214f, 215t
in primary care, 160
in protocols, 160–161
research, 297–298
success strategies in, 162–166
supervision v., 149, 159

Collaboration barrier
  educational isolation as, 155–156
  organizational hierarchy as, 157–158
  professional elitism as, 156
  role/language confusion as, 158–161
  unrecognized diversity as, 158, 162
Collaboration success strategy(ies),
    162–163
  effective team creation as, 163–164
  joint growth/development acceptance
    as, 164
  language use in, 165–166
  protocols/guidelines wisdom as, 164
  students' communication skills for, 166
Collaborative models
  collaborative practice model as, 167
  differentiated practice model in, 167
  for LTC, 167–168
  primary nursing model in, 166
Collaborative practice. *See also* Nurse-
    physician collaboration; Physician-nurse
    collaboration framework
  history of, 143–144
  intensity continuum in, 152–154, 153f
  levels/types of, 153–154
  malpractice insurance, 498–499
  status for, 146–150
Colorado, 180
Columbia University, inaugural doctor of
    nursing practice program, 63t
Commission on Collegiate Nursing
    Education (CCNE), 59
Committee on the Grading of Nursing
    Schools, 144
Common goals, in physician-nurse
    collaboration framework, 151
Communication. *See also* Dialogue;
    Language
  adolescent services aided through,
    416b–417b
  assessment and importance of,
    374–375
  inadequate/inappropriate patterns of,
    161
  with MCPs, 174–175
  students' skills for, 166
Community
  APNs, outreach to, 415–416
  business and transportation considera-
    tions of, 411–412
  describing, 410b
  dialogue with, 408–410
Community Chest Movement, 278
Community Choice Counseling (CCC),
    268–271
Community Health Accreditation
    Program, Medicare and, 466
Community health nurse practitioners
    (CHNPs), 96
Community-based case management
    model, 282t

Compensation, contracts and, 457–458
Competition, independent practice and, 437
Competitive analysis, independent practice
    and, 437
Complementary-alternative medicine
    (CAM), 309, 310t
  development of, 311–313
  educational considerations for, 321,
    322b, 323t
  ethical considerations in, 325–326
  expanding/advancing of, 326b
  modalities, 315–320
    aromatherapy, 319
    biological remedies, 318–319
    energy therapies, 317
    guided images, 316–317
    healing environment, 320
    healing touch, 309, 312b, 317–318
    mind-body therapies, 316
    reiki, 317–318
    spirituality, 319–320
    therapeutic touch, 309, 312b,
      317–318
  models for, 324–325, 325b
  in regulated nursing practice, 321, 323b
  role development in, 324–325
Computer Training Services (CTS), 442
Concordia College, Moorhead, MN,
    inaugural doctor of nursing practice
    program, 63t
Conditions of participation, for Medicare,
    466
Confidence interval, 253t
Confidentiality
  case management with, 284t
  in contracts, 457
Conflict. *See also* Alternative dispute
    resolution
  APNs and, 382
  integrating/dominance approaches to,
    383
  nursing, management strategies for,
    382–383
Conflict of interest, contracts and, 457
Conflict of laws, of contracts, 460
Connector, 408–409
Consensus Model for *APRNAPN*
    Regulation, 180
Consensus Standards Advisory Committee
    (CSAC), 180
Constructive knowledge, 476
Consultant selection, for independent
    practice, 431–432
Consultation, 234
Consumer support
  marketing for, 187
  for MCPs' APNs, 179, 186–187
Consumers, marketing, dialogue of APNs
    with, 408–411
Contemporary medicine, research on,
    313–315

Context, in practice-based bioethics,
    516–518
Continuous quality improvement, APN's
    disease management in, 288–289
Contract(s)
  for APNs, 454–463
  assignment of, 460
  breach, 454
  breach remedies in, 459
  compensation and, 457–458
  confidentiality in, 457
  conflict of interest and, 457
  conflict of laws in, 460
  dispute resolution in, 458
  effective date of, 455
  force majeure in, 461
  indemnification/subrogation in, 458
  legal authority in, 460
  modification of, 460
  not to compete covenant in, 461
  notices in, 459–460
  party relationships in, 455–456
  party responsibilities in, 456–457
  scope of, 455
  severability of, 460
  signatures in, 461
  term/renewal/termination in, 459
  terms of, 455–461
  types, 454–455
Contracting, with MCPs, 175–176, 176b
Contractual obligations, of malpractice
    insurance, 501–503
Controlled dangerous substances (CDS), 423
Conventional allopathic medical and
    nursing practice, 310t
Cooperation, in physician-nurse
    collaboration framework, 152
Coordination, in physician-nurse
    collaboration framework, 152
Core competencies, APNs and, 211–214,
    212f
Corporation, for independent practice, 433
Cost concepts
  direct v. indirect, 195–196f
  incremental v. opportunity, 196–197
  total v. unit, 196
  variable v. fixed, 195, 196f
Cost containment
  clinical practices' inefficiency in, 206
  cost-benefit analysis in, 209
  efficiency v., 208–209
  incentives for, 210
  input v. output in, 208–209
  intensity/price in, 205–206
  overtime in, 206–207
  as patients' benefit, 210
  productivity in, 208–209
  reimbursement v., 209–210
  in resource management, 205–209
  salaries in, 206
  supplies/equipment in, 207–208

turnover in, 207
UAPs for, 207
Cost-benefit analysis, 209
case management with, 284t
Council for Case Management
Accountability (CCMA), 285–286
five care domains for, 285
Council of Primary Care Nurse
Practitioners, 17
Court actions, 466
Court of appeals, 469
Court system, 469–470
APNs in, 472–474
legal opinions in, 470
precedent in, 470
structure of, 469–470
CPR. See Coalition for Patients' Rights
CPT. See Current procedural terminology;
Current procedure terminology
Crataegus hawthorn, 318
Credentialing, 76–78, 130
application, 131
analysis of, 132
organizational standard sources,
133
verification, 131–132
data procurement, 131b
with organizational venues, 141
Credentials component, in career
portfolio, 140
Crile, George, 8
Critical thinking, 245. See also Clinical
judgment
case management with, 284t
CRNA. See Certified registered nurse
anesthetist
Croix de Guerre, 8
Crossing the quality chasm (IOM),
163–164, 365
CSAC. See Consensus Standards Advisory
Committee
CTS. See Computer Training Services
Cultural competence, 355–357. See also
Health literacy
accreditation for APNs and, 376–377
AHA's products for, 372–373
honesty and, 373
HRSA defining, 360
internet research used for, 371–373
legalities for APNs and, 375–376
MCHB defining, 359–360
theoretical basis for, 357–359
for treatment plans, 370
Cultural Competence Health Practitioner
Assessment (CCHPA), 367–368
Cultural congruent care, nursing
assessment and, 359
Cultural diversity, 158
Cultural expression, language as, 368
Cumulative Database of Systematic Reviews,
254

Cumulative Index to Nursing and Allied
Health Literature, 254
Current procedural terminology (CPT), 204
case management services in, 289
coded services, 104, 106
Current procedure terminology (CPT),
codes, 439, 440
Customization, of supplies/equipment, 208

D

Data collection, on MCPs' APNs, 178
Dean Mundinger of the Columbia
University School of Nursing, 62
"The Debilitator," 374
Decision-making, 245. See also Clinical
judgment
organizational, 191
"payor-blind" care in, 210
Defendants, 469
Deficit Reduction Act of 2005 (DRA),
177
Deontology, 513t, 514
Department of Health and Human
Services (DHHS), 487
Depreciation, as expense, 195
DHHS. See Department of Health and
Human Services
Diabetes, BMI for assessment of, 370
Diagnosis related group (DRG), 193
in budgeting process, 200
payment, 103
Dialogue
of APN with consumers for marketing,
408–411
with community, 408–410
discussion v., 154
schools and, 409
technology improving, 411
Dickenson-Hazard, Dr. Nancy, 378
Direct billing, 203
Discharge planner, case management with,
284t
Discussion, dialogue v., 154
Disease management, case management v.,
287–288
Dispute resolution, in contracts, 458
Disruption process, 407
Diversity. See Unrecognized diversity
DNP. See Doctor of Nursing Practice
DNS. See Doctor of nursing service
Doctor of education (EdD), 59
Doctor of Nursing Practice (DNP), 12,
19–20, 61–62, 65, 295
approval of, 59
arguments for/against, 65–67
doctor of philosophy vs., 66–67
programs, 63t–64t
Doctor of nursing science (DNS), 59, 66
Doctor of philosophy (PhD), 59, 60–61
doctor of nursing practice vs., 66–67
enrollment and, 60

graduation rates for, 60
research-focused programs, 60f
Doctor of science in nursing (DSN),
59
Doctoral nursing education, future of,
67–68
Documentation process, for independent
practice, 443–444
Documentation, reimbursement and, 205
DRA. See Deficit Reduction Act of 2005
Drexel University, inaugural doctor of
nursing practice program, 63t
DRG. See Diagnosis related group;
Diagnosis-related group payment
DrNP (hybrid doctoral degree), 66
Dru, Jean-Marie, 407
Drug Enforcement Agency, 456
DSN. See Doctor of science in nursing
Dublin, Louis, 6–7

E

East Missouri Action Agency (EMAA),
473
Eastern Mediterranean, global perspectives
on ANP, 84–85, 84t
EBMR. See Evidence-Based Medicine
Reviews
Economic demographics, for independent
practice, 435
EdD. See Doctor of education
Education. See also Sex education
APN and, 390
child health impacted by, 355
income impacted by, 354
Educational isolation, as collaboration
barrier, 155–156
EEOC. See Equal Employment
Opportunity Commission
Effective date, of contract, 455
EFT. See Electronic funds transfer
EIN. See Employer identification
number
Elderly, acute care nurse practitioner
and, 36
Electronic funds transfer (EFT), 428
Elitism. See Professional elitism
EMAA. See East Missouri Action
Agency
Emotivism, 513t, 515
Employee, 449
APNs as, 452–453
Employee practice, malpractice insurance
in, 496–497
Employee Retirement Income Security Act
(ERISA), 173, 466
Employer identification number (EIN),
430
Energy therapies, 317
England, global perspectives on ANP,
89–90
English language

health literacy linked to proficiency in, 361–362
limited English proficiency, 376
patient teaching and, 374
Equal Employment Opportunity Commission (EEOC), 442
Equipment
cost containment in, 207–208
purchase, for independent practice, 441–442
Equitable relief, 454
ERISA. *See* Employee Retirement Income Security Act
Ether, 7
Ethical agreement, 520
APN and, 520
necessity of, 522–525
between nurse/patient, 519–520
with oneself, 520
Ethics, 510–528. *See also* Bioethics; Practice-based bioethics
contemporary theories of, 513–516, 513t
justice and, 356
Ethnicity. *See also* Asian Americans; Hispanics
health insurance disparities by, 355
mortality rates impacted by, 353–354
in U.S. population, 353t
Ethnocentrism, 369
Europe, global perspectives on ANP, 86
Evercare company, collaboration in, 167–168
Evidence-Based Medicine Reviews (EBMR), 256
Evidence-Based Medicine Toolkit (Badenoch & Heneghan), 254
Evidence-based practice, 244–258
absolute risk reduction in, 253t
APN's role in research with, 299–301
helping clinicians, 299
integrating evidence, 300
appraisal of therapy articles for, 254–255, 255b
appraising process in, 257, 258b
appraising summaries in, 255–257
asking answerable questions in, 252
attitude with, 257–258
clinical judgment in relation to, 245–255
clinical literature for, 252–254
clinical outcomes in, 251–252
competencies supporting, 251–255
confidence interval in, 253t
defined, 244–245
evidence from studies for, 254–255
incidence in, 253t
integrative research review in, 256
MEDLINE in, 254, 255
meta-analysis in, 255–256
number needed to treat in, 253t
P value in, 253t

PICOT format for, 252, 254b
positive predictive value in, 253t
practice guidelines in, 256
prevalence in, 253t
research literature in, 255
sensitivity in, 253t
specificity in, 253t
summary sources in, 256–257
Expenses, 194
depreciation as, 195
nonsalary, 195
Expert knowledge, teaching and, 332t
Expression. *See* Cultural expression

F

Fair Labor Standards Act (FLSA), 442
False Claims Act, 477
Family court system, 264–266
Family physicians (FPs), 150
FECA. *See* Federal Employees Compensation Act
Federal Age Discrimination in Employment Act (ADEA), 442
Federal Anti-Kickback Law & Regulatory Safe Harbors, 477
Federal Anti-Kickback Statute, 477
Federal Employees Compensation Act (FECA), 115
Federal funding, 58
Federal health program exclusion, 487
Federal narcotics license, for independent practice, 427–428
Federal Register, 146–147, 439
Federal Trade Commission (FTC), 187–188, 480, 482
Federal Trade Commission (FTC) Act, 479
Fee setting, for independent practice, 439
Fee-for-service, 172, 203
Fein v. Permanente Medical Group, 473
Fidelity, bioethics and, 521, 521t, 522, 527
Fiji, global perspectives on ANP, 92, 93
Finances
reimbursement, 238–240
reporting relationships dictated by, 230–241
Financial incentives, 178
Financial plan, independent practice and, 438
Financial risk
for health-care providers, 172
for MCPs, 173
Financial self-sufficiency, in independent practice, 421
Financial/tax implications, 450
Financing options, for independent practice, 438–439
Finland, global perspectives on ANP, 86
Fisher, Roger, 383–384
FLSA. *See* Fair Labor Standards Act

Force majeure, in contracts, 461
Ford, Loretta, 2, 102
FPs. *See* Family physicians
France, global perspectives on ANP, 87
Fraud and abuse, 475–479
assessing risk of, 478–479
avoiding, 478–479
Freedom, bioethics and, 521, 521t, 527
Fringe benefits, 194
Frontier Nursing Service (FNS), 5, 6
Frost, Robert, 355
FTC. *See* Federal Trade Commission
Future, collaboration for, 168–169
Future Shock (Toffler), 143

G

Gender roles, 13
Genetic Information Non-Discrimination Act of 2008, 453
Getting to Yes: Negotiating Agreement Without Giving In (Fisher and Ury), 383
GI Bill, 10
Gladwell, Malcolm, 408
Global perspectives, on ANP, 73b, 79–97
Africa, 79
Americas, 82–84
Australia, 91–92
Bahrain, 85
Botswana, 79
Canada, 82–83, 82b
Cayman Islands, 92–93
Eastern Mediterranean, 84–85, 84t
England, 89–90
Europe, 86
Fiji, 92, 93
Finland, 86
France, 87
Hong Kong, China, 92
Iran, 85–86
Ireland, 87
Islands of Western Pacific, 92
Israel, 87–88
Jamaica, 83–84
Netherlands, 88
New Zealand, 94–96, 95f, 96t
Northern Ireland, 89–90
Oman, 86
Republic of South Africa, 79–81, 81b
Samoa, 92, 93–94
Scotland, 89–90
Singapore, 97
South Korea, 96–97
South-East Asia, 90–91
Sweden, 89
Switzerland, 89
Taiwan, 97
Thailand, 90–91
United Kingdom, 89–90
Wales, 89–90
Western Africa, 81–82
Western Pacific, 91–92

Goldfarb v. Virginia State Bar, 480

GPSR. *See* Gross patient services revenue

Grand rounds, teaching plan, development of, 344, 346

Great Conversations, 418

Great Society entitlement programs, 15–16

Gross patient services revenue (GPSR), 194

Guide in Grassroots Activism, 274

Guide to Medical Practice Management Software (CTS), 442

Guided images, 316–317

Gwathmey, James T., 8

H

Hansen v. Caring Professionals, Inc., 453

Haute Autorité De Santé (HAS), 87

Hawaiian health practitioners, 324

HCPCS. *See* Healthcare Common Procedure Coding System

Healing environment, 320

Healing touch, 309, 312b, 317–318

Health and Human Services (HHS), 366

Health care
  ADR and, 381
  APNs and policy for, 367
  changes/challenges in, 392–393
  September 11, 2001, lessons for, 418b–419b
  U.S.A. current dissatisfaction with, 403

Health-Care Antitrust Improvements Act, 482

Health-care providers, financial risk for, 172

The health care workforce in ten states: Education, practice and policy (AFT Healthcare), 165

Health insurance, ethnicity and disparities in, 355

Health Insurance Portability and Accountability Act (HIPAA), 468, 476, 477, 488

Health literacy
  AHRQ defining, 362
  Asian Americans and, 364
  assessment tools for, 360–361, 361t
  English language proficiency linked to, 361–362
  Healthy People 2010 defining, 360
  Hispanics and, 364
  IOM's findings on, 362–363, 363b
  organizations addressing, 374
  translators and, 362–363

Health maintenance organizations (HMO), 107–108, 174b
  APN's disease management in, 287
  case management with, 279

Health plan employer data and information set (HEDIS), 445

Health professional shortage area (HPSA), 436

Health Resources and Services Administration (HRSA), 359
  cultural competence defined by, 360
  mission statement of, 366b

Health services
  professionalism in, 157
  supervision in, 157

Health status, determinants of, 354f

Healthcare Common Procedure Coding System (HCPCS), 440

Healthcare Integrity and Protection Data Bank (HIPDB), 488

Healthy People 2010, 355
  goals of, 352–353
  health literacy defined by, 360

Heart to Heart: For Girls Only, 417b–418b

HEDIS. *See* Health plan employer data and information set

Henderson, Florence, 8

Henry Street Settlement, 4

HHS. *See* Health and Human Services

HIPAA. *See* Health Insurance Portability and Accountability Act

HIPDB. *See* Healthcare Integrity and Protection Data Bank

Hispanics, health literacy and, 364

History of nursing, advocacy in, 261

HIV. *See* Human immunodeficiency virus

HMO. *See* Health maintenance organizations

Hodgins, Agatha Cobourg, 8

Hogan v. Mississippi Board of Nursing, 475

Holism, 310t

Holistic care. *See* Complementary-alternative medicine

Holistic nursing, 311

Home Health Care Planning Improvement Act of 2007, 115

Honesty, cultural competence and, 373

Hong Kong, China, global perspectives on ANP, 92

Hospital Compare, 181

Hospital-based case management model, 282t

Hospital-to-community-based case management model, 282t

HPSA. *See* Health professional shortage area

HRSA. *See* Health Resources and Services Administration

Human immunodeficiency virus (HIV), 80

Husted's symphonological bioethical decision making guide, 523f

Hybrid doctorates, 65

I

I & E. *See* Income and expense

ICD-9. *See* International classification of diseases, ninth modification

ICD-9-CM. *See* International Classification of Disease, 9th Revision, Clinical Modification

"Iceberg" effect, in physician-nurse collaborative relationship, 154–155, 155f

ICN. *See* International Council of Nurses

ICNM. *See* International Confederation of Nurse-Midwives

ICU. *See* Intensive care unit

Identity, APNs and challenges with, 398

Improving Access to Workers' Compensation for Injured Federal Workers Act, 115

Incentives
  for cost containment, 210
  financial, 178
  for reimbursement, 178
  for revenue's maximization, 203

Incidence, 253t

Incident-to-billing, 108–109

Income, education impacting, 354

Income and expense (I & E), 192

Indemnification/subrogation, in contracts, 458

Indemnity insurance companies, 109

Independent contractor, 449
  APNs as, 453

Independent practice, 234
  accountant services for, 431–432
  advanced practice license for, 427
  advantages to, 421
  area service needs assessment, 424
  attorney services for, 431
  barriers to, 421–422
  billing procedures for, 440–441, 441b
  business concept for, 436
  business decisions for, 423b, 424
  business location for, 435
  business name/image for, 434
  business plan for, 436–438
  business start-up time line, 425b–427b
  business structure for, 432–434
  clinical laboratory license for, 429–430
  competition and, 437
  competitive analysis and, 437
  consultant selection for, 431–432
  corporation for, 433
  documentation process for, 443–444
  economic demographics for, 435
  EIN for, 430
  equipment purchase for, 441–442
  establishing fees for, 439
  federal narcotics license for, 427–428
  financial plan and, 438
  financial self-sufficiency in, 421
  licensure for, 427–428

LLC for, 433–434
malpractice insurance in, 497–498
management team/personnel and, 437–438
market analysis for, 436–437
marketing plan and, 437
marketing strategies for, 446–447
MCO and, 428, 439
Medicaid managed care for, 428
Medicaid provider number for, 428
medical biller for, 432
Medicare and, 428–429
NPI for, 429
operations and, 438
opportunities with, 422b
partnership for, 433
personnel hiring/management for, 442–443
policies/procedures for, 446, 447b
practice manager for, 432
professional climate for, 436
professional liability insurance for, 430–431
professional relationships in, 435–436
quality assurance process for, 444–446
reimbursement procedures for, 440
repayment projections and, 438
sole proprietorship for, 432–433
starting an, 423
state narcotics license for, 427
state nursing license for, 427
state tax identification number for, 430
strategy development for, 424
suppliers for, 441–442
UPIN for, 429
Individual rights, 511–512, 512t
Infant death rate, 5
Informational diversity, 158
Informed consent, 300
Ingles, Thelma, 12
INP/APNN. See International Nurse Practitioner/Advanced Practice Nursing Network
Inpatient Prospective Payment System (IPPS), 177
Institute of Medicine (IOM), 362
health literacy findings of, 362–363, 363b
Insurance. See also Malpractice insurance
health, 355
knowledge of structures/benefits of, 284t
Insurer's response, in malpractice lawsuits, 502–503
Integrative medicine, 310t
Integrative research review, 256
Intensive care unit (ICU), 152
Interdisciplinary relationship
from multidisciplinary practice, 153
to transdisciplinary relationship, 153–154

Interdisciplinary teaming, 217–220, 218f, 219f
Internal revenue service (IRS), 430, 449
International Classification of Disease, 9th Revision, Clinical Modification (ICD-9-CM), 440
International classification of diseases, ninth modification (ICD-9), 204
International Confederation of Nurse-Midwives (ICNM), 7
International Council of Nurses (ICN)
advocacy in, 261
APN's role according to, 390–391
role of, 73–74
International Council of Nurses/International Nurse Practitioner/Advanced Practice Nursing Network
characteristics for, 75t
goal of, 74b
International Nurse Practitioner/Advanced Practice Nursing Network (INP/APNN), 73
International perspective. See Global perspectives, on ANP
Internet
cultural competence, research using, 371–373
marketing utilizing, 414–415
Intuition, 248, 250f
IOM. See Institute of Medicine
IPPS. See Inpatient Prospective Payment System
Iran, global perspectives on ANP, 85–86
Ireland, global perspectives on ANP, 87
IRS. See Internal revenue service
Islands of Western Pacific, global perspectives on ANP, 92
Israel, global perspectives on ANP, 87–88

J

Jamaica, global perspectives on ANP, 82, 83–84
JCAHO. See Joint Commission on the Accreditation of Healthcare Organizations
The Joint Commission (TJC), 181, 362, 376, 495
Medicare and, 466
Joint Commission on the Accreditation of Healthcare Organizations (JCAHO), 133
Joint problem solving, 230
Journal of Nurse-Midwifery, 6
Justice, ethics and, 356

K

Keeping Patients Safe: Transforming the Work Environment of Nurses (Institute of Medicine), 144

King, Martin Luther, Jr., 356
Kirk v. Mercy Hospital Tri-County, 452
Knowledge, 371–373, 373b
skills v., 398

L

LAN. See Local area network
Language
of collaboration, 158–159
in collaboration success strategies, 165–166
confusion, as collaboration barrier, 158–161
as cultural expression, 368
marketing and, 414
Laws
antifraud, 476
antitrust, 479–482
conflict of, 460
context for, 465–470
sources of, 466
state, and malpractice lawsuits, 494
Lawsuits. See also Malpractice lawsuits
civil, 486
Lay healers, 3, 4
Leadership
CNM, 236–238
with reporting relationships, 236–238
with research, 298, 301–302
Learner
assessment of, 331–337, 333b
active domain, 337
cognitive domain, 336, 337t
objective development, 335–337
observations, 335
pretests, 335
psychomotor domain, 336–337
questioning, 335
questionnaires, 335
readiness of, 333–334, 334b
strategies for, 335
evaluation of, 348–349
supportive environment for, 331
Lecture, teaching plan, development of, 340–342, 341b
Legal authority, in contracts, 460
Legal counsel, in malpractice lawsuits, 503
Legal issues, 470–475
in scope of practice, 470–472
Legal opinions, in court system, 470
Legalities
APNs, cultural competence and, 375–376
on MCPs' APNs, 178, 179, 188
Legislation, 466–469
Leininger, M. M., 357–359
LEP. See Limited English proficiency
Licensure

exposure, 486–487
for independent practice, 427–428
Limited English proficiency (LEP), 376
Limited liability corporation (LLC), for independent practice, 433–434
Literacy. *See* Health literacy
LLC. *See* Limited liability corporation
Lobenstine Midwifery Clinic, 5, 6
Local area network (LAN), 441
Long-range budgets, 197
Long-term care (LTC), 167–168
LTC. *See* Long-term care

M

Madden, Maurice, 374
Magaw, Alice, 7, 146
Mail-order pharmacies, 127
Male nurses, 8
Malpractice, 486
    APNs and, 487–496
    claims, 488–489
    crisis, 494–496
Malpractice insurance, 485–508
    carrier identification in, 499
    in CNM/physician relationship, 148
    in collaborative practice, 498–499
    contractual obligations of, 501–503
    costs, 501
    coverage selection criteria for, 499–500
    for employed APNs, 496–497
    for independent practice APNs, 497–498
    as risk management tool, 499–501
Malpractice lawsuits
    fostering positive relationships and, 505–507
        with patient/family, 505–506
        with physicians, 507
        with staff, 506–507
    insurer's response in, 502–503
    legal counsel in, 503
    procedure of, 501–503
    settlement in, 503
    state laws and, 494
    trial, 503–507
    witness testimony and, 503–505
Malpractice payments
    by amount, 491t, 492t
    by nurse type, 490t
    by reason, 490t
    by state, 493t–494t
Managed care
    APN's disease management in, 288–289
    definition of, 173
    necessary competencies for, 174–175
Managed care organizations (MCOs), 107–108, 108t, 133, 193
    health maintenance organizations, 107–108

physician-hospital organizations, 107–108
    preferred provider organizations, 107–108
    provider sponsored organizations, 107–108
Managed care panels, 141
Managed care plans (MCPs)
    communication with, 174–175
    contracting with, 175–176, 176b
    definition of, 173
    financial risk for, 173
    HMO as, 174b
    PNs in, 173, 179
    POS plans as, 174b
    PPO as, 174b
    types of, 175
Managed care plans' APNs, 173, 180
    consumer support for, 179, 186–187
    data collection on, 178
    legalities of, 178, 179, 188
    self-assessment process, 174–175
Management team/personnel, independent practice and, 437–438
Market analysis, for independent practice, 436–437
Market segment, 187
Marketing. *See also* Business; Mission statement; Statement of philosophy; Testimonials
    APN promotions for, 412–413, 413b
    APNs' operational definition of, 405b
    APNs problems with, 403
    buzz created in, 413–414
    for consumer support, 187
    defining, 404
    dialogue with consumers for APNs and, 408–411
    disruption process for, 407
    evaluating success/missteps of, 416
    feedback loop for, 406t
    five Ps, 404t
    goals/objectives for, 407
    internet and, 414–415
    language precision for, 414
    needs assessment for, 408
    plan, 405–406, 437
    principles of, 187, 404–405, 404t
    promotion as principle of, 187
    strategies, 446–447
    vision for, 407
Massachusetts General Hospital, 7
Master's degree, 11, 58
Maternal and Child Health Bureau (MCHB), 359
Maternal death rate, 5
Mayo Clinic, 7
MCHB. *See* Maternal and Child Health Bureau
McIsaac, Isabel, 144
MCO. *See* Managed care organizations;

Medicaid managed care organizations
MCPs. *See* Managed care plans
Mediation, narrative, 384
Medicaid, 102, 103, 105, 107, 113, 176–177, 476
    revenue, 193
Medicaid Advanced Practice Nurse and Physician Assistants Access Act of 2007, 115
Medicaid managed care organizations (MCO), independent practice and, 428, 439
Medicaid provider number, for independent practice, 428
Medical biller, for independent practice, 432
Medicare, 102, 103, 104, 106–107, 176–177, 476
    Community Health Accreditation Program and, 466
    conditions of participation, 466
    independent practice and, 428–429
    reimbursement, 239, 240
        APNs and, 397–398
    revenue, 193
    TJC and, 466
Medicare and Medicaid Patient Protection Act, 477
MEDLINE, 254, 255
Meta-analysis, 255–256
    on NP, 172–173
Metzger, Julie, 417b–418b
Midwives, 3
Mind-body therapies, 316
Minnesota Center for Spirituality and Healing, 313
Minnesota State University, inaugural doctor of nursing practice program, 63t
Mission statement
    creating, 407
    of HRSA, 366b
Mobile hospital, 8
Models, of collaboration, 214–216, 214f, 215t
Modification, of contracts, 460
Mortality rates, ethnicity impacting, 353–354
Morton, William T. G., 7
Motivation, of learner, 333–334
Multidisciplinary practice
    interdisciplinary relationship from, 153
    from unidisciplinary base, 153
Multimedia, teaching plan, development of, 346
Mutual assent, 454

N

NACNS. *See* National Association of Clinical Nurse Specialists

NAPNAP. *See* National Association of Pediatric Nurse Associates and Practitioners
Narrative mediation, 384
Narrative thinking, 248–249
National Association of Clinical Nurse Specialists (NACNS), 392
National Association of Pediatric Nurse Associates and Practitioners (NAPNAP), 15
National Cancer Institute (NCI), 364
National Center for Contemporary and Alternative Medicine (NCCAM), 313–315, 315b
National Center for Cultural Competence (NCCC), 367
  self-assessment tool of, 369
National Commission of Nurse Anesthesia Education (NCNAE), 394–395
National Committee for Quality Assurance (NCQA), 445
National Conference of State Legislatures (NCSL), 495
National Council of State Boards of Nursing (NCSBN), 18, 58
National HealthCare Disparities Report (NHDR), 352–353, 355
  2007 report data, 356b
National Institute of Nursing Research (NINR), 61
National Institutes of Health (NIH), 61
National Labor Relations Act, 467
National League for Nursing (NLN), 6
National League for Nursing Accrediting Commission (NLNAC), 59
National League for Nursing Education (NLNE), 144–145
National Organization of Public Health Nurses (NOPHN), 6
National Practitioner Data Bank (NPDB), 488
National provider identifier (NPI), for independent practice, 429
National quality
  Hospital Compare for, 181
  Joint Commission for, 181
  NQF for, 180–181
National Quality Forum (NQF), 180–181
  national voluntary consensus standards and, 184b
  for nursing care measurement, 182b–183b
National Strategy for Suicide Prevention: Goals and Objectives for Action (U.S. DHHS), 272
National Technology Transfer and Advancement Act of 1995, 181
National voluntary consensus standards
  NQF and, 184b
  nursing-centered intervention measures in, 184b
  patient-centered outcome measures in, 184b
  system-centered measures in, 184b
Navigator programs. *See* Patient navigator programs
NCCAM. *See* National Center for Contemporary and Alternative Medicine
NCCC. *See* National Center for Cultural Competence
NCI. *See* National Cancer Institute
NCNAE. *See* National Commission of Nurse Anesthesia Education
NCQA. *See* National Committee for Quality Assurance
NCSBN. *See* National Council of State Boards of Nursing
NCSL. *See* National Conference of State Legislatures
Needs assessment, marketing, 408
Negligence, 486
Net patient services revenue (NPSR), 194
Netherlands, global perspectives on ANP, 88
Networking, 415–416
New Jersey Conscientious Employee Protection Act, 452
New Jersey Department of Health and Senior Services (NJDHSS), 269–270
New York State Medical Society, 146
New Zealand, global perspectives on ANP, 94–96, 95f, 96t
NHDR. *See* National HealthCare Disparities Report
NIC. *See* Nursing Intervention Classifications
Nightingale, Florence, 3, 144, 261, 309
NIH. *See* National Institutes of Health
NINR. *See* National Institute of Nursing Research
Nitrous oxide, 7
NJDHSS. *See* New Jersey Department of Health and Senior Services
NLN. *See* National League for Nursing
NLNAC. *See* National League for Nursing Accrediting Commission
NLNE. *See* National League for Nursing Education
NOC. *See* Nursing Outcomes Classifications
NOPHN. *See* National Organization of Public Health Nurses
North Dakota State, inaugural doctor of nursing practice program, 63t
Northern Ireland, global perspectives on ANP, 89–90
Northern Pacific Railway v. United States, 480
Not to compete covenant, in contracts, 461
Notices, in contracts, 459–460
NP. *See* Nurse practitioner
NPDB. *See* National Practitioner Data Bank
NPI. *See* National provider identifier
NPSR. *See* Net patient services revenue
NQF. *See* National Quality Forum
Number needed to treat, 253t
Nurse anesthetists, 7–9, 39–41, 471
  prescriptive authority and, 123–124
  profile of, 41b
Nurse Midwifery Associates v. Hibbett, 481
Nurse practitioner (NP), 23, 29–33, 390
  care outcomes and, 395–396
  case management by, 281
  CNS merge with, 12
  community and, 31–32
  with FPs, 150
  in MCPs, 173, 179
  meta-analyses on, 172–173
  physician-nurse relationship for, 149–150
  practice settings for, 232, 232t
  prescriptive authority and, 119–120, 121f
  psychiatric mental health, 33
  reimbursement in, 238–239
  reporting relationships for, 230–241
  responsibilities increasing for, 399
  role change of, 30–31
  role negotiation for, 149–150
  role of, 12–19
  role/development of, 391–392
  specialization and, 392
  in transitional care setting, 32–33
Nurse Training Act of 1964, 11
Nurse Training Acts of 1971 and 1975, 17
Nurse-clinician, 9
Nurse-midwives, 4–7, 9, 37–39. *See also* Certified nurse-midwife
  cesarean section and, 39
  historical perspective of, 37–38
  licensing/supervision of, 5
  prescriptive authority and, 122, 123f
  primary care focus in, 38
  profile of, 39b
  tracking progress of, 6–7
Nurse/patient agreement, 519–520
Nurse-physician collaboration, 126. *See also* Physician-nurse collaboration framework
  ANA code of 1950 on, 145
  CNM in, 146, 147–148
  CNS in, 148–149
  CRNA in, 146–147
  "iceberg" effect in, 154–155, 155f
  malpractice insurance in, 148
  NP in, 149–150
  over time, 144–145
  power control in, 162
  responsibility for practice and, 162

Nursing. *See also* Advanced practice nurse
care as central to, 357–358
conflict management strategies for,
382–383
cultural congruent care and assessment
for, 359
history of, 261
promoting retention in, 399–400,
400b
tradition, paradigm shift and, 485–486
Nursing care measurement
evidence in, 182b–183b
meta-analyses as, 172–173
NQF for, 182
value of, 182–183
Nursing Intervention Classifications
(NIC), 285–286
Nursing Outcomes Classifications (NOC),
285–286
Nursing Policy Statement, 143
Nursing: scope and standards of practice
(ANA), 375
Nursing-centered intervention measures,
184b

O

Objectivity, bioethics and, 521, 521t, 527
OBRA. *See* Omnibus Budget
Reconciliation Act
*Observatoire National De La Demographie
Des Professions De Sanfè* (ONDPS), 87
Occupational Safety and Health Act, 467
Occupational Safety and Health
Administration (OSHA), 443
OECD. *See* Organization for Economic
Co-operation and Development
Office environment, business impacted by,
412
Office of Inspector General (OIG), 488
Office of Minority Health (OMH), 360
Office of Technology Assessment (OTA),
179, 495
OIG. *See* Office of Inspector General
Oklahoma, 180
Oltz v. St. Peter's Community Hospital,
481–482
OM. *See* Outcomes management
Oman, global perspectives on ANP, 86
OMH. *See* Office of Minority Health
Omnibus Budget Reconciliation Act
(OBRA), 176, 478
Omnibus Reconciliation Act of 1989,
110
*Online Journal of Knowledge Synthesis for
Nursing*, 257
Operational budgets, 197–198
Operational trust, 163
Operations, independent practice and,
438
Oral fluid intake, temperature changes
with, 305

Organization
accounts chart for, 191–193
decisions, input and, 191
hierarchy, collaboration barrier and,
157–158
P & L for, 192, 192t
profit and, 191, 202
structure of, 191–193
Organization for Economic Co-operation
and Development (OECD), 72
OSHA. *See* Occupational Safety and
Health Administration
OTA. *See* Office of Technology Assessment
Outcomes management (OM), 444
Ozimek, Dorothy, 16

P

P & L. *See* Profit and loss
P value, 253t
Panax notogensing, 318
Paradigm shift, nursing tradition and,
485–486
Partners in delivering culturally competent
research-based care for diverse
populations (PIDCCRCFDP),
371–372, 372b
Partnership, 230, 359
advanced practice and, 211
of APNs, 378
for independent practice, 433
Party relationships, in contract,
455–456
Party responsibilities, in contract,
456–457
Patient care coordinator (PCC), 167
Patient Care Partnership (AHA), 360,
360b
Patient Navigator, Outreach and Chronic
Disease Prevention Act, 366–367
Patient navigator programs, 365–367
Patient services revenue, 192
Patient-centered outcome measures, 184b
Patients
APNs empowering, 368, 368b
APNs imagining perspective of, 357,
369
English language and teaching, 374
learning from, 352
Patient's Bill of Rights (AHA), 360
Payor denials/delays, 205
"Payor-blind" care, 210
PCC. *See* Patient care coordinator
PCP. *See* Primary clinical practitioner
PCPs. *See* Primary care providers
Peabody, Francis, 13
Pediatric setting, acute care nurse
practitioner and, 34–35
PEO. *See* Professional employer
organization
Peplau, Hildegard, 10
Performance improvements (PI), 444

Peripheral intravenous line securement,
306
Personal characteristics, teaching and,
332t
Personnel hiring/management, for
independent practice, 442–443
PharmD, 62
PHC. *See* Primary health care
PhD. *See* Doctor of philosophy
PHOs. *See* Physician-hospital
organizations
Physical readiness, of learner, 333
Physician assistant, 13
Physician Payment Review Commission
(PPRC), 104
Physician-hospital organizations (PHOs),
107–108
Physician-nurse collaboration framework
assertiveness in, 152
common goals in, 151
components for, 150–152, 151t
concept for, 150
cooperation in, 152
coordination in, 152
mutual concerns in, 152
separate and unique practice spheres in,
151
shared power control, 151–152
PI. *See* Performance improvements
PICOT. *See* Population/problem,
intervention, comparison, outcome,
time format
PIDCCRCFDP. *See* Partners in delivering
culturally competent research-based care
for diverse populations
Plaintiffs, 469
Planned Parenthood v. Vines, 473
PNSO. *See* Professional Nursing Staff
Organization
Point of service (POS) plans, 174b
Policies/procedures, for independent
practice, 446, 447b
Population/problem, intervention,
comparison, outcome, time format
(PICOT), 252, 254b
Positive predictive value, 253t
Positive relationships, teaching and,
332t
Power control
in nurse-physician relationship, 162
in physician-nurse collaboration frame-
work, 151–152
PPO. *See* Preferred provider organization
PPRC. *See* Physician Payment Review
Commission
PPS. *See* Prospective payment system
PQRI, 177
Practice guidelines, 161, 256. *See also*
Scope of practice
Practice manager, for independent
practice, 432

Practice settings, specialty practice risks and, 496
Practice-based bioethics, 511. *See also* Bioethics; Ethics
advanced practice and, 512–513
of APN, 518–519
case study analysis of, 525, 526b
context in, 516–518
elements of, 517t
levels of, 517–518
rational decision making for, 515–516
Practice-based evidence component, in career portfolio, 138, 139f, 140
Practitioner contact information, in career portfolio, 138
Precedent, in court system, 470
Preemption, 466
Preferred provider organization (PPO), 107–108, 174b
case management with, 279
Prescriptions, 77–78
Prescriptions, authority, 17
barriers to, 126–127
clinical nurse specialists and, 122
nurse anesthetists and, 123–124
nurse practitioner and, 119–120, 121f
nurse-midwives and, 122, 123f
prescribing patterns, 128
statutory and regulatory change in, 124–126
collaborative formulary, 126
negative/exclusionary formulary, 125
nurse-physician relationships in, 126
open formulary, 126
patterns of, 125
regulator established formulary, 125
Prevalence, 253t
Price-fixing, 480
Primary care, 13–14
collaboration in, 160
teamwork in, 160
Primary care practice, 38–39
Primary care providers (PCPs), 423–424
nonphysicians and, 160
UAPs and, 207
Primary clinical practitioner (PCP), 79
Primary health care (PHC), 72
Privileging, 133–137
background, 133–136
categories, 134b
active, 134b
affiliate, 134b
allied health professional, 134b
courtesy, 134b
honorary, 134b
house, 134b
outpatient, 134b
process, 136–137
rationale, 133–136
temporary, 136–137

Problem solving, 245. *See also* Clinical judgment
Productivity, 208–209
Professional climate, for independent practice, 436
Professional discipline, 474–475
Professional elitism, as collaboration barrier, 156
Professional employer organization (PEO), 443
Professional liability, 485
of APNs, 449–450
Professional liability insurance, for independent practice, 430–431
Professional Nursing Practice, 165
Professional Nursing Staff Organization (PNSO)
research mentors at, 305
research program of, 304–306
blood pressure measurement in, 305–306
peripheral intravenous/central venous line securement in, 306
temperature changes with oral fluid intake in, 305
sustainable objective of, 305
Professional relationships, for independent practice, 435–436
Professionalism, in health services, 157
Profit and loss (P & L), 192, 192t
Profit, organization and, 191, 202
Program budgets, 198–199
Projected workload volume, for budgeting process, 200–201
Promoting. *See* Marketing
Prospective payment system (PPS), 103
Protocols
collaboration in, 160–161
in collaboration success strategies, 164
practice guidelines v., 161
Provider sponsored organizations (PSOs), 107–108
PSOs. *See* Provider sponsored organizations
Psychological readiness, of learner, 333
Psychomotor domain, learner, assessment of, 336–337
Public health nursing, 4
Civil Rights Movement influencing, 279
Community Chest Movement influencing, 278
Social Security Act influencing, 278
Wald's work with, 277–278
Public Law 105-33, 111
Public relations, 404, 404t

Q

Quality assurance process, for independent practice, 444–446
Quality compass, 445

Quality Health-Care Coalition Act, 482
Quality initiatives. *See also* National quality
APNs in, 181–186
Qui tam relator, 477

R

Rapid estimate of adult literacy in medicine (REALM), 360
Rauwolfia serpentina, 318
RBRVS. *See* Resource-based relative value scale
REALM. *See* Rapid estimate of adult literacy in medicine
REALM-Teen, 360
Reason, rule of, 480
Recognition, 186–187, 188. *See also* Consumer support
Reflection, 249, 250
Registered nurse (RN), case management by, 280–281
Registered nurse practitioner (RNP), 161
Regulations, 466
Reid, Duncan, 15
Reiki, 317–318
Reimbursement, 109–112, 110b
barriers to, 176–177
BBA for, 176–177
case management, 289
clinical nurse specialist, 238–240
cost containment v., 209–210
documentation and, 205
DRA for, 177
future of, 112–115, 112b
incentives for, 178
for independent practice, 440
inequities in, 177
IPPS for, 177
Medicare, 239–240, 397–398
nurse practitioner, 238–239
OBRA for, 176
payor denials/delays and, 205
PQRI for, 177
reporting relationships and, 238–241
for revenue's maximization, 204
revenue's maximization with, 204
salaries as, 194–195, 206
VBP for, 177
Reiter, Frances, 9
Repayment projections, independent practice and, 438
Reporting accountability, 157–158
Reporting relationships, 230–241
internal/external forces influencing, 234–235
leadership with, 236–238
money determining, 231–233
reimbursement in, 238–241
specialty alignments with, 235
themes for, 230–231

Republic of South Africa, global perspectives on ANP, 79–81, 81b
Research
  APN's attributes for, 296–297
    in-depth knowledge for, 296
    scholarly habits for, 297
    self-direction for, 296
    working relationships for, 296
  APN's behavior for, 298–302
    leadership, 301–302
    mentoring, 301–302
    problem solving, 299–301
    systems approach, 302
  APNs' problems with, 398–399
  APN's role in, 295–306
    attributes of, 296–297
    collaboration with, 297–298
    facilitative role for, 297–298
    leadership with, 298
    research skill development for, 297
  APNs utilizing, 375
  barriers to evidence use for, 301
  completing, 304
  on contemporary medicine, 313–315
  cultural competence, internet for, 371–373
  evidence-based practice with, 299–301
  funding of, 300–301
  informed consent for, 300
  leadership with, 298, 301–302
  PNSO program for, 304–306
    blood pressure measurement in, 305–306
    peripheral intravenous/central venous line securement in, 306
    temperature changes with oral fluid intake in, 305
  questions for feasibility of, 300–301
  removing barriers to APN, 302–304
    administrative support for, 303–304
    clinical access for, 303
    clinician buy-in for, 303
    time/money for, 304
  time for, 300, 304
Research mentors (RM), 305
Resource management
  activities' volume in, 203–204
  cost containment in, 205–209
  CPT for, 204
  ICD-9 for, 204
  implications of, 209–210
  revenue's maximization in, 202–205
Resource-based relative value scale (RBRVS), 104, 439
Respect, 359
Responsibility for practice, nurse-physician collaboration and, 162
Résumé, 137

Retention, in nursing, promoting, 399–400, 400b
Revenue
  activities' volume for, 203–204
  basis of, 193
  deductions from, 192
  DRG and, 193
  expenses v., 192
  GPSR as, 194
  Medicaid, 193
  Medicare, 193
  nongovernmental, 193–194
  NPSR as, 194
  patient services, 192
  total, in budgeting process, 201
Revenue's maximization
  activities' volume for, 203–204
  direct billing in, 203
  incentive practices in, 203
  reimbursement rates for, 204
  volume v. price in, 202–203
Risk management tool. *See also* Financial risk
  malpractice insurance as, 499–501
RM. *See* Research mentors
RNP. *See* Registered nurse practitioner
Rogers, Martha, 15, 149
Role confusion, as collaboration barrier, 158–161
Rule of reason, 480
Rule-making, 467–469
Rush University, inaugural doctor of nursing practice program, 63t
Russell, Bill, 154

S

Safe harbors, 477
Safe Harbors Provisions, 477
Saint Peter's College, master's degree in case management from, 291b
Salamone, Mary Ellen, 419
Salaries, 194–195
  of APNs, 397
  in cost containment, 206
Samoa, global perspectives on ANP, 92, 93–94
Sanger, Margaret, 261
Saphania tendra, 318
SBA. *See* Small Business Administration
School for Association for the Promotion and Standardization of Midwifery, 5
School nursing, 4
Schools. *See also* Education
  dialogue and, 409
Scope and Standards of Advanced Practice Registered Nursing (ANA), 455, 471
Scope and Standards of Practice (ANA), 295–296
Scope of contract, 455
Scope of practice, 24–41, 25t

  clinical nurse specialist, 26–29
  legal issues in, 470–472
  nurse practitioner, 29–33
Scotland, global perspectives on ANP, 89–90
Second licensure models, of advanced practice nurse, 141–142
Self-assertion, bioethics and, 521, 521t, 522, 527
Self-assessment process, for MCPs' APNs, 174–175
Self-directed instructional methods, teaching plan, development of, 347
Sensitivity, 253t
September 11, 2001, health care lessons from, 418b–419b
Sermchief v. Gonzales, 473
Settlement, in malpractice lawsuits, 503
Settlement House Movement, 4
Severability, of contracts, 460
Sex education, APNs and success with, 417b–418b
Shared power control, in physician-nurse collaboration framework, 151–152
Shared visits, 109
Shell, Richard, 382
Sheppard-Towner Maternity and Infancy Act, 5
Sherman Act, 479, 480, 481
Shuler Nurse Practitioner Model, 324
Signatures, in contracts, 461
Silver, Henry, 14, 102
Simulations, teaching plan, development of, 348
Singapore, global perspectives on ANP, 97
Skills, knowledge v., 398
Small Business Administration (SBA), 439
Social category diversity, 158
Social childbirth, 3
Social Security Act, 278
Social/cultural relativism, 513t, 514–515
Sole proprietorship, for independent practice, 432–433
South Korea, global perspectives on ANP, 96–97
South-East Asia, global perspectives on ANP, 90–91
SPAN. *See* Suicide Prevention Advocacy Network, Inc.
Specialty practice risks, practice settings and, 496
Specificity, 253t
Spiritual assessment, 377b
Spirituality, 319–320
Standards of care for advanced practice nurses, 471t
Standards of professional performance for advanced practice nurses, 472t
Stark I/II regulations, 477
State certification, exposure, 486–487

State laws, malpractice lawsuits, 494
State narcotics license, for independent practice, 427
State nursing license, for independent practice, 427
State tax identification number, for independent practice, 430
Statement of philosophy, 406–407
Statements of Antitrust Enforcement Policy in Health Care (ATD & FTC), 482
Statutory and regulatory change, in prescriptive authority, 124–126
   collaborative formulary, 126
   negative/exclusionary formulary, 125
   nurse-physician relationships in, 126
   open formulary, 126
   patterns of, 125
   regulator established formulary, 125
Stead, Eugene A., 12
Stravic, Mac, 412
Strength/Weakness/Opportunities/Threats (SWOT), 74
Suicide prevention, 271–273
Suicide Prevention Advocacy Network, Inc. (SPAN), 271–272
Sunrise Model, 358f
Supervision, 234
   collaboration v., 149, 159
   in health services, 157
Suppliers, for independent practice, 441–442
Supplies
   cost containment in, 207–208
   variable projection, for budgeting process, 200–201
Surgical anesthesia, 7
Sweden, global perspectives on ANP, 89
Switzerland, global perspectives on ANP, 89
SWOT. *See* Strength/Weakness/Opportunities/Threats
Symposium, Samueli, 311
System-centered measures, 184b

T

Taiwan, global perspectives on ANP, 97
Taussig, Fred, 37
Tax Equity and Fiscal Responsibility Act (TEFRA), 40–41
Tax Relief and Health Care Act of 2006 (TRHCA), 177
Teaching, 331
   effective qualities, 331, 332t
   English language and patient, 374
   skills, 332t
Teaching plan, development of, 337–349, 339f
   case study, 344
   clinical case, 344, 345b
   clinical conference, 343–344
   demonstration, 348
   discussion, 342, 343t

   grand rounds, 344, 346
   lecture, 340–342, 341b
   methods, 340–344
   multimedia, 346
   readability, 347
   sample, 339f
   self-directed instructional methods, 347
   unfolding cases, 344
Teamwork, 230
   attitudes toward, 162
   care impacted by, 381
   components for, 163–164
   in primary care, 160
Technology, dialogue improved through, 411
TEFRA. *See* Tax Equity and Fiscal Responsibility Act
Temporary privileges, 136–137
Term/renewal/termination, in contracts, 459
Test of functional health literacy in adults (TOFHLA), 361, 364
Testimonials, for APNs, 405
Thailand, global perspectives on ANP, 90–91
Therapeutic prescriptions, 77–78
Therapeutic touch, 309, 312b, 317–318
Thomas-Kilmann Index (TKI), 382
The Tipping Point (Gladwell), 408–409
TJC. *See* The Joint Commission; Joint Commission on the Accreditation of Healthcare Organizations
TKI. *See* Thomas-Kilmann Index
Toffler, Alvin, 143
TOFHLA. *See* Test of functional health literacy in adults
Tort reform, 495
Towers, Jan, 15
Training across boundaries, 230
Transdisciplinary relationship, 153–154
Transformative practice, 384
Translators, health literacy and, 362–363
Transportation, business, community considerations regarding, 411–412
Treatment plans, cultural competence for, 370
Tresolini and Pew-Fetzer Task Force, 154
TRHCA. *See* Tax Relief and Health Care Act of 2006
Trial, for malpractice lawsuits, 503–507
TRICARE, 109
Tricare Extra, 109
Tricare Prime, 109
Tricare Standard, 109
Tri-College University, inaugural doctor of nursing practice program, 63t
Trust
   operational, 163
   in physician-nurse collaboration, 151
Truth, Sojourner, 261
20th Annual Legislative Update, 159

U

UAPs. *See* Unlicensed assistive personnel
UCR. *See* Usual and customary reimbursement
Ultimate selling point (USP), 405–406
Understanding, eliciting and negotiating multicultural health beliefs (Jackson), 369, 369b
Unidisciplinary base, multidisciplinary practice from, 153
United Kingdom, global perspectives on ANP, 89–90
United States Department of Justice (USDOJ), 376
United States of America (U.S.A.), health care dissatisfaction in, 403
United States v. Topco Associates, 480
Universal provider identification number (UPIN), for independent practice, 429
University of Alabama at Birmingham, 67
University of Colorado at Denver and Health Sciences Center, inaugural doctor of nursing practice program, 63t
University of Iowa College of Nursing, 285
University of Kentucky, inaugural doctor of nursing practice program, 63t
University of South Carolina, inaugural doctor of nursing practice program, 64t
University of Tennessee Health Science Center, inaugural doctor of nursing practice program, 64t
Unlicensed assistive personnel (UAPs), 207
Unrecognized diversity, as collaboration barrier, 158, 162
UPIN. *See* Universal provider identification number
Ury, Bill, 383–384
U.S. Department of Health and Human Services (USDHHS), 352, 468
USDHHS. *See* U.S. Department of Health and Human Services
USDOJ. *See* United States Department of Justice
USP. *See* Ultimate selling point
Usual and customary reimbursement (UCR), 440
Utilitarianism, 513t, 514

V

Value
   APNs increasing, 412–413
   defining, 412
Value-based purchasing (VBP), 177
Variable supplies projection, for budgeting process, 200–201
VBP. *See* Value-based purchasing
VHA. *See* Voluntary Hospitals of America

Villanova University College of Nursing, case management study at, 290
Virtues, of APNs, 522–525
Vision (marketing), 407
Vizcaino v. Microsoft Corporation, 451
Voluntary Hospitals of America (VHA), 381

W

Wald, Lillian, 4, 261, 277–278
Wales, global perspectives on ANP, 89–90
"Walk a mile in someone else's shoes," 357

Western Africa, global perspectives on ANP, 81–82
Western Pacific, global perspectives on ANP, 91–92
White House Commission on Contemporary and Alternate Medicine Policy, 312–313, 313b
WHO-AFRO, 79
WHO-EMRO, 84–85, 84t
WHO-EURO, 86
WHO-SEARO, 90–91

WHO-WPRO, 91–92
Wilk v. American Medical Association, 481
Wilson, Sophie Gran, 8
Winston, Sophie, 8
Witness testimony, malpractice lawsuits and, 503–505
Work status determination factors, for APNs, 450–452
Workload, cost containment and, 206
Written agreements, 461–463